VITAMINS AND HORMONES

VOLUME 36

VITAMINS AND HORMONES

ADVANCES IN RESEARCH AND APPLICATIONS

Edited by

PAUL L. MUNSON
University of North Carolina
Chapel Hill, North Carolina

EGON DICZFALUSY
Karolinska Sjukhuset
Stockholm, Sweden

JOHN GLOVER
University of Liverpool
Liverpool, England

ROBERT E. OLSON
St. Louis University
St. Louis, Missouri

Consulting Editors

ROBERT S. HARRIS
32 Dwhinda Road
Newton, Massachusetts

KENNETH V. THIMANN
University of California, Santa Cruz
Santa Cruz, California

JOHN A. LORAINE
University of Edinburgh
Edinburgh, Scotland

IRA G. WOOL
University of Chicago
Chicago, Illinois

Volume 36
1978

ACADEMIC PRESS   **New York   San Francisco   London**
A Subsidiary of Harcourt Brace Jovanovich, Publishers

ACADEMIC PRESS, INC.
111 Fifth Avenue, New York, New York 10003

United Kingdom Edition published by
ACADEMIC PRESS, INC. (LONDON) LTD.
24/28 Oval Road, London NW1 7DX

LIBRARY OF CONGRESS CATALOG CARD NUMBER: 43–10535

ISBN 0–12–709836–4

PRINTED IN THE UNITED STATES OF AMERICA

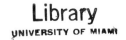

Contents

Cellular Vitamin A Binding Proteins

FRANK CHYTIL AND DAVID E. ONG

Studies on Ascorbic Acid Related to the Genetic Basis of Scurvy

PAUL SATO AND SIDNEY UDENFRIEND

The Interactions between Vitamin B_6 and Hormones

DAVID P. ROSE

Hormonal Factors in Lipogenesis in Mammary Gland

R. J. MAYER

Biological Effects of Antibodies to Gonadal Steroids

EBERHARD NIESCHLAG AND E. JEAN WICKINGS

Effects of Cannabinoids on Reproduction and Development

ERIC BLOCH, BENJAMIN THYSEN, GENE A. MORRILL, ELIOT GARDNER, AND GEORGE FUJIMOTO

Steroid Hormone Regulation of Specific Gene Expression

LAWRENCE CHAN, ANTHONY R. MEANS, AND BERT W. O'MALLEY

Enkephalins and Endorphins

RICHARD J. MILLER AND PEDRO CUATRECASAS

Hormonal Control of Hepatic Gluconeogenesis

S. J. PILKIS, C. R. PARK, AND T. H. CLAUS

Gonadotropin Receptors and Regulation of Steroidogenesis in the Testis and Ovary

MARIA L. DUFAU AND KEVIN J. CATT

Contributors to Volume 36

Numbers in parentheses indicate the pages on which the authors' contributions begin.

ERIC BLOCH, *Departments of Biochemistry, Gynecology-Obstetrics, Albert Einstein College of Medicine, Yeshiva University, Bronx, New York 10461* (203)

KEVIN J. CATT, *Endocrinology and Reproduction Research Branch, National Institute of Child Health and Human Development, National Institutes of Health, Bethesda, Maryland 20014* (461)

LAWRENCE CHAN, *Departments of Cell Biology and Medicine, Baylor College of Medicine, Houston, Texas 77030* (259)

FRANK CHYTIL, *Department of Biochemistry, Vanderbilt University, Nashville, Tennessee 37232* (1)

T. H. CLAUS, *Department of Physiology, Vanderbilt University School of Medicine, Nashville, Tennessee 37232* (383)

PEDRO CUATRECASAS, *Wellcome Research Laboratories, Research Triangle Park, North Carolina, 27709* (297)

MARIA L. DUFAU, *Endocrinology and Reproduction Research Branch, National Institute of Child Health and Human Development, National Institutes of Health, Bethesda, Maryland 20014* (461)

GEORGE FUJIMOTO, *Department of Biochemistry, Albert Einstein College of Medicine, Yeshiva University, Bronx, New York 10461* (203)

ELIOT GARDNER, *Departments of Neuroscience and Psychiatry, Albert Einstein College of Medicine, Yeshiva University, Bronx, New York 10461* (203)

R. J. MAYER, *Department of Biochemistry, Queen's Medical Centre, University of Nottingham, Nottingham NG7 2UH, England* (101)

ANTHONY R. MEANS, *Department of Cell Biology, Baylor College of Medicine, Houston, Texas 77030* (259)

RICHARD J. MILLER, *Department of Pharmacological and Physiological Sciences, The University of Chicago, Chicago, Illinois 60637* (297)

GENE A. MORRILL, *Department of Physiology, Albert Einstein College of Medicine, Yeshiva University, Bronx, New York 10461* (203)

EBERHARD NIESCHLAG, *Abteilung für Experimentelle Endokrinologie, Universitäts-Frauenklinik, Westring 11, D-4400 Münster, Federal Republic of Germany* (165)

BERT W. O'MALLEY, *Department of Cell Biology, Baylor College of Medicine, Houston, Texas 77030* (259)

DAVID E. ONG, *Department of Biochemistry, Vanderbilt University, Nashville, Tennessee 37232* (1)

C. R. PARK, *Department of Physiology, Vanderbilt University School of Medicine, Nashville, Tennessee 37232* (383)

S. J. PILKIS, *Department of Physiology, Vanderbilt University School of Medicine, Nashville, Tennessee 37232* (383)

DAVID P. ROSE, *Division of Clinical Oncology, Wisconsin Clinical Cancer Center, University of Wisconsin, Madison, Wisconsin 53706* (53)

PAUL SATO, *Department of Pharmacology, Life Sciences Building, Michigan State University, East Lansing, Michigan 48824* (33)

BENJAMIN THYSEN, *Departments of Biochemistry, Gynecology-Obstetrics, and Laboratory Medicine, Albert Einstein College of Medicine, Yeshiva University, Bronx, New York 10461* (203)

SIDNEY UDENFRIEND, *Roche Institute of Molecular Biology, Nutley, New Jersey 07110* (33)

E. JEAN WICKINGS, *Abteilung für Experimentelle Endokrinologie, Universitäts-Frauenklinik, Westring 11, D-4400 Münster, Federal Republic of Germany* (165)

Preface

Volume 36 of "Vitamins and Hormones" contains ten reviews, a larger number than has usually appeared in this serial publication in recent years. There are three reviews on vitamins, including one on vitamin–hormone interactions, and seven on other endocrinological topics.

In the last decade, it has become increasingly clear that the fat-soluble vitamins as well as the water-soluble vitamins are intimately involved with cellular proteins in expressing their functions. The review by Frank Chytil and David E. Ong on the binding of retinol and retinoic acid to cellular proteins reveals interesting functional similarities between the unique cytoplasmic binding proteins for retinol and retinoic acid and those for the steroid hormones. In the second vitamin review, Paul Sato and Sidney Udenfriend describe recent research that shows clearly the biochemical and genetic basis for the failure of some species to synthesize vitamin C. The review by David P. Rose deals with the interactions between vitamin B_6 and a variety of hormones, including estrogens, glucocorticosteroids, and hormones of the thyroid, hypothalamus, and anterior pituitary. This remarkable vitamin, which is a precursor of pyridoxal phosphate required as a cofactor by a number of amino acid-metabolizing enzymes, is also surprisingly active in modifying endocrine responses at physiological as well as higher doses.

The majority of the other reviews in this volume deal with gonadal steroids, reproductive biology, and lactation. R. J. Mayer reviews hormonal factors in mammary gland lipogenesis with special emphasis on changes in lipogenic enzyme profiles during gland development as well as lactation. The chapter by Eberhard Nieschlag and E. Jean Wickings reviews investigations of the biological effects of antibodies to gonadal steroids on male and female reproductive functions and the application of steroid antisera as tools in reproduction research. Lawrence Chan, Anthony R. Means, and Bert W. O'Malley review steroid hormone regulation of specific gene expression, concluding that, in general, this regulation of specific protein synthesis is at the pretranslational level. The comprehensive review by Maria L. Dufau and Kevin J. Catt on receptors for gonadotropins and regulation of steroidogenesis in the testis and ovary includes discussions of assay procedures for the hormones, hormone binding to receptors, solubilization and purification of receptors for gonadotropins and gonadal adenylate cyclase, and regulation of the receptors and of gonadal cell responses. The extensive literature on the effects of cannabinoids on reproduction and development is critically reviewed by Eric Bloch, Benjamin Thysen, Gene A. Morrill, Eliot Gardner, and George Fujimoto. Definite effects have been observed, and the authors recommend more intensive study of the subject.

The remaining two chapters extend the scope of this volume. The review of the complex subject of the hormonal control of hepatic gluconeogenesis by S. J. Pilkis, C. R. Park, and T. H. Claus focuses on the minute-to-minute regulation of gluconeogenesis by glucagon, catecholamines, and insulin. Finally, we are indebted to Richard J. Miller and Pedro Cuatrecasas for a thorough review of an exciting new subject, the enkephalins and endorphins, which have important implications for neuroendocrinology and peptide hormone biosynthesis.

The Editors wish to express their indebtedness to the authors of these reviews for maintaining the high standards of our publication. We are confident that this volume will be of interest and service to scientists in biology, chemistry, and medicine.

PAUL L. MUNSON
EGON DICZFALUSY
JOHN GLOVER
ROBERT E. OLSON

VITAMINS AND HORMONES

VOLUME 36

Cellular Vitamin A Binding Proteins

FRANK CHYTIL AND DAVID E. ONG

Department of Biochemistry, Vanderbilt University, Nashville, Tennessee

I. Introduction

It is a virtual requirement to begin any paper or review on vitamin A with a statement such as: Little is known about the mechanism of action of vitamin A except in the visual process. But one may say with certainty that the "action" of vitamin A is shown most dramatically in its ability to control and direct differentiation of epithelial tissues. This ability was perhaps revealed most clearly from the striking histological studies by Wolbach and Howe (1925) of morphological changes in rat occurring during vitamin A deficiency and during refeeding with the vitamin (Wolbach and Howe, 1933). This ability to control and direct differentiation led Wolbach (1954) to suggest that vitamin A shows "hormone-like properties." Consequently any proposed role or

1

mechanism of action cannot be considered complete unless it can explain this ability.

Work on the mechanism of action has been complicated to some extent by inability to identify the "active form" of the vitamin. Ingestion of all-*trans*-retinol will meet all requirements for the vitamin. All-*trans*-retinol is also the form of vitamin A that circulates in the blood, in ternary complex with serum retinol-binding protein and prealbumin (Goodman, 1974; Peterson *et al.*, 1974). However, the possibility that an active form of vitamin A other than, or in addition to, all-*trans*-retinol is generated at the cellular level must be considered. Considerable work has been done and is being directed toward this question of the active form of the vitamin. This search was perhaps stimulated most by the synthesis of retinoic acid (Ahrens and Van Dorp, 1946) and subsequent discovery that it supports growth in the retinol-deprived animal. However, although epithelia seemed to be normal in retinol-deficient, retinoic acid-fed rats, vision was impaired (Dowling and Wald, 1960). Moreover, Thompson *et al.* (1964) found that dietary retinoic acid cannot substitute for retinol in maintaining spermiogenesis or pregnancy. This led to the suggestion that retinoic acid may be the active form in a "systemic" role and retinol the active form in the "reproductive" role (Thompson *et al.*, 1964). The failure of retinoic acid to maintain vision suggested that it could not be reduced to the aldehyde or alcohol *in vivo* (Dowling and Wald, 1960) and so was inactive in reproduction. Retinoic acid is formed *in vivo* from small quantitites of injected retinol (Emerick *et al.*, 1967; Ito *et al.*, 1974).

Another possibility considered was that retinol and retinoic acid may be metabolized to a common active intermediate in some tissues. This has led to the discovery of many metabolites (Olson, 1967, 1968) and is continuing with recent discoveries of several new metabolites in urine and feces (Hänni *et al.*, 1976; Hänni and Bigler, 1977). In spite of considerable efforts, conclusive evidence that one form of the vitamin is the active form is still missing (Sundaresan, 1972). The failure of retinoic acid to substitute for retinol in all physiological functions of vitamin A led us to use the working hypothesis that the effects of retinol and retinoic acid were probably not mediated by a single common intermediate but that retinol and retinoic acid act as separate metabolic entities.

Our primary assumption, however, was that the mechanism of action of vitamin A might be similar to that of steroid hormones (Bashor *et al.*, 1973). Steroid hormones are believed to act in their target cells by first binding to specific proteins, called "receptors," present in the cytosol. Each protein has high affinity and specificity for its steroid hormone. The ligand–protein complex translocates into the nucleus, where it interacts with the chromatin, changing the expression of the genome. This is manifested by alterations in nuclear RNA synthesis resulting in changed differentiation. And, indeed, altered nuclear RNA, synthesis has been described in vitamin A-deficient and -repleted animals (Zachman, 1967; Johnson et al., 1969; Zile and DeLuca, 1970).

These assumptions led to the discovery of two intracellular binding proteins, one specific for retinol (Bashor et al., 1973) and the other specific for retinoic acid (Ong and Chytil, 1975a). However, the necessary evidence that these proteins are indeed "receptors," analogous to those described for steroid hormones, is still incomplete. At present, it seems best to leave assignment of any role(s) to these proteins open.

Progress has certainly been limited by the lack of a "marker" for vitamin A action. We believe that the rapid developments in the field of steroid hormone action as well as of vitamin D were made possible by the discovery that synthesis of specific proteins was influenced by these compounds (O'Malley and Means, 1974). For instance, tryptophan pyrrolase is a perfect marker for glucocorticoid action in liver (Knox, 1951). Ovalbumin synthesis in chick oviduct induced by estrogen (O'Malley, 1967) or synthesis of calcium-binding protein induced by vitamin D are other examples (Wasserman et al., 1974). Progress in delineating the mechanism of vitamin A action and the function of the binding proteins would be certainly aided by knowledge of whether specific gene products arise from its action.

The aim of this chapter is to review the advances in the work on vitamin A that relate to intracellular binding proteins. In evaluating the work in this area, we recognize that our personal biases may have affected our analysis of the published evidence. A review covering only the work in our laboratory appeared recently (Chytil and Ong, 1978). Opsinlike proteins that are part of the photoreceptor system will not be discussed here (for a review, see Fisher et al., 1970). Work on the serum transport protein for retinol, known as retinol-binding protein (RBP) has been reviewed recently (Glover et al., 1974; Goodman, 1974; Peterson et al., 1974).

II. Uptake of Retinol into the Cell

The mechanism of uptake of retinol by the cell from the circulating complex of retinol–RBP–prealbumin is of obvious importance because the plasma membrane is very likely one of the points of regulation of vitamin A action. Two systems have been used for studying the mechanism of uptake of retinol into cells: (1) intestinal mucosa cells from monkey (Peterson et al., 1974; Rask and Peterson, 1976), (2) pigment epithelium cells from bovine retina (Heller, 1975).

In the system of Peterson and co-workers, isolated intestinal mucosal cells readily accumulated [³H]retinol from its complex with RBP (holo-RBP), without concomitant cellular uptake of the protein itself. The uptake process appeared to be mediated by a membrane receptor. This was suggested by the observations that the uptake of [³H]retinol showed saturable kinetics and was competitively inhibited by the presence of holo-RBP (with unlabeled retinol). Inhibition was also observed with apo-RBP, suggesting that the membrane receptor was recognizing the protein, but not the retinol. During the uptake process an altered form of RBP was generated. It appeared similar to a form of apo-RBP found in serum. This variant cannot bind retinol, and consequently cannot bind with prealbumin. It differs from holo-RBP in that it lacks the terminal arginine residue (Rask et al., 1974). The arginineless RBP does not inhibit uptake of retinol by the intestinal cells.

Direct evidence for the existence of a plasma membrane receptor for RBP comes from the work of Heller (1975) using pigment epithelium of the eye. The retina receives retinol from the blood via the choroidal surface of these cells. They contain a high amount of retinol and lie in a single layer next to the outer segment of the photoreceptor cells. A primary function of the pigment epithelium appears to be the uptake and transport of retinol to the photoreceptors. The uptake of retinol by the pigment epithelium is dependent upon retinol being bound to RBP (Maraini and Gozzoli, 1975; Chen and Heller, 1977), as was found for the intestinal cells.

Heller used RBP labeled with ^{125}I to show that isolated pigment epithelial cells (bovine) could specifically bind holo-RBP. It was shown that binding was at the cell surface without penetration of RBP into the cell and that the process was saturable. From 3.7 to 5.2×10^4 binding sites per pigment epithelium cell were observed. Apo-RBP was also bound, but with lower affinity than holo-RBP. Using autoradiographic techniques, Heller and Bok (1976a) showed that the holo-RBP binds only to the choroidal surface of the bovine epithelial cells, indicating specificity of the arrangement of the pigment epithelial plasma membranes.

The dissociation constant for the binding of holo-RBP to the cell was estimated to be $5 \times 10^{-12} M$, similar to values obtained for the interaction of peptide hormones with membrane receptors. Heller suggested that after delivery of the retinol to the cell the apo-RBP (having a smaller affinity to the receptor) is displaced from the membrane surface by fresh holo-RBP (Heller, 1975). Whether the RBP was altered after interaction with the receptor was not examined.

The results obtained from these two systems allow the generalization that the first step in the entry of retinol into a target cell is interaction of the transport protein RBP, charged with retinol, with its specific receptor on the plasma membrane. Furthermore these data suggest complexity of the receptor site, containing a carboxypeptidase responsible for "inactivation" of RBP by removing the terminal arginine, which renders it incapable of interacting with retinol, prealbumin, and the receptor. Moreover, RBP not only appears to be important for transport of retinol in blood, but is also the indispensable entity for recognition by the target cell and consequently for penetration of retinol through the plasma membrane. It is of interest that many genetic variations of plasma proteins have been discovered (Gitlin and Gitlin, 1975), but thus far none for RBP. It is conceivable that most errors in the expression of the gene coding for RBP would be lethal.

The mode of transition of retinol through the plasma membrane is not clear. Recently Maraini et al. (1977) reported that after incubating bovine eye pigment epithelium preparation with [³H]retinol holo-RBP and extraction of the isolated plasma membranes with sodium dodecyl sulfate (SDS), polyacrylamide gel electrophoresis showed radioactivity in the region of 14,500 daltons, suggesting a covalent attachment of retinol to a macromolecule.

III. Cellular Retinol-Binding Protein (CRBP)

The first discovery of a cellular binding protein for compounds with vitamin A activity was that for retinol described by Bashor et al. (1973). This protein, called cellular retinol-binding protein or CRBP, has attracted considerable attention.

The detection of CRBP was achieved by sucrose gradient centrifugation (Bashor et al., 1973). Cytosol from rat testis was incubated with [³H]retinol and then layered on a 5 to 20% sucrose gradient and centrifuged for 18 hours at 189,000 g. After centrifugation the profile of radioactivity showed a peak in the 2 S region of the gradient indicating binding of retinol to a macromolecule (Fig. 1). The binding component was shown to be a protein because treatment of the cytosol with Pronase, but not with RNase or DNase, reduced the binding. The binding protein is very specific: only excess retinol, not retinal or retinoic acid, reduced the binding (see Fig. 1). A slight competition found occasion-

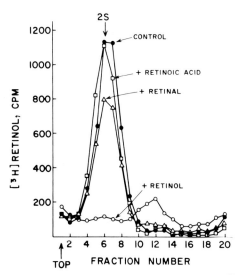

FIG. 1. Demonstration of the existence and specificity of the cellular retinol-binding protein by sucrose gradient centrifugation of testis cytosol after incubation with 40 pmol of [³H]retinol in the presence or in the absence of a 200-fold excess of unlabeled retinol, retinal, or retinoic acid. From Bashor *et al.* (1973).

ally with retinal is apparently due to the reduction of retinal to retinol (Bashor *et al.*, 1973).

Incubation of serum with radioactive retinol and subsequent sucrose gradient centrifugation gives rise to a single peak in the 5 S region of the gradient. Excess nonradioactive retinol, retinal, or retinoic acid did not abolish the peak, indicating that retinol binds to this component nonspecifically (Bashor *et al.*, 1973). The binding component was identified as albumin by immunochemical methods (Bashor and Chytil, 1975; Abe *et al.* 1977). Serum contamination of cytosols occasionally leads to the appearance of such a peak when CRBP is being assayed.

A. DETECTION AND ESTIMATION

The binding protein has been detected and estimated by sucrose gradient centrifugation, as above, by gel filtration on Sephadex G-100 (Bashor *et al.*, 1973), Sephadex G-75 (Futterman *et al.*, 1976), and Sepharose 4B (Wiggert *et al.*, 1977b) shown in Fig. 2. DEAE-cellulose chromatography has also been used (Ong and Chytil, 1975a; Saari and Futterman, 1976a). We routinely use sucrose gradient centrifugation for its estimation (Ong and Chytil, 1976a).

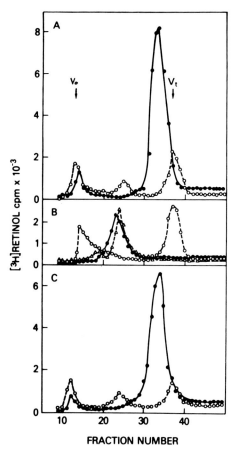

Fig. 2. Detection of cellular retinol-binding protein (CRBP) in the retina by gel filtration. Shown are Sepharose 4B gel filtration patterns of [³H]retinol binding: (A) Chick retinal cytosol incubated with 10^{-7} M [³H]retinol alone (●——●) or with 10^{-5} M nonradiolabeled retinol (○---○). (B) △---△, chick serum (diluted 1:1) incubated with 10^{-7} M [³H]retinol; ●——●, bovine serum albumin (16 mg/ml) incubated with 10^{-7} M [³H]retinol; ○---○, 3×10^{-6} M [³H]retinol alone. (C) Chick pigment epithelium cytosol incubated with 10^{-7} M [³H]retinol alone (●——●) or with 10^{-5} M nonradiolabeled retinol (○---○). From Wiggert et al. (1977b). Reproduced with permission.

B. Tissue and Species Distribution

The protein is widely distributed in the adult rat. It has been detected in brain, eye, skin, spleen, testis, lung, kidney, liver, ovary, and uterus (Bashor et al., 1973; Ong and Chytil, 1975a; Bashor and Chytil, 1975). The cytosols prepared from whole small intestine contain CRBP, but preliminary experiments in this laboratory (Kylberg *et al.*, 1978) suggest that the protein is present only in the jejunum, not in the ileum, of adult rats. Adult rat muscle (heart and gastrocnemius) and serum also are negative for CRBP. No species differences have yet been observed in the tissue distribution of this protein. The protein has been detected in the following species: rat, mouse, rabbit, cow, sheep, human, and chick; thus, occurrence is widespread in higher animals. It is conceivable that in any animal where vitamin A is known to influence the formation of epithelia such binding proteins might exist, fulfilling similar if not identical metabolic functions.

C. CHARACTERISTICS

The binding specificities of CRBP have been extensively studied. In this discussion we will treat CRBP as a single protein without concern for tissue or species origin. With the use of partially purified CRBP, the ability of various retinol derivatives to compete for the binding of [³H]retinol was determined (Ong and Chytil, 1975a). The results are summarized in Table I.

TABLE I

PERCENTAGE INHIBITION OF BINDING OF ALL-*trans*-[³H]RETINOL TO CELLULAR
RETINOL-BINDING PROTEIN FROM RAT TESTIS BY VITAMIN A ACTIVE COMPOUNDS[a]

Compound	Percent inhibition of binding	*In vivo* activity (rat) (%)	Reference
all-*trans*-Retinol	100	100	—
Cis isomers			
13-*cis*-Retinol	95	75	Ames *et al.* (1955a)
9-*cis*-Retinol	51	22	Ames *et al.* (1955a)
9,13-Di-*cis*-retinol	64	24	Ames *et al.* (1955a)
Ring isomers			
α-Retinol	100	2	Ames *et al.* (1955b)
3-Dehydroretinol (vitamin A₂)	100	40	Shantz and Brinkman (1950)
C-15 modifications			
Retinal	0	91	Ames *et al.* (1955b)
Retinoic acid	0	100	Van Dorp and Ahrens (1946)
Retinyl acetate	0	100	Ames *et al.* (1955a)
Retinyl palmitate	0	100	Baxter and Robeson (1942)

[a] Added in 200-fold molar excess over all-*trans*-[³H]retinol (8×10^{-8} M). Adapted from Ong and Chytil (1975b).

Of the *cis* isomers tested, 13-*cis*-retinol was the most effective competitor although less effective than all-*trans*-retinol; 9-*cis*- and 9,13-di-*cis*-retinol had significantly less, but approximately equal, abilities to compete, compared with all-*trans*-retinol. It is compelling that these results parallel the ability of the *cis* isomers to stimulate growth in the vitamin A-deficient rat. The most effective is 13-*cis*-retinol, and 9-*cis*- and 9,13-di-*cis*-retinol have lower but approximately equal activities, compared with all-*trans*-retinol. These data suggest that the ability to interact with the cellular binding protein is one of the factors that determines whether a compound possesses vitamin A activity.

In apparent contradiction to this point is the fact that both α-retinol and 3-dehydroretinol competed as well as all-*trans*-retinol in our binding assay, whereas their *in vivo* activities have been established to be 2% (Ames *et al.*, 1955b) and 40% (Shantz and Brinkman, 1950), respectively, compared with all-*trans*-retinol. When administered to the rat, however, α-retinol is stored in the liver with high efficiency (Ames *et al.*, 1955a) and, at high doses, fully supports growth and development (Goodman *et al.*, 1974). Goodman *et al.* (1974) observed that α-retinol could not enter into the normal serum transport system, so delivery to target tissues is probably inefficient. Clamon *et al.* (1974) have shown that when α-retinyl acetate is added directly to serum-free organ cultures of hamster trachea with keratinized squamous lesions induced by vitamin A deficiency, it is virtually as effective as all-*trans*-retinyl acetate in reversing the metaplasia. Apparently, the change in ring structure prevents the release of α-retinol from the liver to the serum transport system, leading to a low activity *in vivo*, and does not necessarily reflect its potency in a target tissue or conflict with its demonstrated ability to bind to CRBP. This sensitivity to ring conformation may also explain why 3-dehydroretinol exhibits less activity than all-*trans*-retinol *in vivo*.

The partially purified binding protein showed a stringent requirement for the alcohol function at C-15, as neither retinal, retinoic acid, nor esters of the alcohol competed for binding. In crude cytosols, however, an excess of retinyl acetate or palmitate competed effectively (Bashor and Chytil, 1975). It is most likely that the competition observed was due to free retinol generated by esterases. Since retinal can be reduced to retinol *in vivo* (Glover *et al.*, 1948) and the esters hydrolyzed to retinol (Mahadevan *et al.*, 1963), their biological activity may represent their conversion to all-*trans*-retinol, which is bound so effectively by the binding protein. The exception is retinoic acid, which will be discussed below.

This demonstrated binding specificity was consistent with, but not proof of, all-*trans*-retinol being the physiological ligand that interacts with the binding protein. Consequently the partial purification of CRBP with its endogenous ligand allowed the development of evidence that the ligand was indeed all-*trans*-retinol (Ong *et al.*, 1976). It was also shown that CRBP is depleted of retinol during vitamin A deficiency, but the tissue level (in testis) of CRBP did not change. Consequently the level of the protein is apparently not regulated by availability of retinol. In the same experiment the CRBP in the testis from animals pair-fed with a vitamin A-fortified diet was about 40% saturated with retinol. It is conceivable that the degree of saturation may be of importance in the action of this protein.

Recently CRBP from rat liver was purified to homogeneity (Ong and Chytil, 1978a). The binding protein was purified approximately 3500-fold, based on total soluble liver protein. The protein is a single polypeptide chain with a molecular weight of 14,600, based on information obtained by the techniques of sedimentation equilibrium analysis, gel filtration, and SDS polyacrylamide electrophoresis. The protein binds retinol with high affinity; the apparent dissociation constant was determined by fluorometric titration to be $1.6 \times 10^{-8} M$.

The absorption spectrum of pure CRBP with bound retinol is shown in Fig. 3. The portion of the spectrum attributable to retinol (centered at 350 nm) is of particular interest because it shows fine structure not observed for retinol in organic solution. This can be explained if the protein binds retinol in a configuration more nearly planar than the

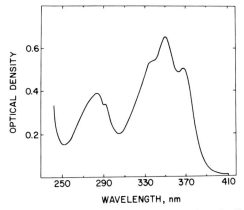

FIG. 3. Absorption spectrum of a homogeneous preparation of cellular retinol-binding protein, $1.35 \times 10^{-5} M$ in $0.05 M$ Tris · HCl, pH 7.5.

average orientation of retinol in organic solution (for discussion of this point see Ong and Chytil, 1978a).

Considerable attention has been given to CRBP in the various specialized epithelia of the eye (see Table II) after the first report of its presence in chick embryo retina and pigment epithelium (Wiggert and Chader, 1975). In general the properties observed for CRBP in these tissues agree with those reported for CRBP in rat tissues. A partial purification and characterization of CRBP from bovine retina has been accomplished by Saari and Futterman (1976a) and Saari et al. (1977).

With crude cytosol and sucrose gradient centrifugation, Scatchard calculations gave an association constant of 5.26×10^7 for retinol and CRBP of stroma and endothelium (Wiggert et al., 1977a). However, in cytosol from retina two types of retinol-binding sites (dissociation constants about $10^{-9} M$ and $4 \times 10^{-8} M$) have been postulated (Wiggert et al. 1977b).

A recent report suggested an "important difference in the receptor in retina and pigment epithelium" (Wiggert et al., 1977b). This was based on competition experiments for binding of [^{3}H]retinol performed with crude cytosol, which showed that retinyl acetate competes in both retina and pigment epithelium, but retinyl palmitate competes only in pigment epithelium. As mentioned before, we have observed that com-

TABLE II

CELLULAR RETINOL-BINDING PROTEIN IN THE EYE

Localization	Source	Reference
Retina	Chicken (embryo)	Wiggert and Chader (1975); Abe et al. (1977)
	Guinea pig	Wiggert et al. (1976)
	Rat	Wiggert et al. (1976)
	Bovine	Saari and Futterman (1976a); Saari et al. (1977)
	Human	Swanson et al. (1976); Bergsma et al. (1977)
Pigment epithelium	Chicken (embryo)	Wiggert and Chader (1975); Abe et al. (1977)
	Guinea pig, rat, bovine	Wiggert et al. (1976); Saari et al. (1977)
	Human	Bergsma et al. (1977)
Corneal epithelium	Calf, bovine	Helmsen et al. (1977)
	Porcine, chicken	Wiggert et al. (1977a)
Corneal stroma	Bovine, porcine, chicken	Wiggert et al. (1977a)
Corneal endothelium	Bovine, porcine, chicken	Wiggert et al. (1977a)

petition by esters is difficult to determine in crude cytosols because of the action of esterases. Consequently this difference needs to be clarified, perhaps by using partially purified preparations of CRBP from both sources. For example, a partially purified preparation of CRBP from bovine retina did not show competition by retinyl acetate or palmitate (Saari and Futterman, 1976b).

Exposure of rat testis cytosol to p-chloromercuribenzoate (M. M. Bashor, unpublished) and chick retina cytosols to N-ethylmaleimide (Wiggert and Chadur, 1975) had little if any effect on binding of retinol to CRBP. It would appear, therefore, that the binding does not depend upon intact sulfhydryl groups. On the other hand, it was recently reported that the addition of dithiothreitol "maximizes" the binding of retinol to CRBP (Wiggert et al., 1977b). Perhaps this effect may be explained by protection of the oxygen-sensitive retinol rather than by stabilization of the protein.

D. Differences between Cellular and Serum Retinol-Binding Protein

Major effort has been given to the demonstration that CRBP is distinct from RBP. Table III contrasts some basic characteristics of the two proteins. With the evidence reviewed here and with the recent amino

TABLE III

Differences between Serum Retinol-Binding Protein (RBP) and Cellular Retinol-Binding Protein (CRBP)

Characteristics	RBP	CRBP
Molecular weight	20,000[a]	14,600[b]
Binding of retinoic acid	Yes[c]	No[d]
Binding of retinal	Yes[c]	No[d]
Binding to prealbumin	Yes[c]	No[f]
Antigenic toward anti-RBP serum	Yes[g]	No[h]
Fluorescence excitation spectrum (maximum nm)	334[a]	350[b]

[a] Muto and Goodman (1972).
[b] Ong and Chytil (1978a).
[c] Glover et al. (1974).
[d] Bashor et al. (1973); Ong and Chytil (1975a).
[e] Kanai et al. (1968); Peterson (1971).
[f] Saari and Futterman (1976b); Abe et al. (1977).
[g] Muto et al. (1972).
[h] Bashor and Chytil (1975).

acid analysis of the homogeneous preparation of liver CRBP (Ong and Chytil, 1978a), it is evident CRBP is a protein distinct from RBP. The antigenic difference, i.e., the nonreactivity of CRBP with antisera to RBP (Bashor and Chytil, 1975), together with the evidence that RBP does not enter the target cells, seems to eliminate the possibility that RBP is a precursor of CRBP.

The work on CRBP in the eye has also confirmed that this protein is different from RBP. This is based again on the difference in size, electrophoretic mobility, and inability of CRBP to bind to serum prealbumin (Saari and Futterman, 1976b; Abe *et al.*, 1977) and by the difference in antigenicity (Abe *et al.*, 1977).

IV. CELLULAR RETINOIC ACID-BINDING PROTEIN

With the discovery that retinoic acid could support the growth of a retinol-deprived animal, retinoic acid became a serious candidate for the "active form" of vitamin A (for review, see Sundaresan, 1972). That it was the only active form was eliminated, however, by the fact that it would not maintain reproduction (Thompson *et al.*, 1964). The apparent inability of CRBP to bind retinoic acid also would seem to exclude the possibility that it acts by substituting for retinol insofar as the action of vitamin A can be accounted for by interaction with CRBP. However, it was soon discovered that some tissues appeared to have a second binding protein specific for retinoic acid (Ong and Chytil, 1975a), subsequently named cellular retinoic acid-binding protein (CRABP). The existence of this separate binding protein for retinoic acid strengthens the idea that retinoic acid acts as a physiological compound, separate from, not in place of, retinol.

A. DETECTION AND ESTIMATION

Sucrose gradient centrifugation of tissue cytosol after incubation with tritiated retinoic acid is the only method now in use (Ong and Chytil, 1975a). Here again presence of CRABP is indicated by a peak of radioactivity in the 2 S region of the gradient (Fig. 4). This binding is saturable and specific; only retinoic acid, but not retinal, retinol, or long-chain fatty acid, competes for binding of tritiated retinoic acid. Esters of retinol also did not compete (Saari and Futterman, 1976b). Nonsaturable binding of retinoic acid is also observed in the 5 S region of the gradient. This has been shown to be binding to serum albumin, known to bind fatty acids (Sani and Hill, 1974). Consequently the

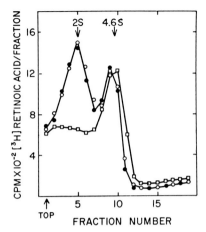

Fig. 4. Detection of cellular retinoic acid-binding protein. Testis cytosol was analyzed by sucrose gradient centrifugation after incubation with [³H]retinoic acid (●———●) and with the addition of a 100-fold excess of unlabeled retinoic acid (□———□) or retinol (○———○).

determination of the specific binding capacity due to CRABP requires that the method chosen separate CRABP from albumin, a common contaminant of cytosols.

B. Tissue and Species Distribution

In adult animals the tissue distribution of CRABP is different from that of CRBP. Wheras CRBP is detectable in all organs studied, with the exception of serum and muscle (heart and gastrocnemius), CRABP has a more limited distribution. It is absent from serum and muscle, but also from kidney, small intestine, liver, lung, and spleen. Positive organs include bladder, brain, eye, mammary gland, ovary, prostate gland, skin, testis, trachea, and uterus (Ong and Chytil, 1975a; Chytil et al., 1975; Futterman et al., 1976; Chytil and Ong, 1976; Sani and Corbett, 1977; Swanson et al., 1976; Wiggert et al., 1977d). CRABP was detected in extracts of epithelial cell layers of chick embryo skin, but not in extracts of the underlying connective tissue (Sani and Hill, 1974; Sani and Corbett, 1977).

No apparent species differences have been observed.

C. Characteristics

All reports on CRABP agree that it is a protein that sediments as a 2 S component on sucrose gradients. The molecular weight by gel filtration has been established as 14,000. The binding protein from embryonic chick skin has a p*I* value of 4.6 (Sani and Hill, 1976).

The binding specificity of CRABP has been determined using two different preparations: CRABP purified 1000-fold from rat testis (Chytil and Ong, 1976) and crude cytosol prepared from chick embryo skin (Sani and Hill, 1976). In both laboratories the binding protein was detected and its affinity for various compounds determined in the manner first described for CRBP (Bashor *et al.*, 1973), using radioactive retinoic acid and sucrose gradient centrifugation. The binding affinity was assessed by competition experiments and, in the case of the testicular preparation, expressed as percentage inhibition (percentage decrease) of binding of radioactive all-*trans* retinoic acid observed when the competing analog was present in a 100-fold molar excess over [³H]retinoic acid (Chytil and Ong, 1976).

Figure 5 shows the structure of the analogs of retinoic acid tested. The relative ability of these compounds to compete for the binding of [³H]retinoic acid by CRABP from rat testis is shown in Table IV. As for CRBP, we see again a striking correlation between the abilities to interact with CRABP and biological activity, as assessed by Sporn *et al.* 1975). The biological activity assessed was growth promotion of epidermal cell cultures (derived from mouse skin) as indicated by increases in RNA, DNA, and protein levels after addition of the test compound. Although no quantitative data are available from experiments using chick skin cytosol (Sani and Hill, 1976), no striking discrepancies in the binding properties of CRABP from these sources have been ob-

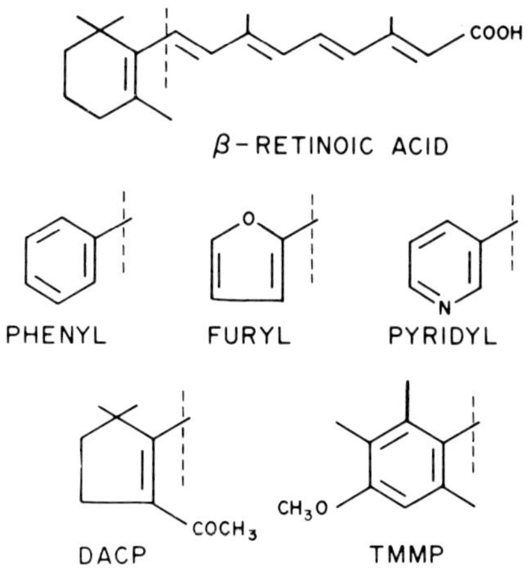

FIG. 5. Structure of β-retinoic acid and analogs with ring modifications. DACP, dimethylacetyl-cyclopentenyl; TMMP, trimethyl-methoxyphenyl.

TABLE IV

PERCENTAGE INHIBITION OF BINDING OF ALL-*trans*-[³H]RETINOIC ACID TO CELLULAR
RETINOIC ACID-BINDING PROTEIN FROM RAT TESTIS AND GROWTH-PROMOTING ACTIVITY
IN THE MOUSE SKIN EPIDERMAL CELL CULTURES BY ANALOGS OF RETINOIC ACID

Compound	Percent inhibition of binding	Growth-promoting ability[a] (% of increase in DNA)
all-*trans*-Retinoic acid	100	46
DACP analog	100	54
TMMP analog	100	65
Phenyl analog	42	23
Furyl analog	34	1[b]
Pyridyl analog	22	9

[a] Sporn *et al.* (1975), when concentration of the analog was $10^{-7} M$.
[b] Concentration of the analog $10^{-6} M$.

served. This correlation suggests that CRABP is mediating the action of these analogs.

On the basis of these results as well as those concerning CRBP, it was suggested that evaluating analogs of retinol and retinoic acid for their ability to bind to CRABP and CRBP might be a useful preliminary screening test to identify those with potential growth activity (Chytil and Ong, 1976).

Recently CRABP has been purified to homogeneity from rat testes (Ong and Chytil, 1978b). The binding protein was purified approxi-

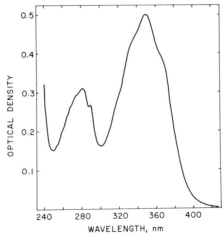

FIG. 6. Absorption spectrum of a homogeneous preparation of CRABP, $1.0 \times 10^{-5} M$ in $0.05 M$ Tris · HCl, pH 8.3.

mately 12,000-fold relative to total soluble testicular protein. The protein is a single polypeptide chain with a molecular weight of 14,600, determined by gel filtration and SDS polyacrylamide electrophoresis. The protein binds retinoic acid with high affinity; the apparent dissociation constant was determined by fluorometric titration to be 4.2 × 10^{-9} M. The absorption spectrum of CRABP saturated with retinoic acid is shown in Fig. 6. The spectrum is dominated by the large peak at 350 nm due to the absorbance of the bound retinoic acid. Testis contains both CRABP and CRBP. CRBP was also purified from this source. Figure 7 shows disc gel electrophoresis of the two binding proteins purified from the same batch of testis, clearly indicating their separation.

Although homogeneous CRABP is now in hand, it might be well to indicate several caveats. Although we firmly believe that CRABP is involved in important aspects of vitamin A action, the endogenous compound that interacts with CRABP has not yet been identified in contrast to CRBP (Ong and Chytil, 1975a). In addition, the observed tissue distribution of CRABP does not fully correlate with those tissues that are properly maintained by administration of retinoic acid to retinol-deprived animals. The failure of administered retinoic acid to maintain reproduction in these animals, coupled with the fact that the reproductive organs (testis, uterus) contain both CRBP and CRABP, may indicate that both retinol and retinoic acid are required, fulfilling different roles (Chytil *et al.*, 1975; Ong and Chytil, 1975a).

V. Cellular Retinol- and Retinoic Acid-Binding Proteins and the Nucleus

The possible interaction of CRBP, CRABP, and their respective ligands with intracellular particles is probably the most exciting area to be investigated now. At the moment of finishing this review we have been successful in detecting specific interaction of the complex [³H]retinol–CRBP with nuclei isolated from livers of vitamin A-deficient rats. The CRBP used was a homogeneous preparation from rat liver. The binding was specific and saturable, with about 1 × 10^{5} sites per nucleus. No specific binding of free [³H]retinol was observed, indicating the necessity of CRBP for the interaction to occur. Whether the binding is to the nuclear membrane, chromatin, or some other nuclear component has not yet been determined. In addition, it will be of interest to follow the interaction by using ¹²⁵I-labeled CRBP. This is

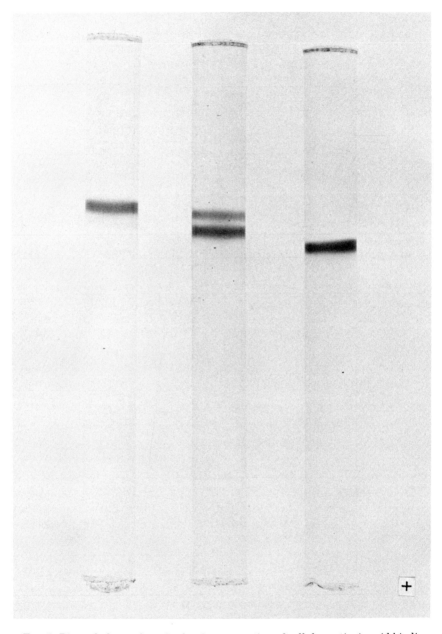

Fig. 7. Disc gel electrophoresis showing separation of cellular retinoic acid-binding protein (CRABP) and cellular retinol-binding protein (CRBP). CRABP was applied to the left and center gel; CRBP was applied to the center and right gel. Both proteins were purified from rat testis.

an important point because we have previously been unable to extract from liver nuclei any 2 S component that will bind retinol. That would suggest that if CRBP enters the nucleus it may be subsequently altered.

In contrast, a recent preliminary note reported that in extracts of nuclei of chick embryo skin, transplantable colon tumor, and Lewis lung carcinoma a 2 S component binding retinoic acid was detected and its "physiochemical properties are in agreement with those of the cellular binding protein for retinoic acid from tissue cytosol" (Sani, 1977). It is of interest that the nuclear extracts also contained serum albumin. This suggests rather considerable contamination of the nuclei with extranuclear proteins. All tissues tested are known to contain CRABP in their cytosols. We have been unable to detect CRABP (or albumin) in extracts of nuclei preparations from fetal liver, adult testes, and brain tissues, all of whose cytosols contain CRABP. We have used [^{3}H]retinoic acid with a specific activity approximately 10-fold greater than that reported by Sani (1977). Moreover, another laboratory was not able to detect a retinoic acid-binding component in extracts of nuclei from human tumors shown to contain CRABP (P. Huber, personal communication, 1977).

Recently preliminary data of Wiggert et al. (1977c) showed the detection by sucrose gradient centrifugation of CRBP and CRABP in the cytosols of cultured retinoblastoma cells. Here again the authors were unable to find in the extracts of nuclei of these cells a component binding either radioactive retinol or retinoic acid. On the other hand, when these cells were preincubated with [^{3}H]retinoic acid a 2 S retinoic acid-binding component was detected in the nuclear extract. The comparison experiment with [^{3}H]retinol was negative.

Whether the occurrence of a nuclear type of CRABP is limited to the embryonic colon tumor and Lewis carcinoma or to all tissue containing CRABP remains to be shown.

VI. PERINATAL DEVELOPMENT OF CELLULAR RETINOL- AND RETINOIC ACID-BINDING PROTEINS

Vitamin A was soon recognized as a factor necessary for reproduction (Evans and Bishop, 1922). Severely deficient females will not conceive; uterine and vaginal keratinization occurs (Moore, 1967). With lesser deficiency, conception may occur, but pregnancy usually ends with fetuses, some of them malformed, being aborted or resorbed. The involvement of vitamin A during pregnancy was recently reexamined and discussed by Goodman's group (Takahashi *et al.*, 1975, 1977). Very little is known about the requirements for vitamin A during the perinatal period.

The observation that fetal but not adult lung contained CRABP suggests that significant alterations may occur in the levels of the binding proteins during organ development (Ong *et al.*, 1975). And in fact a survey of the fetal organs of the rat revealed that both CRBP and CRABP could be detected in all organs examined with the exception of serum (Ong and Chytil, 1976a). Some tissues of the chick embryo have been reported to contain CRABP (Sani and Corbett, 1977). If one assumes that the binding proteins have some relationship to the utilization of vitamin A by the various tissues, then any alterations observed in the levels of these proteins would reflect changing utilizations of retinol or retinoic acid. The time of perinatal development was chosen for closer study. For the initial studies, attention was restricted to liver and lung. Lung epithelium is known to be affected very early in the course of vitamin A deficiency (Wolbach and Howe, 1925), and a high incidence of respiratory problems in vitamin A-deficient human infants has been described (Wolbach, 1954). This suggested that vitamin A may be one of the factors involved in the maturation of the lung. Liver, although less affected in vitamin A deficiency than lung, has been well studied by investigators of perinatal development.

The results obtained in our study are shown in Fig. 8. Both CRBP and CRABP show striking changes during organ maturation. The patterns for liver are distinctly different from those for lung. There is no apparent linkage between levels of CRBP and CRABP in either organ, suggesting that the binding proteins are regulated independently. The changes in the level of the binding proteins imply to us that the requirements for retinol and for retinoic acid during development of each organ change dramatically. Certainly the picture presented is difficult to reconcile with a concept of only one active form for the vitamin. Although we are unable to assign exact significance to the changes observed, several points may be of interest. For example, the disappearance of CRABP in liver generally parallels disappearance of the hematopoietic cells (Greengard *et al.*, 1972). The peak in CRABP level in lung correlates with the time period in which the alveoli are formed in the rat (Burri *et al.*, 1974) suggesting a role for retinoic acid in the processes that led to the formation of new morphological structures. However, the sudden rise in CRBP in liver does not reflect any morphological change of which we are aware. Obviously this area offers interesting research opportunities.

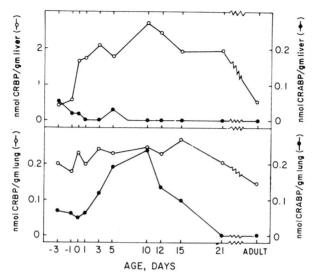

FIG. 8. Perinatal development of cellular retinol-binding protein (CRBP) and cellular retinoic acid-binding protein (CRABP) of rat liver (top) and lung (bottom). Content of binding proteins was determined by specific binding of [³H]retinol and [³H]retinoic acid evaluated by sucrose gradient centrifugation. From Ong and Chytil (1976a).

VII. CELLULAR RETINOL- AND RETINOIC ACID-BINDING PROTEINS IN CANCER

Recent developments in the prevention of chemical carcinogenesis by vitamin A and its synthetic analog (Bollag, 1970; Sporn *et al*., 1976) are logical extensions of the efforts that started very soon after the discovery of vitamin A. That diet may be an important factor when malignant processes are initiated has been considered in the past (reviewed by Burk and Winzler, 1944). Only four years after the discovery of vitamin A as a growth factor, an attempt was made to use a vitamin A-deficient diet for the treatment of patients suffering from cancer (Wyard, 1922), without success. Over the years considerable effort had been given to examining possible relationships of vitamin A to cancer, allowing Burk and Winzler (1944) to conclude: ". . . sufficient evidence has accumulated which makes it desirable to seek further a peculiar and perhaps specific relationship between vitamin A and malignant growth. This evidence consists of the demonstration of hyperplastic lesions of epithelial linings in vitamin A deficiency, possible alteration of vitamin A metabolism in tumor bearing patients, the effect of carcinogens on vitamin A metabolism and occasional experiments indicating that the dietary vitamin A level may influence the growth and incidence of experimental cancer."

More recent evidence, reviewed by Sporn (1977), has shown that dietary deficiency of vitamin A leads to increased incidence of spontaneous and carcinogen or virus-induced epithelial metaplasias and tumors in experimental animals and possibly in man. High doses of retinol esters, retinoic acid and some of its analogs have been reported to be effective in reducing the incidence of chemically induced epithelial metaplasia and tumors in experimental animals. They also appear to have the ability to cause the regression of some preneoplastic lesions in experimental animals and in man. Some transplantable rodent tumors do not show inhibition (Bollag, 1970).

With this body of evidence pointing to a relationship between vitamin A and some premalignant and malignant lesions, it was logical to examine tumors for the presence or absence of the binding proteins for vitamin A. The available data for experimental tumors are collected in Table V. As can be seen, many contain both proteins, some contain none or only CRABP, only one so far contains CRBP alone. We have also examined a limited sample of malignant human tumors (Table VI) all of which contain CRABP.

An interesting point we have observed for several human tumors from lung, breast, skin, and stomach is that CRABP is detectable only in the tumor not in the adjacent, histologically normal tissue (Fig. 9). We reported earlier that CRABP is much more widespread in fetal organs compared to adult and its expression is lost during development. The reappearance of fetal proteins in certain tumors is a phenomenon frequently observed (Abelev, 1971; Shapira, 1973).

The binding affinity of CRABP in extracts of DMBA-induced mouse papilloma and of human breast carcinoma was examined as previously done for CRABP from rat testis. Table VII show results of these experiments. It is of interest that the binding affinity is very similar for CRABP in both tumors and also to that observed with the protein partially purified from rat testis (see Section IV, C). Here again, DACP and TMMP analogs are good competitors, as well as all-*trans*- and 13-*cis*-retinoic acid. Phenyl and furyl analogs compete less well, and no competition was observed with the pyridyl derivative. This correlates well with the ability of these compounds to reverse metaplasia of hamster trachea induced by vitamin A deficiency as shown by Sporn *et al.* (1975), suggesting that the ability of retinoic acid and its derivatives to control differentiation may be mediated through CRABP. In addition, those compounds shown to be effective as prophylactic or

TABLE V

CELLULAR RETINOIC ACID- (CRABP) AND RETINOL-BINDING (CRBP) PROTEINS
IN EXPERIMENTAL TUMORS

Tumor	CRBP	CRABP
At20 mouse pituitary tumor cell line[a,b]	−	+
B16 melanoma[c]	?	+
Chondrosarcoma[d]	−	+
Colon adenocarcinoma[b]	+	−
Colon tumors 26 and 51 (metastatic)[c]	?	+
Colon tumors 36 and 58 (nonmetastatic)[c]	?	−
Dunning leukemia[d]	+	+
Ehrlich ascites[b]	−	−
Ehrlich carcinoma (solid)[d]	−	−
Hepatoma AS-30D[a]	−	?
Human adenocarcinoma HAD-1[d]	+	+
Lewis lung tumor[c]	?	+
L1210 leukemia[d]	−	−
Mammary adenocarcinoma MAC-1[d]	+	+
Mammary tumor C3H 13/C/24 (metastatic)[c]	?	+
Mammary tumor C3H 04/A/64 (metastatic)[c]	?	−
Mammary tumor C3H 16/C/13 (metastatic)[c]	?	+
Mouse skin papilloma[d]	+	+
Novikoff hepatoma[a,b]	−	−
Ridgway osteogenic sarcoma[c]	?	+
Sarcoma 180[d,e]	−	+
SV40-transformed 3T3 mouse fibroblast[b]	−	+
Walker 256 carcinosarcoma[d]	+	+

[a] Bashor and Chytil (1975).
[b] D. E. Ong, unpublished observation.
[c] Sani and Corbett (1977) or Sani and Titus (1977).
[d] Ong and Chytil (1976b).
[e] Not detected by Sani and Titus (1977).

TABLE VI

CELLULAR RETINOL AND RETINOIC ACID-BINDING PROTEINS
IN MALIGNANT HUMAN TUMORS

Tumor origin	CRBP	CRABP
Breast	−	+
Lung	−	+
Thyroid	?	+
Kidney (Wilms)	+	+
Uterus	+	+
Skin	?	+
Stomach	?	+

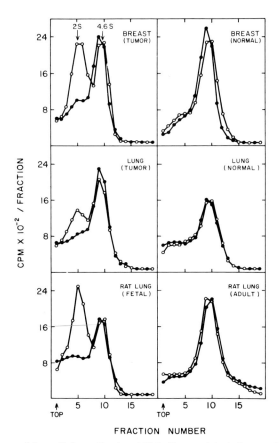

FRACTION NUMBER

FIG. 9. Presence of the cellular retinoic acid-binding protein in human lung and breast tumors and rat fetal lung. Portions of the tissue extracts were incubated with 40 pmol of [³H]retinoic acid (O) and with an additional 8 nmol of unlabeled retinoic acid(●). Portions of the incubation mixtures were subjected to sucrose gradient centrifugation for 20 hours at 148,000 g. From Ong *et al.* (1975). Copyright 1975 by the American Association for the Advancement of Science.

therapeutic agents against DMBA-induced papillomas (Bollag, 1970) or a transplantable chondrosarcoma (Heilman and Swarm, 1975), both of which contain CRABP, are bound well by this protein. These compounds are retinoic acid, 13-*cis*-retinoic acid, and the TMMP analog of retinoic acid. To our knowledge no analog of retinoic acid with low affinity for CRABP has shown activity in such systems. This led to the suggestion that the presence of the appropriate binding protein may be a required, although not necessarily sufficient, condition for a tumor to

TABLE VII

PERCENTAGE INHIBITION OF BINDING OF ALL-*trans*-[³H]RETINOIC ACID TO CELLULAR
RETINOIC ACID-BINDING PROTEIN BY ANALOGS OF RETINOIC ACID AND THE ABILITY
TO REVERSE METAPLASIA IN TRACHEAL ORGAN CULTURE

Compound	Mouse papilloma binding protein (%)	Human breast tumor binding protein (%)	Reversal of metaplasia[a]
all-*trans*-Retinoic acid	100	100	Marked
13-*cis*-Retinoic acid	75	90	—
DACP analog[b]	100	100	Marked
TMMP analog[b]	100	100	Marked
Phenyl analog	36	36	Minimal
Furyl analog	16	24	Almost none
Pyridyl analog	0	0	Almost none

[a] Sporn *et al.* (1975).
[b] DACP, dimethylacetyl-cyclopentenyl; TMMP, trimethyl-methoxyphenyl.

be sensitive to treatment with vitamin A and its analogs (Ong and Chytil, 1976b).

VIII. OTHER CELLULAR VITAMIN A BINDING PROTEINS

There have been reports of compounds with vitamin A activity interacting with other cellular macromolecules. In contrast to CRBP and CRABP the studies of these interactions have not yet been extended beyond a limited range of tissue type and species. For several the specificity of the interaction needs further investigation.

A. CELLULAR RETINAL (11-*cis*)-BINDING PROTEIN

Recently Futterman *et al.* (1977) detected a protein in bovine retina which binds 11-*cis*-retinal but not retinol or retinoic acid. Figure 10 shows the gel filtration experiment that led to the discovery of this protein. The apparent molecular weight is 50,000, quite distinct from CRBP and CRABP. As this protein was not capable of reducing or oxidizing retinal in the presence of NAD or NADH, the authors concluded that it was not a dehydrogenase. However, the bound retinal could be reduced to retinol in the presence of added alcohol dehydrogenase and NADH, indicating the aldehyde group of retinal is still accessible when bound to the protein. As the protein apparently does not bind retinol or retinoic acid the specificity may be determined by

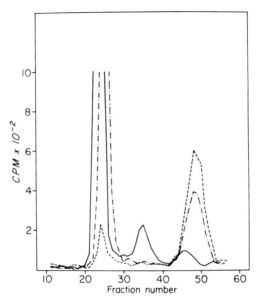

FIG. 10. Demonstration of cellular 11-*cis*-retinal-binding protein. Comparison of binding of tritium-labeled retinol (– · – ·), retinoic acid (---), and retinal (——) to the soluble protein fraction from bovine retina. [³H]Retinol, [³H]retinoic acid, or [³H]retinal was incubated with the soluble protein fraction from bovine retina for 1 hour at room temperature and analyzed by gel filtration using Sephadex G-100. Fractions were collected and samples were counted. From Futterman *et al.* (1977). Reproduced with permission.

the configuration of the double-bond system rather than the oxidation state of C-15. The 11-*cis* isomer of retinal had the highest affinity of those examined for binding. The authors suggest that the protein might be involved in the formation and utilization of 11-*cis*-retinal for regeneration of bleached rhodopsin. If this is the case, the presence of this protein should then be limited to retina.

B. CELLULAR RETINOL-BINDING LIPOGLYCOPROTEIN

Heller (1976) and Heller and Bok (1976b) have reported that bovine pigment epithelial cells and rod photoreceptor outer segment fractions each contain a lipoglycoprotein (molecular weight greater than 1×10^6) with which retinol associates. Here again gel filtration (shown in Fig. 11) was used for detection of these components. In addition to the high molecular weight protein labeled with retinol, the figure also shows a smaller peak, just past the arrow indicating position of the RBP. It is quite possible that the peak indicates the presence of CRBP,

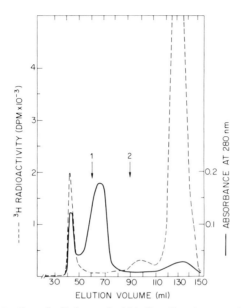

FIG. 11. Demonstration of cellular retinol-binding lipoglycoprotein. Gel filtration of [³H]retinol-labeled pigment epithelial (PE) cytosol. Cytosol was applied to a Sephadex G-100 column equilibrated with 0.033 M sodium phosphate buffer, pH 7.0, containing 0.1 M NaCl. Arrow 1 indicates the elution position from the same column, under the same experimental conditions of retinol–RBP–prealbumin complex; and arrow 2, that of free retinol–RBP. From Heller (1976). Reproduced with permission.

known to be present in bovine retina (Wiggert *et al.*, 1976; Saari and Futterman, 1976a). There is no evidence presently available as to the specificity of the binding of the high molecular weight lipoglycoproteins. Further work will be necessary to decide whether these proteins have any relationship to the other binding proteins. It should be mentioned that Wiggert *et al.* (1977b) were not able to detect these proteins in bovine retina.

C. ESTROGEN-BINDING PROTEIN FROM THE PREPUTIAL GLAND

Recently an extract of rat preputial gland was found to contain a protein that binds estrone and estradiol (Feldman *et al.*, 1977). The protein had an apparent molecular weight of 15,000 and was obtained as a homogeneous preparation after 26-fold purification. The association constant for estrone as determined by equilibrium dialysis, was $1.2 \times 10^7 M$. Interestingly, the authors observed that retinoic acid, but not retinol, reduced the binding of estrone. However, the low binding specificity of the protein makes it an unlikely candidate for mediation of retinoic acid action.

D. The 7 S or 8 S Retinol-Binding Protein

Sucrose gradient centrifugation of bovine retinal cytosol preincubated with [³H]retinol indicated the presence of a binding component that sedimented in the 7–8 S region of the gradient (Wiggert et al., 1976). The peak is abolished in the presence of either excess unlabeled retinol or retinoic acid (Wiggert et al., 1977e). It has been detected in newborn and adult retina and pigment epithelium and adult bovine brain, but not in the corresponding fetal tissues (Wiggert et al., 1976). The protein is apparently present in the retina of bovine, porcine, monkey, and human origin, but not in that of chicken or rat. Interestingly, the binding cannot be demonstrated by gel filtration on Sepharose 4B (Wiggert et al., 1977e; 1978). In a recent note Bergsma et al. (1977) reported that normal human retina contained both a 2 S and an 8 S retinol-binding component, but only the 2 S component (CRBP) was observed in retina from a patient with retinitis pigmentosa.

Cytosols from corneal stroma and endothelium also exhibited an 8 S retinol-binding component. However no competition with excess retinol was observed (Wiggert et al., 1977a). Further work will be required before one can draw any conclusions about the specificity, distribution, or function of these 7–8 S species.

E. Low Molecular Weight Retinol-Binding Protein

It has been reported that the cytosol of rat seminiferous tubules contains a component of molecular weight 4800 that binds retinol (Gambhir and Ahluwalia, 1974a,b). However, retinyl acetate was used to detect binding. The component was reportedly purified to homogeneity in two steps using ammonium sulfate precipitation and gel filtration. After close examination of the reports, we feel that the nature of this component needs clarification.

IX. Conclusions

Of the intracellular binding components for compounds with vitamin A activity discussed in this review, cellular retinol-binding protein and cellular retinoic acid-binding protein appear to be of special interest. Their existence has been confirmed in a number of laboratories without serious discrepancy in published reports of their properties. Consideration of the characteristics of these proteins allows new insights into the role(s) of vitamin A in cellular metabolism.

1. Strong (although circumstantial) evidence has been presented that these two proteins mediate important aspects of vitamin A action.

2. The existence of a protein that specifically binds retinoic acid gives strong support to the idea that retinoic acid is one of the physiological forms of vitamin A.

3. The fact that retinol and retinoic acid have separate binding proteins indicates, however, that these two compounds are not interchangeable in cellular metabolism.

4. That these proteins are apparently regulated independently suggests that there are changing requirements for the different roles of retinol and retinoic acid during growth and differentiation.

5. The discovery of differences in the presence or absence of the binding proteins in malignant and normal tissue might be related to the observed effects of vitamin A-like compounds in cancer.

6. Both binding proteins have now been purified and characterized; this may soon allow the development of direct evidence for their separate roles in vitamin A action in normal as well as malignant processes.

ACKNOWLEDGMENTS

Supported by grants from the U.S. Public Health Service HD-05348, HD-09195, HL-14214, HL-15341, and CA-20850. The generous assistance of the Hoffmann-La Roche Company is acknowledged.

REFERENCES

Abe, T., Wiggert, B., Bergsma, D. R., and Chader, G. J. (1977). *Biochim. Biophys. Acta* **498**, 355.
Abelev, G. I. (1971). *Adv. Cancer Res.* **14**, 295.
Ahrens, J. F., and Van Dorp, D. A. (1946). *Nature (London)* **157**, 190.
Ames, S. R., Swanson, W. J., and Harris, P. L. (1955a). *J. Am. Chem. Soc.* **77**, 4134.
Ames, S. R., Swanson, W. J., and Harris, P. L. (1955b). *J. Am. Chem. Soc.* **77**, 4136.
Bashor, M. M., and Chytil, F. (1975). *Biochim. Biophys. Acta* **411**, 87.
Bashor, M. M., Toft, D. O., and Chytil, F. (1973). *Proc. Natl. Acad. Sci. U.S.A.* **70**, 3483.
Baxter, J. G., and Robeson, C. D. (1942). J. Am. Chem. Soc. **64**, 2407.
Bergsma, D. R., Wiggert, B. N., Funahashi, M., Kuwabara, T., and Chader, G. J. (1977). *Nature (London)* **265**, 66.
Bollag, W. (1970). *Int. J. Vitam. Res.* **40**, 299.
Burk, D., and Winzler, R. J. (1944). *Vitam. Horm. (N.Y.)* **2**, 305.
Burri, P. H., Dbaly, J., and Weibel, E. R. (1974). *Anat. Rec.* **178**, 711.
Chen, C. C., and Heller, J. (1977). *J. Biol. Chem.* **252**, 5216.
Chytil, F., and Ong, D. E. (1976). *Nature (London)* **260**, 5546.

Chytil, F., and Ong, D. E. (1978). In "Receptors and Hormone Action" (B. W. O'Malley and L. Birnbaumer, eds.), Vol. 2, p. 573. Academic Press, New York.

Chytil, F., Page, D. L., and Ong, D. E. (1975). Int. J. Vitam. Nutr. Res. 45, 293.

Clamon, G. H., Sporn, M. B., Smith, J. M., and Saffiotti, U. (1974). Nature (London) 250, 64.

Dowling, J. E., and Wald, G. (1960). Proc. Natl. Acad. Sci. U.S.A. 46, 587.

Emerick, R. J., Zile, M., and DeLuca, H. F. (1967). Biochem. J. 102, 606.

Evans, H. M., and Bishop, K. S. (1922). J. Metab. Res. 1, 335.

Feldman, M., Voigt, W., and Hsia, S. L. (1977). J. Biol. Chem. 252, 3324.

Fisher, K. D., Carr, C. J., Huff, J. E., and Huber, T. E. (1970). Fed. Proc., Fed. Am. Soc. Exp. Biol. 29, 1605.

Futterman, S., Saari, J. C., and Swanson, D. E. (1976). Exp. Eye Res. 22, 419.

Futterman, S., Saari, J. C., and Blair, S. (1977). J. Biol. Chem. 252, 3267.

Gambhir, K. K., and Ahluwalia, B. S. (1974a), Fed. Proc., Fed. Am. Soc. Exp. Biol. 33, 688.

Gambhir, K. K., and Ahluwalia, B. S. (1974b). Biochem. Biophys. Res. Commun. 61, 501.

Gitlin, D., and Gitlin, J. (1975). In "The Plasma Proteins" (F. W. Putnam, ed.), 2nd ed., Vol. 2, p. 264. Academic Press, New York.

Glover, J., Goodwin, T. W., and Morton, R. A. (1948). Biochem. J. 43, 109.

Glover, J., Jay, C., and White, G. H. (1974). Vitam. Horm. (N.Y.) 32, 215.

Goodman, D. S. (1974). Vitam. Horm. (N.Y.) 32, 167.

Goodman, D. S., Smith, J. E., Hembry, R. M., and Dingle, J. T. (1974). J. Lipid Res. 15, 406.

Greengard, O., Federman, M., and Knox, W. E. (1972). J. Cell Biol. 52, 261.

Hänni, R., and Bigler, F. (1977). Helv. Chim. Acta 60, 881.

Hänni, R., Bigler, F., Meister, W., and Englert, G. (1976). Helv. Chim. Acta 59, 2221.

Heilman, C., and Swarm, R. L. (1975). Fed. Proc. Fed. Am. Soc. Exp. Biol. 34, 822.

Heller, J. (1975). J. Biol. Chem. 250, 6549.

Heller, J. (1976). J. Biol. Chem. 251, 2952.

Heller, J., and Bok, D. (1976a). Am. J. Ophthalmol. 81, 93.

Heller, J., and Bok, D. (1976b). Exp. Eye Res. 22, 403.

Helmsen, R., Wiggert, B., and Chader, G. J. (1977). Exp. Eye Res. 24, 213.

Ito, Y., Zile, M., DeLuca, H. F., and Ahrens, H. M. (1974). Biochim. Biophys. Acta 369, 338.

Johnson, B. C., Kennedy, M., and Chiba, N. (1969). Am. J. Clin. Nutr. 22, 1048.

Kanai, M., Raz, A., and Goodman, D. S. (1968). J. Clin. Invest. 47, 2025.

Knox, W. E. (1951). J. Exp. Pathol. 32, 462.

Kylberg, H., Ong, D. E., and Chytil, F. (1978). Fed. Proc. Fed. Am. Soc. Exp. Biol. 37, 708.

Mahadevan, S., Seshadri Sastry, P., and Ganguly, J. (1963). Biochem. J. 88, 531.

Maraini, G., and Gozzolli, F. (1975). Invest. Ophthalmol. 14, 785.

Maraini, G., Ottonello, S., Gozzolli, F., and Merli, A. (1977). Nature (London) 265, 68.

Moore, T. (1967). In "The Vitamins" (W. H. Sebrell and R. S. Harris, eds.), 2nd ed., Vol. 1, p. 245. Academic Press, New York.

Muto, Y., and Goodman, D. S. (1972). J. Biol. Chem. 247, 2533.

Muto, Y., Smith, J. E., Milch, P. O., and Goodman, D. S. (1972). J. Biol. Chem. 247, 2542.

Olson, J. A. (1967). Pharmacol. Rev. 19, 559.

Olson, J. A. (1968). Vitam. Horm. (N.Y.) 26, 1.

O'Malley, B. W. (1967). Biochemistry 6, 2546.

O'Malley, B. W., and Means, A. P. (1974). *Science* **183**, 610.

Ong, D. E., and Chytil, F. (1975a). *J. Biol. Chem.* **250**, 6113.

Ong, D. E., and Chytil, F. (1975b). *Nature (London)* **255**, 74.

Ong, D. E., and Chytil, F. (1976a). *Proc. Natl. Acad. Sci. U.S.A.* **73**, 3976.

Ong, D. E., and Chytil, F. (1976b). *Cancer Lett.* **2**, 25.

Ong, D. E., and Chytil, F. (1978a). *J. Biol. Chem.* **253**, 828.

Ong, D. E., and Chytil, F. (1978b). J. Biol. Chem. **253**, 4551.

Ong, D. E., Page, D. L., and Chytil, F. (1975). *Science* **190**, 60.

Ong, D. E., Tsai, C. H., and Chytil, F. (1976). *J. Nutr.* **106**, 204.

Peterson, P. A. (1971). *J. Biol. Chem.* **245**. 34.

Peterson, P. A., Nilsson, S. F., Ostberg, L., and Vahlquist, A. (1974). *Vitam. Horm. (N.Y.)* **32**, 181.

Rask, L., and Peterson, P. A. (1976). *J. Biol. Chem.* **251**, 6360.

Rask, L., Vahlquist, A., and Peterson, P. A. (1974). *J. Biol. Chem.* **246**, 6638.

Saari, J. C., and Futterman, S. (1976a). *Exp. Eye Res.* **22**, 425.

Saari, J. C., and Futterman, S. (1976b). *Biochim. Biophys. Acta* **444**, 789.

Saari, J. C., Bunt, A. H., Futterman, S., and Berman, E. R. (1977). *Invest. Ophthalmol.* **16**, 797.

Sani, B. P. (1977). *Biochem. Biophys. Res. Commun.* **75**, 7.

Sani, B. P., and Corbett, T. H. (1977). *Cancer Res.* **37**, 209.

Sani, B. P., and Hill, D. L. (1974). *Biochim. Biophys. Res. Commun.* **61**, 1276.

Sani, B. P., and Hill, D. L. (1976). *Cancer Res.* **36**, 409.

Sani, B. P., and Titus, B. C. (1977). *Cancer Res.* **37**, 4031.

Shantz, E. M., and Brinkman, J. H. (1950). *J. Biol. Chem.* **183**, 467.

Shapira, F. (1973). *Adv. Cancer Res.* **18**, 77.

Sporn, M. B. (1977). *Nutr. Rev.* **35**, 65.

Sporn, M. B., Clamon, G. H., Dunlop, N. M., Newton, D. L., Smith, J. M., and Saffiotti, U. (1975). *Nature (London)* **253**, 47.

Sporn, M. B., Dunlop, N. M., Newton, L., and Smith, S. M. (1976). *Fed. Proc., Fed. Am. Soc. Exp. Biol.* **35**, 1332.

Sundaresan, P. R. (1972). *J. Sci. Ind. Res.* **31**, 581.

Swanson, D., Futterman, S., and Saari, J. C. (1976). *Invest. Ophthalmol.* **15**, 1017.

Takahashi, Y. I., Smith, J. E., Winick, M., and Goodman, D. S. (1975). *J. Nutr.* **105**, 1299.

Takahashi, Y. I., Smith, J. E., and Goodman, D. S. (1977). *Am. J. Physiol.* **232**, E263.

Thompson, J. N., Howell, J. McC., and Pitt, G. A. (1964). *Proc. R. Soc. London, Ser. B* **159**, 510.

Van Dorp, D. A., and Ahrens, J. F. (1946). *Nature (London)* **158**, 60.

Wasserman, R. H., Carradino, R. A., Fullmer, C. S., and Taylor, A. N. (1974). *Vitam. Horm. (N.Y.)* **32**, 299.

Wiggert, B., and Chader, G. J. (1975). *Exp. Eye Res.* **21**, 143.

Wiggert, B., Bergsma, D. R., and Chader, G. J. (1976). *Exp. Eye Res.* **22**, 411.

Wiggert, B., Bergsma, D. R., Helmsen, R. J., Alligood, J., Lewis, M., and Chader, G. J. (1977a). *Biochim. Biophys. Acta* **491**, 104.

Wiggert, B., Bergsma, D. R., Lewis, M., Abe, T., and Chader, G. J. (1977b). *Biochim. Biophys. Acta* **498**, 336.

Wiggert, B., Russel, P., Lewis, M., and Chader, J. G. (1977c). *Biochem. Biophys. Res. Commun.* **79**, 218.

Wiggert, B., Bergsma, D. R., Helmsen, R., and Chader, G. J. (1977d). *Biochem. J.* **169**, 87.

Wiggert, B., Mizukawa, A., Kuwabara, T., and Chader, J. G. (1977e). *J. Neurochem.* **29,** 947.

Wiggert, B., Bergsma, D. R., Lewis, M., and Chader, G. J. (1978). *J. Neurochem.* **30,** 653.

Wolbach, S. B. (1954). *In* "The Vitamins" (W. H. Sebrell, Jr. and R. S. Harris, eds.), 1st ed., Vol. 1, p. 106. Academic Press, New York.

Wolbach, S. B., and Howe, P. R. (1925). *J. Exp. Med.* **42,** 753.

Wolbach, S. B., and Howe, P. R. (1933). *J. Exp. Med.* **57,** 511.

Wyard, S. (1922). *Lancet* 840.

Zachman, R. D. (1967). *Life Sci.* **6** 2207.

Zile, M., and DeLuca, H. F. (1970). *Arch. Biochem. Biophys.* **140,** 210.

VITAMINS AND HORMONES, VOL. 36

Studies on Ascorbic Acid
Related to the Genetic Basis of Scurvy

PAUL SATO AND SIDNEY UDENFRIEND

Michigan State University, Department of Pharmacology, East Lansing, Michigan, and Roche Institute of Molecular Biology, Nutley, New Jersey

I. INTRODUCTION

The importance of ascorbic acid has long been known, scurvy being the first recognized deficiency disease in man. The vitamin has been shown to be involved in biological hydroxylation reactions of a number of metabolic pathways. Many of the areas of current research on the metabolism as well as on the physiological functions of the vitamin have been reviewed recently (King and Burns, 1975). Ascorbic acid is produced by nearly all living organisms, plant and animal. However, in the course of evolution primates, guinea pigs (Burns *et al.*, 1956; Burns, 1957; Chatterjee *et al.*, 1961a), bats (Birney *et al.*, 1976), and several other species including certain fish (Chatterjee, 1973a,b) suffered a mutation making them dependent upon an exogenous source of ascorbic acid. As a result they are susceptible to a serious deficiency disease, scurvy, if the vitamin is not supplied. The fact that these species have survived through evolution with so serious an enzyme defect indicates that they were generally highly successful in obtaining adequate amounts of ascorbic acid from the environment. In this review we will summarize recent findings on the biosynthesis of ascorbic acid in mammals, in particular on the biochemical and genetic basis for the failure of some species to synthesize the vitamin.

II. Biosynthesis of Ascorbic Acid in Mammals

Studies with radioactive tracers have shown that ascorbic acid is derived from glucose as part of the glucuronic acid pathway. Reviews of the biosynthesis of ascorbic have appeared recently (King, 1973; Burns, 1975; Chatterjee et al., 1975). As shown in Fig. 1, glucose is oxidized to D-glucuronic acid, which is reduced to L-gulonic acid by an NADPH-requiring enzyme (Hassan and Lehninger, 1956; Ashwell et al., 1961; Mano et al., 1961). L-Gulonic acid is then lactonized to L-gulonolactone (Winkelman and Lehninger, 1958; Yamada et al., 1959). These reactions occur in the soluble fraction of liver. L-Gulonolactone is then oxidized to ascorbic acid through the intermediate 2-keto-L-gulonolactone. This step is catalyzed by a liver microsomal enzyme, L-gulonolactone oxidase (Kanfer et al., 1959; Chatterjee et al., 1961b).

III. The Missing Enzyme in Mammals Subject to Scurvy

After the elucidation of the biosynthetic pathway of ascorbic acid in mammals, it was shown that tissues of animals subject to scurvy (guinea pigs, bats, and primates) contain no L-gulonolactone oxidase activity (Burns et al., 1956; Burns, 1957; Chatterjee et al., 1961b; Chatterjee, 1973a,b). Since all the other enzyme activities shown above were present, it was concluded that the genetic defect in scurvy-prone animals was due to a deficiency of the enzyme L-gulonolactone oxidase. The lactonase that catalyzes conversion of L-gulonic acid to L-gulonolactone is a reversible enzyme, and the equilibrium of the reaction favors the acid form (Chatterjee et al., 1960). Thus L-gulonolactone does not accumulate in the tissues of scurvy-prone animals.

Subsequent to those studies, Chatterjee and co-workers (1957, 1961a; Chatterjee, 1970; Dutta Gupta et al., 1973) speculated that animals that develop scurvy might lack a second enzyme in the pathway of ascorbic acid synthesis. They reasoned that since L-gulonolactone oxidase is a microsomal enzyme, the other enzymes involved in the formation of ascorbic acid should also be microsomal,

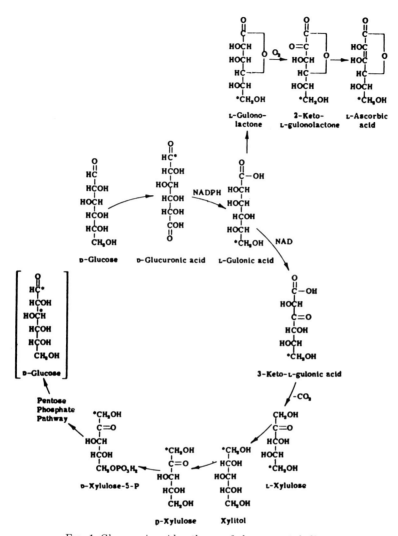

FIG. 1. Glucuronic acid pathway of glucose metabolism.

and that the enzyme in cytosol which converts D-glucuronic acid to L-gulonic acid is not an adequate source of L-gulonolactone for the biosynthesis of the vitamin. They thus questioned the accepted pathway for ascorbic acid biosynthesis and proposed a second pathway involving a microsomal enzyme that converts D-glucuronolactone to L-gulonolactone (Fig. 2).

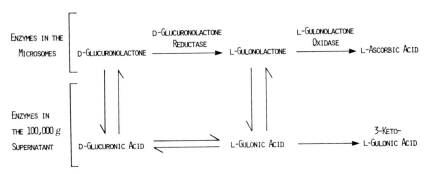

FIG. 2. Proposed second pathway of ascorbic acid biosynthesis.

Evidence for this was found by showing the two-step conversion of D-glucuronolactone to ascorbic acid by washed rat liver microsomes. This conversion, however, was unusual in that it required carbonyl reagents, such as hydroxylamine, semicarbazide, or cyanide, for activity. Since conversion of L-gulonolactone to ascorbic acid by L-gulonolactone oxidase did not require a carbonyl reagent, it was concluded by Chatterjee that a specific microsomal D-glucuronolactone reductase, which requires carbonyl reagents for activation, was involved in the biosynthesis of ascorbic acid. When liver microsomes from scurvy-prone animals were examined, they were also found to be deficient in this carbonyl reagent-requiring D-glucuronolactone reductase. This led Chatterjee to conclude that two enzymes in the ascorbic acid pathway were deficient in scurvy.

In evaluating these findings we considered that the presence of these carbonyl reagents would produce derivatives of D-glucuronolactone that resemble L-gulonolactone (Sato et al., 1976). That is, the furanose ring of D-glucuronolactone would be opened on combination with the carbonyl reagent (Fig. 3). If this were so, then L-gulonolactone oxidase might itself oxidize D-glucuronolactone. It was found that in the presence of hydroxylamine or semicarbazide L-gulonolactone oxidase, which had been purified nearly to homogeneity, did indeed convert D-glucuronolactone to "ascorbic acid" as measured by the method of Zannoni et al. (1974). It was also shown that the oxime and semicarbazone derivatives of D-glucuronolactone were themselves substrates of purified L-gulonolactone oxidase from both rat and goat liver. Both compounds were found to be converted to "ascorbic acid."

If our hypothesis, that L-gulonolactone oxidase is directly oxidizing the D-glucuronolactone derivatives, is true, then the product(s) of these

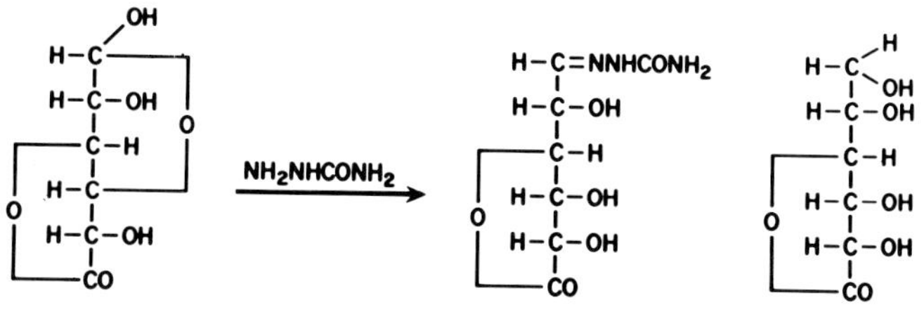

D-Glucurono-6,3-lactone

D-Glucurono-6,3-lactone semicarbazone

L-Gulono-1,4-lactone

FIG. 3. Proposed derivative of D-glucuronolactone produced on interaction with a carbonyl reagent.

reactions should be not ascorbic acid itself, but the corresponding conjugates of ascorbic acid and the carbonyl reagent. In fact, the products of the reactions, when subjected to thin-layer chromatography, were shown to differ from ascorbic acid. When the semicarbazone of D-glucuronolactone, labeled in the semicarbazone moiety, was treated with purified goat liver L-gulonolactone oxidase, the product isolated on thin-layer chromatography was shown to be radioactive. This showed that pure L-gulonolactone oxidase catalyzes the conversion of D-glucuronolactone semicarbazone to the semicarbazone of ascorbic acid. The affinity of L-gulonolactone oxidase for the carbonyl derivatives of D-glucuronolactone was found to be lower than for L-gulonolactone. Furthermore, L-gulonolactone effectively inhibited the reaction with D-glucuronolactone [14C]semicarbazone.

The possibility remained that a form of D-glucuronolactone reductase, which requires a carbonyl reagent for activation, is present in microsomes and that this was removed during purification. This possibility was ruled out by carrying out the purification procedure and monitoring the activities at each step using L-gulonolactone, D-glucuronolactone semicarbazone, or D-glucuronolactone oxime as substrates. The specific activities obtained with each of the three substrates increased equally at each step in the procedure, over a 70-fold range of purification, starting with intact goat liver microsomes (Table I), and over a 120-fold purification during the preparation of rat L-gulonolactone oxidase.

It must be concluded that the conversion of D-glucuronolactone to "ascorbic acid" is not indicative of another microsomal enzyme in the ascorbic acid pathway. Rather, L-gulonolactone oxidase itself is capable of oxidizing the semicarbazone and oxime of D-glucuronolactone to

TABLE I

COMPARISON OF ACTIVITIES OF THREE SUBSTRATES DURING THE PURIFICATION OF
GOAT L-GULONOLACTONE OXIDASE[a,b]

	L-Gulonolactone		D-Glucuronolactone semicarbazone		D-Glucuronolactone oxime	
	Specific activity	Purification	Specific activity	Purification	Specific activity	Purification
Microsomes	6.75	—	6.63	—	6.02	—
Tryptic digestion	10.79	1.6	8.52	1.3	8.21	1.4
Tween 20	9.30	1.4	11.48	1.7	7.22	1.2
$(NH_4)_2SO_4$	18.73	2.8	17.25	2.6	14.19	2.4
BioGel A 1.5 m	42.91	6.4	39.80	6.0	37.64	6.3
DEAE-Sephadex	201.35	29.8	212.99	32.1	208.27	34.6
Hydroxyapatite	463.28	68.6	503.12	75.9	407.10	67.6

[a] From Sato et al. (1976), with permission.
[b] Specific activity in milliunits per milligram of protein; purification relative to microsomes.

their corresponding ascorbic acid derivatives. Since all the other enzymes in the pathway are present, L-gulonolactone oxidase is the only missing enzyme activity in mammals subject to scurvy.

IV. L-GULONOLACTONE OXIDASE

The final step in the pathway from glucose to ascorbic acid is catalyzed by L-gulonolactone oxidase (EC 1.1.3.8). The requirement for ascorbic acid by some mammals, results from an inherited lack of an active form of this enzyme. The first step to understanding the genetic basis of scurvy was the purification and characterization of this enzyme.

A number of assays for L-gulonolactone oxidase activity have been described (Nakagawa and Asano, 1970; Sato et al., 1976; Ayaz et al., 1976). In the method generally used in our studies, the reaction mixture (1 ml) contained 50 mM potassium phosphate buffer, pH 7.5, 2.5 mM L-gulonolactone, 1 mM EDTA, and enzyme. The mixture was incubated for 15 minutes at 37°C, and the reaction was stopped by the addition of 0.1 ml of 50% trichloroacetic acid. After centrifuging to remove protein, ascorbic acid in the supernatant solution was assayed by the method of Zannoni et al. (1974). Since ascorbic acid autoxidizes (about 20%) during the incubation, the amount of ascorbic acid found must be corrected in the determination of enzyme activity.

A. Purification and Characterization

Nishikimi *et al.* (1976) have recently purified L-gulonolactone oxidase almost to homogeneity from liver microsomes of two species, rat and goat. Summaries of the purification procedures are presented in Table II. As can be seen, the preparations were purified 135-fold compared to liver microsomes, about 2-fold more pure than was previously reported (Nakagawa *et al.*, 1975). Although the yields from this procedure were low (about 5%), the preparations were pure enough to produce apparently monospecific antisera to goat enzyme. After further purification by polyacrylamide gel electrophoresis, the same was true for rat enzyme. Furthermore, these preparations showed only one major protein band on sodium dodecyl sulfate (SDS)–polyacrylamide gel electrophoresis (greater than 95% pure).

B. Kinetics

The kinetics of L-gulonolactone oxidase have been extensively studied by Brush and May (1966). From their studies on solubilized rat liver microsomes, they propose the following sequence of reactions for L-gulonolactone oxidase: (a) combination of the enzyme with L-gulonolactone; (b) reduction of the enzyme to produce ascorbic acid; (c) combination of the reduced enzyme with oxidant, which can be either oxygen or 2,6-dichloroindophenol; and (d) oxidation of the enzyme to its original state. These authors also reported that the affinity

TABLE II
SUMMARY OF PURIFICATION OF L-GULONOLACTONE OXIDASE[a]

	Rat liver		Goat liver	
Step	Total activity (mU)	Specific activity (mU/mg protein)	Total activity (mU)	Specific activity (mU/mg protein)
Microsomes	11,600	3.9	33,500	17
Tryptic digestion	10,100	7.3	24,300	27
Tween 20	5,970	15	13,300	36
$(NH_4)_2SO_4$	4,600	31	8,730	51
Sephadex G-150	4,570	53	8,730	88
DEAE-Sephadex	1,380	86	2,740	375
Hydroxyapatite	649	540	1,150	2050

[a] From Nishikimi *et al.* (1976), with permission.

constant obtained for oxygen is 12.5 atmospheres, which is over 300 times the partial pressure in tissues. They speculated that, as a consequence, ascorbic acid synthesis would be very nearly proportional to oxygen levels in the intact liver and would be relatively unaffected by the concentration of L-gulonolactone. This is of particular interest, since ascorbic acid has been proposed as a defense against oxygen toxicity (Nishikimi, 1975; Willis and Kratzing, 1976; Nishikimi and Udenfriend, 1977).

The apparent K_m of purified rat enzyme for L-gulonolactone at atmospheric conditions is 0.066 mM, and that of the goat enzyme for this substrate is about 2-fold higher, 0.15 mM. The V_{max} of the rat enzyme is 0.63 μmol/min per milligram of protein, and that of the goat enzyme is 2.7 μmol/min per milligram of protein (Nishikimi et al., 1976).

C. Molecular Weight

Gel filtration of the purified native enzyme of both rat and goat showed that L-gulonolactone oxidase exists as large aggregates with an apparent molecular weight in the order of 500,000. Eliceiri et al. (1969), using sodium deoxycholate-solubilized rat liver microsomes, found 2 peaks of enzyme activity on gel filtration chromatography and estimated aggregate molecular weights of 450,000 and 200,000. They concluded that the enzyme was probably attached to a submicrosomal particle. In contrast, Nakagawa and Asano (1970), using a partially purified preparation, estimated the apparent molecular weight of rat enzyme to be approximately 100,000 by gel filtration. In all cases, the detergents used for solubilization of the enzyme were not completely eliminated from the preparation, and the discrepancies in the molecular weights may, in part, result from differences in the nature of detergents used or, for that matter, from differences in the buffer systems used. Further investigations are required to obtain the precise molecular weight of the native enzyme.

Rat and goat enzymes were found to have essentially the same monomer molecular weights (51,000) by SDS–polyacrylamide gel electrophoresis (Nishikimi et al., 1976).

D. Flavin Prosthetic Group

The rat enzyme has been shown to contain an L-gulonolactone reducible flavin as a prosthetic group (Nakagawa et al., 1975). This flavin is not liberated from the protein on denaturation, but is released by proteolytic digestion. The purified flavin peptide liberated by Pronase digestion and acid hydrolysis yields 8-α-[$N^{(1)}$-histidyl]riboflavin as the structure of the covalently bound flavin of this enzyme (Kenney et al., 1976). Purified goat enzyme also exhibits the typical absorbance spectrum of a simple flavoprotein (Nishikimi et al., 1976). More recently, Nishikimi et al. (1977) have shown that the microsomal L-gulonolactone oxidase isolated from various mammals, birds, and amphibians is a covalently bound flavinyl polypeptide of molecular weight 51,000, the same as rat and goat L-gulonolactone oxidase.

E. FACTORS THAT AFFECT SYNTHESIS OF ASCORBIC ACID

Sulfhydryl reducing agents have been found to stimulate L-gulonolactone oxidase activity of purified rat and goat enzyme (Sato et al., 1976). For example, after correcting the rate of reaction for autoxidation of ascorbate, homocysteine (4.9 mM) caused a 2.5-fold increase in ascorbate formed. The apparent K_m of the enzyme for L-gulonolactone, however, was unchanged. Glutathione has been reported to stimulate L-gulonolactone oxidase activity 20% in rat liver microsomes (Chatterjee et al., 1960; Kar et al., 1962). Kar et al. (1965) reported inhibition of L-gulonolactone oxidase by p-chloromercuribenzoate, and that glutathione or mercaptoethanol overcame this inhibition. They explain these results by proposing that L-gulonolactone oxidase is a sulfhydryl enzyme. It is of interest that homocysteine (4.0 mM) does not lead to detectable L-gulonolactone oxidase activity in guinea pig liver microsomes (unpublished observation).

In addition to p-chloromercuribenzoate L-gulonolactone oxidase can be inhibited by the alkaloid lycorine (Mineshita et al., 1959; Conney et al., 1961; Arrigoni et al., 1975), adenosine triphosphate (Ganguli et al., 1956), as well as by microsomal phospholipids (McCay, 1966). The possibility that guinea pig, monkey, or human liver microsomes contain inhibitors of L-gulonolactone oxidase has been ruled out by mixing experiments (Chatterjee et al., 1961a). In ascorbate-producing animals almost any type of nutritional deficiency, such as vitamin A or D (Malathi and Ganguly, 1964; Ghosh et al., 1965), α-tocopherol (Caputto et al., 1958; McCay et al., 1959), total calories (Stubbs et al., 1973a), or protein (Mukherjee et al., 1968; Stubbs et al., 1973b), leads to a decrease in excretion and presumably in synthesis of the vitamin. The inhibition of ascorbic acid synthesis resulting from α-tocopherol deficiency has been found to involve phospholipids (McCay, 1966). Specifically, it has been proposed that α-tocopherol by inhibiting lipid peroxidation changes the orientation of endogenous phospholipids on the surface of

L-gulonolactone oxidase. Variations in ascorbate synthesis are also produced by an excess or deficiency of various hormones, in particular pituitary, thyroid, or sex hormones (Vanha, 1963; Dieter, 1969; Biswas, 1970). Stirpe and Comporti (1965) observed that liver preparations from alloxan-diabetic rats carry out synthesis of ascorbic acid poorly and that after insulin therapy normal ascorbic acid synthesis is restored.

A pronounced increase in ascorbic acid biosynthesis occurs after administration of certain drugs and carcinogens. This effect has been extensively studied (Longenecker et al., 1940; Conney et al., 1961; Aarts, 1966). Although the mechanism of this induction is not clearly understood, Burns et al. (1960) have shown that it is not due to an effect on L-gulonolactone oxidase. Inducers do not activate ascorbic acid synthesis in guinea pigs (Samuels et al., 1940) or humans (Enklewitz and Lasker 1935). Chatterjee et al. (1975) have recently reported that agents that stimulate histamine formation also stimulate ascorbic acid synthesis. They suggested that stimulation of ascorbic acid biosynthesis may be mediated by histamine.

V. MAN, MONKEYS, AND GUINEA PIGS DO NOT EXPRESS THE GENE FOR L-GULONOLACTONE OXIDASE

Since scurvy is so easily prevented by including ascorbic acid in the diet, there has been little interest in the genetics of the disease. What has been overlooked, however, is that scurvy provides an unusually convenient model for studies of a human inborn error of metabolism. The enzymic as well as the genetic basis for it are constant, and defined. Furthermore, enzyme-deficient tissue is readily available in a common laboratory animal, the guinea pig, and does not require careful breeding of animals or involved therapeutic treatment. Studies on L-gulonolactone oxidase in the guinea pig should yield information and methods for the study of less treatable and more complex enzyme deficiency diseases in man.

It is known that tissues from animals that cannot make ascorbic acid are devoid of L-gulonolactone oxidase activity. What has not been known is whether the deficiency in enzymic activity is due to a total failure of gene expression. Recently, we utilized immunological methods, immunoprecipitation, microcomplement fixation, and radioimmunoassay to determine whether antigenic material related to L-gulonolactone oxidase is present in the guinea pig, monkey, or man (Sato and Udenfriend, 1978; Nishikimi and Udenfriend, 1976). Liver microsomes, as well as other tissues and cell fractions, from humans,

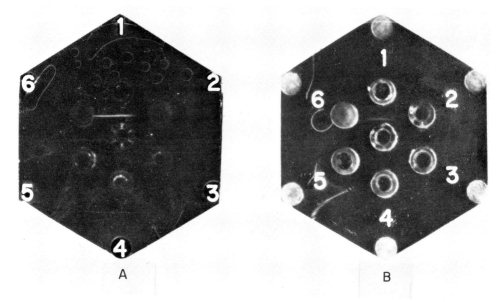

Fɪɢ. 4. Ouchterlony double immunodiffusion analysis of rabbit antiserum to rat and goat ʟ-gulonolactone oxidase with tissue extracts of scurvy-prone species. In both plates well 1 contains detergent-solubilized rat liver microsomes; well 2, solubilized human liver microsomes; well 3, human liver 100,000 g supernatant; well 4, solubilized guinea pig liver microsomes; well 5, solubilized monkey kidney microsomes; well 6, solubilized monkey liver microsomes. The center well of plate A contains undiluted antiserum to rat ʟ-gulonolactone oxidase; and the center well of B contains antiserum to goat ʟ-gulonolactone oxidase diluted 2-fold. Approximately 200 μg of tissue protein were used in each well. From Sato and Udenfriend (1978).

African green monkeys, and guinea pigs did not contain material that crossreacted with antibodies directed against either rat or goat ʟ-gulonolactone oxidase when measured by the Ouchterlony immuno-precipitin test (Fig. 4). On the other hand, liver microsomal extracts of all mammals tested (10 species, 4 orders) which contain ʟ-gulonolactone oxidase activity were shown to contain crossreactive enzyme (Figs. 5 and 6).

Microcomplement fixation tests also failed to detect crossreacting material (CRM) in any of the enzymically inactive tissues. Although this method is inherently more sensitive than the Ouchterlony immuno-precipitin test and is able to detect soluble antigen–antibody complexes, its sensitivity was limited by interference of the large amounts of tissue required. In order to determine whether small amounts of antigen were present in scurvy-prone species, a radioimmunoassay for

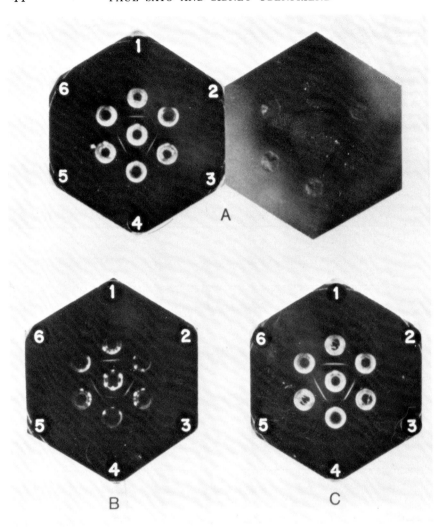

FIG. 5. Ouchterlony test patterns of rabbit antiserum to rat L-gulonolactone oxidase with detergent-solubilized microsomes from various animals. Wells 1, 3, and 5 of all plates contained the purified rat L-gulonolactone oxidase (0.4 mg/ml), and the center wells of each plate contained undiluted rabbit antiserum to rat enzyme. (A) Well 2, rat; well 4, guinea pig; and well 6, mouse. The right-hand picture is the plate stained by enzymic activity. (B) Well 2, monkey; well 4, hamster; and well 6, gerbil. (C) Well 2, sheep; well 4, goat; and well 6, cattle. From Nishikimi and Udenfriend (1976).

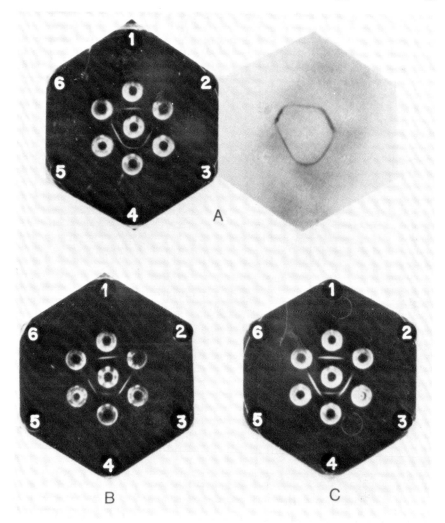

FIG. 6. Ouchterlony test patterns of rabbit antiserum to goat L-gulonolactone oxidase with detergent-solubilized microsomes from various animals. Wells 1, 3, and 5 of all the plates contained the purified goat enzyme (0.2 mg/ml), and the center wells of each plate contained rabbit antiserum to goat enzyme, diluted 2-fold. (A) Well 2, sheep; well 4, goat; and well 6, cattle. The right-hand picture is the plate stained by enzymic activity. (B) Well 2, monkey; well 4, hamster; and well 6, gerbil. (C) Well 2, rat; well 4, mouse; and well 6, guinea pig. From Nishikimi and Udenfriend (1976).

L-gulonolactone oxidase was developed using tritium-labeled rat
L-gulonolactone oxidase and antiserum directed against the rat enzyme. This assay is approximately 20 times more sensitive than the
other immunoassays. To demonstrate crossreactivity to rat antibody
with tissues from other species that synthesize ascorbic acid, microsomal extracts were assayed both for enzyme activity and by the
radioimmunoassay. As shown in Table III, the extracts from all the
species examined were active antigenically as well as enzymically.
Even the enzyme from the chicken, a species far removed from the rat,
yielded an activity of 2.6 units per milligram of solubilized microsomal
protein. When tissues from scurvy-prone animals were examined, no
enzyme activity was detected. However, when subjected to radioimmunoassay, all these tissues, including rat kidney, which contains no
L-gulonolactone oxidase activity, did yield very low values (Table IV).
Although these values were small, they could not rule out the presence
of traces of protein that truly crossreacted with antibody to rat enzyme.

On further investigation it was shown, first of all, that none of these
extracts inhibited formation of the antigen–antibody complex. Then, in
order to determine whether the small amounts of CRM in the livers of
scurvy-prone animals and rat kidney were related to L-gulonolactone
oxidase, or were some nonspecific material resulting from the large
amounts of tissue used in the assays, we attempted to concentrate the
immunoreactive material from large amounts of tissue. When guinea
pig microsomes were extracted and treated as in the procedure for
purification of rat enzyme (ammonium sulfate precipitation, gel filtration, and DEAE anion-exchange chromatography) crossreacting material appeared in all fractions and there was no increase in concentration in any fraction. It became apparent that the small amounts of

TABLE III
IMMUNOLOGIC AND ENZYMIC ACTIVITIES IN ASCORBIC ACID-FORMING ANIMALS[a]

Microsomal extract from	Immunologic activity[b] (U/mg)	Enzymic activity (nmol/min/mg)
Rat liver	56.5	4.7
Goat liver	3.5	7.6
Gerbil liver	1.5	2.6
Mouse liver	2.1	4.4
Rabbit liver	1.2	2.1
Chicken kidney	2.6	12.0

[a] From Sato and Udenfriend (1978).
[b] Immunologic activity was determined by radioimmunoassay, using rat liver antigen
and antibody.

TABLE IV

IMMUNOLOGIC ACTIVITY IN TISSUES CONTAINING NO DETECTABLE[a]
L-GULONOLACTONE OXIDASE[b]

Animal and tissue	Immunologic activity[c] (U/mg)
Guinea pig	
Liver microsomes	0.21
Kidney microsomes	0.08
Fetal guinea pig	
Liver microsomes	0.16
Rat	
Kidney microsomes	0.11
Monkey	
Liver microsomes	0.16
Kidney microsomes	0.15
Spleen microsomes	0.12
Brain microsomes	0.08
Human	
Liver microsomes	0.23

[a] Enzyme specific activity <0.05 nmol/min/mg.
[b] From Sato and Udenfriend (1978).
[c] Immunologic activity was determined by radioimmunoassay.

CRM from these tissues is not a single substance. This suggested that the CRM in enzyme-deficient tissues represents nonspecific interference in the radioimmunoassay rather than an aberrant form of the enzyme.

Another approach was employed to determine whether the small amounts of apparent CRM present in guinea pig, monkey, and human tissue was antigenically related to L-gulonolactone oxidase. Assuming the material that reacted in the radioimmunoassay to be specifically related to the enzyme, it must be limited in quantity and must bind to antibody. It should then be possible to adsorb it quantitatively out of tissue extracts with excess antibody. To determine if this were so, antibody against rat enzyme was bound to cyanogen bromide-activated Sepharose, and tissues were treated with this preparation. As shown in Table V, L-gulonolactone oxidase activity could be removed quantitatively from rat, goat, rabbit, and chicken microsomal extracts by adsorption onto the antibody. On the other hand, none of the apparent CRM from extracts of livers from scurvy-prone animals or from rat kidney was removed by this treatment. Even when the unadsorbed fractions were treated again with the immobilized antibody, there was no detectable loss of immunoreactive material. To ensure that guinea pig, monkey, or human tissue extracts did not inhibit immunoadsorp-

TABLE V
ANTIBODY AFFINITY CHROMATOGRAPHY OF L-GULONOLACTONE OXIDASE[a]

Microsomal extract source[c]	Immunologic activity (U/mg)[b]		
	Before adsorption	After adsorption	Fraction adsorbed
Goat liver	3.9	0.15	96%
Rabbit liver	1.2	0.10	92%
Rat liver	54.5	0.11	100%
Chicken kidney	2.6	0.07	97%
Guinea pig liver	0.21	0.24	−14%
Human liver	0.23	0.23	0%
Monkey liver	0.16	0.19	−19%
Rat kidney	0.11	0.10	9%

[a] From Sato and Udenfriend (1978).

[b] Immunologic activity was determined by radioimmunoassay.

[c] The first four tissues listed contain L-gulonolactone oxidase activity; the last four do not.

tion, purified rat enzyme was added to liver extracts from these animals prior to immunoadsorption. The antibody-Sepharose was able to remove all the added rat enzyme from the tissue extracts even in the presence of these extracts. Therefore, even the small amount of apparent CRM found in the direct radioimmunoassay does not represent a protein related to L-gulonolactone oxidase.

In conclusion, three different immunological methods failed to detect even traces of antigen in liver microsomes from man, monkey, or guinea pig, which specifically reacts with antibody directed against L-gulonolactone oxidase. In view of the wide crossreactivity of the antiserum with the enzyme from other species that synthesize ascorbic acid, these studies show rather conclusively that the gene for L-gulonolactone oxidase is not expressed in scurvy-prone animals. Of course, the possibility cannot be entirely excluded that the gene product is so altered that it is not recognized by antiserum to the enzyme, but this would be unlikely for all three species, particularly since even the chicken enzyme does crossreact.

Nishikimi et al. (1977) have recently tested for the occurrence of a flavin band on SDS-polyacrylamide gels of crude microsomal preparations from animals. They found that by acidification of the gels with acetic acid the flavin band could be detected by fluorescence when the gels were observed under ultraviolet illumination at 365 nm. Tissues with L-gulonolactone oxidase activity were shown to contain a flavinyl polypeptide of molecular weight about 51,000. However, no fluorescent band was detected in liver microsomal extracts from scurvy-prone animals. This study further supports the immunological evidence that scurvy-prone animals do not contain an aberrant form of L-gulonolactone oxidase by showing that they do not contain a flavinyl polypeptide homologous to L-gluconolactone oxidase.

VI. Studies on Ascorbic Acid Synthesis in Scurvy-Prone Species

Although we find no evidence for L-gulonolactone oxidase in man, monkeys, or guinea pigs, some reports have appeared claiming that under certain circumstances ascorbic acid synthesis does in fact occur in these animals (Baker *et al.*, 1962). Evidence was presented that in the guinea pig L-gulonolactone oxidase is present in the fetus but disappears before birth (DeFabro, 1968). However, in our laboratory we have not been able to detect the enzyme in fetal guinea pig tissues (Sato and Udenfriend, 1978). J. Gross (personal communication) has also investigated this and finds "no L-gulonolactone oxidase by enzymatic assay in guinea pig liver at several stages of fetal development." Human fetuses have also been found to be deficient in L-gulonolactone oxidase (Hollmann and Neubaur, 1966). Synthesis of ascorbic acid has been reported to take place in the human placenta (Rajalakshmi *et al.*, 1967). Odumosu and Wilson (1973) have claimed that a small proportion of female guinea pigs possess the ability to synthesize ascorbic acid. However, they based their claim on finding longer survival times than usual on a scorbutogenic diet. Recently, Ginter (1976) reported that he found three guinea pigs out of several thousand that were capable of synthesizing sufficient ascorbic acid for their needs. This study is based on a urinary excretion of the vitamin which exceeded the dietary intake, and an unusually long survival time on an ascorbic acid-deficient diet. L-Gulonolactone oxidase activity was not determined in these animals. In fact, the report is based on a reevaluation of Ginter's studies, which were carried out in 1956, 20 years prior to publication of his 1976 paper. We are somewhat skeptical of all these reports and feel that the production of ascorbic acid by certain individuals of a scurvy-prone species has yet to be demonstrated.

VII. Summary

1. This review is concerned with the biosynthesis of ascorbic acid, primarily with the biochemical and genetic basis for the inability of certain species to synthesize the vitamin.

2. It had been generally accepted that the biochemical alteration in species that are unable to synthesize ascorbic acid was a lack of the liver microsomal enzyme L-gulonolactone oxidase, the terminal enzyme in the biosynthetic pathway of the vitamin. More recently, a second pathway to the vitamin was proposed, involving an enzyme, D-glucuronolactone reductase. Scurvy-prone species appeared to lack this enzyme as well as L-gulonolactone oxidase. We have found, however, that purified L-gulonolactone oxidase can convert certain D-glucuronolactone derivatives to ascorbic acid-like products. We conclude that there is no evidence for the enzyme D-glucuronolactone reductase and that L-gulonolactone oxidase is the only enzyme missing in animals subject to scurvy.

3. Using immunoprecipitation, microcomplement fixation, and radioimmunoassay, antibody directed against L-gulonolactone oxidase from the rat and goat was shown to crossreact with the enzyme from all other animal species tested that possess enzymic activity. Tissue extracts from man, monkey, and guinea pig did not crossreact with either antibody. The conclusion is that man, monkeys, and guinea pigs do not express the gene for L-gulonolactone oxidase.

4. A few reports of ascorbic acid synthesis by man and guinea pigs have appeared. The possibility exists that certain members of a scurvy-prone species possess the biosynthetic ability to produce ascorbate. None of these finds have yet been substantiated.

REFERENCES

Aarts, E. M. (1966). *Biochem. Pharmacol.* **15**, 1469.

Arrigoni, O., Liso, R. A., and Calabrese, G. (1975). *Nature (London)* **256**, 513.

Ashwell, G., Kanfer, J., Smiley, J. D., and Burns, J. J. (1961). *Ann. N.Y. Acad. Sci.* **92**, 105.

Ayaz, K. M., Jenness, R., and Birney, E. C. (1976). *Anal. Biochem.* **72**, 161.

Baker, E. M., Sauberlich, H. E., Wolfskill, S. J., Wallace, W. T., and Dean, E. E. (1962). *Proc. Soc. Exp. Biol. Med.* **109**, 737.

Birney, E. C., Jenness, R., and Ayaz, K. M. (1976). *Nature (London)* **260**, 626.

Biswas, N. M. (1970). *Endokrinologie* **56**, 248.

Brush, J. S., and May, H. E. (1966). *J. Biol. Chem.* **241**, 2907.

Burns, J. J. (1957). *Nature (London)* **180**, 553.

Burns, J. J. (1975). *Ann. N.Y. Acad. Sci.* **258**, 5.

Burns, J. J., Peyser, P., and Moltz, A. (1956). *Science* **124**, 1148.

Burns, J. J., Conney, A. H., Dayton, P. G., Evans, C., Martin, G. R., and Taller, D. (1960). *J. Pharmacol. Exp. Ther.* **129**, 132.

Caputto, R., McCay, P. B., and Carpenter, M. P. (1958). *J. Biol. Chem.* **233**, 1025.

Chatterjee, I. B. (1970). *In* "Methods in Enzymology" (D. B. McCormick and L. D. Wright, eds.), Vol. 18, Part A, p. 28. Academic Press, New York.

Chatterjee, I. B. (1973a). *Sci. Cult.* **39**, 210.

Chatterjee, I. B. (1973b). *Science* **182**, 1271.

Chatterjee, I. B., Ghosh, N. C., Ghosh, J. J., and Guha, B. C. (1957). *Science* **126**, 608.

Chatterjee, I. B., Chatterjee, G. C., Ghosh, N. C., Ghosh, J. J., and Guha, B. C. (1960). *Biochem. J.* **74**, 193.

Chatterjee, I. B., Kar, N. C., Ghosh, N. C., and Guha, B. C., (1961a). *Ann. N.Y. Acad. Sci.* **92**, 36.

Chatterjee, I. B., Kar, N. C., Ghosh, N. C., and Guha, B. C. (1961b). *Nature (London)* **192**, 163.

Chatterjee, I. B., Majumder, A. K., Nandi, B. K., and Subramanian, N. (1975). *Ann. N.Y. Acad. Sci.* **258**, 24.

Conney, A. H., Bray, G. A., Evans, C., and Burns, J. J. (1961). *Ann. N.Y. Acad. Sci.* **92**, 115.

DeFabro, S. P. (1978). *C. R. Seances Soc. Biol. Ses Fil.* **162**, 284.

Dieter, M. P. (1969). *Proc. Soc. Exp. Biol. Med.* **130**, 210.

Dutta Gupta, S., Choudhury, P. K., and Chatterjee, I. B. (1973). *Int. J. Biochem.* **4**, 309.

Eliceiri, G. L., Lai, E. L., and McCay, P. B. (1969). *J. Biol. Chem.* **244**, 2641.

Enklewitz, M., and Lasker, M. (1935). *J. Biol. Chem.* **110**, 443.

Ganguli, N. C., Roy, S. C., and Guha, B. C. (1956). *Arch. Biochem. Biophys.* **61**, 211.

Ghosh, N. C., Chatterjee, I., and Chatterjee, G. C. (1965). *Biochem. J.* **97**, 247.

Ginter, E. (1976). *Int. J. Vitam. Nutr. Res.* **46**, 173.

Hassan, M. ul, and Lehninger, A. L. (1956). *J. Biol. Chem.* **223**, 123.

Hollmann, S., and Neubaur, J. (1966). *Klin. Wochenschr.* **44**, 722.

Kanfer, J., Burns, J. J., and Ashwell, G. (1959). *Biochim. Biophys. Acta* **31**, 556.

Kar, N. C., Chatterjee, I. B., Ghosh, N. C., and Guha, B. C. (1962). *Biochem. J.* **84**, 16.

Kar, N. C., Ghosh, N. C., and Chatterjee, G. C. (1965). *Arch. Biochem. Biophys.* **112**, 207.

Kenney, W. C., Edmondson, D. E., Singer, T. P., Nakagawa, H., Asano, A., and Sato, R. (1976). *Biochem. Biophys. Res. Commun.* **71**, 1194.

King, C. G. (1973). *World Rev. Nutr. Diet.* **18**, 47.

King, C. G., and Burns, J. J. (1975). *Ann. N.Y. Acad. Sci.* **258**.

Longenecker, H. E., Fricke, H. H., and King, C. (1940). *J. Biol. Chem.* **135**, 497.

McCay, P. B. (1966). *J. Biol. Chem.* **241**, 2333.

McCay, P. B., Carpenter, M. P., Kitabachi, A. E., and Caputto, R. (1959). *Arch. Biochem. Biophys.* **82**, 452.

Malathi, P., and Ganguly, J. (1964). *Biochem. J.* **92**, 521.

Mano, Y., Suzuki, K., Yamada, K., and Shimazono, N. (1961). *J. Biochem. (Tokyo)* **49**, 618.

Mineshita, T., Yamaguchi, K., and Yamamoto, K. (1959). *Proc. Jpn. Acad.* **35**, 405.

Mukherjee, D., Kar, N. C., Sasmal, N., and Chatterjee, G. C. (1968). *Biochem. J.* **106**, 627.

Nakagawa, H., and Asano, A. (1970). *J. Biochem. (Tokyo)* **68**, 737.

Nakagawa, H., Asano, A., and Sato, R. (1975). *J. Biochem. (Tokyo)* **77**, 221.

Nishikimi, M. (1975). *Biochem. Biophys. Res. Commun.* **63**, 463.

Nishikimi, M., and Udenfriend, S. (1976). *Proc. Natl. Acad. Sci. U.S.A.* **73**, 2066.

Nishikimi, M., and Udenfriend, S. (1977). *Trends Biochem. Sci.* **2**, 111.

Nishikimi, M., Tolbert, B. M., and Udenfriend, S. (1976). *Arch. Biochem. Biophys.* **175**, 427.

Nishikimi, M., Kiuchi, K., and Yagi, K. (1977). *FEBS Lett.* **81**, 323.

Odumosu, A., and Wilson, C. W. M. (1973). *Nature (London)* **242**, 519.

Rajalakshmi, R., Subbulakshmi, G., Ramakrishnan, C V., Joshi, S. K., and Bhatt, R. V. (1967). *Curr. Sci.* **36**, 45.

Samuels, L. T., Ritz, N. D., and Poyet, E. B. (1940). *J. Pharmacol. Exp. Ther.* **68**, 465.

Sato, P., and Udenfriend, S. (1978). *Arch. Biochem. Biophys.* **187,** 158.
Sato, P., Nishikimi, M., and Udenfriend, S. (1976). *Biochem. Biophys. Res. Commun.* **71,** 293.
Stirpe, F., and Comporti, M. (1965). *Biochem. J.* **97,** 561.
Stubbs, D. W., Griffin, J. F., and Guest, M. M. (1973a). *Proc. Soc. Exp. Biol. Med.* **144,** 195.
Stubbs, D. W., Griffin, J. F., and Guest, M. M. (1973b). *Proc. Soc. Exp. Biol. Med.* **144,** 199.
Vanha, P. T. P. (1963). *Experientia* **19,** 426.
Willis, R. J., and Kratzing, C. C. (1976). *Biochim. Biophys. Acta* **444,** 108.
Winkelman, J., and Lehninger, A. L. (1958). *J. Biol. Chem* **233,** 794.
Yamada, K., Ishikawa, S., and Shimazono, N. (1959). *Biochim. Biophys. Acta* **32,** 253.
Zannoni, V., Lynch, M., Goldstein, S., and Sato, P. (1974). *Biochem. Med.* **11,** 41.

The Interactions between Vitamin B_6 and Hormones

DAVID P. ROSE

*Division of Clinical Oncology, Wisconsin Clinical Cancer Center,
University of Wisconsin, Madison, Wisconsin*

I. INTRODUCTION

In 1963, Dr. Jeng M. Hsu wrote a chapter entitled "Interrelations between Vitamin B_6 and Hormones" for the twenty-first volume of this series. The 15 years since that time have seen rapid growth in some areas, but relative inactivity in others.

Clinical interest in the relationship between hormones and vitamin B_6 function dates back to the early studies of tryptophan metabolism in man. Abnormal urinary excretions of tryptophan metabolites, similar to those seen in experimental vitamin B_6 deficiency, were observed during pregnancy and in patients with hyperthyroidism. Later, altered tryptophan metabolism was demonstrated in women taking oral contraceptives or treated with estrogens. In all of these clinical situations, the abnormal tryptophan metabolism was corrected by pyridoxine administration, which suggested the presence of a vitamin B_6 deficiency or an increased requirement for the vitamin.

53

While these human studies were progressing, investigations were being made of the biochemical interactions between steroid hormones and pyridoxal phosphate-dependent enzymes. These were shown to fall into two broad categories; enzyme induction as an expression of steroidal action, and inhibition of enzyme activity due to competition between the steroid and pyridoxal phosphate for the apoenzyme. In the 1960s, stimulated in large part by concern that the use of oral contraceptives might cause vitamin deficiencies, attempts were made to apply these biochemical findings to the clinical situation.

Another, and most recent, area of research interest concerning hormones and vitamin B_6 is the role that this vitamin may play in the regulation of pituitary hormones. The secretion of hypothalamic factors, which, in turn, stimulate or inhibit the release of hormones from the adenohypophysis, is modulated by two neurotransmitters, dopamine and 5-hydroxytryptamine (serotonin). Pyridoxal phosphate is the coenzyme involved in decarboxylation reactions that yield these amines, and recent studies have shown that the administration of large doses of pyridoxine alters the pituitary secretion of prolactin and growth hormone in man.

These three topics, the influence of hormones on vitamin B_6 nutrition in man, the interaction between steroid hormones and pyridoxal phosphate-dependent enzymes, and the role of vitamin B_6 in regulating hypothalamopituitary functions are the areas to be covered in this chapter.

II. Estrogens and Contraceptive Steroids

A. Estrogens and Tryptophan Metabolism in Man

1. The Tryptophan–Nicotinic Acid Ribonucleotide Metabolic Pathway

The first indication that estrogen administration may influence vitamin B_6 was the report by Rose (1966a) that women using estrogen-containing oral contraceptives excrete excessively large amounts of xanthurenic acid in their urine after an oral tryptophan load. This abnormality of tryptophan metabolism, which is similar to that seen in vitamin B_6 deficiency, was corrected by treatment with large doses of pyridoxine.

The metabolic pathway by which L-tryptophan is converted to nicotinic acid ribonucleotide is shown in Fig. 1. The first step, opening of the pyrrole ring of the indole nucleus, takes place in two stages: an

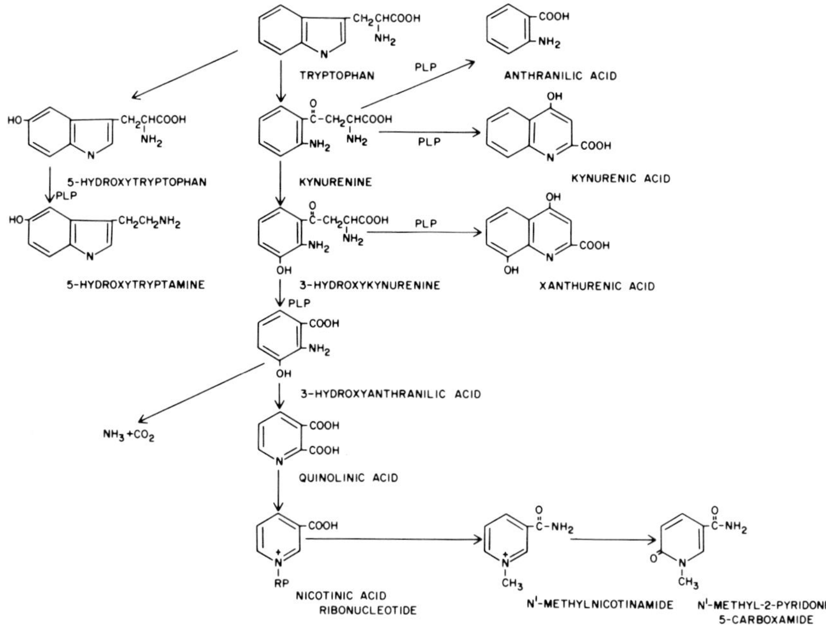

FIG. 1. The metabolism of tryptophan to nicotinic acid ribonucleotide and 5-hydroxytryptamine.

initial oxidation reaction to give formylkynurenine, followed by hydrolysis to yield kynurenine. The oxidation, which involves the direct incorporation of gaseous oxygen into the molecule (Hayaishi et al., 1957) is catalyzed by an iron-porphyrin protein, tryptophan oxygenase.

Formylkynurenine is hydrolyzed by a hepatic formamidase, which is always present in excess relative to tryptophan oxygenase. In consequence, when liver preparations are studied, formylkynurenine does not accumulate and "tryptophan oxygenase" is assayed by following the rate of kynurenine production from the tryptophan substrate. Elevated levels of tryptophan oxygenase are induced by adrenal glucocorticoids, and treatment with hydrocortisone increases both hepatic tryptophan oxygenase activity and urinary kynurenine excretion in man (Altman and Greengard, 1966).

Several of the other enzymic reactions on the tryptophan-nicotinic acid ribonucleotide pathway require pyridoxal phosphate as a coenzyme (Fig. 1). Vitamin B_6 deficiency in man is characterized by elevated excretions of kynurenine, 3-hydroxykynurenine, and xanthurenic acid in urine collected after an oral dose of tryptophan, indicating that a "metabolic block" occurs at the level of the conversion of

3-hydroxykynurenine to 3-hydroxyanthranilic acid. This reaction, which involves the removal of alanine from the 3-hydroxykynurenine side chain is catalyzed by vitamin B_6-dependent kynureninase. Ogasawara et al. (1962) showed that the activity of this supernatant enzyme is markedly reduced in vitamin B_6-deficient rats, whereas Ueda (1967) found the mitochondrial kynurenine aminotransferase, which produces xanthurenic acid from 3-hydroxykynurenine, to be little affected. This difference in sensitivity to a lack of pyridoxal phosphate explains why the urinary excretion of xanthurenic acid is elevated in vitamin B_6 deficiency.

One abnormality that remains unexplained is the increased urinary excretion of quinolinic acid that has been demonstrated both in experimentally induced dietary vitamin B_6 deficiency (Brown et al., 1965) and after treatment with the antagonist deoxypyridoxine (Rose and Toseland, 1973). Although this suggests that there is a pyridoxal phosphate-requiring step beyond 3-hydroxyanthranilic acid, such a reaction has never been demonstrated.

The principal urinary excretion products of nicotinic acid are N^1-methylnicotinamide and N^1-methyl-2-pyridone-5-carboxamide. Although a proportion of these metabolites is derived from dietary nicotinyl compounds, the extent to which their excretion is increased after an oral tryptophan load does give an indication of the capacity for conversion of the amino acid to nicotinic acid ribonucleotide. Despite the evidence of a metabolic block on the pathway in vitamin B_6 deficiency, human subjects fed a high-protein, low-vitamin B_6 diet showed no change in the yields of nicotinic acid or its metabolites during the period of deficiency (Brown et al., 1965).

2. Effect of Estrogens on Tryptophan Metabolism

Treatment with estrogen-containing oral contraceptives causes elevated urinary excretions of xanthurenic acid, kynurenine, 3-hydroxykynurenine, and 3-hydroxyanthranilic acid (Rose, 1966b; Price et al., 1967; Luhby et al., 1971; Coelingh Bennink et al., 1974) and of quinolinic acid (Rose and Toseland, 1973). A 2-gm L-tryptophan load usually demonstrates an increased xanthurenic acid excretion within 21 days of starting treatment; after 3 months the urinary levels of the other metabolites are also elevated. When the oral contraceptive is discontinued, it may be 3 months or more before tryptophan metabolism returns to normal (Rose and Adams, 1972).

In addition to tryptophan metabolites, women taking estrogen-containing oral contraceptives excrete increased levels of N^1-methylnicotinamide, but not N^1-methyl-2-pyridone-5-carboxamide, in urine collected with or without tryptophan loading (Rose *et al.*, 1968; Leklem *et al.*, 1975a). It was suggested that estrogens increase the turnover of the tryptophan-nicotinic acid ribonucleotide pathway, perhaps because they cause an elevation in circulating corticosteroids with consequent induction of tryptophan oxygenase. When a tryptophan load is given, more substrate may then be presented to the partially inhibited kynureninase than can be metabolized; the result would be an increase in the urinary excretion of those intermediate compounds proximal to the block (Rose and Braidman, 1971; Rose *et al.*, 1972).

The most widely used oral contraceptives are a combination of a synthetic estrogen and a progestogen. There is no doubt that the estrogenic component is responsible for the abnormalities in tryptophan metabolism; identical changes occur when an estrogen is given alone (Rose, 1966b), and progestogens, in fact, reduce the severity of the disturbance in tryptophan metabolism when the two steroids are used in combination (Rose *et al.*, 1973a). Megestrol acetate, which in the past was used as a single-agent oral contraceptive, has no effect on tryptophan metabolism (Rose and Adams, 1972).

The precise mechanism by which estrogens alter tryptophan metabolism has not been determined with certainty, although vitamin B₆ is clearly involved. The crucial question from a clinical viewpoint is whether or not a true deficiency of vitamin B₆ is present, and whether the abnormal tryptophan metabolism provides sufficient grounds for the routine administration of pyridoxine supplements to oral contraceptive users. This problem will be discussed in depth in Section II, C).

B. Estrogens and Pyridoxal Phosphate-Dependent Enzyme Systems

1. *Enzyme Inhibition*

A direct interaction between estrogens, pyridoxal phosphate, and one of the enzymes involved in tryptophan metabolism was first demonstrated by Mason and Gullekson (1960a). They performed *in vitro* studies of the effect of estrogens on the supernatant form of kynurenine aminotransferase, which is responsible for the transamination of kynurenine to kynurenic acid. It was found that some esters of estrogens have an inhibitory action. Estradiol disulfate and diethylstilbestrol sulfate, the ester of a nonsteroidal estrogen, were the most potent inhibitors, the former being effective at a concentration as low as 0.5

μM. Nonanionic steroids, including estradiol and estrone, were without effect even in saturated solution. The inhibition was reversed by dialysis and appeared to result from the formation of a reversible complex between the apoenzyme and estrogen sulfate such that there was competition between the steroid and pyridoxal phosphate for the apoprotein.

There is indirect evidence that a similar inhibition may take place *in vivo*. Thus, the level of kidney kynurenine aminotransferase activity is higher in mature male rats than in females (Mason and Gullekson, 1960b), and ovariectomy causes an increase in the enzyme level (Mason *et al.*, 1969). Treatment with estradiol causes a reduction in kidney kynurenine aminotransferase in both male and female animals.

At first sight, these data appeared to provide a straightforward explanation for the effect of synthetic estrogens on tryptophan metabolism in man. Supernatant enzymes, such as the kynurenine aminotransferase studied by Mason and his co-workers, may be more susceptible to inhibition by estrogen esters than those contained within the mitochondria. And, as noted earlier, there is evidence that pyridoxal phosphate is more tightly bound to *mitochondrial* kynurenine aminotransferase than to the supernatant kynureninase. Competitive inhibition of the pyridoxal phosphate-dependent kynureninase might, therefore, result in accumulation of 3-hydroxykynurenine in the liver, which could then be preferentially metabolized to xanthurenic acid by mitochondrial kynurenine aminotransferase. Treatment with large doses of pyridoxine could reverse the inhibition, because the high concentration of pyridoxal phosphate in the liver would displace the estrogen conjugates from the apokynureninase.

There are several difficulties in accepting this explanation, although it may still be the right one. Mature male rats have higher levels of kynureninase activity in liver than mature females, and when male rats are treated with estradiol the enzyme level is reduced to that of untreated females (Mason and Gullekson, 1960b; Rose and Brown, 1969). Unfortunately, however, kynureninase is not impaired in female rats receiving estradiol, and females treated with mestranol and norethynodrel (a synthetic estrogen–progestogen combination used as an oral contraceptive; Enovid) actually show an increase in the activity of this enzyme (Rose and Brown, 1969).

The situation is complicated further by differences in the effect of estrogen esters on kidney supernatant kynurenine aminotransferase compared with the hepatic supernatant enzyme; there is no sex difference in the activity of liver kynurenine aminotransferase in the rat, and no change occurs after ovariectomy or treatment with estrogens (Mason et al., 1969; Rose and Brown, 1969). This potential source of confusion may extend to kynureninase. Rose and Brown (1969) used the rate of formation of anthranilic acid from kynurenine in their assay. But, bearing in mind the differences in the susceptibility of kidney and liver kynurenine aminotransferases to estrogen esters, it should be noted that the isoenzyme with which we are primarily concerned is the one that catalyzes the formation of 3-hydroxyanthranilic acid from 3-hydroxykynurenine.

Finally, as always, one must take care in transferring observations made in one species to another. Whereas in the human, vitamin B$_6$ deficiency, pregnancy, and oral contraceptive administration all produce an identical abnormality of tryptophan metabolism, the pregnant rat excretes normal amounts of urinary xanthurenic acid (Mainardi, 1947). The two species also differ in the relative distribution of estrogen conjugate excretions between urine and bile, and the extent to which there is enterohepatic recirculation of these compounds; these factors will influence the steady-state hepatic concentration of the estrogen sulfates (Sandberg et al., 1967).

2. Enzyme Induction

The term "induction" was originally introduced to indicate an increase in the rate of synthesis of a specific apoenzyme. When applied to conclusions based on animal tissue enzyme assays, however, it needs to be redefined as "an increase in the amount of a specific apoprotein due to an increase in the ratio of its rates of synthesis and degradation" (Greengard, 1967). This may arise from an elevation in apoenzyme synthesis, decreased degradation ("stabilization"), or a combination of these two factors.

A number of vitamin B$_6$-dependent enzymes are inducible by estrogens, either directly or because estrogen treatment causes an increase in the level of circulating glucocorticoids, which in turn stimulates enzyme protein synthesis.

Alanine aminotransferase activity is increased in the livers of estrogen-treated rats (Rosen et al., 1959; Keller et al., 1969; Braidman and Rose, 1971). Estrogen administration increased the plasma corticosteroid concentration, but much of the hormone is bound to transcortin (corticosteroid-binding globulin), and is considered to be biologically inert (Sandberg et al., 1960). Keller et al. (1969) found that when the level of plasma corticosterone was increased in the male rat by estrogens there was an elevation in the activity of hepatic, but not pancreatic, alanine aminotransferase. They suggested that the protein-bound corticosterone can gain access to the enzyme-synthesizing systems within the hepatocytes by pinocytosis, and dissociate there to yield the free steroid, which induces increased alanine aminotransferase production. It was hypothesized that because the pancreatic cell membrane is much thicker, entry of the transcortin-bound steroid was blocked and so enzyme induction could not take place within pancreatic tissue.

This attractive experiment has been widely quoted (by the present author, among others) to support the concept that increases in estrogens, induced by elevated plasma corticosteroids, can modify hepatic enzyme activity. One difficulty with this interpretation is that estrogens also increase liver alanine aminotransferase levels in female rats (Braidman and Rose, 1971), even though they do not alter the concentrations of corticosteroid-binding globulin (Gala and Westphal, 1965) or total plasma corticosterone (D'Angelo, 1968). Adrenal steroids do, however, have some role in the induction of female rat liver alanine aminotransferase by estrogens. Thus, bilateral adrenalectomy causes a decline in the level of enzyme activity, which is unaffected by estradiol administration (Braidman and Rose, 1971). This problem has not been pursued in recent years and merits further investigation.

Erythrocyte alanine aminotransferase and aspartate amino-transferase activities are widely used indicators of vitamin B_6 nutritional status in man (Section II, C). Erythrocyte alanine amino-transferase is unchanged in women taking estrogen-containing oral contraceptives, whereas there is an elevation in aspartate amino-transferase (Aly et al., 1971; Rose et al., 1972, 1973b; Miller et al., 1975). In the mature female rat, ethynylestradiol given alone causes an increase in both erythrocyte and hepatic alanine aminotransferases, but only in erythrocyte aspartate aminotransferase; a similar effect occurs after ACTH administration (Li Chung C. Chen and D. P. Rose, unpublished data).

Corticosteroids increase hepatic alanine aminotransferase activity by a mRNA-mediated induction of apoenzyme synthesis (Segal and Kim, 1963), but if this is the mechanism for the observed elevations in erythrocyte aminotransferases it must occur in the red cell precursors because mature erythrocytes have lost the capacity for protein synthesis.

An alternative explanation is that the sulfate esters formed from the administered estrogen reduce the rate of enzyme degradation. In their *in vitro* studies of kynurenine aminotransferase, Mason and Gullekson (1960a) found that the formation of a complex between the apoenzyme and an estrogen sulfate protected the protein from thermal inactivation. If a similar phenomenon occurs in the circulating erythrocyte, the apoenzyme–estrogen ester complex could conceivably dissociate when the hemolyzate is prepared for the enzyme assay. The increased amount of total enzyme would then be included in the final determination.

Rose *et al*. (1976) performed some experiments suggesting that induction of hepatic alanine aminotransferase occurs in women using oral contraceptives. The metabolism of an orally administered alanine load was studied in women taking an estrogen-containing oral contraceptive and in female controls of similar age. After ingestion of the amino acid, the increases in plasma alanine above the fasting concentrations were significantly less for the oral contraceptive users than for the controls (Fig. 2). But, the fasting blood pyruvate levels were higher in these women, and further increases, suggesting a rapid rate of transamination, occurred after alanine loading (Fig. 3). These results are consistent with the postulate that the estrogenic component of the oral contraceptives, by raising alanine aminotransferase activity, enhances the rate of clearance of alanine from the blood and the production of pyruvate.

Tyrosine aminotransferase is another vitamin B$_6$-dependent enzyme, the activity of which is stimulated by glucocorticoids (Lin and Knox, 1957) and estrogens (Braidman and Rose, 1971). The effect of estradiol on rat liver tyrosine aminotransferase is not entirely dependent on intact adrenal function; the reduction in enzyme activity that occurs

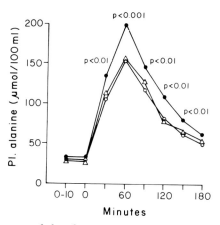

FIG. 2. Mean responses of the plasma alanine concentration to a 200 mg/kg body weight oral amino acid load for 30 oral contraceptive users (○), 11 oral contraceptive users after pyridoxine administration (△), and 14 controls (●). The *p* values refer to the significance levels of differences between the 30 oral contraceptive users and 14 controls. From Rose *et al*. (1976).

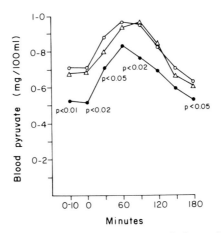

F<small>IG</small>. 3. Mean blood pyruvate concentrations before and after oral alanine loads for oral contraceptive users (○), oral contraceptive users treated with pyridoxine (△), and controls (●). The p values refer to the significance of differences between the 30 oral contraceptive users and 14 controls. From Rose *et al.* (1976).

after bilateral adrenalectomy is partially, but not completely, reversed by estrogen administration (Braidman and Rose, 1971).

In man, treatment with glucocorticoids causes a reduction in plasma tyrosine, which was attributed to enzyme induction with an increased rate of amino acid degradation by tyrosine aminotransferase (Rivlin and Melmon, 1965). The low plasma tyrosine concentrations that occur in users of oral contraceptives and estrogen-treated women were attributed to a similar mechanism (Rose and Cramp, 1970).

3. *Comment*

It is clear that the interaction that takes place between estrogens and vitamin B_6-dependent enzymes is a complex one. The activity of some enzymes is stimulated by an induction mechanism, whereas others are inhibited by competition between estrogen conjugates and pyridoxal phosphate for receptor sites on the apoenzyme molecule. Yet, occupation of these receptor sites by the steroid ester protects the enzyme from degradation *in vitro*, and, if the same effect occurs *in vivo*, this may also result in induction as defined here. Under these circumstances, treatment with large doses of pyridoxine, by producing a high coenzyme concentration, may displace the estrogen conjugate from the apoprotein and produce a very high level of the previously inhibited enzyme.

The estrogen-induced elevation in the amounts of certain apoen-zymes, by selectively increasing pyridoxal phosphate binding and al-tering its tissue distribution, may contribute to a "relative deficiency" of the vitamin (Section II, C).

C. Vitamin B$_6$ Requirements in Users of Oral Contraceptives

1. Evidence for Vitamin B$_6$ Deficiency

The reports that oral contraceptive users frequently have an abnor-mality of tryptophan metabolism, which is similar to that of vitamin B$_6$ deficiency, inevitably raised questions concerning their nutritional status for this vitamin. The term "relative deficiency" was introduced because it was thought that their total body concentration of the vita-min was probably normal, but that its function as a coenzyme was impaired (Rose, 1966b).

However, as we have seen, estrogens may have at least two effects on tryptophan metabolism in man. First, induction of tryptophan oxygenase may increase the turnover of the entire tryptophan–nicotinic acid ribonucleotide pathway, and in so doing increase the pyridoxal phosphate requirement. Second, the estrogen esters formed in the liver may compete with pyridoxal phosphate for the kynureninase apoenzyme, and, by inhibition of the metabolism of 3-hydroxykynurenine to 3-hydroxyanthranilic acid, produce most (but not all) of the features of abnormal tryptophan metabolism in vitamin B$_6$-deficient subjects and oral contraceptive users.

Because of the complexity of the effects of contraceptive steroids on tryptophan metabolism, more direct tests were applied to evaluate the vitamin B$_6$ nutritional status of women taking these preparations.

Erythrocyte alanine aminotransferase and aspartate amino-transferase activities are decreased in dietary vitamin B$_6$ deficiency; an even more sensitive index of depletion is to determine the degree of stimulation of activity which is obtained *in vitro* by adding pyridoxal phosphate to the assay system (Raica and Sauberlich, 1964; Cinnamon and Beaton, 1970).

Doberenz *et al.* (1971) measured erythrocyte alanine amino-transferase activity with and without stimulation *in vitro* by pyridoxal phosphate in 13 oral contraceptive users and 11 controls. The mean basal enzyme activity was significantly lower, and the percentage of stimulation obtained by pyridoxal phosphate greater, in the oral con-traceptive group. There was, however, considerable overlap in the indi-vidual results for the two groups. Rose *et al.* (1973b) could find no difference in the basal erythrocyte alanine aminotransferase activities of 80 oral contraceptive users compared with 50 untreated controls. There was an increased stimulation of the enzyme *in vitro* by pyridoxal phosphate, but this was present in only 12 oral contraceptive users (15%), whereas approximately 80% had abnormal tryptophan metabolism.

Salkeld *et al*. (1973) employed the stimulation *in vitro* of erythrocyte aspartate aminotransferase by pyridoxal phosphate as an index of vitamin B_6 deficiency. There were 233 oral contraceptive users and 76 age-matched controls, all of whom were attending a gynecology clinic; normal values for the assay had been determined in samples from more than 300 blood donors. Abnormal stimulation tests, regarded as indicative of frank vitamin B_6 deficiency, were found in 37% of the oral contraceptive-treated women and 13% of the controls. A further 11 % and 5%, respectively, were considered to have only marginally adequate vitamin B_6 reserves.

It is difficult to interpret these results because, as has been discussed previously (Section II, B, 2), the synthetic estrogens used in oral contraceptives have a direct effect on aspartate aminotransferase. Other workers concluded that the erythrocyte aspartate aminotransferase assay is of no value in assessing the vitamin B_6 nutritional status of oral contraceptive users (Shane and Contractor, 1975).

An alternative approach is to measure vitamin B_6 or its metabolites in plasma, whole blood, or urine. Rose *et al*. (1972) determined the excretion of 4-pyridoxic acid and tryptophan metabolites in the urine of 31 oral contraceptive users; 26 had abnormal tryptophan metabolism, but the 4-pyridoxic acid excretion was decreased in only seven. Miller *et al*. (1974) fed a controlled diet containing 1.9 mg of vitamin B_6 daily to three women taking an oral contraceptive and two nonusers of similar age for 11 days. The oral contraceptive-treated women excreted approximately 30% less microbiological assayable urinary vitamin B_6 than the controls. There was no difference in the urinary 4-pyridoxic acid excretions.

Miller and co-workers (1974) measured blood pyridoxine, pyridoxamine, and pyridoxal by differential microbiological assays. Only slight reductions were found in the 3 oral contraceptive users compared with 2 controls, but, as the authors themselves pointed out, trichloroacetic acid was used to prepare the samples for analysis, and this may have excluded protein-bound pyridoxal phosphate from the assay.

Several groups of investigators have now published data on the plasma pyridoxal phosphate levels in oral contraceptive-treated women. Lumeng *et al.* (1974) found that 20% of 55 women who had been taking an oral contraceptive for at least 6 months had subnormal levels. A longitudinal study of 10 others showed that after an initial fall the plasma pyridoxal phosphate tended to rise toward normal over a 6-month period of oral contraception. This effect may have been due to altered dietary intake of the vitamin, to an adaptive change in its absorption from the intestine, or to a redistribution of pyridoxal phosphate between tissues and plasma.

Miller *et al.* (1975) found no abnormality in the plasma pyridoxal phosphate concentrations of 10 women who had been taking an oral contraceptive for 4–27 months. However, 7 of these women were in the 20- to 24-year age range, and Lumeng *et al.* (1974) had also observed that the plasma pyridoxal phosphate is normal in younger women; significant reductions were found only in those who were between 25 and 34 years old.

Shane and Contractor (1975) measured the whole-blood pyridoxal phosphate in 21 women aged 18 to 38 years, 9 of whom were taking an oral contraceptive, the other 12 acting as controls. The level of the vitamer in the oral contraceptive users (7.6 ± 1.1 ng/ml) was significantly lower than that of the control group (9.6 ± 1.7 ng/ml).

One study suggests that the socioeconomic status may be a modifying factor. Prasad *et al.* (1976) found that in women from higher socioeconomic groups the plasma pyridoxal phosphate was significantly lower in oral contraceptive users compared with controls. This difference was not evident in women with low socioeconomic backgrounds, suggesting that they were already marginally deficient in vitamin and that this obscured any effect of the contraceptive steroids. It seems curious that the presumed dietary deficiency and the adverse influence of oral contraceptives on vitamin B$_6$ nutrition did not summate to produce even more severe changes in the women drawn from the low socioeconomic population. Driskell *et al.* (1976) obtained evidence that the dietary intake of the vitamin in female university students was considerably below the recommended daily allowance; oral contraceptive users in this population did have a subclinical vitamin B$_6$ deficiency, as evidenced by an elevated *in vitro* stimulation of erythrocyte alanine aminotransferase with pyridoxal phosphate.

A study at the University of Wisconsin was designed to investigate the combined effects of vitamin B$_6$ deficiency and oral contraceptive use on tryptophan metabolism, and various parameters of vitamin B$_6$ nutritional status. The results were published in a series of papers, but have also been summarized in a review article (Leklem *et al.*, 1975b). The rates at which a group of 15 oral contraceptive users and 9

matched controls became depleted of vitamin B_6 were followed when
they consumed a diet providing only 0.19 mg of pyridoxine equivalents
per day. Rates of repletion were then observed with different supplemental doses of pyridoxine hydrochloride (0.8 mg, 2.0 mg, and 20
mg).

The urinary excretion of tryptophan metabolites after a 2-gm oral
load of the amino acid, urinary cystathionine levels after a 3.0-gm
L-methionine load, 4-pyridoxic acid excretion, plasma pyridoxal phosphate, and erythrocyte alanine aminotransferase and aspartate
aminotransferase were used as indicators of vitamin B_6 deficiency.

The oral contraceptive users had abnormal tryptophan metabolism
before commencing the vitamin B_6-deficient diet, but urinary cystathionine excretion, which is elevated in dietary vitamin B_6 deficiency
(Park and Linkswiler, 1970), was not affected. During the 4-week
period of low vitamin B_6 ingestion the excretion of tryptophan metabolites and cystathionine increased in both groups of subjects, but the
rates at which the abnormalities evolved were greater in the oral contraceptive users (Figs. 4 and 5).

The predepletion levels for 4-pyridoxic acid did not differ between
groups, and no significant variations occurred during the depletion
period; in both oral contraceptive users and controls, there were rapid
declines in the urinary excretion of this vitamin B_6 metabolite, with
only slightly lower levels in the former group.

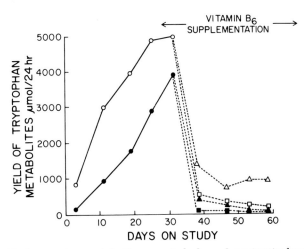

FIG. 4. Yield of tryptophan metabolites excreted after a 2-gm tryptophan load by oral
contraceptive users (○) and controls (●) during a vitamin B_6-depletion period and subsequent repletion. Pyridoxine hydrochloride supplementation was at 0.8 mg/day (oral
contraceptive users, △) or 2.0 mg/day (oral contraceptive users, □; controls, ■).

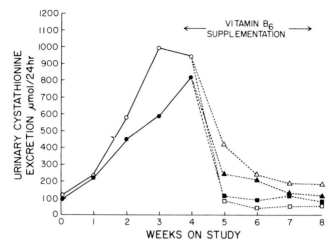

FIG. 5. Yield of cystathionine excreted after an oral 3-gm L-methionine load by oral contraceptive users (○) and controls (●) during a vitamin B$_6$-depletion period and subsequent repletion. Pyridoxine hydrochloride supplementation was as indicated in Fig. 4.

Initially, the mean plasma pyridoxal phosphate concentration was lower in the oral contraceptive-treated women than the controls, although the difference was not statistically significant. The levels remained lower in the oral contraceptive users during the deficiency period, although, because of a more rapid decline in the control group, the values were almost identical by 4 weeks (Fig. 6). This observation appears to support the suggestion of Prasad *et al*. (1976) that a marginal dietary deficiency of vitamin B$_6$ may obscure any effect of oral

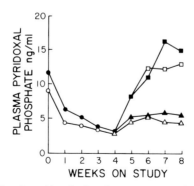

FIG. 6. Plasma pyridoxal pyridoxal phosphate concentrations in oral contraceptive users (○) and controls (●) during vitamin B$_6$ depletion and subsequent repletion. Pyridoxine hydrochloride supplementation was as indicated in Fig. 4.

contraceptives on plasma pyridoxal phosphate levels. However, it should be noted that the sets of values came together only when there had been a 73% average reduction in the control group plasma pyridoxal phosphate concentration.

Erythrocyte alanine aminotransferase and aspartate amino-transferase activities, and the degree of stimulation *in vitro* by pyridoxal phosphate, were similar in oral contraceptive users and controls before consumption of the vitamin B_6-deficient diet, and, as depletion progressed, the two groups showed similar changes in the two enzymes.

The abnormalities of tryptophan and methionine metabolism were reversed promptly when the vitamin B_6-deficient diet for the control group was supplemented with 0.8 mg of pyridoxine hydrochloride daily (Figs. 4 and 5). Although the oral contraceptive users also showed a marked reduction in urinary tryptophan metabolite excretions with the 0.8 mg pyridoxine hydrochloride supplement, the levels were still above predepletion values after 4 weeks of treatment. Similarly, the oral contraceptive users continued to excrete higher levels of urinary cystathionine after supplementation with this dose of the vitamin.

When the dietary intake of vitamin B_6 was supplemented with 2.0 mg of pyridoxine hydrochloride a day, the oral contraceptive-treated group showed a rapid decline in tryptophan metabolite excretion to levels below the predepletion values, although they remained higher than those of the controls (Fig. 4). Supplementation of the oral contraceptive users with 20 mg of pyridoxine hydrochloride daily promptly restored tryptophan metabolism to normal. Similar changes occurred in urinary cystathionine excretion (Fig. 5).

Although an 0.8 mg pyridoxine hydrochloride supplement for 4 weeks produced some increase in the pyridoxal phosphate levels, they remained at approximately half of predepletion values in both groups of women. With a 2.0 mg supplement, the plasma vitamer increased to predepletion levels over a 2-week period; the controls continued to increase until the end of the experiment, whereas the oral contraceptive users showed a plateau (Fig. 6).

Interpretation of the results from this study must be approached with caution. Apart from abnormal tryptophan metabolism, the 15 users of oral contraceptives had no evidence of vitamin B_6 deficiency before the dietary depletion period. Their mean plasma pyridoxal phosphate concentration, urinary 4-pyridoxic acid excretion, and cystathione excretion, and the erythrocyte aminotransferase activities, were all similar to those of the nine controls. But, the overall experience reviewed earlier in this section suggests that direct evidence of vitamin B$_6$ deficiency is found in approximately 15–20% of women taking estrogen-containing oral contraceptives; the majority show only abnormal tryptophan metabolism. Because of the complexity of the experimental design, notably the use of a strictly controlled vitamin B$_6$-deficient diet and repeated blood and urine sample collections, the number of subjects in each group was small. In consequence, the pre-depletion data should not be regarded as arguing against the occurrence of vitamin B$_6$ deficiency in some oral contraceptive users. While the differences between the two groups in the rates at which the various parameters of vitamin B$_6$ deficiency changed during the depletion and repletion periods were small, they do suggest that oral contraceptives increase the vitamin B$_6$ requirement.

The author's belief is that at least two mechanisms are at work that could affect vitamin B$_6$ nutrition. First, induction of certain amino acid-metabolizing enzymes, some requiring pyridoxal phosphate as a coenzyme, may divert vitamin B$_6$ from equally essential metabolic activities, and decrease the total available body pool. Second, conjugates formed in the liver from the relatively large amounts of administered estrogenic steroids may compete with pyridoxal phosphate for apoenzymes, and so cause inhibition of the type described in Section II, B.

2. Oral Contraceptives, Vitamin B$_6$, and Carbohydrate Metabolism

A deterioration in glucose tolerance occurs in many women taking estrogen-containing oral contraceptives (Gershberg et al., 1964; Wynn and Doar, 1966, 1969; Spellacy, 1969; Beck and Wells, 1969). Impaired glucose tolerance may be demonstrated by either oral or intravenous tests, although the former usually yields a higher incidence of abnormal responses (Wynn and Doar, 1966; Buchler and Warren, 1966).

In one longitudinal study (Wynn and Doar, 1969), relative impairment of glucose tolerance after taking an oral contraceptive, in comparison to the pretreatment results, was observed in 78% and 70% of oral and intravenous glucose-tolerance tests, respectively; 13% had frankly abnormal glucose tolerance of a degree equal to that seen in subclinical ("chemical") diabetes. Spellacy et al. (1968) carried out a longitudinal study of 93 women who were tested before and after one year of treatment with an estrogen–progestogen preparation. There were only slight increases in the peak blood glucose concentrations during an intravenous glucose-tolerance test, but pronounced elevations in the plasma insulin levels. The greatest changes in glucose and insulin were seen in older women, those who gained weight excessively during treatment, and those who had had infants weighing more than nine pounds.

The clinical significance of impaired glucose tolerance in oral contraceptive users is still unclear. Javier *et al.* (1968) found that the plasma insulin rose in the early stages of oral contraceptive use, but that with prolonged administration the plasma insulin levels during oral glucose-tolerance tests tended to be low in some patients despite further deterioration in glucose tolerance. These observations suggested that initial peripheral insulin resistance may lead in time to exhaustion of the pancreatic islets' capacity to secrete insulin. Wynn and Doar (1970) pointed out that it will require an extensive study of several hundreds of patients over many years before the risk of pancreatic islet exhaustion, and the onset of clinically overt diabetes mellitus, can be properly assessed. The risk of permanent damage to pancreatic endocrine function has also been discussed by Kalkhoff *et al.* (1969) and Spellacy (1969).

There are a number of similarities between the metabolic effects of oral contraceptives and of pregnancy. In normal pregnancy, the high levels of hormones, such as estrogens, chorionic somatomammotropin and corticosteroids, antagonize the actions of insulin on carbohydrate uptake and utilization. The result is that although normal glucose tolerance may be maintained, this is achieved by increasing insulin secretion (Kalkhoff *et al.*, 1964). Gestational diabetes appears to be due to an exacerbation of insulin resistance, which, as in oral contraceptive-treated women with "chemical" diabetes, is reflected by high plasma insulin levels (Kalkhoff *et al.*, 1964; Carrington and McWilliams, 1966).

Normal pregnancy is associated with a similar disturbance in tryptophan metabolism to that seen in oral contraceptive users. Elevated excretions of xanthurenic acid and other metabolites are present in urine collected after a tryptophan load, and these abnormalities are reversed by treatment with pyridoxine. In the later stages of pregnancy there is a decline in tissue and plasma vitamin B_6 levels because of transplacental diversion to the fetus (Section II, D).

The hypothesis that impaired glucose tolerance in oral contraceptive users and pregnant women might be related to their abnormal tryptophan metabolism was based on the work of Kotake (1955) and Kotake *et al.* (1968, 1975). They had found that feeding rats a high tryptophan–vitamin B_6-deficient (or excess fatty acid) diet caused xanthurenic aciduria, hyperglycemia, glycosuria, and damage to the β-cells of the pancreatic islets. A similar diabetic state could be induced by the intraperitoneal injection of xanthurenic acid into rats receiving a normal diet. Later, it was shown that xanthurenic acid and insulin will form *in vitro* a complex that has considerably less hypoglycemic activity than the native hormone (Kotake *et al.*, 1968, 1975).

A preliminary report published by Spellacy *et al.* (1972) suggested that treatment with vitamin B$_6$ might improve the glucose tolerance of oral contraceptive users. Twelve women were studied whose glucose tolerance had deteriorated while taking contraceptive steroids. Although an overall improvement in glucose tolerance was achieved by treatment with pyridoxine, 25 mg daily for 1 month, this, in fact, occurred in only 8 of the patients. No attempt was made to determine the vitamin B$_6$ nutritional status in this study.

Adams *et al.* (1976) studied the oral glucose tolerance and vitamin B$_6$ nutrition of 46 women who were taking an estrogen-containing oral contraceptive. Eighteen were classified as vitamin B$_6$ deficient on the basis of an elevated ratio of 3-hydroxykynurenine to 3-hydroxyanthranilic acid excreted after a 2-gm tryptophan load, urinary 4-pyridoxic acid excretion, and erythrocyte alanine and aspartate aminotransferase activities. From earlier discussion in this chapter, it will be noted that these tests, with the exception of the alanine aminotransferase assay with and without pyridoxal phosphate stimulation *in vitro*, are poor indicators of vitamin B$_6$ nutritional status. Nevertheless, glucose tolerance was improved by pyridoxine supplementation, 20 mg twice daily for 4 weeks, only in the 18 who were regarded as deficient in vitamin B$_6$.

Fourteen patients with gestational diabetes were studied by Coelingh Bennink and Schreurs (1975); 13 had excessive xanthurenic acid excretion after a tryptophan load, and 8 had low blood vitamin B$_6$ levels. Treatment with pyridoxine hydrochloride, 100 mg daily for 2 weeks, corrected the abnormal xanthurenic acid and vitamin B$_6$ levels, and in 13 of the 14 there was a considerable improvement in glucose tolerance. This is an important finding because, although not everyone agrees on the importance of closely regulated blood glucose levels in other areas of diabetic management, the outcome for the fetus may depend on the control of carbohydrate metabolism during pregnancy. Thus, even mild untreated gestational diabetes may cause increased morbidity and mortality (Beischer and Lowry, 1965; Dandrow and O'Sullivan, 1966; Campbell *et al.*, 1971).

Whether the basic abnormality responsible for unimpaired glucose tolerance with insulin resistance in oral contraceptive users and pregnant women is truly the formation of an insulin–xanthurenic acid complex remains uncertain. In an unpublished study, D. P. Rose attempted to demonstrate a deleterious effect of high levels of circulating xanthurenic acid on carbohydrate metabolism. Oral glucose-tolerance tests were performed on 13 women who had been using an oral contraceptive for at least 6 months. Twenty-one days later they began a 7-day period of tryptophan supplementation, 1 gm of L-tryptophan at breakfast and 1 gm at suppertime. Glucose tolerance was then reassessed. Twenty-four-hour urine collections were made on the day before each glucose-tolerance test and assayed for xanthurenic acid. The supplementation of dietary tryptophan so as to give approximately a 3-fold increase in intake did cause a significant elevation in urinary xanthurenic acid, but no changes in either plasma glucose or insulin responses were observed during the oral glucose-tolerance tests. It was concluded that the formation of an insulin–xanthurenic acid complex was unlikely to be the explanation for impaired glucose tolerance in oral contraceptive users.

A similar conclusion was reached by Adams et al. (1976) from their study of vitamin B_6 and carbohydrate metabolism. As an alternative, they referred to the fact that the tryptophan metabolites 3-hydroxyanthranilic acid and quinolinic acid can inhibit gluconeogenesis by suppressing phosphoenolpyruvate carboxykinase activity (Veneziale et al., 1967). It was suggested that impaired glucose tolerance in vitamin B_6-deficient oral contraceptive users arises because the levels of these metabolites are subnormal, with a consequent elevation in the activity of this enzyme and enhanced gluconeogenesis. It is difficult to reconcile this proposal with reports that both 3-hydroxyanthranilic acid (Rose, 1966b; Price et al., 1972) and quinolinic acid (Rose and Toseland, 1973) are elevated in both experimental vitamin B_6 deficiency and oral contraceptive users.

Finally, it should be noted that Cornish and Tesoriero (1975) were unable to render rats hyperglycemic with xanthurenic acid, even when they were fed a high-fat diet.

3. Oral Contraceptive-Related Mental Depression and Vitamin B_6

Some women become severely depressed when taking an oral contraceptive (Daly et al., 1967; Grounds et al., 1970; Herzberg et al., 1970); this complication is particularly likely to occur in those with a previous history of depressive illness or premenstrual tension (Lewis and Hoghughi, 1969; Nilsson et al., 1968; Herzberg et al., 1971). The incidence of depression due to oral contraceptive use has been hotly debated, but in one study 6.6% of users were more severely depressed than any of the women in the control group (Herzberg et al., 1970). Certainly, it appears to be a common reason for women discontinuing this form of contraception (Dennis and Jeffery, 1968).

In endogenous depression, there is quite strong evidence that at least one biochemical abnormality concerned with the etiology of the disease is a defect in the synthesis of 5-hydroxytryptamine (5-HT) from tryptophan. This transformation occurs in two steps, a hydroxylation reaction to yield 5-hydroxytryptophan, followed by a decarboxylation that requires pyridoxal phosphate as a coenzyme. 5-HT is synthesized at several sites, including the liver and kidney, but, because the amine cannot cross the blood–brain barrier (Schanberg, 1963), that present in the brain has to be produced *in situ*.

Reserpine, which decreases the level of amines in the brain, is not an infrequent cause of depression (Bunney and Davis, 1965), while monoamine oxidase inhibitors, which increase brain amine levels, are valuable drugs in the treatment of the endogenous disease. Tryptophan, when given in large doses, enhances the effectiveness of the monoamine oxidase inhibitors (Coppen *et al.*, 1967), and alone may be as effective as electroconvulsive therapy (Broadhurst, 1970). 5-Hydroxytryptophan, which does cross the blood–brain barrier, has been used successfully to obtain remission from a prolonged episode of depression (Persson and Roos, 1967).

Further evidence involving disordered tryptophan metabolism in the etiology of depression includes the demonstration of low levels of 5-hydroxyindoleacetic acid, the excretory metabolite of 5-HT, in the cerebrospinal fluid of depressed patients (Ashcroft *et al.*, 1966), and reduced brain 5-HT concentrations in suicide victims who had suffered from endogenous depression (Shaw *et al.*, 1967). Finally, the plasma free tryptophan, which determines the level of the amino acid in brain tissue, and hence 5-HT synthesis (Gessa *et al.*, 1972; Curzon, 1975), is reduced in depressed patients (Coppen *et al.*, 1973; Baumann *et al.*, 1975).

The demonstration of abnormal tryptophan metabolism in oral contraceptive users suggested that impaired 5-HT synthesis might explain the occurrence of depression in some of these women. Three possible mechanisms were considered: diversion of available tryptophan away from 5-HT formation and into the nicotinic acid ribonucleotide synthesizing pathway, interference with tryptophan uptake by brain tissue, and impairment of 5-hydroxytryptophan decarboxylase activity.

High early-morning 11-hydroxycorticosteroid concentrations have been reported in the plasma of patients with endogenous depression (Knapp *et al.*, 1967), as have elevated urinary excretions of kynurenine (Curzon and Bridges, 1970). Green and Curzon (1968) postulated that a cortisol-induced rise in tryptophan oxygenase activity, by promoting the entry of substrate into the tryptophan-nicotinic acid ribonucleotide pathway, could reduce brain 5-HT synthesis and so precipitate a depressive state. They did show that tryptophan oxygenase induction caused a decline in rat brain 5-HT, which was prevented when allopurinol, an inhibitor of the enzyme, was injected along with the steroid. These data led Rose and Braidman (1970) to speculate that a similar induction of tryptophan oxygenase in oral contraceptive users might explain the development of depression. In the rat, treatment with a combination of an estrogen and a progestogen did reduce the brain 5-HT level (Nisticò and Preziosi, 1970).

Two alternative mechanisms by which the altered tryptophan metabolism of oral contraceptive users could reduce brain 5-HT levels, and so cause depression, suggested a therapeutic role for vitamin B_6. First, Green and Curzon (1970) found that injected kynurenine or 3-hydroxykynurenine reduced the 5-HT content of rat brain; *in vitro* these metabolites decreased the uptake of tryptophan by brain slices. An accumulation of tryptophan metabolites in oral contraceptive-treated women could conceivably have a similar effect, which would be reversed by the administration of large doses of vitamin B_6.

Second, there is evidence that the enzymic decarboxylation of 5-hydroxytryptophan may be rate-limiting in the synthesis of 5-HT by human brain tissue (Robins *et al.*, 1967). 5-Hydroxytryptophan decarboxylase activity is inhibited *in vitro* by estrogen conjugates competing with pyridoxal phosphate for the apoenzyme (Mason and Schirch, 1961); a similar phenomenon may occur *in vivo*, as is thought to be true of hepatic kynureninase (Section II, B, 1). A simple vitamin B_6 deficiency might also be responsible for loss of enzyme activity and 5-HT production.

Baumblatt and Winston (1970) were the first to report that treatment with 50 mg of pyridoxine daily was effective in oral contraceptive-related depression. Their finding was challenged because the study was uncontrolled, and not subjected to statistical evaluation.

Later, a formal, double-blind crossover-design clinical trial was performed by Adams *et al.* (1973). Thirty-two women who had developed depression for the first time while taking an oral contraceptive were included in the study. Pyridoxine hydrochloride, 20 mg twice daily, or a placebo, was administered for 2 months, followed by the alternative preparation for the same period of time. The ratio of 3-hydroxykynurenine to 3-hydroxyanthranilic acid excreted after a 2-gm tryptophan load, urinary 4-pyridoxic acid, and erythrocyte aminotransferases activities were used as indicators of vitamin B$_6$ nutritional status. Therapeutic efficacy was evaluated by a Beck self-rating depression questionnaire.

Eleven of the 32 patients were regarded as vitamin B$_6$ deficient, and only this group showed a statistically validated benefit from pyridoxine administration. When the placebo was given first, some patients, both those who were and those who were not vitamin B$_6$ deficient, showed a temporary improvement in their depression. This "placebo effect," which is commonly seen in such clinical trials, was not maintained throughout the treatment period. A further report, in which the series was enlarged to 30 women, confirmed the original finding (Adams *et al.*, 1974).

4. Oral Contraceptive-Induced Hypertriglyceridemia and Vitamin B$_6$

Hyperlipidemia, notably an increase in the serum triglycerides, is a well recognized complication of the use of oral contraceptives (Gershberg *et al.*, 1968; Wynn *et al.*, 1969; Stokes and Wynn, 1971). The clinical importance of this metabolic abnormality is that in other situations it is associated with the development of occlusive vascular disease, and increased risk of myocardial infarction, both of which are known complications of oral contraceptive use (Inman *et al.*, 1970; Mann and Inman, 1975).

Amino acids which yield pyruvate during their metabolism are potential sources for increased triglyceride synthesis by way of the intramitochondrial oxidation of pyruvate to acetyl-SCoA. Rose *et al.* (1977) studied the changes in the serum triglyceride levels after alanine ingestion in oral contraceptive users and controls. Little effect was observed in 13 controls, but marked increases occurred in 23 oral contraceptive-treated women. Ten of the oral contraceptive users were then treated with 25 mg of pyridoxine hydrochloride daily for 28 days. The vitamin appeared to cause a reduction in both the fasting serum triglycerides, and the response to alanine loading.

These preliminary observations prompted a crossover therapeutic trial in which the same daily dose of pyridoxine hydrochloride, or a placebo, was given for 2 months, followed by a further 2 months' treatment with the alternative treatment. Fifty oral contraceptive users, who as a group were hypertriglyceridemic, and 25 controls took part in the study. Unfortunately, no effect of pyridoxine was observed on the fasting serum triglycerides of either group, indicating that the earlier finding was an unexplained artifact (D. P. Rose, unpublished data).

5. *Comment*

From the published work it appears that approximately 70–80% of women taking an oral contraceptive develop abnormal tryptophan metabolism. This incidence may be declining as the use of preparations containing 50 μg or less of estrogen increases; women taking some oral contraceptives with a 50-μg dose excrete normal, or only slightly elevated, levels of urinary tryptophan metabolites (Rose *et al.*, 1973a; Leklem *et al.*, 1973). True vitamin B_6 deficiency, as judged by biochemical tests, occurs in only 15% or so of oral contraceptive users, and most of these show no clinical abnormalities. One important unknown, however, is the number of women who develop changes of mood due to altered tryptophan–vitamin B_6 metabolism, and in consequence discontinue this form of contraception after only a few treatment cycles.

Some workers have recommended that women using estrogen-containing oral contraceptives should routinely receive a 20- to 30-mg supplement of pyridoxine each day in order to correct their abnormal tryptophan metabolism (Toseland and Price, 1969; Luhby *et al.*, 1971). The author has opposed this proposal because of concern that, by stimulating the entry of amino acids in degradative pathways, vitamin B_6 supplementation might accentuate preexisting hypoaminoacidemias (Rose *et al.*, 1973b; Rose, 1978). This would be particularly undesirable when oral contraceptives are employed for population control programs in areas of the world where protein-calorie malnutrition is endemic. The only experimental evidence, one way or the other, was an investigation referred to earlier (Section II, B, 2) in which alanine metabolism was studied in oral contraceptive users and control women. Supplementation with pyridoxine hydrochloride, 25 mg daily for 28 weeks, while sufficient to produce very high levels of erythrocyte alanine aminotransferase, had no discernible effect on metabolism of the amino acid.

D. Pregnancy, Endogenous Estrogens, and Vitamin B_6

1. *Pregnancy*

The excretions of xanthurenic acid, kynurenine, 3-hydroxykynurenine, and kynurenic acid (Brown *et al.*, 1961), and 3-hydroxyanthranilic acid (Hernandez, 1964) are all elevated to an abnormal degree in urine collected from pregnant women after a tryptophan load. These changes are reversed by treatment with pyridoxine. Increased amounts of N^1-methylnicotinamide (Hernandez, 1964) and

N-methyl-2-pyridone-5-carboxamide (Brown *et al.*, 1961) are also excreted during pregnancy. This pattern is consistent with there being two factors responsible for the abnormal tryptophan metabolism of pregnancy: a vitamin B_6 deficiency produced by a redistribution of the vitamin to the fetus, and a direct influence of endogenously produced hormones, presumably estrogens, on the tryptophan–nicotinic acid ribonucleotide pathway. Supporting evidence for this interpretation was provided by Hamfelt and Hahn (1969); they showed that whereas xanthurenic acid excretion is elevated early in pregnancy, the plasma pyridoxal phosphate concentration is reduced only in the last trimester, at which time there is a significant loss to the fetus.

Several early studies suggested that a true vitamin B_6 deficiency does develop during pregnancy. Wachstein and Gudaitis (1953) found that there is a low excretion of 4-pyridoxic acid in urine collected after a loading dose of pyridoxine. Women at term had low leukocyte and plasma pyridoxal phosphate concentrations, with a subnormal rise in the plasma level after pyridoxine administration (Wachstein *et al.*, 1960). Brin (1971) showed that, compared with cord blood levels, the vitamers of B_6 and erythrocyte aminotransferase activities are reduced in maternal blood at term. These observations reflect the transplacental loss of vitamin B_6 to the fetus. In addition to utilization of the vitamin by the fetus, the very high levels of circulating estrogens in pregnancy may contribute to an increased vitamin B_6 requirement by stimulating amino acid catabolic, pyridoxal phosphate-dependent, pathways, just as do the synthetic estrogens in oral contraceptive users.

More recent investigations were designed to determine the vitamin B_6 requirements of the normal pregnant woman. In one study, the average plasma pyridoxal phosphate level for 58 nonpregnant women was 10.5 ± 4.1 ng/ml, whereas for 13 pregnant women ingesting 2.0–2.5 mg of pyridoxine a day it was 3.7 ± 1.5 ng/ml. Eleven other pregnant women receiving 10 mg of pyridoxine daily had a mean level of 7.5 ± 4.5 ng/ml (Cleary *et al.*, 1975). Lumeng *et al.* (1976) confirmed these findings, but in addition showed that a daily intake of 4.0 mg of pyridoxine during pregnancy is insufficient to maintain a normal level of plasma pyridoxal phosphate. Thus, the currently recommended dietary allowance of vitamin B_6 for pregnant women, 2.5 mg/day (Food and Nutrition Board, 1974), fails to maintain the circulating pyridoxal phosphate level at that of the healthy nonpregnant woman.

There is evidence that low tissue pyridoxal phosphate levels may be implicated in the etiology of toxemia of pregnancy (preeclampsia). Sprince *et al.* (1951) originally reported that the urinary xanthurenic acid excretion after a tryptophan load was higher in preeclamptic patients than in normal pregnant women. Much more recently, Brophy and Siiteri (1975) assayed pyridoxal phosphate in maternal and cord blood. Although the levels in preeclamptic patients did not differ significantly from those of healthy women, the mean concentration in their newborn infants (12.2 ng/ml) was lower than that in healthy neonates (28.4 ng/ml).

Vitamin B_6-related biochemical abnormalities have been observed in the placentas of preeclamptic women. Klieger et al. (1969) found that the levels of vitamin B_6 vitamers and pyridoxal kinase activity were less than half those of normal placentas, and Gaynor and Dempsey (1972) reported reductions in both pyridoxal kinase and pyridoxine phosphate oxidase activity. Two therapeutic trials of pyridoxine supplementation in pregnancy produced conflicting results. Wachstein and Graffeo (1956) observed that the incidence of preeclampsia was lower in pregnant women treated with 10 mg of pyridoxine hydrochloride a day than in a group of untreated controls. But this was not confirmed by Hillman et al. (1963) in a double-blind clinical trial involving 956 pregnant women treated with 20 mg of pyridoxine hydrochloride daily and 576 untreated women.

Dempsey (1978) has discussed the vitamin B_6 requirements of the preeclamptic patient and of the healthy pregnant woman. From his own work and a review of the literature he concluded that altered vitamin B_6 metabolism probably does have a role in the etiology of preeclampsia. He suggested that vitamin B_6 be given in sufficient quantity to maintain the pyridoxal phosphate levels in cord blood at those found in normal pregnancies, and that, in view of the low pyridoxine phosphate oxidase activity in preeclamptic placentas, the supplement should be pyridoxal rather than pyridoxine. After 20 years of debate, it is clearly time that this important issue be resolved by a carefully designed therapeutic trial with pyridoxine, pyridoxal, and placebo-treated groups of patients.

As far as the healthy pregnant woman is concerned, there appears to be a case for ensuring a daily vitamin B_6 intake, as pyridoxine equivalents of between 4 an 10 mg, rather than the 2.5 mg recommended at present (Dempsey, 1978).

2. Endogenous Estrogens in the Nonpregnant Woman

There is a limited amount of data suggesting that endogenous estrogen levels per se influence tryptophan metabolism, but probably not vitamin B_6 requirements, in man.

Michael et al. (1964) found that young adult women excrete a higher percentage of a 100 mg/kg body weight dose of tryptophan as urinary metabolites than men, and this was confirmed by two other studies using a fixed 5-gm load (Mainardi and Tenconi, 1964; Rose, 1967a). After the menopause, this sex difference was not evident, post-menopausal women excreting similar levels to adult men (Rose, 1967a).

Fluctuations in the levels of tryptophan metabolite excretion were observed with the stage of the menstrual cycle; significantly higher 3-hydroxykynurenine, 3-hydroxyanthranilic acid, and xanthurenic acid excretions occur at ovulation, when plasma estrogens are at their peak, than immediately after menstruation (Brown et al., 1961; Rose, 1967a). Some breast cancer patients treated by bilateral oophorectomy excrete reduced amounts of metabolites compared with the levels seen in premenopausal patients of similar age (Rose, 1967b).

The mechanism responsible for the observed sex difference and changes in tryptophan metabolism with the menstrual cycle remains uncertain. Variations in tryptophan oxygenase may be responsible; adult female rats have a higher level of activity of this hepatic enzyme than males (Pinto and Rosenthal, 1965; Braidman and Rose, 1971). This enzyme is inducible by corticosteroids (Section III, A), and both plasma ACTH and cortisol levels vary with the stage of the menstrual cycle. ACTH concentrations are low during the follicular phase and increase to a peak on the day of the LH peak; plasma cortisol is also at its lowest level in the follicular phase and peaks immediately before ovulation (Genazzani et al., 1975). These menstrual cycle-related changes are consistent with an elevation in tryptophan oxygenase activity being responsible for increased urinary excretion of tryptophan metabolites at the time of ovulation.

A sex difference in plasma cortisol cannot, however, explain the larger excretion of tryptophan metabolites by premenopausal women compared with men; Zumoff et al. (1974) found that the mean 24-hour value for plasma cortisol was significantly higher in adult males. An alternative is that the altered tryptophan metabolism is due directly to differences in circulating estrogen levels. Braidman and Rose (1971) found that tryptophan oxygenase activity was increased in adrenalec-tomized female rats by treatment with estrogens.

With the possible exception of the very high levels in pregnancy, there is no convincing evidence that endogenous estrogens alter vita-min B_6 requirements. Erythrocyte alanine aminotransferase activity is higher in adult men than women, but there is no difference in the stimulation by pyridoxal phosphate in vitro (Rose et al., 1973b). There does not appear to be a sex difference in plasma pyridoxal phosphate levels. The values obtained for healthy adult males (Li, 1978) were similar to those of young women who were not taking an oral contraceptive (Brown et al., 1975).

III. Corticosteroids and ACTH

A. Effects on Pyridoxal Phosphate-Dependent Enzymes

A number of amino acid-metabolizing, pyridoxal phosphate-dependent, enzymes are inducible by adrenocorticosteroids. Typically, there is a prolonged delay between steroid administration and the attainment of maximal enzyme activity. Hepatic alanine aminotransferase, for example, reaches its peak 48 hours after hydrocortisone injection, and the increased activity then persists for 5 days (Rosen et al., 1963). The maximal level of serine dehydrase occurs 24 hours after glucocorticoid treatment (Pitot and Peraino, 1964), and aspartate aminotransferase activity is increased in male rats only after daily injections of 2.5 mg of hydrocortisone per 100 gm body weight given for 5 days (Herzfeld and Greengard, 1971).

The slow response of these enzymes to glucocorticoids contrasts with the effect on tryptophan oxygenase, which exhibits a maximal response 4–5 hours after a single dose of hydrocortisone (Feigelson et al., 1962). The delayed effect may be because the mechanism of induction is related to glucocorticoid-mediated uptake of amino acids into the liver, which permits regulation of gluconeogenesis. When dietary carbohydrate intake is low and protein uptake relatively high, amino acids are thus able to promote their own degradation for utilization in gluconeogenesis. Conversely, a high carbohydrate intake may depress glucocorticoid and amino acid induction of amino acid-metabolizing enzymes and so reduce gluconeogenic activity.

B. Vitamin B_6 Function and Tryptophan Metabolism

Although adrenocorticosteroids stimulate the turnover of amino acid degradative pathways which utilize pyridoxal phosphate-dependent enzymes, very few studies have been performed to determine their influence on vitamin B_6 nutrition. Hsu (1963) quoted a study by Yeh in which rats treated with 2 units of ACTH daily for 10 days were found to have normal levels of pyridoxal phosphate in liver and other organs. However, in view of the slow response of most of the amino acid-metabolizing enzymes to corticosteroids, the duration of treatment may have been inadequate to cause depletion of tissue vitamin B_6 levels.

Li Chung C. Chen and D. P. Rose (unpublished data) administered hydrocortisone in daily doses of 1 mg or 6 mg to adult female rats. Although both erythrocyte and hepatic alanine aminotransferase levels were elevated after 14 days there was no change in the *in vitro* stimulation by pyridoxal phosphate.

Rose and McGinty (1968) studied the effect of hydrocortisone on the urinary excretion of metabolites of the tryptophan-nicotinic acid ribonucleotide pathway in man. A single intramuscular injection of the steroid was administered 5 hours before the ingestion of a tryptophan load. Corticosteroid induction of tryptophan oxygenase produced increased excretions of kynurenine, 3-hydroxykynurenine, xanthurenic acid, and 3-hydroxyanthranilic acid. This accumulation of metabolites was prevented when large doses of pyridoxine were given before the tryptophan load, presumably, in part, because of activation of kynureninase apoenzyme. But, the urinary excretion of 3-hydroxyanthranilic acid was also reduced, indicating that pyridoxine supplementation facilitated the metabolism of tryptophan at a step beyond the formation of this metabolite.

Tryptophan oxygenase and tyrosine aminotransferase activities are increased in the livers of tumor-bearing rats; both enzyme levels return to normal after bilateral adrenalectomy (Greengard et al., 1967). These changes occur at a late stage in tumor growth and are most likely a consequence of the pituitary–adrenal axis response to stress. In man, the trauma of major surgery causes a rapid rise in the level of plasma ACTH and cortisol, and these endocrine responses are associated with elevated urinary tryptophan metabolite excretions (Rose and McGinty, 1968).

There do not appear to be any reported studies of the effect of physical stress on vitamin B_6 nutrition in man. Potera et al. (1977) found that low plasma pyridoxal phosphate levels are common in patients with advanced cancer, but not in those with early disease. A poor dietary intake of vitamin B_6 was excluded by normal urinary 4-pyridoxic acid excretions. Among the explanations to be considered is an excessive utilization of vitamin B_6 in stress-induced amino acid catabolic reactions. Studies of the vitamin B_6 nutritional status of patients undergoing major surgical procedures, or with chronic debilitating disease, have become important now that total parenteral nutrition is gaining in acceptability as a support technique. There is a need to define the daily supplemental doses of vitamin B_6, and other vitamins, in this situation.

IV. THYROID HORMONES

A. EFFECTS ON PYRIDOXAL PHOSPHATE-DEPENDENT ENZYMES

The early studies of the effect of thyroid hormones on tissue vitamin B_6 levels and pyridoxal phosphate-dependent enzymes were reviewed by Hsu (1963), and so will be only briefly summarized here.

The biosynthesis of pyridoxal phosphate from pyridoxal is catalyzed by a kinase and requires ATP as a cofactor. Mascitelli-Coriandoli and Boldrini (1959) showed that thyroxine-treated rats had reduced levels of hepatic and, to a lesser extent, myocardial pyridoxine and pyridoxal phosphate. Pyridoxine concentrations were not affected to the same degree as the active coenzyme, suggesting that there was both excessive vitamin B_6 utilization and a reduction in oxidative phosphorylation. This was confirmed by the demonstration that injected pyridoxine hydrochloride increased tissue pyridoxine, but not pyridoxal phosphate levels, whereas ATP increased the pyridoxal phosphate concentration. Whether or not the formation of pyridoxal phosphate was depressed because of a lack of available ATP is uncertain; the K_m for the kinases is very much lower than the 2–5 mM levels of ATP in cells.

Animals rendered hyperthyroid by thyroxine injections show a loss of activity of many pyridoxal phosphate-dependent enzymes, although as in dietary vitamin B_6 deficiency, they are affected to varying degrees. Thus, cysteine desulfhydrase is very sensitive to vitamin B_6 depletion (Dietrich and Borries, 1956), and activity of this enzyme is rapidly impaired during thyroxine administration (Horvath, 1957). Liver aspartate aminotransferase, which is relatively resistant to the effects of vitamin B_6 deficiency (Wiss and Weber, 1964), is actually elevated in hyperthyroid rats (Canal and Maffei-Faccioli, 1960).

Prolonged vitamin B_6 deficiency causes a loss of apoenzyme, so that complete reactivation of the enzyme is not achieved by the addition of pyridoxal phosphate *in vitro* to the assay system (Hope, 1955). Similarly, hepatic dopadecarboxylase activity is lost in thyroid hormone-treated rats and is not reactivated by the coenzyme (Holtz *et al.*, 1956).

In more recent years, studies have been made of the effect of thyroid hormones on some of the enzymes of the tryptophan-nicotinic acid ribonucleotide pathway. This work was stimulated by the observation that the concentration of pyridine nucleotides is subnormal in the livers of hyperthyroid rats (Bosch and Harper, 1959). Okamoto *et al.* (1971) assayed kynurenine 3-hydroxylase, kynurenine hydrolase, which removes the alanine side chain from kynurenine to yield anthranilic acid, and the mitochondrial kynurenine aminotransferase, which catalyzes the production of kynurenic acid, in thyroxine-treated and control rats. The hyperthyroid animals had elevated levels of kynurenine aminotransferase and reduced kynurenine 3-hydroxylase activity, changes shown to be due to altered rates of enzyme synthesis. Kynurenine hydrolase, the only one of the three enzymes located in the cytosol fraction, was unaffected by thyroxine administration. This study indicates that thyroid hormone may have a role in the synthesis of nicotinyl cofactors from tryptophan.

Abdel-Tawab *et al.* (1975) studied the effect of thyroxine on kynurenine hydrolase and mitochondrial kynurenine aminotransferase *in vitro*. At a concentration of 10^{-6} *M*, L-thyroxine inhibited aminotransferase activity, but had no effect on kynurenine hydrolase. With increasing concentrations, the degree of inhibition of kynurenine aminotransferase increased and there was stimulation of kynurenine hydrolase activity.

These results are contradictory to those obtained in the *in vivo* study by Okamoto *et al.* (1971) described above. In the *in vitro* study, inhibition of kynurenine aminotransferase activity was partially reversed by pyridoxal phosphate. Indeed, with a thyroxine concentration of 10^{-6} *M* the ratios of basal activity to those obtained in the presence of 50, 100, or 200 μg of pyridoxal phosphate per gram of liver were the same as the corresponding ratios in the absence of thyroxine. Higher concentrations of thyroxine produced total inhibition of the enzyme, but, again, activity was recovered to approximately 30% of the corresponding control in the presence of 100 μg of pyridoxal phosphate per gram of liver.

One explanation for these findings is that at a concentration of 10^{-6} *M* thyroxine was competing with pyridoxal phosphate for the kynurenine aminotransferase apoenzyme; a similar effect of estrogen conjugates was described in Section II, B, 1. Higher thyroxine concentrations may have caused either partial degradation of the enzyme directly, or enzyme loss may have resulted from the high pH necessary to keep the hormone in solution. Further studies of this phenomenon are indicated, including the effect of dialysis on the thyroxine-inhibited enzyme.

B. TRYPTOPHAN METABOLISM IN MAN

There do not appear to be any published studies of tryptophan metabolism in hyperthyroid or hypothyroid patients comparable with the "in-depth" investigations of pregnant women and oral contraceptive users. Wachstein and Lobel (1956) found excessively elevated urinary xanthurenic acid excretions after a 10-gm DL-tryptophan load by 4 patients with hyperthyroidism. Kotake *et al.* (1958) reported 3 cases in which the urinary xanthurenic acid excretion was reduced by thyroidectomy. Wohl *et al.* (1960) studied xanthurenic acid excretion after 10-gm DL-tryptophan loads in 14 clinically and biochemically hyperthyroid patients. High excretions of the metabolite were corrected by a single intramuscular injection of 50 mg of pyridoxine hydrochloride, given 30 min before the tryptophan. As the dietary intakes of vitamin B_6 in these patients were equal to, or above, the recommended daily allowance (2 mg) it appeared that the hypermetabolic state had increased the requirement, with a resulting "relative deficiency."

In light of the animal studies described by Okamoto *et al.* (1971), it would be of interest to measure urinary N^1-methylnicotinamide and N^1-methyl-2-pyridone-5-carboxamide. They did measure urinary kynurenine, 3-hydroxykynurenine, kynurenic acid, and xanthurenic acid excretions after tryptophan loading in their hyperthyroid rats. Kynurenine excretion was greatly elevated, with lesser increases in kynurenic acid and xanthurenic acid. As was to be expected in view of the low kynurenine 3-hydroxylase activity, urinary 3-hydroxykynurenine excretion was subnormal. The effect of pyridoxine supplementation was not examined in this study.

The hypermetabolic state of thyrotoxicosis increases the requirements for all nutrients, but there is little indication that any of the clinical features of the disease are attributable to a deficiency of vitamin B_6. Soskin and Levine (1944) did suggest that the muscle weakness of hyperthyroidism is due to a "relative" vitamin B_6 deficiency, and in 3 patients this symptom was eliminated by daily injections of pyridoxine (Rosenbaum *et al.*, 1942).

Although it might be of interest to reinvestigate this question by a combination of modern techniques for evaluating muscle function and biopsy examinations, the indications are that low levels of tissue pyridoxal phosphate and impaired muscle power in hyperthyroidism are not causally related, but share a common mechanism, the lack of available ATP.

The muscles affected in thyrotoxicosis are predominantly those with a high percentage of mitochondria-rich red fibers (Ramsay, 1966). Because of their high content of mitochondria, they have a high capacity for ATP production and derive their energy for muscle contraction from this source (Lawrie, 1953). Satoyashi *et al.* (1963) have shown that the loss of muscle power in hyperthyroidism is related to a decreased ATP concentration in biopsy specimens.

V. PITUITARY HORMONES

A. BRAIN AMINES AND THE HYPOPHYSIAL TROPIC HORMONES

The secretion of several pituitary hormones is influenced by the concentrations of hypothalamic dopamine and 5-hydroxytryptamine (5-HT). Because the amines cannot cross the blood–brain barrier, those present in the brain have to be synthesized *in situ*.

Dopamine is formed by the decarboxylation of L-dopa (L-3,4-dihydroxyphenylalanine), and 5-HT by the decarboxylation of 5-hydroxytryptophan. These reactions are catalyzed by the same enzyme, aromatic L-amino acid decarboxylase, for which pyridoxal phosphate functions as the coenzyme. There is a high level of the decarboxylase activity in liver, and this may divert dopa away from brain amine synthesis; thus, pyridoxine administration reverses the side effects, but also reduces the efficacy, of L-dopa in the treatment of Parkinson's disease because it promotes the extraneural formation of dopamine (Papavasiliou *et al.*, 1972).

Dopamine and 5-HT are essentially antagonistic in their effects upon pituitary hormone regulation. This may represent a direct action of 5-HT, or the amine may exert its effect by displacing dopamine from dopaminergic neurons (Flux *et al.*, 1971). In the rat, it has been shown that brain 5-HT concentrations are decreased by L-dopa administration (Bartholini *et al.*, 1969).

Cozzolino *et al.* (1975) determined the urinary excretions of several metabolites of the tryptophan-nicotinic acid ribonucleotide pathway, including kynurenine, 3-hydroxykynurenine, and 3-hydroxyanthranilic acid, in 7 Parkinsonian patients before and during L-dopa therapy. Treatment with L-dopa was complicated by anorexia, glossitis, dysphagia, and abdominal pain, and produced increases in urinary kynurenine and 3-hydroxykynurenine with reciprocal declines in 3-hydroxyanthranilic acid excretions. The effect of pyridoxine administration in this situation was not tested, but the authors did suggest that the clinical side effects were due to a loss of pyridoxal phosphate-dependent kynureninase, with a resulting decrease in the synthesis of nicotinyl coenzymes.

B. PROLACTIN AND THYROID STIMULATING HORMONE (TSH)

Prolactin secretion is predominantly under inhibitory control from the hypothalamus. Prolactin-inhibitory factor (PIF), which originates in the hypothalamus, has not been characterized. Its release is either mediated via afferent dopaminergic impulses, or dopamine may actually prove to be PIF. Treatment with L-dopa reduces the plasma prolactin concentration in normal subjects, and patients with nonpuerperal galactorrhea (Kleinberg et al., 1971, 1977), and the injection of dopamine into the third ventricle of the rat increases PIF activity in pituitary stalk portal blood and decreases serum prolactin levels (Kamberi et al., 1970a). But, in addition to its action via the hypothalamus, dopamine also appears to act directly on the pituitary, since it inhibits prolactin secretion in vitro (Koch et al., 1970; MacLeod and Lehmeyer, 1974).

5-HT stimulates the release of prolactin from the adenohypophysial lactotrophs. Kamberi et al. (1971b) showed that when 5-HT was injected into the third ventricle of a rat it stimulated prolactin secretion and inhibited that of FSH. Melatonin, which is related structurally to 5-HT, also caused an increase in plasma prolactin and a decline in plasma FSH.

The experimental data in man have been less satisfactory. MacIndoe and Turkington (1973) reported that the intravenous infusion of 10 gm of L-tryptophan, but not 4 gm, consistently produced elevations of bioassayable plasma prolactin in normal subjects, but Wiebe et al. (1977) observed no effect of the amino acid on radioimmunoassayable prolactin when administered in doses of 90 mg/kg body weight. This discrepancy may have been due to differences in dose and route of administration, or to a greater response in bioassayable, as compared with radioimmunoassayable, hormone. But, a similar conflict holds for 5-hydroxytryptophan, the immediate precursor of 5-HT, which, like the parent amino acid, can cross the blood–brain barrier. Kato et al. (1974) claimed that a 200-mg oral dose increased the plasma prolactin significantly in 18 of 21 normal subjects and that the stimulation could be blocked by the simultaneous infusion of a 5-HT antagonist. In contrast, Handwerger et al. (1975) found no effect of the same dose of 5-hydroxytryptophan compared with a placebo. They suggested that the dose was inadequate to influence brain 5-HT when given by the oral route, and that Kato et al. (1974) inadvertently observed a nonspecific stress effect.

Recently, experiments were conducted that permitted higher concentrations of 5-hydroxytryptophan to be achieved in human brain. Lancranjan et al. (1977) used a soluble ester of 1,5-hydroxytryptophan prepared for intravenous administration, and benserazide, an inhibitor of peripheral decarboxylase activity, to investigate prolactin and growth hormone release in man. Plasma prolactin showed some increase with the enzyme inhibitor alone, and a further elevation after infusion of 1,5-hydroxytryptophan. These studies indicate that with peripheral decarboxylation blocked, 1,5-hydroxytryptophan can cross the blood–brain barrier and be converted to 5-HT in sufficient quantity to influence prolactin release.

The secretion of TSH is regulated mainly by hypothalamic thyrotropin-releasing hormone (TRH). Although TRH also stimulates prolactin release, current evidence suggests that it is not an important regulator of this hormone under physiological conditions (Franz, 1978).

Grimm and Reichlin (1973) proposed that the release of TRH from the hypothalamus is regulated by a dual-opposing monoaminergic system, again with dopamine and 5-HT having antagonistic roles. Doubt was cast on this concept by Chen and Meites (1975); they found no effect of single doses of L-dopa on either basal rat serum TSH levels, or TSH responses to TRH, even though the prolactin levels were suppressed. However, this may have been a question of different degrees of sensitivity for the two hormones. Thus, although L-dopa does not affect the basal TSH concentrations in euthyroid subjects (Eddy et al., 1971), chronic administration of the drug to patients with Parkinson's disease suppresses the response of plasma TSH to TRH stimulation (Spaulding et al., 1972), and so also does the acute infusion of dopamine in normal subjects (Besses et al., 1975). Refetoff et al. (1974) showed that L-dopa suppresses the elevated plasma TSH concentrations in patients with primary hypothyroidism.

In 1973 Foukas reported that oral treatment with 200 mg of pyridoxine hydrochloride, three times a day, was as effective as diethylstilbestrol for the suppression of puerperal lactation. This was a formal double-blind, placebo-controlled trial of 254 patients. Lactation was suppressed within 1 week in 95% of pyridoxine-treated women, 83% of those receiving diethylstilbestrol, and only 17% of the placebo-treated group. The mechanism was presumed to be an increase in hypothalamic dopamine, via stimulation of dopa decarboxylase, and hence, enhanced PIF activity.

Conflicting results were obtained from a later study. MacDonald et al. (1976) also performed a double-blind controlled therapeutic trial. Pyridoxine hydrochloride, in the same dose as that used by Foukas (1973), or a placebo, was administered for 6 days, commencing within 24 hours of delivery. No difference was observed between the two preparations, as judged by the interval from delivery to cessation of lactation and the degree of breast discomfort and engorgement. Plasma prolactin concentrations were not determined in either of these investigations, and the reason for the discrepancy in the results from the two studies is unclear.

Delitala *et al.* (1976) measured plasma prolactin and TSH in four female healthy adults. Pyridoxine hydrochloride, 300 mg, was administered intravenously as a single bolus; all the subjects showed a decline in plasma prolactin that was maintained for the 3-hour sampling period.

These same authors reported that pyridoxine, like L-dopa, suppresses prolactin release in the galactorrhea–amenorrhea syndrome (Delitala *et al.*, 1975). McIntosh (1976) studied three women with hyperprolactinemia and the galactorrhea–amenorrhea syndrome, and observed a return to normal ovulatory cycles within 37 to 94 days of starting treatment with 200–600 mg of pyridoxine hydrochloride daily. In addition, the serum prolactin levels became normal, and the galactorrhea ceased, during pyridoxine administration. When the pyridoxine was discontinued, the serum prolactin levels rose, and there was a reappearance of both the galactorrhea and amenorrhea.

Vitamin B_6 therapy is not uniformly effective in the galactorrhea–amenorrhea syndrome. Tolis *et al.* (1977) found that a single 300-mg intravenous bolus of pyridoxine hydrochloride had no effect on the serum prolactin in 5 hyperprolactinemic patients, and daily oral doses of 400 mg for 2 months had no effect on their disease. They did show a satisfactory response to the ergot derivative bromocryptine. In this same study, four healthy women with regular menstrual cycles were treated first with a single intravenous injection of 300 mg of pyridoxine hydrochloride, and then with 200 mg a day orally for 2 months. Neither mode of administration affected the serum prolactin levels.

Harris *et al.* (1977) studied the effect of pyridoxine on prolactin release in the female rat. A single intraperitoneal injection on the day of proestrus delayed the normal prolactin surge; the LH surge did take place, and the animals ovulated the next day. Pyridoxine also decreased the response of serum prolactin to TRH stimulation in rats treated with α-methylparatyrosine, an inhibitor of dopamine synthesis. This effect is analogous to that of dopamine on the isolated pituitary (MacLeod and Lehmeyer, 1974) and indicates that vitamin B_6 may act, at least in part, by blocking prolactin release from the pituitary lactotrophs.

There is little information on the effect of vitamin B_6 on TRH regulation of plasma TSH levels. Delitala *et al.* (1976) reported that a single 300-mg dose of pyridoxine hydrochloride administered intravenously had no effect on the serum TSH concentrations in eight normal subjects, but that both plasma TSH and prolactin levels were suppressed in patients with primary hypothyroidism (Delitala *et al.*, 1977). This action of pyridoxine duplicates that of L-dopa administration in patients with elevated plasma TSH concentrations due to hypothyroidism. Burrow *et al.* (1977) found that 300 mg of pyridoxine hydrochloride given intravenously to normal subjects 60 min before a TRH stimulation test had no effect on the serum TSH response; this is in keeping with the observation by Delitala *et al.* (1977) that the vitamin did not influence basal serum TSH concentrations in euthyroid subjects.

C. GROWTH HORMONE AND GONADOTROPINS

The secretion of growth hormone (GH) is regulated at the hypothalamic level by both a growth hormone-releasing factor (GH-RF) and a growth hormone-release inhibiting hormone (GH-RIH; somatostatin). The structure of GH-RIH was elucidated by Brazeau *et al.* (1973), who also synthesized the hormone, a tetradecapeptide, and established its biological activity.

GH-RIH suppresses the normal responses in plasma GH levels to various stimuli, including exercise (Prange Hansen *et al.*, 1973), insulin-induced hypoglycemia (Hall *et al.*, 1973), L-dopa and arginine (Siler *et al.*, 1973). The normal suppression of plasma prolactin by L-dopa is unaffected by GH-RIH (Siler *et al.*, 1973). In addition, GH-RIH inhibits the plasma TSH response to TRH, but does not affect the increase in plasma prolactin (Hall *et al.*, 1973). The suppressive effect of GH-RIH on TRH stimulated TSH release and L-dopa stimulated GH release on the one hand, and the lack of suppression of the effects of these factors on prolactin on the other, is consistent with there being a separate receptor site in the pituitary for prolactin regulation.

Although it was generally accepted that a hypothalamic releasing factor existed for the control of GH release, as it does for TSH and the gonadotropins, its demonstration was prevented by the large amounts of GH-RIH present in hypothalamic extracts. Recently, the purification of a GH-RF from porcine hypothalamic tissue was achieved by immunologically neutralizing GH-RIH activity (Redding and Schally, 1977).

The hypothalamic regulation of gonadotropin release appears to be more straightforward. A single decapeptide is responsible for the release of both LH and FSH from the pituitary (Matsuo *et al.*, 1971; Redding *et al.*, 1972). These hypothalamic factors concerned in GH, LH, and FSH regulation are controlled, in turn, by dopaminergic activity originating in the median eminence of the hypothalamus. Thus, direct infusions of catecholamines into the lateral ventricles of the rat stimulate GH release (Müller *et al.*, 1968), and the introduction of dopamine into the third ventricle causes a release of LH and FSH (Kamberi *et al.*, 1970b, 1971a).

In man, GH release is normally stimulated by treatment with L-dopa (Boyd *et al.*, 1970), but it is frequently suppressed in acromegalic patients (Liuzzi *et al.*, 1972; Hoyte and Martin, 1975). Varying reports have been published concerning the effect of L-dopa on gonadotropin levels. Dickey *et al.* (1971) observed elevations in both FSH and LH in women with normal menstrual cycles, anovulatory women, and normal men after an oral dose of 250 mg of L-dopa, while others found only an inconsistent effect (Zarate *et al.*, 1973; Delitala *et al.*, 1974).

Imura *et al.* (1973) reported that the oral administration of 150 mg of 5-hydroxytryptophan to healthy adult males caused a rise in plasma GH in 6 of 8 subjects. Plasma ACTH increased in 6 and plasma cortisol in 7, but it was not stated whether these were the same subjects who showed a GH response. In a similar study, Handwerger *et al.* (1975) found no significant effect of a 200-mg oral dose of 5-hydroxytryptophan on plasma GH compared with a placebo. Both preparations caused a small increase, which was probably due to a nonspecific stress response. Müller *et al.* (1974) also reported that 5-hydroxytryptophan had no consistent effect on plasma GH in 7 female subjects; L-tryptophan, given orally in a dose of 70 mg/kg, produced a slight rise in 21 normal women and 11 normal men.

As in the case of prolactin, these conflicting results were probably due to insufficient concentrations of 5-hydroxytryptophan passing across the blood–brain barrier. Thus, Lancranjan *et al.* (1977) were able to demonstrate a marked increase in plasma GH levels after combined treatment with 1,5-hydroxytryptophan, given intravenously, and benserazide. A nonspecific stress effect was excluded by the lack of response to saline infusion. Pyridoxine administration has been reported to influence both GH and gonadotropin release in man. Delitala *et al.* (1976) observed an increase in plasma GH after the intravenous injection of 300 mg of pyridoxine hydrochloride; there was no change in LH or FSH levels. In keeping with the paradoxical effect of dopamine on plasma GH in acromegaly, the levels of this hormone were suppressed in 5 pyridoxine-treated acromegalics.

In contrast to its own stimulatory effect on GH release, pyridoxine inhibits the action of L-dopa. Mims *et al.* (1975) determined the serum GH response to a 1.0-gm dose of L-dopa in normal subjects. Pyridoxine was then given as a single 100-mg intravenous injection 60 min before repeating the L-dopa test, and by infusion of a further 100 mg over a 1-hour period commencing 30 minutes prior to L-dopa ingestion. The vitamin either blunted, or prevented completely, the GH response to L-dopa. In additional experiments, pyridoxine had no effect on the GH response to insulin-induced hypoglycemia.

The most likely explanation for these findings is that the high concentration of pyridoxal phosphate stimulated dopa decarboxylase activity in the liver, so that it was rapidly converted to dopamine, which, as noted earlier, cannot cross the blood–brain barrier. Less L-dopa would then be available for the intraneural production of dopamine. Similar studies concerning the prolactin response to simultaneous treatment with L-dopa and pyridoxine in hyperprolactinemic and normal subjects would be of interest.

Again, it must be acknowledged that others have failed to observe an effect of pyridoxine on growth hormone release. Tolis *et al.* (1977), in their study of healthy subjects and patients with the galactorrhea–amenorrhea syndrome referred to earlier (Section V, A), assayed GH as well as prolactin. Neither group showed a change in plasma GH in response to pyridoxine administration, although the hyperprolactinemic patients, who were the only ones tested, did have a normal pituitary GH reserve as judged by their response to apomorphine or insulin-induced hypoglycemia.

There are no published data concerning the effect of vitamin B$_6$ deficiency on pituitary function in man. Makris and Gershoff (1973) found that vitamin B$_6$-deficient weanling rats have low pituitary and serum GH levels compared with ad libitum fed controls. However, pair-fed controls had similar GH levels to the deficient animals, suggesting that inanition, rather than the vitamin B$_6$ deficiency, was responsible for the hormonal changes. Failure to control for impaired food intake invalidated earlier studies on the effect of vitamin B$_6$ deficiency on gonadotropins (Hsu, 1963).

D. COMMENT

The experiments described in this section all involved the administration of massive doses of pyridoxine hydrochloride, much of which would have been metabolized to 4-pyridoxic acid and excreted in the urine. In the acute experiments, when the vitamin was given as a single intravenous injection, any stimulation of brain decarboxylase would result solely from activation of preexisting apoenzyme by pyridoxal phosphate. But, when pyridoxine was taken orally over an extended period of time, as in the study of women with the galactorrhea–amenorrhea syndrome performed by McIntosh (1976), cofactor induction of enzyme synthesis (Greengard and Gordon, 1963;

Holten *et al.*, 1967) may have produced an actual increase in the level of apoenzyme protein.

While there is no doubt that the stimulation of aromatic L-amino acid decarboxylase by pyridoxine increases the metabolism of exogenous L-dopa to dopamine, it is less certain that this would result in enhanced dopamine production from the amino acid precursor, tyrosine. In animal tissues the rate-limiting step in catecholamine synthesis is the hydroxylation of tyrosine to yield L-dopa (Udenfriend, 1964), not the decarboxylation reaction. Similarly, 5-HT synthesis in the brain is normally controlled by the availability of L-tryptophan, the concentration of which is well below the K_m of the first enzyme on the biosynthetic pathway, tryptophan hydroxylase (Jéquier *et al.*, 1967). There may be, however, an important species difference in the rate-limiting reaction for catecholamine and 5-HT synthesis. Robins *et al.* (1967) reported that the decarboxylation of 5-hydroxytryptophan, not the hydroxylase reaction, is rate limiting for the synthesis of brain 5-HT in man. This may also hold for dopamine synthesis, since the two amines are formed by a common enzyme.

Because dopamine and 5-HT have opposing actions on the regulation of prolactin, any effect of pyridoxine administration on the plasma prolactin concentration must depend on the relative changes that it produces in synthesis of the two amines. The governing factor here may be the amounts of amino acid substrates present in hypothalamic tissue. Tryptophan is unique among the amino acids in that it circulates largely bound to plasma albumin (McMenamy and Oncley, 1958); the level in the brain, and hence 5-HT synthesis, is determined by the plasma free tryptophan (Tagliamonte *et al.*, 1973). Unlike tryptophan, for which the brain concentration is less than twice the K_m for tryptophan hydroxylase, there is no restriction placed on dopamine synthesis because of a limitation of available tyrosine; brain levels of tyrosine are approximately 22 times higher than the K_m of tyrosine hydroxylase (McGeer *et al.*, 1968). As a consequence of these differences, increasing the activity of aromatic L-amino acid decarboxylase may favor dopamine synthesis and the inhibition of prolactin release.

The conflicting reports concerning the effect of pyridoxine administration on prolactin and GH release could have arisen from differences in the amounts of available tryptophan and tyrosine within the brain. The high K_m for tryptophan indicates that tryptophan hydroxylase may not be fully saturated with substrate under normal conditions. Studies in which the dietary intake of tryptophan and tyrosine are supplemented, with and without the simultaneous administration of pyridoxine hydrochloride, might provide additional useful data.

VI. Summary

Both endogenous and exogenous hormones interact with vitamin B$_6$. There is a considerable body of data concerning the estrogens. These steroids compete with pyridoxal phosphate-dependent apoenzymes for the cofactor *in vitro*, and a similar effect probably occurs *in vivo*. The use of estrogen-containing oral contraceptives is associated with an abnormality of tryptophan metabolism similar to that seen in dietary vitamin B$_6$ deficiency, and corrected by pyridoxine administration. However, plasma pyridoxal phosphate concentrations, and other indices of vitamin B$_6$ nutritional status, are abnormal in only a minority of these patients. Vitamin B$_6$ deficiency occurs also in pregnancy, and it has been proposed as at least one of the factors concerned in the etiology of preeclampsia.

Although there is some indication that both corticosteroids and thyroid hormones increase the requirement for vitamin B$_6$, and modify the activities of pyridoxal phosphate-dependent enzymes, these relationships have received only limited attention in recent years. Current work is, however, revealing some interesting associations between vitamin B$_6$ and the regulation of anterior pituitary hormones. These effects appear to be mediated at the hypothalamic level via the two neurotransmitters 5-hydroxytryptamine and dopamine, both of which are synthesized by vitamin B$_6$-dependent metabolic pathways. A potential clinical application of these observations is in the management of hyperprolactinemia, but there continues to be controversy concerning the efficacy of pyridoxine therapy in this situation.

REFERENCES

Abdel-Tawab, G. A., El-Zoghby, S. M., and Saad, A. A. (1975). *Acta Vitaminol. Enzymol.* **29**, 326.

Adams, P. W., Wynn, V., Rose, D. P., Seed, M., Folkard, J., and Strong, R. (1973). *Lancet* **1**, 897.

Adams, P. W., Wynn, V., Seed, M., and Folkard, J. (1974). *Lancet* **2**, 516.

Adams, P. W., Wynn, V., Folkard, J., and Seed, M. (1976). *Lancet* **1**, 759.

Altman, K., and Greengard, O. (1966). *J. Clin. Invest.* **45**, 1527.

Aly, H. E., Donald, E. A., and Simpson, M. H. W. (1971). *Am. J. Clin. Nutr.* **24**, 297.

Ashcroft, G. W., Crawford, T. B. B., Eccleston, D., Sharman, D. F., MacDougall, E. J., Stanton, J. B., and Binns, J. K. (1966). *Lancet* **2**, 1049.

Bartholini, G., Da Prada, M., and Pletscher, A. J. (1969). *J. Pharm. Pharmacol.* **20**, 228.

Baumann, P., Schmocker, M., Reyero, F., and Heimann, H. (1975). *Acta Vitaminol. Enzymol.* **29**, 255.

Baumblatt, M. J., and Winston, F. (1970). *Lancet* **1**, 832.

Beck, P., and Wells, S. A. (1969). *J. Clin. Endocrinol. Metab.* **29**, 807.

Beischer, N. A., and Lowry, J. (1965). *J. Obstet. Gynaecol. Br. Commonw.* **70**, 685.

Besses, G. S., Burrow, G. N., Spaulding, S. W., and Donabedian, R. K. (1975). *J. Clin. Endocrinol. Metab.* **41**, 985.

Bosch, A. J., and Harper, A. E. (1959). *J. Biol. Chem.* **234**, 929.

Boyd, A. E., III, Lebovitz, H. E., and Pfeiffer, J. B. (1970). *N. Engl. J. Med.* **283**, 1425.

Braidman, I. P., and Rose, D. P. (1971). *Endocrinology* **89**, 1250.

Brazeau, P., Vale, W., Burgus, R., Ling, N., Butcher, M., Rivier, J., and Guillemin, R. (1973). *Science* **179**, 77.

Brin, M. (1971). *Am. J. Clin. Nutr.* **24**, 704.

Broadhurst, A. D. (1970). *Lancet* **1**, 1392.

Brophy, M. H., and Siiteri, P. K. (1975). *Am. J. Obstet. Gynecol.* **121**, 1075.

Brown, R. R., Thornton, M. J., and Price, J. M. (1961). *J. Clin. Invest.* **40**, 617.

Brown, R. R., Yess, N., Price, J. M., Linkswiler, H., Swan, P., and Hankes, L. V. (1965). *J. Nutr.* **87**, 419.

Brown, R. R., Rose, D. P., Leklem, J. E., Linkswiler, H., and Anand, R. (1975). *Am. J. Clin. Nutr.* **28**, 10.

Buchler, D., and Warren, J. C. (1966). *Am. J. Obstet. Gynecol.* **95**, 479.

Bunney, W. E., and Davis, J. M. (1965). *Arch. Gen. Psychiatry* **13**, 483.

Burrow, G. N., May, P. B., Spaulding, S. W., and Donabedian, R. K. (1977). *J. Clin. Endocrinol. Metab.* **45**, 65.

Campbell, N., Dyke, D. A., and Taylor, K. W. (1971). *J. Obstet. Gynaecol. Br. Commonw.* **78**, 498.

Canal, N., and Maffei-Faccioli, A. (1960). *Chem. Abstr.* **54**, 16631.

Carrington, E. R., and McWilliams, N. B. (1966). *Am. J. Obstet. Gynecol.* **96**, 922.

Chen, H. J., and Meites, J. (1975). *Endocrinology* **96**, 10.

Cinnamon, A. D., and Beaton, J. R. (1970). *Am. J. Clin. Nutr.* **23**, 696.

Cleary, R. E., Lumeng, L., and Li, T.-K. (1975). *Am. J. Obstet. Gynecol.* **121**, 25.

Coelingh Bennink, H. J. T., and Schreurs, W. H. P. (1974). *Contraception* **9**, 347.

Coelingh Bennink, H. J. T., and Schreurs, W. H. P. (1975). *Br. Med. J.* **3**, 13.

Coppen, A., Shaw, D. M., Herzberg, B., and Maggs, R. (1967). *Lancet* **2**, 1178.

Coppen, A., Eccleston, E. G., and Peet, M. (1973). *Lancet* **2**, 60.

Cornish, E. J., and Tesoriero, W. (1975). *Br. Med. J.* **3**, 649.

Cozzolino, G., Campriani, S., and Campanelli, C. (1975). *Acta Vitaminol. Enzymol.* **29**, 202.

Curzon, G. (1975). *Acta Vitaminol. Enzymol.* **29**, 69.

Curzon, G., and Bridges, P. K. (1970). *J. Neurol., Neurosurg. Psychiatry* **33**, 698.

Daly, R. J., Kane, F. J., Jr., and Ewing, J. A. (1967). *Lancet* **2**, 444.

Dandrow, R. V., and O'Sullivan, J. B. (1966). *Am. J. Obstet. Gynecol.* **96**, 1144.

D'Angelo, S. A. (1968). *Endocrinology* **82**, 1035.

Delitala, G., Masala, A., Alagna, S., and Rolandi, E. (1974). *Folia Endocrinol.* **27**, 279.

Delitala, G., Masala, A., Alagna, S., and Devilla, L. (1975). *IRCS Libr. Compend.* **3**, 525.

Delitala, G., Masala, A., Alagna, S., and Devilla, L. (1976). *J. Clin. Endocrinol. Metab.* **42**, 603.

Delitala, G., Rovasio, P., and Lotti, G. (1977). *J. Clin. Endocrinol. Metab.* **45**, 1019.

Dempsey, W. B. (1978). *In* "Human Vitamin B_6 Requirements" (H. E. Sauberlich and M. L. Brown, eds.), pp. 202–209. Natl. Acad. Sci., Washington, D.C.

Dennis, K. J., and Jeffery, J. d'A. (1968). *Lancet* **2**, 454.

Dickey, R. P., Marks, B., and Stevens, V. C. (1971). *Program 53rd Annu. Meet., Am. Endocr. Soc. Abstract*, p. 183.

Dietrich, L. S., and Borries, E. (1956). *Arch. Biochem. Biophys.* **64**, 512.

Doberenz, A. R., Van Miller, J. P., Green, J. R., and Beaton, J. R. (1971). *Proc. Soc. Exp. Biol. Med.* **137,** 1100.

Driskell, J A., Geders, J. M., and Urban, M. C. (1976). *J. Lab. Clin. Med.* **87,** 813.

Eddy, R. L., Jones, A. L., Charmakjian, Z. H., and Silverthorne, M C. (1971). *J. Clin. Endocrinol. Metab.* **33,** 709.

Feigelson, P., Feigelson, M., and Greengard, O. (1962). *Recent Prog. Horm. Res.* **18,** 491.

Flux, K., Butcher, L. L., and Engel, J. (1971). *J. Pharm. Pharmacol.* **23,** 420.

Food and Nutrition Board. (1974). "Recommended Dietary Allowances," 8th ed. Nat. Acad. Sci., Washington, D.C.

Foukas, M. D. (1973). *J. Obstet. Gynaecol. Br. Commonw.* **80,** 718.

Franz, A. G. (1978). *N. Engl. J. Med.* **298,** 201.

Gala, R. R., and Westphal, U. (1965). *Endocrinology* **77,** 841.

Gaynor, R., and Dempsey, W. B. (1972). *Clin. Chim. Acta* **37,** 411.

Genazzani, A. R., Lemarchand-Béraud, T., Aubert, M. L., and Felber, J. P. (1975). *J. Clin. Endocrinol. Metab.* **41,** 431.

Gershberg, H., Javier, Z., and Hulse, M. (1964). *Diabetes* **13,** 378.

Gershberg, H., Hulse, M., and Javier, Z. (1968). *Obstet. Gynecol.* **31,** 186.

Gessa, G. L., Biggio, G., and Tagliamonte, A. (1972). *Fed. Proc., Fed. Am. Soc. Exp. Biol.* **31,** 599.

Green, A. R., and Curzon, G. (1968). *Nature (London)* **220,** 1095.

Green, A. R., and Curzon, G. (1970). *Biochem. Pharmacol.* **19,** 2061.

Greengard, O. (1967). *Adv. Enzyme Regul.* **5,** 397–405.

Greengard, O., and Gordon, M. (1963). *J. Biol. Chem.* **238,** 3708.

Greengard, O., Baker, G. T., and Friedell, G. H. (1967). *Enzymol. Biol. Clin.* **8,** 241.

Grimm, Y., and Reichlin, S. (1973). *Endocrinology* **93,** 626.

Grounds, D., Davies, B., and Mowbray, R. (1970). *Br. J. Psychiatry* **116,** 169.

Hall, R., Besser, G. M., Schally, A. V., Coy, D. H., Evered, D., Goldie, D. J., Kastin, A. J., McNeilly, A. S., Mortimer, C. H., Phenekos, C., Tunbridge, W. M. G., and Weightman, D. (1973). *Lancet* **2,** 581.

Hamfelt, A., and Hahn, L. (1969). *Clin. Chim. Acta* **25,** 91.

Handwerger, S., Plonk, J. W., Lebovitz, H. E., Bivens, C. H., and Feldman, J. M. (1975). *Horm. Metab. Res.* **7,** 214.

Harris, A. R., Smith, M. S., Alex, S., Salhanick, H. A., Vagenakis, A. G., and Braverman, L. E. (1977). *Program 59th Annu. Meet., Am. Endocr. Soc.* Abstract, p. 63.

Hayaishi, O., Rothberg, S., Mehler, A. H., and Saito, Y. (1957). *J. Biol. Chem.* **229,** 889.

Hernandez, T. (1964). *Fed. Proc., Fed. Am. Soc. Exp. Biol.* **23,** 136.

Herzberg, B. N., Johnson, A. L., and Brown, S. (1970). *Br. Med. J.* **4,** 142.

Herzberg, B. N., Draper, K. C., Johnson, A. L., and Nicol, G. C. (1971). *Br. Med. J.* **3,** 495.

Herzfeld, A., and Greengard, O. (1971). *Biochim. Biophys. Acta* **237,** 88.

Hillman, R. W., Carbaud, P. G., Nilsson, D. E., Arpin, P. D., and Tufano, R. J. (1963). *Am. J. Clin. Nutr.* **12,** 427.

Holten, D., Wicks, W. D., and Kenney, F. T. (1967). *J. Biol. Chem.* **242,** 1053.

Holtz, P., Stock, K., and Westerman, E. (1956). *Arch. Exp. Pathol. Pharmakol.* **228,** 322.

Hope, D. B. (1955). *Biochem. J.* **59,** 497.

Horvath, A. (1957). *Nature (London)* **179,** 968.

Hoyte, K. M., and Martin, J. B. (1975). *J. Clin. Endocrinol. Metab.* **41,** 656.

Hsu, J. M. (1963). *Vitam. Horm. (N.Y.)* **21,** 113.

Imura, H., Nakai, Y., and Yoshimi, T. (1973). *J. Clin. Endocrinol. Metab.* **36,** 204.

Inman, W. H. W., Vessey, M. P., Westerholm, B., and Engelund, A. (1970). *Br. Med. J.* **2,** 203.

Javier, Z., Gershberg, H., and Hulse, M. (1968). *Metab., Clin. Exp.* **17,** 443.

Jéquier, E., Lovenberg, W., and Sjoerdsma, A. (1967). *Mol. Pharmacol.* **3,** 274.

Kalkhoff, R. K., Schalch, D. S., Walker, J. L., Beck, P., Kipnis, D. M., and Daughaday, W. H. (1964). *Trans. Assoc. Am. Physicians* **77,** 270.

Kalkhoff, R. K., Kim, H. J., and Stoddard, F. J. (1969). *In* "Metabolic Effects of Gonadal Hormones and Contraceptive Steroids" (H. A. Salhanick, D. M. Kipnis, and R. L. Vande Wiele, eds.), pp. 193–203. Plenum, New York.

Kamberi, I. A., Mical, R. S., and Porter, J. C. (1970a). *Experientia* **26,** 1150.

Kamberi, I. A., Mical, R. S., and Porter, J. C. (1970b). *Endocrinology* **87,** 1.

Kamberi, I. A., Mical, R. S., and Porter, J. C. (1971a). *Endocrinology* **88,** 1003.

Kamberi, I. A., Mical, R. S., and Porter, J. C. (1971b). *Endocrinology* **88,** 1288.

Kato, Y., Nakai, Y., Imura, H., Chihara, K., and Ohgo, S. (1974). *J. Clin. Endocrinol. Metab.* **38,** 695.

Keller, N., Richardson, U. I., and Yates, F. E. (1969). *Endocrinology* **84,** 49.

Kleinberg, D. L., Noel, G. L., and Frantz, A. G. (1971). *J. Clin. Endocrinol. Metab.* **33,** 873.

Kleinberg, D. L., Noel, G. L., and Frantz, A. G. (1977). *N. Engl. J. Med.* **296,** 589.

Klieger, J. A., Altshuler, C. H., Krakow, G., and Hollister, C. (1969). *Ann. N.Y. Acad. Sci.* **166,** 288.

Knapp, M. S., Keane, P. M., and Wright, J. G. (1967). *Br. Med. J.* **2,** 27.

Koch, Y., Lu, K. H., and Meites, J. (1970). *Endocrinology* **87,** 673.

Kotake, Y. (1955). *J. Vitaminol.* **1,** 157.

Kotake, Y., Takebayashi, H., Matsumura, Y., Takeda, T., and Sakamoto, S. (1958). *Proc. Jpn. Acad.* **34,** 180.

Kotake, Y., Sotokawa, T., Murakami, E., Hisatake, A., Abe, M., and Ikeda, Y. (1968). *J. Biochem. (Tokyo)* **63,** 578.

Kotake, Y., Ueda, T., Mori, T., Igaki, S., and Hattori, M. (1975). *Acta Vitaminol. Enzymol.* **29,** 236.

Lancranjan, I., Wirz-Justice, A., Puhringer, W., and Del Pozo, E. (1977). *J. Clin. Endocrinol. Metab.* **45,** 588.

Lawrie, R. A. (1953). *Biochem. J.* **55,** 305.

Leklem, J. E., Rose, D. P., and Brown, R. R. (1973). *Metab., Clin. Exp.* **22,** 1499.

Leklem, J. E., Brown, R. R., Rose, D. P., Linkswiler, H., and Arend, R. A. (1975a). *Am. J. Clin. Nutr.* **28,** 146.

Leklem, J. E., Brown, R. R., Rose, D. P., and Linkswiler, H. M. (1975b). *Am. J. Clin. Nutr.* **28,** 535.

Lewis, A., and Hoghughi, M. (1969). *Br. J. Psychiatry* **115,** 697.

Li, T. -K. (1978). *In* "Human Vitamin B₆ Requirements" (H. E. Sauberlich and M. L. Brown, eds.), pp. 210–225. Nat. Acad. Sci., Washington, D.C.

Lin, E. C. C., and Knox, W. E. (1957). *Biochim. Biophys. Acta* **26,** 85.

Liuzzi, A., Chiodini, P. G., Botalla, L., Cremascoli, G., and Silvestrini, F. (1972). *J. Clin. Endocrinol. Metab.* **35,** 941.

Luhby, A. L., Brin, M., Gordon, M., Davis, P., Murphy, M., and Spiegel, H. (1971). *Am. J. Clin. Nutr.* **24,** 684.

Lumeng, L., Cleary, R. E., and Li, T. K. (1974). *Am. J. Clin. Nutr.* **27,** 326.

Lumeng, L., Cleary, R. E., Wagner, R., Yu, P.-L., and Li, T.-K. (1976). *Am. J. Clin. Nutr.* **29,** 1376.

MacDonald, H. N., Collins, Y. D., Tobin, M. J. W., and Wijayaratne, D. N. (1976). *Br. J. Obstet. Gynaecol.* **83,** 54.

McGeer, E. G., Peters, D. A. V., and McGear, P. L. (1968). *Life Sci.* **7,** 605.

MacIndoe, J. H., and Turkington, R. W. (1973). *J. Clin. Invest.* **52,** 1972.

MacLeod, R. M., and Lehmeyer, J. E. (1974). *Endocrinology* **94,** 1077.

McIntosh, E. N. (1976). *J. Clin. Endocrinol. Metab.* **42,** 1192.

McMenamy, R. H., and Oncley, J. L. (1958). *J. Biol. Chem.* **233,** 1436.

Mainardi, L. (1947). *Acta Vitaminol.* **3,** 110.

Mainardi, L., and Tenconi, L. T. (1964). *Acta Vitaminol.* **18,** 249.

Makris, A., and Gershoff, S. N. (1973). *Horm. Metab. Res.* **5,** 457.

Mann, J. I., and Inman, W. H. W. (1975). *Br. Med. J.* **2,** 245.

Mascitelli-Coriandoli, E., and Boldrini, R. (1959). *Experientia* **15,** 229.

Mason, M., and Gullekson, E. H. (1960a). *J. Biol. Chem.* **235,** 1312.

Mason, M., and Gullekson, E. H. (1960b). *Fed. Proc., Fed. Am. Soc. Exp. Biol.* **19,** 170.

Mason, M., and Schirch, L. (1961). *Fed. Proc., Fed. Am. Soc. Exp. Biol.* **20,** 200.

Mason, M., Ford, J., and Wu, H. L. C. (1969). *Ann. N.Y. Acad. Sci.* **166,** 170.

Matsuo, H., Baba, Y., Nair, R. M. G., Arimura, A., and Schally, A. V. (1971). *Biochem. Biophys. Res. Commun.* **43,** 1334.

Michael, A. F., Drummond, K. N., Doeden, D., Anderson, J. A., and Good, R. A. (1964). *J. Clin. Invest.* **43,** 1730.

Miller, L. T., Benson, E. M., Edwards, M. A., and Young, J. (1974). *Am. J. Clin. Nutr.* **27,** 797.

Miller, L. T., Johnson, A., Benson, E. M., and Woodring, M. J. (1975). *Am. J. Clin. Nutr.* **28,** 846.

Mims, R. B., Scott, C. L., Modebe, O., and Bethune, J. E. (1975). *J. Clin. Endocrinol. Metab.* **40,** 256.

Müller, E. E., Pra, P. D., and Pecile, A. (1968). *Endocrinology* **83,** 893.

Müller, E. E., Brambilla, F., Cavagnini, F., Peracchi, M., and Panerai, A. (1974). *J. Clin Endocrinol. Metab.* **39,** 1.

Nilsson, Å., Jacobson, L., and Ingemanson, C.-A. (1968). *Acta Psychiatr. Scand.* **44,** Suppl. 203, 259.

Nisticò, G., and Preziosi, P. (1970). *Lancet* **2,** 213.

Ogasawara, N., Hagino, Y., and Kotake, Y. (1962). *J. Biochem. (Tokyo)* **52,** 162.

Okamoto, H., Okada, F., and Hayaishi, O. (1971). *J. Biol. Chem.* **24,** 7759.

Papavasiliou, P. S., Cotzias, G. C., Duby, S. E., Steck, J., Fehling, C., and Bell, M. A. (1972). *N. Engl. J. Med.* **288,** 8.

Park, Y. K., and Linkswiler, H. (1970). *J. Nutr.* **100,** 110.

Persson, T., and Roos, B. E. (1967). *Lancet* **2,** 987.

Pinto, P. V. C., and Rosenthal, H. L. (1965). *Experientia* **21,** 511.

Pitot, H. C., and Peraino, C. (1964). *J. Biol. Chem.* **239,** 1783.

Potera, C., Rose, D. P., and Brown, R. R. (1977). *Am. J. Clin. Nutr.* **30,** 1677.

Prange Hansen, Aa., Ørskov, H., Seyer-Hansen, K., and Lundbaek, K. (1973). *Br. Med. J.* **3,** 523.

Prasad, A. S., Lei, K. Y., Moghissi, K. S., Stryker, J. C., and Oberleas, D. (1976). *Am. J. Obstet. Gynecol.* **125,** 1063.

Price, J. M., Thornton, M. J., and Mueller, L. M. (1967). *Am. J. Clin. Nutr.* **20,** 452.

Price, S. A., Rose, D. P., and Toseland, P. A. (1972). *Am. J. Clin. Nutr.* **25,** 494.

Raica, N., and Sauberlich, H. E. (1964). *Am. J. Clin. Nutr.* **15,** 67.

Ramsay, I. D. (1966). *Lancet* **2,** 931.

Redding, T. W., and Schally, A. V. (1977). *Program 59th Annu. Meet., Am. Endocr. Soc.* Abstract, p. 231.

Redding, T. W., Schally, A. V., Arimura, A., and Matsuo, H. (1972). *Endocrinology* **90,** 764.

98 DAVID P. ROSE

Refetoff, S., Fang, V. S., Rapoport, B., and Friesen, H. G. (1974). *J. Clin. Endocrinol. Metab.* **38,** 450.
Rivlin, R. S., and Melmon, K. L. (1965). *J. Clin. Invest.* **44,** 1960.
Robins, E., Robins, J. M., Croninger, A. B., Moses, S. G., Spencer, S. J., and Hudgens, R. W. (1967). *Biochem. Med.* **1,** 240.
Rose, D. P. (1966a). *Nature (London)* **210,** 196.
Rose, D. P. (1966b). *Clin. Sci.* **31,** 265.
Rose, D. P. (1967a). *Clin. Chim. Acta* **18,** 221.
Rose, D. P. (1967b). *Lancet* **1,** 239.
Rose, D. P. (1978). *In* "Human Vitamin B₆ Requirements" (H. E. Sauberlich and M. L. Brown, eds.), pp. 193–201. Nat. Acad. Sci., Washington, D.C.
Rose, D. P., and Adams, P. W. (1972). *J. Clin. Pathol.* **25,** 252.
Rose, D. P., and Braidman, I. P. (1970). *Lancet* **1,** 1117.
Rose, D. P., and Braidman, I. P. (1971). *Am. J. Clin. Nutr.* **24,** 673.
Rose, D. P., and Brown, R. R. (1969). *Biochim. Biophys. Acta* **184,** 412.
Rose, D. P., and Cramp, D. G. (1970). *Clin. Chim. Acta* **29,** 49.
Rose, D. P., and McGinty, F. (1968). *Clin. Sci.* **35,** 1.
Rose, D. P., and Toseland, P. A. (1973). *Metab., Clin. Exp.* **22,** 165.
Rose, D. P., Brown, R. R., and Price, J. M. (1968). *Nature (London)* **219,** 1259.
Rose, D. P., Strong, R., Adams, P. W., and Harding, P. E. (1972). *Clin. Sci.* **42,** 465.
Rose, D. P., Adams, P. W., and Strong, R. (1973a). *J. Obstet. Gynaecol. Br. Commonw.* **80,** 82.
Rose, D. P., Strong, R., Folkard, J., and Adams, P. W. (1973b). *Am. J. Clin. Nutr.* **26,** 48.
Rose, D. P., Leklem, J. E., Brown, R. R., and Potera, C. (1976). *Am. J. Clin. Nutr.* **29,** 956.
Rose, D. P., Leklem, J. E., Fardal, L., Baron, R. B., and Shrago, E. (1977). *Am. J. Clin. Nutr.* **30,** 691.
Rosen, F., Roberts, N. R., Budnick, L. E., and Nichol, C. A. (1959). *Endocrinology* **65,** 256.
Rosen, F., Harding, H. R., Milholland, R. J., and Nichol, C. A. (1963). *J. Biol. Chem.* **238,** 5725.
Rosenbaum, E. E., Portis, S., and Soskin, S. (1942). *J. Lab. Clin. Med.* **27,** 763.
Salkeld, R. M., Knörr, K., and Körner, W. F. (1973). *Clin. Chim. Acta* **49,** 195.
Sandberg, A. A., Slaunwhite, W. R., Jr., and Carter, A. C. (1960). *J. Clin. Invest.* **39,** 1914.
Sandberg, A. A., Kirdani, R. Y., Back, N., Weyman, P., and Slaunwhite, W. R., Jr. (1967). *Am. J. Physiol.* **213,** 1138.
Satoyashi, E., Murakami, K., Kowa, H., Kinoshita, M., Noguchi, K., Hoshina, S., Nishiyama, Y., and Ito, K. (1963). *Neurology* **13,** 645.
Schanberg, S. M. (1963). *J. Pharmacol. Exp. Ther.* **139,** 191.
Segal, H. L., and Kim, Y. S. (1963). *Proc. Natl. Acad. Sci. U.S.A.* **50,** 912.
Shane, B., and Contractor, S. F. (1975). *Am. J. Clin. Nutr.* **28,** 739.
Shaw, D. M., Camps, F. E., and Eccleston, E. G. (1967). *Br. J. Psychiatry* **113,** 1407.
Siler, T. M., VandenBerg, G., and Yen, S. S. C. (1973). *J. Clin. Endocrinol. Metab.* **37,** 632.
Soskin, S., and Levine, R. (1944). *Arch. Intern. Med.* **74,** 375.
Spaulding, S. W., Burrow, G. N., Donabedian, R., and Van Woert, M. (1972). *J. Clin. Endocrinol. Metab.* **35,** 182.
Spellacy, W. N. (1969). *Am. J. Obstet. Gynecol.* **104,** 448.
Spellacy, W. N., Carlson, K. L., Birk, S. A., and Schade, S. L. (1968). *Metab., Clin. Exp.* **17,** 496.
Spellacy, W. N., Buhi, W. C., and Birk, S. A. (1972). *Contraception* **6,** 265.

Sprince, H., Lowy, R. S., Folsome, C. E., and Behrman, J. S. (1951). *Am. J. Obstet. Gynecol.* **62**, 84.

Stokes, T., and Wynn, V. (1971). *Lancet* **2**, 677.

Tagliamonte, A., Biggio, G., Vargiu, L., and Gessa, G. L. (1973). *J. Neurochem.* **20**, 909.

Tolis, G., Laliberté, R., Guyda, H., and Naftolin, F. (1977). *J. Clin. Endocrinol. Metab.* **44**, 1197.

Toseland, P. A., and Price, S. (1969). *Br. Med. J.* **1**, 777.

Udenfriend, S. (1964). *Vitam. Horm. (N.Y.)* **22**, 445.

Ueda, T. (1967). *Nagoya J. Med. Sci.* **30**, 259.

Veneziale, C. M., Walter, P., Kneer, N., and Lardy, H. A. (1967). *Biochemistry* **6**, 2129.

Wachstein, M., and Graffeo, L. W. (1956). *Obstet. Gynecol.* **8**, 177.

Wachstein, M., and Gudaitis, A. (1953). *Am. J. Obstet. Gynecol.* **66**, 1207.

Wachstein, M., and Lobel, S. (1956). *Am. J. Clin. Pathol.* **26**, 910.

Wachstein, M., Kellner, J. D., and Ortiz, J. M. (1960). *Proc. Soc. Exp. Biol. Med.* **103**, 350.

Wiebe, R. H., Handwerger, S., and Hammond, C. B. (1977). *J. Clin. Endocrinol. Metab.* **45**, 1310.

Wiss, O., and Weber, F. (1964). *Vita. Horm. (N.Y.)* **22**, 495.

Wohl, M. G., Levy, H. A., Szutka, A., and Maldia, G. (1960). *Proc. Soc. Exp. Biol. Med.* **105**, 523.

Wynn, V., and Doar, J. W. H. (1966). *Lancet* **2**, 715.

Wynn, V., and Doar, J. W. H. (1969). *Lancet* **2**, 761.

Wynn, V., and Doar, J. W. H. (1970). *J. Clin. Pathol.* **23**, Suppl. 3, 19.

Wynn, V., Doar, J. W. H., Mills, G. L., and Stokes, T. (1969). *Lancet* **2**, 756.

Zarate, A., Canales, E. S., Soria, J., Maneiro, P. J., and MacGregor, C. (1973). *Neuroendocrinology* **12**, 362.

Zumoff, B., Fukushima, D. K., Weitzman, E. D., Kream, J., and Hellman, L. (1974). *J. Clin. Endocrinol. Metab.* **39**, 805.

Hormonal Factors in Lipogenesis in Mammary Gland

R. J. MAYER

Department of Biochemistry, Queen's Medical Centre, University of Nottingham, Nottingham, England

I. INTRODUCTION

A. BACKGROUND

Mammary gland development results in the production of a lactating tissue that has the capacity for enormous rates of milk production. Milk contains protein, carbohydrate, and fat, which are produced at the highest rates in lactating tissue. The high biosynthetic capacities are a consequence of the differentiation of the mammary lobuloalveolar cells. It is becoming increasingly clear that cell differentiation is hormonally controlled and that the differentiated state of a given cell type can be hormonally maintained (Rutter *et al.*, 1973).

Cell differentiation has been defined as the progressive restriction of developmental potential (Rutter *et al.*, 1973), which in the stages of

101

terminal differentiation is associated with the acquisition of cell-specific enzymes or proteins that produce the morphological and physiological characteristics of the phenotypically differentiated cell. Several studies on the hormonal regulation of the acquisition of lipogenic enzymology in differentiating cells have recently been reviewed (Mayer and Paskin, 1978).

The hormonally regulated differentiation of lobuloalveolar cells in mammary gland involves the acquisition of three biosynthetic capacities: for protein, carbohydrate, and fat. Many of the cell-specific enzymes that accumulate in the differentiating cells participate in the biosynthesis of fat. Therefore the study of the enzymes involved in fat biosynthesis in developing mammary gland provides an excellent opportunity to try to elucidate the mechanisms by which hormones regulate selective gene expression in differentiating cells. Furthermore, postsynthetic regulation of enzyme amounts in differentiating and differentiated cells (by modulation of rates of protein degradation) can be easily studied in mammary gland.

B. Definitions of Terms

The term lipogenesis will be restricted to mean the process of fatty acid biosynthesis from malonyl-CoA and the provision of substrates for the process by the various "satellite" enzyme systems (Gumaa *et al.*, 1973; Brindley, 1978). Lipogenesis is therefore distinct from glycerolipid or phospholipid synthesis with respect to physiological regulation and pathological disturbance (Brindley, 1978).

Hormone actions at the cellular level can be divided into those that are rapidly mediated (acute responses) and those that are slowly mediated (chronic responses). Several acute hormone responses, such as the regulation of glycogen metabolism or lipolysis, have been delineated in detail. These responses to hormones are very rapid and are associated with changes in cellular concentration of cyclic AMP (cAMP) (Butcher, 1970; Hers, 1976). The chronic hormonal regulation of cell metabolism occurs over periods of hours to weeks, and usually involves selective changes in gene expression resulting in the accumulation of enzymes or proteins necessary for some differentiated function (Chan and O'Malley, 1976). Cells may often show a pleiotypic response to acute or chronic hormonal stimulation. Coordinated changes in a variety of cell functions may occur on hormonal stimulation and may result in the required change in cell growth, differentiation, or function (Hersko *et al.*, 1971).

C. Objectives

There have been several excellent reviews on the hormonal regulation of mammary gland development (Anderson, 1974; Tucker, 1974; Mepham, 1976) and on various aspects of lipid metabolism in developing and lactating mammary gland (Bauman and Davis, 1974; Smith and Abraham, 1975; Paton and Jensen, 1975; Dils, 1977). It is therefore not necessary in this review to collate in detail published reports on hormonal synergisms or antagonisms in gland development, or to draw attention to reports on the existence of various lipogenic enzymes in mammary gland.

However, it is necessary to analyze data on the lipogenic response and changes in lipogenic enzyme profiles during mammary gland development and lactation in terms of the putative mechanisms of hormone action. The hormonally regulated changes in the activities of lipogenic enzymes in developing mammary gland will be compared with changes in the activities of nonlipogenic enzymes, with respect to the concept of cell-specific and non-cell-specific enzymes or proteins in differentiating cells (Holtzer and Abbot, 1968; Ephrussi, 1972; Paskin and Mayer, 1977). Where possible, particular attention will be given to the mechanisms of hormonally regulated changes in lipogenic enzyme concentrations. The role of both enzyme synthesis and enzyme degradation in determining the accumulation profiles of lipogenic enzymes in mammary gland will be analyzed. The acute hormonal regulation of the provision of substrates for lipogenesis in lactating mammary gland will be reviewed (Goheer and Coore, 1977; Robinson and Williamson, 1977a,b). Changes in lipogenic enzyme profiles during mammary gland growth and differentiation will be related to the concept of coordinated changes in enzyme concentrations in developing cells, which may be regulated intracellularly by concentrations of cyclic nucleotides (Sapag-Hagar et al., 1974; Sapag-Hagar and Greenbaum, 1974a,b). Finally, the data on lipogenic rates and lipogenic enzymes in mammary tumors will be collated. The hormonal response of lipogenic enzymes in mammary tumors will be analyzed, and an attempt will be made to rationalize changes in lipogenesis and lipogenic enzyme profiles in terms of the theory of transformation-linked or progression-linked determinants of tumor development (Weber, 1977).

D. Phases of Mammary Gland Development

The developmental changes in lipogenesis in mammary gland vary with the stages of mammary growth and differentiation. The hormonal regulation of the phases of mammary development is complex, but is generally considered in terms of synergism and antagonism between the various hormones (Tucker, 1974).

Several authorities have used different terms to define the different phases of mammary development (Tucker, 1974; Anderson, 1974; Smith and Abraham, 1975; Mepham, 1976). The control of mammogenesis (development of the atrophic gland by means of ductal growth up to and after puberty), lactogenesis (development of the capacity to produce milk in association with pronounced lobuloalveolar growth and cytodifferentiation of the lobuloalveolar cells), and lactation (copious milk production, which is maintained by galactopoietic hormones) are thought to be closely related hormonal processes (Tucker, 1974). The hormonal regulators of each phase of development are not clearly defined (Cowie and Tindall, 1971), and there are obviously species differences superimposed on any general considerations. In the rat it has been noted that the principal difference between mammogenic and lactogenic hormones may be the absence of ovarian steroids from the latter group (Mepham, 1976). It has been suggested that there is a synergism with estrogens and progesterone of virtually all the adenohypophysial hormones to stimulate optimal mammary growth (Turner, 1970). In general, progesterone is considered to have an antilactogenic action in that it blocks the biosynthesis of α-lactalbumin (Turkington and Hill, 1969), lactose (Kuhn, 1969), and casein (Houdebine and Gaye, 1975). Prolactin receptors are present on or near the alveolar secretory cell membrane in rabbit mammary gland (Birkinshaw and Falconer, 1972). Circulating prolactin concentration remains low through pregnancy and increases at parturition: the highest levels are reached on day 5 of lactation (Durand and Djiane, 1977). The onset of milk secretion is also paralleled by a large increase (greater than 5-fold) in the number of prolactin receptors (Djiane et al., 1977). It has been suggested that lactogenesis during pregnancy may be triggered by either an increase in the concentration of placental lactogen or, in a species where this hormone is absent, by an early decrease in progesterone concentration (Durand and Djiane, 1977).

Species differences are very apparent in the hormone combinations that can maintain lactation, and they vary from the combination of prolactin, growth hormone, glucocorticoids, and triiodothyronine in the goat to prolactin alone in the rabbit (Cowie, 1969; Cowie et al., 1969). Anderson (1974) considers that the measurement of a continual increase in DNA in mammary gland during pregnancy and early lactation had a profound effect on the concept of mammary development.

Species variation in the extent of mammary lobuloalveolar cell proliferation before and after parturition is considerable (Anderson, 1974) and will be of great importance in determining the relative differences in total biosynthetic capacities of mammary glands (Baldwin and Yang, 1974). It is against this considerable species variation in the nature of the hormonal stimuli and the temporal axis of development that biosynthetic flux profiles, including lipogenic enzyme accumulation profiles, must be considered.

II. Lipogenesis in Developing Mammary Gland *in Vivo*

A. Metabolic Changes Related to Lipogenesis

The metabolic adaptations in the developing mammary gland are predominantly related to the biosynthesis of lactose, fat, and protein. Many of the enzymological adaptations are related to the use of substrates for lipogenesis and the provision of reducing equivalents for the process. The sources of substrates for lipogenesis are obviously related to the nutritional environment of the particular species, whether ruminant or nonruminant. In the ruminant, acetate is a predominant precursor for lipogenesis whereas in nonruminants the major precursor of fatty acids is glucose. Similarly, the source of reducing equivalents for fatty acid biosynthesis is different in ruminants and nonruminants, as might be expected when different carbon sources are available for oxidation to provide NADPH. The enzymes responsible for catalysis of reactions in fatty acid synthesis and the provision of reducing equivalents have been identified and developmental profiles measured for many of them (Bauman and Davis, 1974; Baldwin and Yang, 1974; Smith and Abraham, 1975).

Particular attention has been given to differences in the methods of production of NADPH for lipogenesis in mammary gland of ruminants and nonruminants. Two essentially similar schemes have been proposed for the generation of NADPH (Bauman *et al.*, 1970; Gumaa *et al.*, 1973; Bauman and Davis, 1974). The schemes have been developed from interpretations of measurements of the fate of radiolabeled precursors in lipogenesis and especially from measurements of the activities of enzymes that may be involved in NADPH production during lactogenesis and in lactation.

In the ruminant (Fig. 1A) cytosolic isocitrate dehydrogenase is allocated a key role in NADPH biosynthesis (Bauman *et al.*, 1970; Gumaa *et al.*, 1973), although the pentose phosphate pathway will also play an

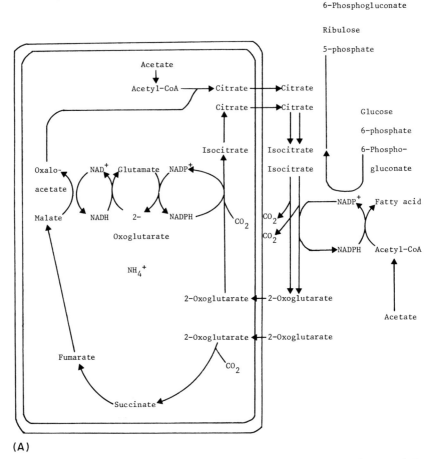

(A)

Fig. 1. Proposed scheme for the generation of reducing equivalents for lipogenesis in (A) sheep and (B) rat mammary gland. The area enclosed in the double border represents the mitochondrial compartment. ——, Major pathways; - - -, minor pathways. Scheme is presented from Gumaa et al. (1973) with permission of authors and publishers.

important role here. The quantitative significance of the pentose phosphate pathway will depend on glucose availability in the ruminant mammary gland. Gumaa et al. (1973) have pointed out that in a tissue such as ruminant mammary gland, which is adapted to conserve glucose, the pentose phosphate pathway is almost an optimal system in relation to lipogenesis.

In the nonruminant (Fig. 1B) the pentose phosphate pathway and the malate transhydrogenation cycle are seen as the potential pro-

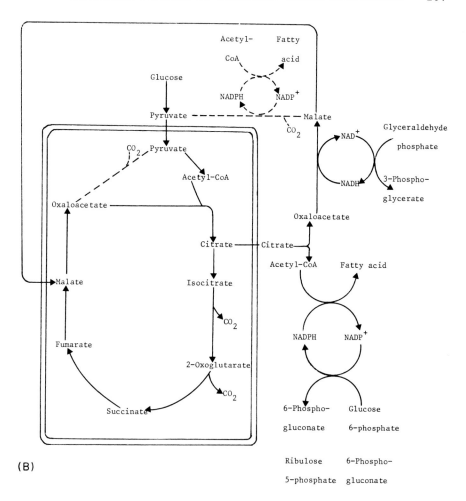

(B)

ducers of NADPH (Bauman and Davis, 1974). It has been postulated that in lactating-rat mammary gland the pentose phosphate pathway is the predominant system. The malate transhydrogenation system plays a lesser role than in adipose tissue, and cytosolic isocitrate dehydrogenase is much less important than in ruminants (Gumaa et al., 1973).

B. Developmental Changes in Lipogenic Flux

Changes in lipogenic flux are associated with lactogenic or lactational hormonal stimuli. Extremely low rates of lipogenesis can be measured in preparations of mammary gland taken before pregnancy or in the early stages of pregnancy. Detailed measurements of the change in lipogenic flux during rabbit mammary gland development have been made by Strong and Dils (1972) and are shown in Fig. 2. The results show a biphasic increase in lipogenic rate with an initial lipogenic stimulus in midpregnancy (16–18 days) and a second lipogenic stimulus occurring just before parturition. Significantly, in midpregnancy there is a coincident abrupt increase in the percentage of medium-chain fatty acids ($C_8 + C_{10}$, characteristic of rabbit milk) which are synthesized by the gland. The biphasic increase in lipogenic

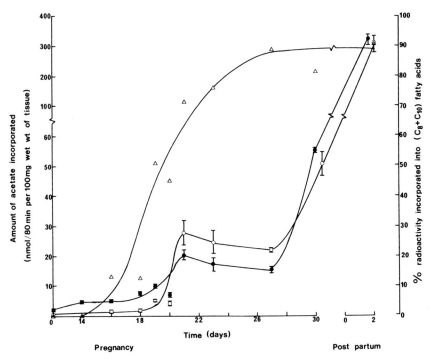

FIG. 2. [^{14}C]Acetate incorporation into lipids ($\triangle$) by mammary explants from rabbits at different stages of pregnancy and at early lactation. Incubations (80 minutes) contained 0.1 mM sodium [1-^{14}C]acetate (1–2 μCi) plus 1.0 mM glucose ($\bullet$). Results from incubations with 1.0 mM sodium [1-^{14}C]acetate (1–2 μCi) plus 10 mM glucose ($\bigcirc$) have been divided by ten. Duplicate incubations were used, and the mean ± half the difference between the two values is given. The percentage radioactivity incorporated into ($C_8 + C_{10}$) fatty acids was measured after incubation (80 minutes) in 1.0 mM sodium [1-^{14}C]acetate (1–2 μCi) plus 10 mM glucose. The combined lipid extract from duplicate incubations was analyzed. Results are presented from Strong and Dils (1972) with permission of authors and publishers.

flux in rabbit mammary gland has also been measured by Mellenberger and Bauman (1974), who found, in contrast to Strong and Dils
(1972), that the second lipogenic stimulus occurred postpartum. The
accumulation profiles for the lipogenic enzymes which have been measured in rabbit mammary gland show a similar biphasic appearance.
Thus acetyl-CoA carboxylase and ATP-citrate lyase (Mellenberger and
Bauman, 1974) and glucose-6-phosphate dehydrogenase, 6-phospho-
gluconate dehydrogenase, and fatty acid synthetase show similar accumulation profiles (B. K. Speake, R. Dils, and R. J. Mayer, unpublished observations).

Comparisons with other species are restricted since the detailed enzymic measurements required are sometimes difficult to obtain, e.g.,
with biopsy samples. However, it is interesting that only low activities
of acetyl-CoA carboxylase (Mackall and Lane, 1977) and isoenzyme 1
of glucose-6-phosphate dehydrogenase (Richards and Hilf, 1972b) could
be measured in rat mammary gland at the end of pregnancy. These
results may indicate species differences in the onset and temporal
development of lipogenesis since mammary tissues from rabbit, cow,
and mouse have the capacity to synthesize milk components several
days prepartum (Strong and Dils, 1972; Mellenberger et al., 1973; Denamur, 1969b; Jones, 1972); in rat mammary tissue the ability to synthesize milk components occurs 12–24 hours before parturition (Kuhn,
1969). The changes in the pattern of chain length of fatty acids synthesized in the developing gland is discussed in Section II, E. As previously
mentioned, progesterone may act in the rat as a repressor of milk
biosynthesis (Kuhn, 1969). Several investigations have been reviewed
(Denamur, 1971), and it has been suggested that in the rabbit the
depressed plasma progesterone on day 21 of pregnancy, combined with
a rise in the concentration of free glucocorticoids, may coincide with the
first lipogenic stimulus in the mammary gland. From studies with
explants of mammary gland from "pseudopregnant" rabbits it is apparent that prolactin and insulin are also required for the first
lipogenic stimulus in rabbit mammary gland (Strong et al., 1972).

A biphasic accumulation of milk proteins has been observed in the
mammary gland (Stockdale and Topper, 1966; Turkington et al., 1968;
Vonderhaar et al., 1973) and the biosynthetic processes in mammary
gland may therefore form part of a two-phase lactogenic program.
Biphasic accumulation of certain enzymes and proteins has been
noticed in several developing systems, including pancreas (Rutter et
al., 1968a) and thyroid (Shain et al., 1972). Based on the simple
biphasic pattern of accumulation of exocrine proteins and insulin in
the developing pancreas, Rutter and colleagues (1968a,b) proposed a

model in which a single programmatic change (the primary transition) leads to the "protodifferentiated" state of a cell, with a low rate of synthesis of cell-specific protein(s), and a secondary transition causes a much higher rate of synthesis of cell-specific protein(s). Whether this type of model is applicable to the events during lactogenesis in mammary gland is open to conjecture and must await much more detailed analyses of the transcriptional, translational, and posttranslational events involved in the accumulation of intracellular and secretory mammary enzymes and proteins.

The data presently available on changes in the rate of fatty acid biosynthesis during lactogenesis in rabbit and bovine mammary glands show a very good correlation with the accumulation profiles of some lipogenic enzymes (Mellenberger et al., 1973; Mellenberger and Bauman, 1974). This type of analysis shows the importance of understanding the mechanism and regulation of enzyme accumulation in developing cells (Paskin and Mayer, 1977; Mayer and Paskin, 1978).

C. Models for Enzymic Changes in Developing Mammary Gland

In the preceding section, the changes in lipogenic flux in lactogenesis and lactation have been described together with the concomitant changes in the activities of some lipogenic enzymes. Attempts have been made to account for the accumulation profiles of lipogenic and other enzymes in terms of models that describe the general characteristics of changes in enzyme activities in differentiating lobuloalveolar cells during lactogenesis and lactation. This approach is fundamental to understanding the hormonal regulation of mammary differentiation, since it allows putative enzyme subgroups to be identified in differentiating cells.

Groups of enzymes could be identified that might be expected to have different turnover (synthesis and degradation) characteristics in response to hormonal stimulation of the tissue. Such an approach may identify the products of selective gene expression and should help to explain how specific genes or groups of genes may be activated during hormonal stimulation of differentiation. Furthermore, identification of such subgroups may define proteins with different susceptibilities to degradation during their accumulation in developing mammary epithelial cells. This may help to elucidate the mechanism and regulation of enzyme degradation in differentiating cells (Paskin and Mayer, 1977; Mayer and Paskin, 1978). Two attempts have been made to analyze changes in enzyme activities in developing mammary gland.

Baldwin and Yang (1974) have presented a model in which enzymes are placed into three groups depending on the nature of the changes in their activities during secretory cell development: (1) constitutive enzymes whose activities are not hormone dependent, or are hormone dependent in only the most general way, requiring only a hormonal environment consistent with cell survival for their synthesis; (2) enzymes whose synthesis or amounts are in part constitutive and in part hormone dependent; (3) enzymes whose synthesis is almost entirely subject to specific hormonal regulation. Although there are not enough data for clear definitions of these enzyme groups, there is sufficient information to distinguish between them. Baldwin and Yang (1974) noted that the general increases in enzyme activities in the rat mammary gland are complete by day 3 to 5 of lactation, and in other species either by late pregnancy or early lactation. Constitutive enzymes (controlling general metabolic activities, e.g., aspartate aminotransferase) do not change their activities significantly after this time (on a DNA basis). By contrast, the activities of enzymes involved in milk biosynthesis continue to increase to reach maxima (on a DNA basis) at peak lactation (e.g., glucose-6-phosphate dehydrogenase and UDP-glucose pyrophosphorylase). The synthesis of enzymes involved in milk synthesis is considered to be under partial or complete hormone control (Baldwin and Yang, 1974). These authors also draw attention to the dramatic decline in enzyme activities on weaning, which may be related to milk accumulation, cell damage, or ischemia (McLean, 1964; Levy, 1964); however, dramatic decreases in enzyme activities occur on hormone removal from mammary explants *in vitro* (Section III, E).

The concept of the existence of constant and specific proportions in groups of enzymes (Pette *et al.*, 1962a,b) has been used to analyze changes in enzyme activities in developing mammary gland (McLean *et al.*, 1972; Gumaa *et al.*, 1973). This concept was developed to identify enzymes of special importance in the metabolism of different tissues (Pette *et al.*, 1962a,b) and was extended by McLean *et al.* (1972) to investigate the changes in enzyme activities in mammary gland as the tissue progresses through late pregnancy into lactation. The activities of many enzymes in the mammary gland were measured and expressed relative to that of the rate-limiting enzyme in glycolysis, phosphofructokinase. The relative activities show a distinct pattern, the enzymes falling into three groups that appear to be functionally related. All the enzymes measured responded in lactogenesis by increases in activity, but the activities changed in different ways. The groups of enzymes are: (1) the enzymes of glycolysis and the majority of the pentose phosphate pathway, which behave as a constant proportion group and relative to phosphofructokinase do not change their correspondence during lactogenesis and lactation; (2) enzymes of the tricarboxylic acid cycle, which, relative to phosphofructokinase, decline in activities during the initiation and progression of lactation; (3) enzymes related to fatty acid synthesis, which show a pattern opposite to that of the second group— i.e., they increase in activities more rapidly than phosphofructokinase. In the rat the enzymes of this third group are citrate synthetase, citrate cleavage enzyme, acetyl-CoA carboxylase, fatty acid synthetase, and glucose-6-phosphate dehydrogenase. Analysis of the work of Baldwin and Milligan (1966) shows that lactose-synthesizing enzymes fall into the third group, increasing in activities faster than those of the glycolytic sequence.

This type of analysis shows that whereas certain enzymes behave as a group and change their activities with remarkable consistency (constant-proportion enzymes) other groups of enzymes may change activities independently. Gumaa et al. (1973) have used this type of analysis to identify enzymes involved in the provision of NADPH for fatty acid biosynthesis by the consistent patterns of change in activities in mammary gland development. Their approach is an extension of, and alternative to, that proposed by Baldwin and Yang (1974). The treatment of enzyme activity data by the procedure of McLean et al. (1972) identifies enzyme groups that might be expected to be independent, partially dependent, or totally dependent on hormonal stimulation of the tissue by their relative changes in activities in lactogenesis and lactation.

Such enzyme activity profiles are of even greater value if it can be shown that the changes in activities are due to changes in enzyme amounts. This can be conveniently established by immunochemical methods (Walker and Mayer, 1978). If it is shown that enzyme-activity profiles are enzyme-amount profiles (Section III, E), then these analyses are extremely valuable in defining enzyme groups that might be expected to have different hormonally regulated changes in their turnover (synthesis and degradation) during mammary gland differentiation.

An alternative and general model in which intracellular proteins are divided into non-cell-specific ("household") proteins, which are ubiquitous in a multicellular organism, and cell-specific ("luxury") proteins, which are produced in specific cell types, has been proposed by Holtzer and Abbot (1968) and Ephrussi (1972). Changes in the turnover characteristics of proteins in the two groups might be expected to be considerably different in differentiating cells.

None of these models consider completely all the groups of proteins that can presently be recognized in phenotypically differentiated cells. Currently these groups are non-cell-specific intracellular proteins, cell-specific intracellular proteins, and secretory proteins (which, although cell-specific, are removed from the cell in which they are produced). The turnover characteristics of these protein subgroups could be different and have been considered in a model (Table I) suggested by Paskin and Mayer (1977). With reference to the enzyme groups considered in the previous models (Baldwin and Yang, 1974; McLean *et al.*, 1972), enzymes of lactose and lipid biosynthesis can be seen as cell-specific and intracellular, enzymes of the tricarboxylic acid cycle and glycolysis as non-cell-specific enzymes, and casein is a secreted protein. Current investigations in this laboratory are aimed at determining how closely the turnover characteristics of the lipogenic enzymes fatty acid synthetase, 6-phosphogluconate dehydrogenase, and acetyl-CoA carboxylase and the secretory protein casein may fit with the model shown in Table I.

D. HORMONAL FACTORS AND LIPOGENIC RATE IN MAMMARY GLAND

Hormones are involved in mammary gland *in vivo* in regulating two distinguishable parts of lipogenesis, the rate of fatty acid biosynthesis and the chain-length composition of the fatty acids produced.

The developmental changes in lipogenesis and the accumulation profiles for lipogenic enzymes have been described in Section II, B, and some of the putative roles of hormones at midpregnancy and in lactogenesis and lactation have been discussed. As with other biosynthetic processes in the mammary gland, many studies of hormonal regulation of lipogenic processes have used mammary explants *in vitro*. However,

TABLE I

PROTEIN SUBGROUP TURNOVER DURING CYTODIFFERENTIATION

Subgroup	Rate of protein synthesis	Rate of protein degradation
Cell-specific intracellular proteins	Large increase	Transitory decrease during protein accumulation
Non-cell-specific intracellular proteins	Some increase	No change
Secretory proteins	Large increase	Little degradation during accumulation, none during secretion

Abraham *et al*. (1960) investigated the effects of pituitary and adrenal cortex hormones on processes in milk fat biosynthesis and showed that, if hypophysectomized rats were supplied with prolactin and hydrocortisone at parturition and subsequently postpartum, then slices of mammary gland displayed the same metabolic activity (glycolysis, pentose phosphate pathway, and fatty acid synthesis) as in normal rats. In addition to hormonal factors necessary for lipogenesis, other influences, such as the suckling stimulus and the removal of milk from the gland, may be involved in regulating the second lipogenic stimulus (Section II, B).

Experiments have been conducted to measure the hormone response, by the rate of fatty acid biosynthesis, fatty acid pattern, and activities of lipogenic enzymes, in explants of mammary gland obtained at different stages of pregnancy and lactation in the rabbit (Speake *et al.*, 1976a). The data are shown in Table II. The results indicate that whereas the midpregnant tissue responds well to insulin, prolactin, and cortisol, tissue from just before or just after parturition shows a much poorer stimulation of lipogenesis or none at all. In explants from lactating tissue there are decreases in the rate of fatty acid biosynthesis, the percentage of medium-chain fatty acids synthesized, and the activity of fatty acid synthetase compared to that in the earlier stages of development. However, the decreases observed in the absence of hormones are significantly greater than in the presence of hormones. Experiments of this type show that the response of the mammary gland to hormones progressively decreases during pregnancy and in lactation. However, the interpretation of these responses is complex, since it undoubtedly results from several factors including the accumulation of milk within the alveolar lumina in explants, which simply prevents further response to hormones in the tissue by hydrodynamic feedback similar to that which is believed to occur during mammary involution *in vivo*. During involution there is certainly a very rapid decrease in the activities of many mammary enzymes in the initial stages of the process (Jones, 1967).

Obviously, hormones exquisitely regulate the biosynthetic capacities of the lactating gland *in vivo* (Sections I, D and IV), but it has not been possible to mimic these effects with explants from lactating mammary gland from rabbits *in vitro*.

The understanding of the hormonal regulation of fatty acid biosynthesis can only be increased when experiments on the hormonal control of the transcription of lipogenic enzymes (e.g., fatty acid synthetase) have been carried out, similar to those performed on casein synthesis (Rosen *et al.*, 1975; Houdebine, 1976; Terry *et al.*, 1977).

TABLE II

EFFECT OF HORMONES ON THE LIPOGENIC CAPACITY OF MAMMARY EXPLANTS OBTAINED FROM RABBITS AT VARIOUS STAGES OF PREGNANCY AND LACTATION[a]

State of pregnancy or lactation at which mammary explants obtained	Time in culture (hr)	Culture conditions	Rate of fatty acid synthesis (nmol of acetate incorporated into fatty acids/hr per mg of tissue)	Medium-chain ($C_{8:0}$ + $C_{10:0}$) fatty acids synthesized (%)	Specific activity of fatty acid synthetase (nmol of NADPH oxidized/min per mg of cytosol protein)	Specific activity of glucose-6-phosphate dehydrogenase (nmol of NADP$^+$ reduced/min per mg of cytosol protein)
Day 16 of pregnancy	0	—	0.04 ± 0.01	0	1.1 ± 0.2	12.3 ± 2.0
	45	No hormones	0.09 ± 0.01	0	0.0	14.2 ± 5.1
	45	Hormones	1.31 ± 0.5	40 ± 12	14.0 ± 0.5	38.7 ± 4.6
Day 27 of pregnancy	0	—	0.72 ± 0.10	ND	33.1 ± 2.2	42.2 ± 1.0
	45	No hormones	0.30 ± 0.10	ND	17.0 ± 2.8	41.7 ± 3.3
	45	Hormones	2.91 ± 0.20	ND	26.8 ± 5.0	53.0 ± 8.7
Day 3 of lactation	0	—	3.72 ± 0.02	96 ± 3	37.9 ± 2.0	ND
	45	No hormones	0.30 ± 0.11	64 ± 21	2.0 ± 0.3	ND
	45	Hormones	0.82 ± 0.30	62 ± 26	8.3 ± 1.3	ND

[a] Mammary explants were cultured at 37°C in an atmosphere in O_2 + CO_2 (95:5) in medium 199. Insulin (5 μg/ml), cortisol (1 μg/ml), and prolactin (1 μg/ml) were present where indicated. Rates of fatty acid synthesis, fatty acid synthetase specific activities, and the percentages of medium-chain fatty acids synthesized were determined as described by Speake et al. (1975). Glucose-6-phosphate dehydrogenase was assayed by the method of Gul and Dils (1969). Results are expressed as means ± half the difference between two separate determinations. ND, Not determined. Results are presented with permission of publishers and authors from Speake et al. (1976a).

E. REGULATION OF PATTERN OF FATTY ACIDS

Short-chain ($C_{4:0}$ and $C_{8:0}$) and medium-chain ($C_{8:0}$–$C_{12:0}$) fatty acids predominate in the fat of most, but not all, milks. Primate milk fat contains 10–25% medium-chain fatty acids; lagomorph milk fat contains up to 70%; milk fat of Proboscidea contains up to 93%; and in carnivores the milk fat contains only small amounts of medium-chain fatty acids (Smith and Abraham, 1975).

Abraham et al. (1961) and Smith and Dils (1966) demonstrated that a wide range of fatty acids ($C_{4:0}$–$C_{18:0}$) were synthesized by particle-free supernatant fractions prepared from homogenates of rat and rabbit mammary gland, respectively. A significant proportion of medium-chain ($C_{8:0}$–$C_{12:0}$) acids were formed. The addition of the microsomal fraction from these tissues, together with cofactors, increased the rate of fatty acid synthesis from acetate and also resulted in an increased rate of synthesis of long-chain ($C_{14:0}$ and $C_{16:0}$) fatty acids. Subsequently, Carey and Dils (1973a,b) and Strong et al. (1973) showed that at high protein concentrations the cell-free homogenate, the microsomes plus supernatant, and the particle-free supernatant fractions prepared from lactating rat and rabbit mammary glands could synthesize medium-chain ($C_{8:0}$–$C_{12:0}$) fatty acids in proportions similar to those synthesized by lactating mammary gland in vivo. When the subcellular fractions were diluted there was a progressive increase in the proportion of long-chain ($C_{14:0}$ and $C_{16:0}$) fatty acids synthesized. With each of the subcellular fractions, the difference in the proportions of fatty acids synthesized at high and at low protein concentration was not dependent on the rate of fatty acid synthesis from acetate.

Evidence has been presented (Carey and Dils, 1973b; Strong et al., 1973) that chain termination at $C_{8:0}$–$C_{12:0}$ acids is controlled by one or more factors present in the particle-free supernatant prepared from lactating rabbit mammary gland. Such factor(s) could be precipitated from the particle-free supernatant at 40–100% saturation with ammonium sulfate. The role of a factor(s) in a 40–100% ammonium sulfate fraction had also been previously implicated by Bartley et al. (1967).

A high-speed supernatant (2.83 × 10⁶ g-hr) prepared from lactating-rabbit mammary gland had two distinct effects on the synthesis of medium-chain fatty acids (Clark, 1976). The preparation caused chain elongation of $C_{4:0}$ to $C_{10:0}$ and $C_{12:0}$ fatty acids with dilute microsome plus particle-free supernatant (6 × 10⁶ g-min) systems which synthesized predominantly butyrate. The preparation also had chain-terminating properties in that it reduced the proportion of $C_{14:0}$ and $C_{16:0}$ and increased the proportion of $C_{10:0}$ and $C_{12:0}$ fatty acids synthesized by dilute microsomal plus particle-free supernatant, which synthesized predominantly long-chain fatty acids.

When the particle-free supernatant from lactating mammary gland was applied to Sephadex G-100, five fractions could be resolved, one of which (fraction IV) contained a protein factor(s) controlling chain termination at $C_{8:0}$–$C_{12:0}$ fatty acids. The factor(s) was able to direct the synthesis of medium-chain fatty acids in a preparation containing the enzymes required for fatty acid synthesis (fraction I) plus a microsomal fraction, or in a preparation of purified fatty acid synthetase (Knudsen and Dils, 1975). Fraction IV also contained acyl-thioester hydrolase(s) active toward medium-chain as well as long-chain acyl-CoA esters. It was proposed that this activity could control chain termination by cleaving medium-chain acyl groups from the acyl carrier protein of fatty acid synthetase (Knudsen et al., 1975).

An acyl-thioester hydrolase has been isolated from the cytosol of lactating rabbit mammary gland. The purified enzyme has a molecular weight of 29,000 and contains a single subunit. The enzyme terminates fatty acid synthesis at medium-chain ($C_{8:0}$–$C_{10:0}$) fatty acids when it is incubated with fatty acid synthetase and rate-limiting concentrations of malonyl-CoA. This limitation is obligatory for chain termination (Knudsen et al., 1976). A similar enzyme has been shown to be present in the cytosol from lactating-rat mammary gland (Libertini et al., 1976). The molecular weight of the purified hydrolase is similar to that of the acyl-thioester hydrolase (32,000) which can be cleaved from fatty acid synthetase prepared from lactating-rat mammary gland. The enzyme has a marked specificity for long-chain acyl-CoA esters (Smith et al., 1976; Agradi et al., 1976).

Knudsen et al. (1976) noted that the presence of a medium-chain acyl-thioester hydrolase in extracts of lactating mammary gland explains, at least in part, previous reports (Carey and Dils, 1973a,b; Strong et al., 1973; Knudsen, 1976) of an unidentified factor(s) in these extracts controlling chain termination. The medium-chain acyl-thioester hydrolase has been shown immunochemically to be distinct from fatty acid synthetase. However, purified fatty acid synthetase gave unexpected immunological reactivity with antiserum to the medium-chain hydrolase. The proportion of the medium-chain hydrolase that is associated with the synthetase is too small to be detected by polyacrylamide gel electrophoresis in the presence of sodium dodecyl sulfate (SDS) or to elicit an immune response in sheep (Chivers *et al.*, 1976). It is tempting to speculate that there may be a specific binding site for the medium-chain hydrolase on the fatty acid synthetase molecule.

Presently there is little information on the accumulation of the medium chain hydrolase in mammary gland during lactogenesis or in lactation. However, preliminary immunochemical data sugest that the enzyme appears in rabbit mammary gland between days 17 and 22 of pregnancy (Chivers *et al.*, 1976), which coincides with the onset of medium-chain fatty acid production in the gland (Fig. 2).

A chain length-modifying protein has also been prepared from rabbit mammary gland, which may loosely but specifically interact with fatty acid synthetase (Carey, 1977). Medium-chain acyl-CoA thioesterases have also been partially purified from lactating-rabbit mammary gland (Waltham and Carey, 1976).

It seems clear that at least one medium-chain acyl-thioester hydrolase is responsible for fatty acid chain-length termination in rabbit mammary gland. However, other factors seem to be involved in fatty acid chain termination *in vivo*. Clark (1976) has shown the existence of chain elongation factors in the high-speed supernatant ($2.83 \times 10^6 g$-hr) which are stable to heat and acid treatment. These factors are not present in fraction IV prepared from a particle-free supernatant from rabbit mammary gland. Clark (1976) has presented a model for the properties of the high speed supernatant and fraction IV (Knudsen and Dils, 1975) based on these observations (Fig. 3).

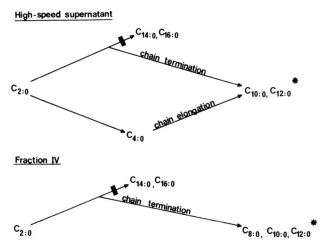

FIG. 3. Regulation of fatty acid chain length in mammary gland. Asterisks indicate fatty acids synthesized.

III. HORMONAL FACTORS IN LIPOGENESIS DURING MAMMARY GLAND
DEVELOPMENT *in Vitro*

A. HORMONAL FACTORS IN MAMMARY GLAND DEVELOPMENT *in Vitro*

Explants of mammary gland from various stages of pregnancy, particularly midpregnancy, have been used to study several aspects of mammary development. The feature that makes the explant system so useful is the exquisite response of the tissue to hormones, shown particularly by the synthesis and accumulation of milk proteins and lactose (see, e.g., Forsyth, 1971). The organ-culture technique, particularly with mammary explants from midpregnant animals, has been used extensively in order to dissect the role of individual hormones in the initiation of lactogenesis. Topper and Oka (1974) have reviewed studies with mammary explants from the mouse, carried out to identify the hormonal involvement in the regulation of cell proliferation and cell differentiation; they note that the intricate interdependencies of the reported hormonal effects are largely descriptive, with little progress in the understanding of the mechanisms of hormone action at the molecular level. Attempts have been made to identify the hormones or hormone combinations that control cell division (mitogenesis) and to identify the role of hormones in the control of the phases of cytodifferentiation in developing lobuloalveolar cells in mouse mammary gland (Topper and Oka, 1974).

Topper and Oka (1974) conclude that prolactin is the hormone required for the sensitization of epithelial cells to the mitogenic effects of insulin and other serum factors that may be mitogenic. Placental lactogen may play a role in some species, such as the rat. Hydrocortisone seems to mediate the accumulation of rough endoplasmic reticulum in these differentiating cells, but prolactin is required for the production of the biosynthetic products of the mammary gland (i.e., casein and α-lactalbumin). For optimal cell development all three hormones (insulin, prolactin, and hydrocortisone) are required, and if an incomplete hormone combination is used to stimulate the tissue then a partial, incompletely sustained response occurs: transient formation of rough endoplasmic reticulum in the presence of insulin or a short burst of RNA synthesis in the presence of insulin and prolactin (Topper and Oka, 1974). Hallowes *et al.* (1973) have demonstrated that insulin, prolactin, and corticosterone are necessary for maximal fatty acid synthesis in mammary explants from midpregnant rat. Similarly insulin, prolactin, and hydrocortisone are required for maximal lactogenic response with explants from cow mammary gland obtained 30–40 days prepartum (Collier *et al.*, 1977). This type of phenomenon is seen for the accumulation of fatty acid synthetase in mammary explants from mid-pregnant rabbits after stimulation with incomplete hormone combinations (Section III, E). It has been suggested that the hormonal requirements may be different for the acquisition of different biosynthetic capacities in mammary gland development; the hormone requirements for formation of nonsecretory proteins by mammary epithelial cells may be different from those for secretory proteins (Topper and Oka, 1974). These suggestions will be verified only when the action of hormones on selective gene expression, specifically of genes coding for the enzymes involved in lactose, lipid, and casein biosynthesis, have been delineated.

Studies on the mode of action of hormones on gene expression in mammary cells have been carried out mainly on casein. It has been shown that the synthesis of casein in explants of mammary gland from pseudopregnant rabbits is increased by prolactin. This increase coincides with the appearance of mRNA for casein. Both this appearance of mRNA and the increase in the rate of casein biosynthesis were prevented when progesterone and prolactin were injected into pseudopregnant rabbits (Houdebine and Gaye, 1975; Houdebine, 1976). From such work it is becoming clear that the acquisition of proteins in developing mammary gland is due to hormonally controlled selective gene expression. The mechanism of hormone action at the transcriptional and translational levels is under intensive study (Rosen *et al.*, 1975; Craig *et al.*, 1976; Terry *et al.*, 1977). The understanding of the hormonal control of lipogenesis in the mammary gland has not progressed to the same extent as that for casein. The problems are much more difficult since lipogenesis is brought about by many enzymic processes; even an enzyme like fatty acid synthetase, which has been extensively studied (Section III, E), is present in much smaller amounts than casein. This makes the methods used to characterize casein mRNA much more difficult to use for studies on the regulation of mRNA production for fatty acid synthetase. However, changes in the content of polysomes for acetyl-CoA carboxylase (Tanabe *et al.*, 1976; Nakanishi *et al.*, 1976) and fatty acid synthetase (Strauss *et al.*, 1975) in liver in various dietary and genetic conditions have been followed.

The hormonal involvement in milk fat synthesis in mammary explants of several species has been studied (Moretti and Abraham, 1966; Mayne and Barry, 1970). The role of hormones in the regulation of the acquisition of high capacities for lipogenesis, in the production and maintenance of the pattern of fatty acids in the tissue, and in regulating the turnover of lipogenic enzymes is discussed below (Sections III, B–E).

B. Lipogenesis and Fatty Acid Pattern in Mammary Explants from Pseudopregnant Rabbits

The hormonal control of the synthesis of milk proteins and lactose has been studied in considerable detail using explants of mammary gland (Forsyth, 1971; Topper and Oka, 1974; Houdebine and Gaye, 1975). Far fewer data are available on the effects of hormones on lipogenesis in mammary explants, although a considerable effort has been invested in this field of research in the last few years.

As previously noted (Section II, D and E) there are two facets to the hormonal regulation of lipogenesis. These are the regulation of the rate of fatty acid synthesis and the regulation of the pattern of fatty acids produced by the tissue. These problems have been considered from several points of view over the last 5 years, including the elucidation of the enzymological means by which the pattern of fatty acids is produced in developing mammary gland (Knudsen and Dils, 1975; Knudsen *et al.*, 1976) (Section II, E) and the regulation of the production of the lipogenic enzymes, particularly fatty acid synthetase, required for the increased rates of lipogenesis in the developing gland (Speake *et al.*, 1975, 1976b; Manning *et al.*, 1976; Paskin and Mayer, 1977; Mayer and Paskin, 1978; Betts and Mayer, 1977). The results on the hormonal regulation of enzyme turnover in mammary gland have suggested a model for enzyme turnover that may be applicable to the turnover of enzymes and proteins in many types of differentiating cells (Speake *et al.*, 1976b; Paskin and Mayer, 1977; Mayer and Paskin, 1978).

In early reports it was shown that insulin could stimulate fatty acid synthesis in mammary explants from midpregnant mice (Moretti and Abraham, 1966) and that the rate of fatty acid synthesis could be better maintained over 2 days by culture with insulin, corticosterone, and prolactin (Mayne and Barry, 1970). The appearance of lipid droplets in mammary explants treated with this hormone combination can be observed histologically in a number of species including the rabbit (Barnawell, 1965; Denamur, 1969a; Mills and Topper, 1970). It was also shown that when explants of mammary gland from pseudopregnant rabbits were cultured for 2 days with insulin, corticosterone, and prolactin, the incorporation of [1-^{14}C]glucose and [6-^{14}C]glucose into total lipids increased severalfold compared to that in explants cultured in the absence of hormones (Bolton, 1971).

After these observations of Bolton (1971) a detailed study of the effects of hormones on the rate of lipogenesis and the pattern of chain length of fatty acids synthesized in mammary explants from pseudopregnant rabbits was carried out (Strong *et al.*, 1972). Rabbit mammary gland was chosen for the work because it is particularly easy to dissect out explants containing large numbers of epithelial cells, and a characteristic pattern of fatty acids is synthesized by rabbit lobuloalveolar cells in lactation, i.e., about 70% ($C_{8:0}$ + $C_{10:0}$) fatty acids (Carey and Dils, 1972).

The experiments of Strong *et al.* (1972) showed that if explants from pseudopregnant rabbits were cultured with insulin, corticosterone, and

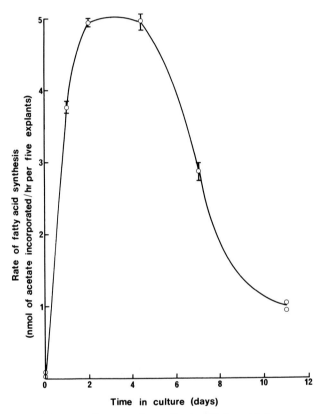

Fig. 4. Effects of time in culture on the synthesis of fatty acids by mammary explants from an 11-day pseudopregnant rabbit. Explants were cultured with insulin and corticosterone for the times shown. Prolactin was present at concentrations of 0.2, 1.0, and 5.0 µg per milliliter of medium. With explants cultured for 11 days, 1.0 µg of prolactin per milliliter of medium was used. Duplicate groups of five explants were then incubated for 1 hour at 37°C in 1.0 ml of Krebs–Henseleit bicarbonate buffer containing 0.1 mM sodium [1-¹⁴C]acetate (2 µCi) plus 1.0 mM glucose. For each period in culture, altering the concentration of prolactin had no effect on the rate of fatty acid synthesis. The mean value, ± standard error of the mean, of the six determinations of acetate incorporation after each period in culture is therefore given. For days 0 and 11 in culture, duplicate results are given. Results are presented from Strong *et al.* (1972) with permission of authors and publishers.

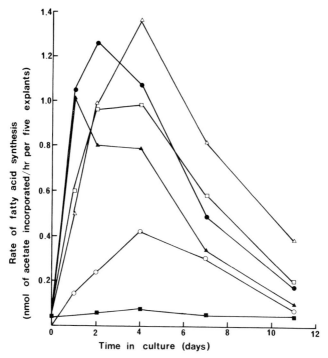

FIG. 5. Rate of synthesis of individual fatty acids by mammary explants from an 11-day-pseudopregnant rabbit as a function of time in culture. The rate of synthesis of individual fatty acids was calculated from the overall rate of fatty acid synthesis (Fig. 4) and the proportions of the fatty acids synthesized. ^{14}C-Labeled fatty acids were extracted from duplicate groups of explants, and the extracts were combined and analyzed by radio-gas-liquid chromatography (GLC). With explants cultured for 11 days, a single radio-GLC analysis was carried out on the combined extracts from duplicate determinations. Fatty acids: $\bigcirc$, $C_{8:0}$; $\triangle$, $C_{10:0}$; $\square$, $C_{12:0}$; $\bullet$, $C_{14:0} + C_{16:1}$; $\blacksquare$, $C_{18:0} + C_{18:1}$. Results are presented from Strong et al. (1972) with permission of authors and publishers.

prolactin for 6–7 days they would synthesize triglycerides enriched in the medium-chain fatty acids characteristic of rabbit milk. Freshly excised explants from pseudopregnant rabbits synthesize triglycerides and phospholipids containing long-chain fatty acids. The maximum rate of fatty acid synthesis observed with such explants after culture with insulin, corticosterone, and prolactin was similar to that seen with freshly excised explants from lactating rabbit mammary gland. The changes in the rate of total fatty acid synthesis and in the rates of synthesis of fatty acids of different chain lengths are shown in Figs. 4 and 5, respectively. The maximal rates of synthesis of medium-chain fatty acids ($C_{8:0} + C_{10:0}$) are achieved after a time in culture (4–6 days;

Fig. 5) that is somewhat later than that required to achieve the maximal rate of total fatty acid synthesis (2–4 days; Fig. 4). It appears that the maximal rate of synthesis of long-chain fatty acids ($C_{14:0}$ + $C_{16:0}$) precedes that of the medium-chain fatty acids. The precipitous decline in the rate of fatty acid synthesis after 6 days in culture may result from the large accumulation of secretory material in the lumina of the lobuloalveolar cells, together with the expected degenerative changes in the explanted tissue, such as disorganization of the alveolar epithelium and tissue necrosis (Strong et al., 1972).

These studies illustrate the usefulness of the explant system for the study of lipogenesis, at least for a period of 4–6 days in culture. Strong et al. (1972) commented that since the pattern of milk fatty acids is so specific (Morrison, 1970) its development could be used to assess the effect of hormones on mammary differentiation, at least in those species that synthesize milk fat containing medium-chain fatty acids (e.g., mouse: Wang et al., 1972). However, the use of fatty acid pattern would be of little use with those species whose milk contains only long-chain fatty acids (e.g., guinea pig: Smith et al., 1968).

C. Lipogenesis and Fatty Acid Pattern in Mammary Explants from Midpregnant Rabbits

Forsyth et al. (1972) have studied the interactions of insulin, corticosterone, and prolactin in promoting milk fat synthesis by mammary explants from pregnant rabbits. The results were compared with findings on the control of lipogenesis in vivo in the rabbit mammary gland and in mammary explants from pseudopregnant rabbits (Section III, A), and contrasted with the known effects of hormones in vitro on mammary explants from midpregnant mice (Wang et al., 1972).

The effects of insulin, cortisol, and prolactin on the rate of lipogenesis and fatty acid pattern in mammary explants from midpregnant rabbits have also been studied by Speake et al. (1975). In this work the effect of removal of hormones at different times during the hormonally stimulated increase in the rate of lipogenesis was studied. Lipogenic rate and the pattern of fatty acids produced were measured after hormone removal. In later work the effect of different hormone combinations on the activity, rate of synthesis and rate of degradation of fatty acid synthetase was measured. This work provides some interesting comparisons of the effects of different hormone combinations on the rate of the overall process of lipogenesis, the pattern of fatty acids produced, and changes in the amount of a lipogenic enzyme involved in the process (Speake et al., 1976b).

The effects of different hormone combinations on the rate of lipogenesis and pattern of fatty acids synthesized in explants from 16-day-pregnant rabbits (Forsyth *et al.*, 1972) are complex and require careful interpretation. When mammary explants are cultured with no hormones or with insulin alone, very low rates of fatty acid biosynthesis take place and long-chain fatty acids are predominantly synthesized. Culture of explants with prolactin or with insulin and prolactin results in an approximately 10–12-fold stimulation of the rate of lipogenesis; approximately 60–72% of the fatty acids synthesized are medium-chain ($C_{8:0} + C_{10:0}$) fatty acids. Culture of explants with prolactin and corticosterone gives similarly high rates of lipogenesis, but only approximately 25% of the fatty acids are of medium-chain length. Culture of explants with insulin and corticosterone results in an approximately 2-fold stimulation of lipogenesis over rates shown in explants cultured with insulin alone, but predominantly long-chain fatty acids were synthesized. Further experiments were carried out in which explants were cultured with insulin and corticosterone for 2 days and then for either 2 or 4 days with prolactin or insulin and prolactin. In these experiments a higher rate of lipogenesis (approximately 2-fold) was obtained than in explants cultured throughout with prolactin or insulin and prolactin, but in no case did the percentage of medium-chain fatty acids reach the proportion synthesized in explants cultured throughout with prolactin or insulin and prolactin (maximum proportion approximately 50% of fatty acids synthesized). Explants cultured with insulin, prolactin and corticosterone gave the highest rates of fatty acid synthesis but even after 6 days in culture the percentage of medium-chain fatty acids synthesized did not exceed about 30%. Thus prolactin appears obligatory for those high rates of production of the medium-chain fatty acids ($C_{8:0} + C_{10:0}$) found in rabbit milk (approximately 70% of the fatty acids synthesized). The results show that a hormone combination giving maximal rates of fatty acid synthesis (insulin, prolactin, and corticosterone), or preculture with a hormone combination that subsequently leads to a high rate of fatty acid synthesis (insulin and corticosterone), causes a reduction in the percentage of medium-chain fatty acids which are synthesized. Although corticosterone is required to achieve maximal rates of fatty acid synthesis (with insulin and prolactin), Forsyth *et al.* (1972) suggested that it might cause the preferential synthesis of long-chain fatty acids or antagonize the effect of prolactin.

Forsyth *et al.* (1972) show that culture of explants for 2 or 4 days with prolactin caused the synthesis of fatty acids with a pattern similar to that observed in freshly prepared explants from rabbits pregnant for 23 days. Therefore the stimulation of lipogenesis in mammary gland between 18 and 23 days of pregnancy observed *in vivo* (Strong and Dils,

1972) can be mimicked in organ culture by prolactin alone. However, in order to obtain rates of fatty acid biosynthesis similar to those seen in early lactation (Strong et al., 1972) culture with insulin, corticosterone, and prolactin was required. Paradoxically, hormone combinations that can produce lactational rates of lipogenesis in explants cannot mimic the in vivo lactational pattern of fatty acids.

These results contrast with those reported for mammary explants from midpregnant mice where synthesis of milk fatty acids was induced by culture with insulin, prolactin, and corticosterone (Wang et al., 1972). Prolactin alone was ineffective in stimulating lipogenesis, and although insulin was stimulatory (Moretti and Abraham, 1966), the pattern of fatty acids synthesized resembled that of tissue rather than milk lipid (Wang et al., 1972).

In mammary explants from 11-day pseudopregnant rabbits, culture for 2 or 4 days with prolactin alone gave a small stimulation of the rate of fatty acid synthesis but caused the production of predominantly (70–80%) medium-chain fatty acids ($C_{8:0}$ + $C_{10:0}$); the increased rate of fatty acid synthesis was not maintained, and it declined from 2 to 6 days in culture with prolactin. Culture of rabbit mammary explants with insulin and prolactin gave a slower stimulus to lipogenic rate, but after 2 days in culture medium-chain fatty acids were predominantly produced (approximately 80% of fatty acids). Over a 6-day culture period the lipogenic rate increased to a maximum and subsequently declined, i.e., an unsustained response to the hormones was obtained. Again, in a way similar to explants from midpregnant rabbits, culture with corticosterone and prolactin resulted in very low rates of fatty acid synthesis, long-chain fatty acids being synthesized predominantly. Finally, culture of mammary explants from pseudopregnant rabbits with insulin, prolactin, and corticosterone resulted in the highest rates of fatty acid biosynthesis, the maximum rate being achieved after 2 days in culture. Although the increase in the proportion of medium-chain fatty acids occurred slowly, eventually, after 6 days in culture, mostly ($C_{8:0}$ + $C_{10:0}$) fatty acids were produced (Forsyth et al., 1972). These results are similar to those obtained previously with mammary explants from pseudopregnant rabbits (Strong et al., 1972). The milk fatty acid pattern in mammary explants from midpregnant rabbits does not seem to develop in response to insulin, prolactin, and corticosterone after 6 days in culture as described for the pattern in explants from the pseudopregnant animals (Forsyth et al., 1972).

The responses of explants from midpregnant rabbits show that insulin, prolactin, and corticosterone are required for the maximum rate of fatty acid synthesis (similar to early lactation). However, this high rate is obtained at the expense of the production of the large amounts of medium-chain fatty acids which are characteristic of rabbit milk fat, at least after 6 days in culture. Insulin may increase the rate of lipogenesis in the presence of prolactin without affecting the fatty acid pattern, while corticosterone seems to antagonize the prolactin action of stimulating medium-chain fatty acid production. The results agree in general with *in vivo* findings. Prolactin will restore milk yield and milk fatty acid composition to normal in the hypophysectomized lactating rabbit (Cowie *et al.*, 1969) and will induce lactation in pseudopregnant rabbits after removal of the ovaries and adrenals (Cowie and Watson, 1966) or of the pituitaries, ovaries, and adrenals (Denamur, 1971). Adrenal corticoids may have a role in normal lactogenesis, since milk secretion is induced by injections of adrenocorticotropic hormone into pseudopregnant rabbits (Chadwick, 1971).

The apparently independent development of lipogenic rate and characteristic fatty acid pattern, suggested by the results of Forsyth *et al.* (1972), is intriguing and may reflect the mechanism of action of the hormones on selective gene expression or perhaps, as suggested by Forsyth *et al.* (1972), may represent hormone effects on different cell populations. In the presence of prolactin alone, the genes expressed may include those for enzymes involved in the production of medium-chain fatty acids. However, maximal tissue development occurs in the presence of insulin, prolactin, and cortisol (as measured by fat and casein production and secretion). This development is presumably accompanied by maximal gene expression in the lobuloalveolar cells. This could result in decreased production of enzymes producing medium-chain fatty acids by a process as simple as competition for protein translational machinery when maximal production of mRNA is occurring. Such a proposal may be applicable in cases where mammary explants are subjected to acute hormonal stimulation resulting in enormous increases in the biosynthetic capacities of the lobuloalveolar cells, to give rates of lipogenesis in a few days (2–4 days) that normally occur in the midpregnant gland over a period of approximately 2 weeks.

The interpretation of the hormonal response of mammary explants is further complicated when the profiles for changes in the rate of fatty acid biosynthesis, and synthesis of medium-chain fatty acids are made (Speake *et al.*, 1975). The picture is made still more complex when the effects of hormones on lipogenesis and fatty acid pattern are compared to the effects of hormones on changes in the activities (amount) and rates of synthesis of a lipogenic enzyme, fatty acid synthetase.

The results presented in Figs. 6 and 7 show the effect of insulin,

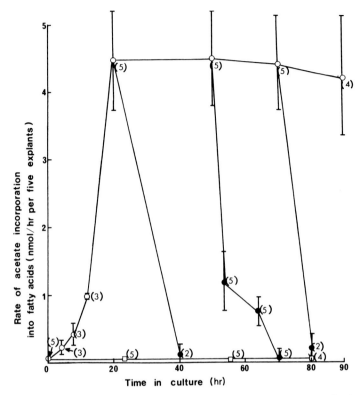

F IG. 6. Effect of hormones on the rate of lipogenesis in mammary explants. After culture with insulin, prolactin, and cortisol for the times indicated, duplicate groups of five explants were removed from the medium. They were then incubated for 1 hour at 37°C with sodium [1-¹⁴C]acetate in Krebs–Henseleit bicarbonate buffer containing glucose. The lipids in each group of explants were extracted and saponified. The fatty acids were extracted, and one-tenth of each extract was used to determine the radioactivity present. The rates of fatty acid synthesis have been calculated by the method of Strong *et al.* (1972). The rate of lipogenesis in explants that had been cultured in the presence of hormones (○), after removal of the hormones from the medium (●), and in explants that had been cultured throughout in the absence of hormones (□). The results are expressed as means ±2 SEM. The values in parentheses indicate the number of observations at each time-point. Results are presented with the permission of the authors and published from Speake *et al.* (1975).

prolactin, and cortisol on the developmental profiles for lipogenesis and fatty-acid pattern in explants prepared from midpregnant rabbits. The increase in the rate of fatty acid synthesis is very rapid, reaching the highest measured value after 20 hours in culture (Fig. 6). The maintenance of the high rate of lipogenesis is dependent on the presence of hormones; removal of hormones from the explants after 1, 2, or 3 days in culture with hormones results in a precipitous decline in the rate of lipogenesis. By contrast with the rate of lipogenesis, the production of medium-chain fatty acids increases more slowly (Fig. 7), in a manner similar to that shown previously (Forsyth *et al.*, 1972). However, the maximum proportion of medium-chain fatty acids synthesized reaches 50% of the total fatty acids produced, approximately double the proportion reported previously (Forsyth *et al.*, 1972). The pattern of fatty acids produced by the explants is again completely dependent on the presence of hormones; on hormone removal the pattern of fatty acids, like the lipogenic rate, falls precipitously. The increase in lipogenic rate (Fig. 6) correlates to some degree with the increases of lipogenic enzyme activities in explants in the presence of insulin, prolactin, and cortisol (Fig. 10; Section III, D). The precipitous decline in the proportion of medium-chain fatty acids synthesized (Fig. 7) on removal of hormones from explants coincides with the decrease in lipogenesis and

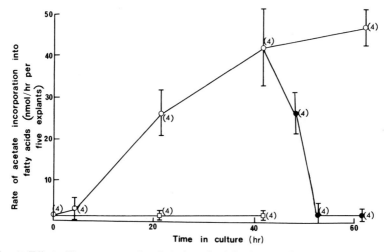

Fig. 7. Effect of hormones on the chain length of the fatty acids synthesized by mammary explants. Portions of the fatty acid samples (obtained as described in the legend to Fig. 6) were analyzed by radio-gas-liquid chromatography (GLC). To obtain sufficient radioactivity for radio-GLC, equal portions of the pentane–diethyl ether extracts prepared from duplicate explant preparations were combined (i.e., 90% of the pentane–diethyl ether extract prepared from each sample was combined). The percentage of the total radioactivity present in medium-chain fatty acids when explants had been cultured in the presence of hormones (○), after removal of the hormones from the medium (●), and when explants had been cultured throughout in the absence of hormones (□). The results are expressed as the means ±2 SEM. The values in parentheses indicate the number of observations at each time-point. Results of Speake *et al.* (1975) are presented with the permission of the authors and publishers.

contrasts with observations made on explants prepared from lactating mammary gland.

The culture of explants from lactating gland results in a precipitous decline in the rate of lipogenesis, but a much smaller decrease in the synthesis of medium-chain fatty acids (Table II). As mentioned previously (Section II, D) there are special factors that influence the metabolic behavior of explants of lactating mammary gland in culture. Alternatively, the development of extra regulators of fatty acid pattern in lactating tissue may override the hormone dependence of fatty acid pattern shown in Fig. 7, in order to preserve that pattern in milk fat during involution of the lactating gland (or in explants after hormone removal). The rates of synthesis and degradation of enzymes involved in maintaining the fatty acid pattern (e.g., medium-chain hydrolase) may be very low in lactating compared to midpregnant tissue; this may explain the relatively slow decrease in the proportion of medium-chain

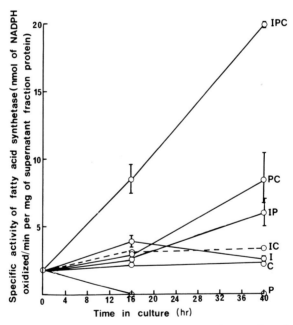

FIG. 8. Fatty acid synthetase activity in mammary explants cultured with different hormone combinations. Explants were cultured with hormone combinations shown for the times indicated. Groups of explants were removed and homogenized. Fatty acid synthetase activity was assayed in the supernatant fraction. Where indicated, the error bars are for the mean value ± half the difference between two independent experiments. I, insulin; P, prolactin; C, cortisol. Results are presented from Speake *et al.* (1976b) with permission of authors and publishers.

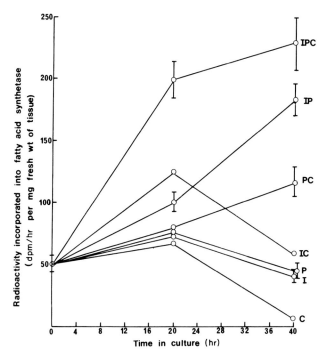

FIG. 9. Apparent rates of synthesis of fatty acid synthetase in mammary explants cultured with different hormone combinations. Explants were cultured with the hormone combinations shown for the times indicated. Groups of explants were removed and were incubated with L-[U-^{14}C]leucine. The explants were homogenized, and supernatant fractions were prepared. The rate of incorporation of radioactivity into immunodetectable fatty acid synthetase was then measured. Where indicated, the error bars are the mean values ± half the difference between two independent experiments. I, insulin; P, prolactin; C, cortisol. Results are presented from Speake *et al.* (1976b) with permission of authors and publishers.

fatty acids when explants from lactating mammary gland are cultured in the absence of hormones.

The data of Forsyth *et al.* (1972) show that culture of mammary explants from midpregnant rabbits with prolactin gives a rapid increase in the proportion of medium-chain fatty acids synthesized, but lipogenic rates are relatively low. The explanation for this could be that prolactin alone stimulates accumulation of the enzymes involved in producing medium-chain fatty acids but makes much less accumulation of other lipogenic enzymes. This explanation is supported by the observation that there is no increase in the activity (Fig. 8) or rate of synthesis (Fig. 9) of the lipogenic enzyme, fatty acid synthetase when

mammary explants from midpregnant rabbits are cultured with prolactin alone (Speake *et al.*, 1976b). However, culture of explants with
insulin, prolactin, and cortisol results in the maximum increase in the
activity and rate of synthesis of fatty acid synthetase. From the data in
Figs. 8 and 9, it is apparent that hormone combinations that contain
prolactin cause some increase in the activity and rate of synthesis of
fatty acid synthetase, whereas hormone combinations that do not contain prolactin produce little or no increase in the activity or rate of
synthesis of this enzyme. It is only in the presence of all three hormones (insulin, prolactin, and cortisol) that there is a general increase
in protein synthesis in the tissue. With two hormone combinations
containing prolactin (i.e., insulin and prolactin, cortisol and prolactin),
a combination not containing prolactin (i.e., insulin and cortisol), or
with the individual hormones, no increase in the general rate of protein
synthesis could be measured in a supernatant fraction (84×10^3
g_{av}-min) prepared from the tissue (Speake *et al.*, 1976b).

These data support the concept that prolactin alone or insulin and
prolactin together cause incomplete differentiation of mammary
explants (as measured by low fatty acid synthetase activity, rate of
enzyme synthesis, or lipogenic rate (Forsyth *et al.*, 1972)). However,
maximal amounts of medium-chain fatty acids are produced by these
hormones. Much greater cytodifferentiation occurs in the tissue in response to insulin, prolactin, and cortisol [as measured by high fatty
acid synthetase activity, rate of enzyme synthesis, or lipogenic rate
(Forsyth *et al.*, 1972)], but the increased cytodifferentiation is accompanied by decreased rates of medium-chain fatty acid synthesis. The
detailed mechanism of hormonal control of these processes is presently
unknown but is probably mediated at the transcriptional or translational levels.

D. HORMONAL REGULATION OF LIPOGENIC ENZYME ACTIVITIES

Mammary explants have been used for several studies on the role of
hormones in the regulation of lipogenic enzyme activities. Detailed
studies have been performed on glucose-6-phosphate dehydrogenase
and 6-phosphogluconate dehydrogenase (Leader and Barry, 1969; Rivera and Cummins, 1971; Green *et al.*, 1971; Oka and Perry, 1974; Betts
and Mayer, 1977), on acetyl-CoA carboxylase (Manning *et al.*, 1976),
and particularly on fatty acid synthetase (Speake *et al.*, 1975, 1976b).

Leader and Barry (1969) studied changes in the activity of glucose-
6-phosphate dehydrogenase in mouse mammary explants cultured
with insulin. Increases in the activity of the enzyme occurred that were

similar to those occurring at parturition. When explants from late-pregnant mice were cultured with insulin for 22 hours, maximal increase in enzyme activity occurred, and this was not further stimulated by addition of prolactin and corticosterone to the culture medium. However, when explants were cultured for 45 hours the activity of glucose-6-phosphate dehydrogenase was significantly greater in the presence of insulin, prolactin, and corticosterone than in explants cultured with insulin alone. With mammary explants from midpregnant mice insulin produced a large increase in the activity of the enzyme after 22 or 45 hours in culture, and this was at both times significantly increased by further addition of prolactin and corticosterone. Actinomycin D, cycloheximide, and puromycin all prevented the normal increase in enzyme activity seen in explants from late pregnant mice after 22 hours in culture, but hydroxyurea at a concentration that inhibited [^{3}H]thymidine incorporation into DNA by 92% had no such effect. Actinomycin D and cycloheximide largely failed to prevent the rise in enzyme activity if added after 3.5 and 12 hours, respectively. It was concluded that all essential RNA and protein synthesis is finished by 3.5 and 12 hours, although most of the enzyme activity increase occurs gradually between 12 and 22 hours in culture. Actinomycin D, cycloheximide, and puromycin blocked the increases in the activity of 6-phosphogluconate dehydrogenase in explants from late-pregnant mice. The authors suggested that the increase in enzyme activity, both in culture and in the living animal at parturition, is produced by an influx of glucose, which may be restrained during pregnancy by the growth hormone-like action of placental lactogen.

Green et al. (1971) further studied the hormonal regulation of glucose-6-phosphate and 6-phosphogluconate dehydrogenase activities in mammary explants from mice. The results showed that insulin, glucose, amino acids, and inorganic salts were the minimal requirement needed to increase enzyme activities in explants from late-pregnant mice. Insulin could be replaced in the incubation medium by cysteine, which may serve to increase glucose uptake into the lobuloalveolar cells. Glucose may be replaced by mannose or fructose. With higher glucose concentrations in the culture media, insulin did not potentiate the glucose-mediated increase in enzyme activity. Glucose was necessary initially in order to trigger the increase in enzyme activity, which occurred after 12 hours in culture (Leader and Barry, 1969). The authors suggested that increases in the activities of glucose-6-phosphate dehydrogenase and 6-phosphogluconate dehydrogenase result from an increased uptake of glucose by the mammary tissue, and that the increases in activity are caused by a metabolic product of glucose that stimulates the formation of mRNA during a 4-hour period after glucose is added to the culture medium. Although glucose is certainly essential for the increase in enzyme activities, the experimental design used by the authors (i.e., choice of a single time at which to measure enzyme activities, and no attempt to use different hormone combinations) precluded a measurement of any potentiating effects of hormones on the glucose effect. Such an effect had previously been measured by Leader and Barry (1969) and subsequently by other authors (Rivera and Cummins, 1971; Betts and Mayer, 1977).

Rivera and Cummins (1971) showed that sustained maximal increases in the activities of glucose-6-phosphate dehydrogenase and 6-phosphogluconate dehydrogenase were obtained when mammary explants from midpregnant mice were cultured with insulin, prolactin, and corticosterone. DNA synthesis and cell division were not required for the increases in dehydrogenase activities, and increased concentrations of glucose in the medium neither replaced nor enhanced the hormonal effects. Hormones were required in the medium for several hours in order to produce the maximal increase in enzyme activities which were measured after 48 hours in culture. After this time the continued presence of hormones was not required to maintain enzyme activities over the following 24 hours. Actinomycin D and cycloheximide prevented enzyme activity increases when present throughout the culture period. Cycloheximide was largely ineffective when added during the late phase (44 hours) of increase in enzyme activity, whereas actinomycin D was still 50% inhibitory at this time. The inhibitors of transcription and translation were added to explants in the presence of insulin and prolactin, which may in part explain the discrepancy between these results and those presented by Leader and Barry (1969).

Oka and Perry (1974) have shown that insulin, prolactin, and cortisol are required for a maximal increase in the activity of glucose-6-phosphate dehydrogenase in mammary explants from midpregnant mice. Cortisol enhanced the effect of insulin in causing an increase in enzyme activity. This effect was mimicked by spermidine, but not by spermine or putrescine. The increase in enzyme activity which was brought about by insulin or insulin and prolactin was not sustained. Insulin and cortisol, or insulin, prolactin, and cortisol, were required for a sustained increase in enzyme activity in a manner similar to that described by Rivera and Cummins (1971). As previously described (Section III, C) hormone combinations containing prolactin (ideally the three-hormone combination, insulin, prolactin, and cortisol) are required for sustained mammary cytodifferentiation.

Several problems are highlighted by these reports on the activities of the dehydrogenases in mammary explants. The mechanism of the change in enzyme activities must be identified—i.e., whether the increase in enzyme activities is due to activation of preexisting enzyme or to an increase in the concentration (amount) of the enzymes in the tissue. The role of hormones and glucose in triggering the increases in enzyme activities in the tissue must be defined.

The changes in the activities of three lipogenic enzymes in mammary explants from midpregnant rabbits are shown in Fig. 10. Increases in the activities of all the enzymes occur in the presence of insulin, prolactin, and cortisol. Removal of hormones from the culture medium after various times in culture results in a fall in enzyme activities. When explants are cultured in the absence of hormones there

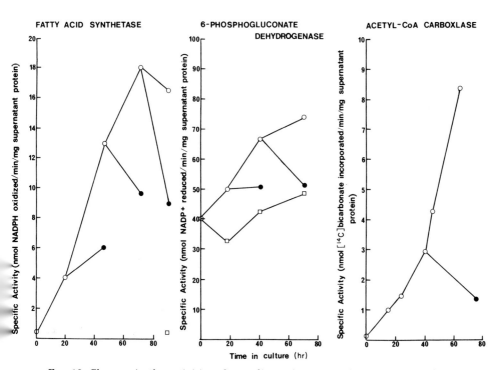

FIG. 10. Changes in the activities of some lipogenic enzymes in mammary explants cultured with hormones. Culture in the presence of insulin, prolactin, and cortisol (○), in the absence of hormones (□), after the removal of hormones from the explants (●). The results are unpublished data of Speake, Dils, and Mayer and Betts and Mayer for fatty acid synthetase and 6-phosphogluconate dehydrogenase. The results of acetyl-CoA carboxylase are presented from Manning et al. (1976) with permission of authors and publishers.

is no increase in the activity of acetyl-CoA carboxylase and fatty acid synthetase. However, the activity of 6-phosphogluconate dehydrogenase does increase in the absence of hormones. As pointed out by Leader and Barry (1969), the understanding of changes in the activities of the dehydrogenases in mammary explants has been hampered by the lack of methods for measuring the amounts of the enzymes. 6-Phosphogluconate dehydrogenase has been purified from rabbit mammary gland (Betts and Mayer, 1975) and a monospecific antiserum produced to the enzyme (Walker *et al.*, 1976). This antiserum has been used to measure the changes in the amount of 6-phosphogluconate dehydrogenase in mammary explants from mid-pregnant rabbits. The results (Fig. 11) conclusively show that changes in the activity of the enzyme in the presence or absence of hormones are due to changes in enzyme amount (Betts and Mayer, 1977). Although the glucose concentration in the medium determines the increase in the activity of the enzyme in the absence of hormones (Leader and Barry, 1969), in the presence of hormones the increase in enzyme amount was independent of the glucose concentration in the culture medium (Fig. 11). It was possible to use the antiserum to show that all changes in the activity of 6-phosphogluconate dehydrogenase were changes in enzyme amount. Although the results were somewhat equivocal, it appeared that a continuous change in the amount of 6-phosphogluconate dehydrogenase occurs on stimulation of the mammary explants, in contrast to the delayed increase in glucose-6-phosphate dehydrogenase activity in mouse mammary explants reported by Leader and Barry (1969) and Oka and Parry (1974).

The role of glucose in triggering the increase in the amount of 6-phosphogluconate dehydrogenase in explants of rabbit mammary gland has been defined (Betts and Mayer, 1977). In the absence of glucose, no increase in the amount of the enzyme occurred in the presence or in the absence of hormones. When explants were cultured in the presence of glucose, increases in the amount of the enzyme occurred with or without hormones (insulin, prolactin, and cortisol). Transfer of explants to glucose-free medium resulted in a decrease in the amount of enzyme, both in the presence and in the absence of hormones. When explants were cultured in the absence of glucose, little increase in the amount of the enzyme occurred in the presence or in the absence of hormones, but if the explants were transferred to a glucose-containing medium an increase occurred in the amount of the enzyme in the presence, but not in the absence, of hormones. The regulation of the amount of 6-phosphogluconate dehydrogenase in mammary explants is evidently complex. However, the results do show the obligatory require-

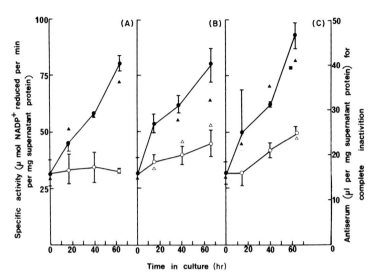

FIG. 11. Effect of glucose concentration and hormones on the activity of 6-phosphogluconate dehydrogenase in mammary explants. Explants were cultured in medium 199 containing glucose. The final glucose concentrations were 1.39 mM (A), 5.55 mM (B), 55.5 mM (C). Where indicated, explants were cultured with insulin (5 μg/ml), prolactin (1 μg/ml), and cortisol (1 μg/ml). At times indicated, groups of 30 explants were taken and homogenized in 0.6 ml of 250 mM sodium phosphate buffer, pH 7.0, containing 0.1 mM dithiothreitol and 50 μM NADP$^+$, then centrifuged for 14,000 g_{av} for 6 min. Samples of the supernatant were taken for measurement of enzyme activity and protein. Where indicated samples (50 μl) were taken for immunotitration. Specific activity of 6-phosphogluconate dehydrogenase in explants cultured throughout in the presence of insulin, prolactin, and cortisol (●) and in the absence of hormones (○). Extrapolated volume of antiserum required for complete inhibition of enzyme activity in the presence (▲) and the absence of hormones (△). The volume of antiserum required for complete precipitation of the enzymes was extrapolated from five values on an immunotitration curve. Where indicated, the results are means ± half the difference for two independent experiments. Results are presented from Betts and Mayer (1977) with permission of the authors and publishers.

ment for glucose to produce an increase in enzyme amount, and the potentiating effect of insulin, prolactin, and cortisol on the glucose-triggered increase in enzyme amount.

The studies on 6-phosphogluconate dehydrogenase (Betts and Mayer, 1977) illustrate the usefulness of the immunochemical approach in order to determine changes in amount, rather than just activity, of an enzyme. This approach can be extended so that immunoisolation procedures may be used to purify an enzyme from a tissue extract. When this can be done, it is possible through the use of pulse radiochemical procedures to measure the apparent rates of synthesis and degradation of an enzyme (Section III, E). As discussed in Section III, C, hormone action can be assessed in terms of the hormonal effects on the rate of synthesis of specific enzymes [e.g., fatty acid synthetase (Fig. 9)]. Therefore with immunochemical methods one can measure hormonally stimulated changes in the amount, rate of synthesis, and rate of degradation of an enzyme. It is only by means of this approach that the effect of hormones on selective gene expression and/or enzyme degradation during the accumulation of lipogenic enzymes in mammary cytodifferentiation can be studied.

E. HORMONAL REGULATION OF THE TURNOVER OF FATTY ACID
   SYNTHETASE

By definition, hypertrophy in differentiating cells must occur when protein synthesis exceeds protein degradation (Goldberg and St. John, 1976). Increases in the amounts of proteins in differentiating cells are a consequence of selective gene expression, which results in specific protein synthesis (Abercrombie, 1967; Chan and O'Malley, 1976). However, the change in the amount of an enzyme or protein will depend not only on the quantitative change in protein synthesis with time, but also on any such changes in protein degradation during the phase of accumulation of the enzyme or protein in the cell. The mechanism and regulation of both specific protein synthesis (selective gene expression) and protein degradation are as yet unknown. The hormonally stimulated differentiation of the mammary lobuloalveolar cells provides an excellent system in which to study all these processes. As previously mentioned (Section II, C), several attempts have been made to produce models that describe the differential changes in groups of enzyme activities. These models are conceptually very important and serve to stress the fact that in differentiating cells it is not sufficient to analyze enzyme activity changes alone; changes in the amounts of enzymes must be measured in the differentiating cells, for it is the amounts of enzymes that usually change in response to some hormonal stimulus.

In mammary gland the regulation of the turnover (synthesis and degradation) of the lipogenic enzymes shown in Table III is currently being studied in detail. All of these lipogenic enzymes accumulate in mammary gland during development, but the precise mechanism by which hormones can regulate their accumulation is not understood. It has been shown that increases in the activities of three of the enzymes are due to increases in their amounts. Thus increases in the activities of 6-phosphogluconate dehydrogenase (Betts and Mayer, 1977), fatty

TABLE III

HORMONAL REGULATION OF ENZYME TURNOVER IN MAMMARY EXPLANTS IN ORGAN CULTURE[a]

Enzyme	Tissue	Stimulus	Activity	Amount	Rate of synthesis	Rate of degradation	
ACC	Mammary gland (MG), rabbit	I, P, C	↑	↑	↑	?	R. J. Mayer (unpublished)
FAS	MG, rabbit	I, P, C	↑	↑	↑	↓ During accumulation	Speake et al. (1975, 1976b)
6PGDH	MG, rabbit	I, P, C	↑	↑	?	?	Betts and Mayer (1977)
G6PDH	MG, rabbit	I, P, C	↑	?	?	?	L. E. Smith and R. J. Mayer (unpublished)
G6PDH	MG, mouse	I	↑	?	↑ (presumed)	?	Leader and Barry (1969)

[a] ↑ and ↓ increase or decrease in parameter, respectively; ACC, acetyl-CoA carboxylase; FAS, fatty acid synthetase; 6PGDH, 6-phosphogluconate dehydrogenase; G6PDH, glucose-6-phosphate dehydrogenase; I, insulin; P, prolactin; C, cortisol.

acid synthetase (Speake *et al.*, 1975, 1976b), and acetyl-CoA carboxylase (R. J. Mayer, unpublished observations) are due to increases in the amounts of the enzymes. Furthermore it is known that the increases in the amounts of acetyl-CoA carboxylase (R. J. Mayer, unpublished) and fatty acid synthetase (Speake *et al.*, 1975, 1976b) are associated with increases in the rate of synthesis of the enzymes. The most intriguing and unexpected observations have been made on the rate of degradation of fatty acid synthetase during mammary explant differentiation. This rate was measured by a pulse-chase radioimmunochemical method with radiolabeled amino acids. It was shown that the apparent rate of degradation of the enzyme decreased or even ceased completely for a transitory period during the phase of most rapid enzyme accumulation, which accompanies the increase in the rate of synthesis of the enzyme in the tissue.

By comparison, measurements of the apparent rates of degradation of cytosol proteins in the same experiments gave somewhat equivocal results, in that the apparent rate of degradation of cytosol protein was either unchanged during cell differentiation or was decreased (Speake *et al.*, 1975). In subsequent experiments (Speake *et al.*, 1976b) the effect of different hormone combinations on the apparent rates of degradation of fatty acid synthetase and protein in a supernatant fraction prepared from explant homogenates were studied. The results are shown in Table IV. The apparent transitory decrease in the rate of degradation of the enzyme was shown only in explants cultured with hormone combinations containing prolactin. These combinations gave the largest increases in enzyme activity and rate of enzyme synthesis (Figs. 8 and 9).

These results suggest that there is a hormonally regulated program of enzyme turnover during mammary cytodifferentiation. Not only may selective gene expression be regulated hormonally, but also the rate of degradation of proteins may be controlled. Protein synthesis and protein degradation are probably mechanistically independent processes, but if patterns of change like those of fatty acid synthetase are of a general nature in differentiating cells, then the two processes may be to some extent interdependent (Volpe and Marasa, 1975).

There have been several reports that decreased rates of enzyme or protein degradation accompany increased rates of enzyme or protein synthesis in differentiating cells (Philippidis *et al.*, 1972; Murphy and Walker, 1974; Scornik, 1972; Swick and Ip, 1974; Hill and Malamud, 1974). Recently, it has become apparent that changes in the rate of protein degradation may be the single most important regulatory factor in the determination of the protein content of liver after dietary change (Conde and Scornik, 1976), after partial hepatectomy (Scornik and

TABLE IV

CHANGES IN THE APPARENT RATE OF DEGRADATION OF FATTY ACID SYNTHETASE AND OF
EXPLANT SUPERNATANT PROTEIN IN MAMMARY EXPLANTS FROM MIDPREGNANT RABBITS
DURING CULTURE WITH COMBINATIONS OF INSULIN, PROLACTIN, AND CORTISOL[a]

Period in culture when degradation was measured (hours)	Culture conditions	Apparent half-lives, $t_{1/2}$ (hours)	
		Explant supernatant protein	Fatty acid synthetase
0–17	No hormones	58	15
15–36	Insulin	15	18
41–61	Insulin	15	19
15–36	Cortisol	20	46
41–61	Cortisol	18	38
15–36	Insulin + cortisol	18	19
41–61	Insulin + cortisol	19	20
18–38	Insulin + prolactin	44	∞
43–66	Insulin + prolactin	30	22
17–40	Prolactin + cortisol	33	216
42–65	Prolactin + cortisol	58	11
18–38	Insulin + prolactin + cortisol	28	172
43–66	Insulin + prolactin + cortisol	32	38
19–43	Insulin + prolactin + cortisol + dibutyryl-cAMP + theophylline	41	37
45–65	Insulin + prolactin + cortisol + dibutyryl-cAMP + theophylline	25	51

[a] The apparent rates of degradation were measured during defined periods in culture by the disappearance of radioactivity from immunodetectable fatty acid synthetase and from trichloroacetic acid-precipitable protein isolated from the explant supernatant fraction. The loss of radioactivity from protein was exponential with respect to time and was assumed to represent the degradation of protein. The apparent degradation coefficients (K_d) were calculated from gradients (i.e., slope $\times$ 2.303) of graphs of log (disintegrations per minute in fatty acid synthetase or in the supernatant protein) versus the time after the administration of L-[U-^{14}C]leucine. Half-lives were calculated from the relationship $t_{1/2} = \ln 2/K_d$. Dibutyryl cyclic AMP (1 mM) plus theophylline (1 mM) were present in the culture medium in some experiments. Results are presented with permission of authors and publishers from Speake *et al.* (1976b).

Botbol, 1976), or during neonatal liver development (Conde and Scornik, 1977). It should be pointed out that considerable care must be taken in the interpretation of measurements of the rates of protein degradation by pulse-chase isotope methods (Rannels *et al.*, 1975), particularly in view of the problem of isotopic reutilization. This process will lead to underestimation of the rate of degradation of a protein. The problem is nowhere as acute as in situations where increases in the rate of protein synthesis are occurring, of which one excellent example is in differentiating cells. Because of this problem, considerable effort has been expended in carrying out experiments to determine whether isotopic reutilization occurs (Speake *et al.*, 1976b) or to try to minimize the effect by an appropriate choice of isotope (Swick and Ip, 1974) or experimental conditions (Conde and Scornik, 1977). However, some authors have used other means to measure the rate of protein degradation. Protein degradation has been estimated by the differences between the amount of protein synthesized and the amount of protein accumulated in a given time (Millward *et al.*, 1975; Conde and Scornik, 1977). Computer modeling has been used to calculate myosin degradation during cardiac hypertrophy in rabbits (Morkin *et al.*, 1972). In this model the rate constant of myosin degradation was calculated from the disappearance of radiolabeled lysine from the tissue and measured estimates of myosin synthesis. Clearly a computer model can be of value in more general cases, i.e., when changes in enzyme quantity or protein mass are occurring. The rate of degradation of enzymes over prolonged periods can be calculated by computer analysis of enzyme synthesis and enzyme accumulation profiles in differentiating cells (Paskin and Mayer, 1977; Mayer and Paskin, 1978).

Berlin and Schimke (1965) have suggested that temporal changes in enzyme amounts are described by Eq. (1).

$$dE/dt = K_S - K_D E \qquad (1)$$

where dE/dt = rate of change in enzyme amount E with respect to time (t); K_S = rate constant of synthesis of enzyme; K_D = rate constant of degradation of enzyme. A steady-state concentration of enzyme is maintained when $K_S/K_D = E$. Berlin and Schimke (1965) showed that if K_S and K_D are assumed to change instantaneously, then Eq. (1) can be integrated to a form that can be used to estimate the amount of enzyme present at any time after the change. However, it is becoming clear that K_S and K_D are themselves functions of time in differentiating cells or indeed during nutritional stimulation of differentiated cells (Chee and Swick, 1976). Equation (1) can be used to determine the rate of change of the amount of an enzyme and therefore the amount of enzyme present at a given time, when K_S and K_D are changing, by taking sufficiently small intervals of time (Δt) and applying the equation in the form:

$$\Delta E/\Delta t = k_S - k_D E \qquad (2)$$

where k_S and k_D are the values of K_S and K_D, respectively, which are defined as constant over the short time interval under consideration. A computer program can easily be devised to calculate an enzyme amount profile, synthesis profile, or degradation profile after some stimulus starting from initial values (Paskin and Mayer, 1977), given two of the three profiles (changes of E, K_S, or K_D with time).

Such a computer analysis has been used to analyze the turnover characteristics of fatty acid synthetase in mammary explants cultured for 2 days in the presence of insulin, prolactin, and cortisol. The degradation profile for the enzyme has been computed from the measured increases in enzyme activity (which are enzyme amounts; Speake *et al.*, 1975) and the measured increases in the rate of enzyme synthesis (absolute rates, determined by pulses of L-[4,5-³H]leucine: L. E. Smith, N. Paskin, and R. J. Mayer, unpublished methods). The results of such an analysis are shown in Fig. 12. Analysis of enzyme accumulation and enzyme synthesis profiles by the method based on Eq. (2) shows a transitory decrease in the rate of degradation of fatty acid synthetase during the phase of most rapid enzyme accumulation (Mayer and Paskin, 1978). Therefore the analysis confirms that there is a transitory

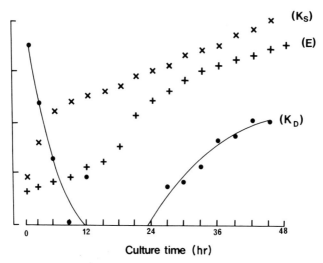

FIG. 12. Turnover characteristics of fatty acid synthetase during accumulation in mammary explants in organ culture. Explants were cultured with insulin (5 μg/ml), prolactin (1 μg/ml), and cortisol (1 μg/ml). The incorporation of L-[4,5-³H]leucine into fatty acid synthetase was measured after isolation of the enzyme by immunoabsorbent chromatography and sodium dodecyl sulfate-polyacrylamide electrophoresis. E (+) = % of initial enzyme amount; K_S (×) = % of initial amount hr⁻¹, and K_D (●) = hr⁻¹. E scale, 0–640; K_S scale, 0–16; K_D scale, 0–0.04.

decrease in the rate of degradation of the enzyme (Speake *et al.*, 1975, 1976b). The computed analysis offers an indirect method of estimation of the rate of enzyme degradation in comparison with direct measurement by pulse-chase radioimmunochemical techniques: both methods show that a transitory fall in the rate of degradation of fatty acid synthetase occurs together with an increase in the rate of enzyme synthesis on hormonal stimulation of mammary explants.

Therefore it seems that a regulated program of turnover (synthesis and degradation) of fatty acid synthetase exists in mammary tissue in response to hormone combinations that contain prolactin (Speake *et al.*, 1976b; Mayer and Paskin, 1978). Such a regulated program of enzyme turnover may particularly apply to cell-specific intracellular proteins (Table I). It has been proposed that changes in enzyme synthesis may trigger changes in enzyme degradation (Volpe and Marasa, 1975). The data presented in Table IV and Fig. 12 support and extend this contention; it seems that transitory changes in enzyme degradation must be related to transcriptional and translational events in protein synthesis. It is difficult to determine whether decreases in general protein degradation in mammary explants occur, particularly since different protein subgroups may have different turnover characteristics (Table I). However, a small decrease in the rate of cytosol protein degradation in mammary explants may perhaps occur on hormonal stimulation of the tissue (Speake *et al.*, 1975, 1976b). In recent experiments. (L. E. Smith and R. J. Mayer, unpublished observations), further evidence has been obtained for some decrease in the rate of degradation of total explant protein on stimulation of the tissue with insulin, prolactin, and cortisol. In these experiments (Fig. 13) the rate of degradation of explant protein seemed to decrease between 22 and 63 hours when explants were cultured with hormones. No significant difference in the rate of protein degradation was seen when explants were cultured in media containing 0.025–4.6 mM leucine, indicating that the extent of isotopic reutilization in the tissue must be minimal (Rannels *et al.*, 1975).

The computer analysis of an enzyme accumulation and synthesis profile in order to estimate the enzyme degradation profile has been used to analyze the turnover characteristics of lipogenic and other enzymes in developing tissues (Mayer and Paskin, 1978). In many cases the measured enzyme accumulation profiles in these tissues could be accounted for by the measured enzyme synthesis profiles only if some transitory decrease in enzyme degradation occurred during the phase of enzyme accumulation. Thus a regulated program of enzyme turnover, where both the rates of synthesis and degradation of an enzyme

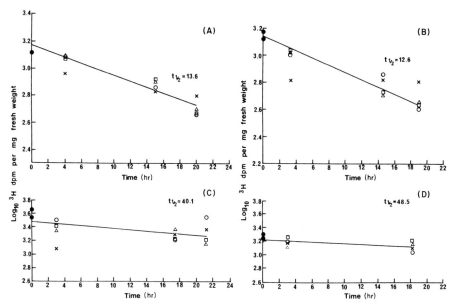

FIG. 13. Apparent rate of degradation of explant protein at different times in culture in the presence or the absence of hormones. Explants were cultured for 0 (A, B), 21.5 (C), and 45 (D) hours with insulin, prolactin, and cortisol. They were then incubated for 30 minutes with 20 μCi of L-[4,5-³H]leucine, very carefully washed, and further cultured for various times. Explants were cultured for 19 hours in the presence (A) and the absence (B) of hormones, or for 21 hours (C) and 18 hours (D) in the presence of hormones. At the times indicated, explants were taken and homogenized; the radioactivity was measured in carefully washed trichloroacetic acid-insoluble protein. The half-lives ($t_{1/2}$) of the protein are computed from the slope of each graph of log disintegrations per minute in protein versus time (i.e., slope × 2.303 = K_D); $t_{1/2}$ = ln2/K_D. Leucine concentration: ×, 0.025 mM; 0, 0.1 mM; △, 0.46 mM; □, 4.6 mM. (L. E. Smith and R. J. Mayer, unpublished results).

may alter as the amount of an enzyme changes in a differentiating cell, may be widespread. The energetic and regulatory advantages of enzyme "sparing" during enzyme accumulation have been discussed (Mayer and Paskin, 1977). It should be noted that approximately 44% of the theoretical energy of synthesis of fatty acid synthetase is saved by the transitory decrease in the rate of enzyme degradation shown in Fig. 12 (calculated relative to the energy required to synthesize the same amount of enzyme over 48 hours if the rate of degradation of the enzyme was not changed). The energetic, temporal and regulatory advantages of modulating protein degradation as well as protein synthesis in response to hormones in developing mammary gland cannot yet be fully assessed. This information will be available only when the turnover characteristics of many mammary proteins have been measured.

It has already been clearly shown that changes in the rate of protein degradation in liver are of singular importance in the regulation of liver protein mass in regenerating, developing or adult liver (Scornik and Botbol, 1976; Conde and Scornik, 1976, 1977). The rates of degradation of an enzyme (Table IV) and of general protein (Fig. 13) in mammary explants in the presence of insulin, prolactin, and cortisol are relatively fast, and the major secretory protein, casein, accounts for only some 30% of the protein synthesized (Speake et al., 1976b). In the rat, casein accounts for only approximately 50% of protein synthesized in the lactating mammary gland (Rosen et al., 1975). Modulation of the rate of protein degradation may be important for the regulation of the amounts of enzymes and proteins (Scornik and Botbol, 1976) in developing, and possibly in the developed (lactating), mammary gland.

IV. LIPOGENESIS AND CYCLIC NUCLEOTIDES

In an attempt to understand the mechanism of hormone action at the cellular level in mammary gland, a comprehensive study of the effects of cyclic nucleotides on differentiation, development, and metabolism of the tissue has been carried out (Sapag-Hagar et al., 1974; Sapag-Hagar and Greenbaum, 1974a,b; Speake et al., 1976b).

Sapag-Hagar et al. (1974) showed that when mammary explants from rats (10 or 20 days pregnant) are cultured with dibutyryl-cAMP (10^{-3} M) the activities of many enzymes are inhibited; in particular, the activities of the enzymes involved in lipogenesis decreased. The rate of DNA, RNA, and fatty acid synthesis was also markedly decreased, whereas the synthesis of casein was slightly increased. The effect of dibutyryl-cAMP was most marked on the enzymes that normally increase during mammary gland development, especially the enzymes of the malonyl-CoA pathway of fatty acid synthesis and "satellite" enzymes of lipogenesis. The maximal effect was shown on the activity of fatty acid synthetase in tissue taken from 10-day and 20-day pregnant rats. The rate of fatty acid synthesis was reduced by 60% when explants were cultured with dibutyryl-cAMP. These observations are similar to some reported previously where lipogenesis was inhibited in liver slices (Bricker and Levey, 1972) and in rat liver (Allred and Roehrig, 1973) by cAMP.

The activities of adenyl cyclase and phosphodiesterase and the content of cAMP have been measured in mammary glands of rats at different stages of development (Sapag-Hagar and Greenbaum, 1974). The results show that there are coordinated changes in the activities of adenyl cyclase and phosphodiesterase and the tissue content of cAMP at different stages of pregnancy and lactation. The activity of adenyl cyclase rises to a peak at the end of pregnancy whereas that of phosphodiesterase does not change significantly; consequently the tissue content of cAMP rises to a peak at the end of pregnancy. A large decrease in the activity of adenyl cyclase, an increase in phosphodiesterase, and therefore a decrease in cAMP in the tissue, occurs in lactation. The authors found that progesterone and β-estradiol caused a stimulation of adenyl cyclase activity in the gland from pregnant animals, whereas hydrocortisone, insulin, and prolactin did not. Only insulin inhibited the adenyl cyclase activity of lactating tissue. Sapag-Hagar and Greenbaum (1974a) argued that in the second half of pregnancy estrogen, progesterone, and hydrocortisone act cooperatively to increase the tissue content of cAMP; this increase, possibly through activation of protein kinases, could lead to the selective modulation of cell physiological processes and therefore control growth and development of the gland. After parturition, the tissue content of cAMP decreases because there is less adenyl cyclase activity, the estrogen and progesterone stimuli are removed, and there is an increase in phosphodiesterase activity. Therefore the decrease in the tissue content of cAMP may stimulate the processes involved in the biosynthesis of milk in the mammary gland, e.g., by increasing the rates of formation of biosynthetic enzymes.

There is evidence that increased cAMP content of liver tends to decrease the synthesis of lipogenic enzymes. Glucagon and cAMP prevent the increase in the synthesis rate of glucose-6-phosphate dehydrogenase which normally occurs on feeding fasting rats with a high carbohydrate diet (Rudack et al., 1971).

Speake et al. (1976b) have shown that dibutyryl-cAMP and theophylline will prevent the normal large increase in the amount of fatty acid synthetase which occurs when mammary explants from midpregnant rabbits are cultured with insulin, prolactin, and cortisol. The increase in the activity of the enzyme is delayed by the presence of dibutyryl-cAMP in the culture medium (Fig. 14A). The mechanism of this effect is shown in Fig. 14B: the cyclic nucleotide prevents the normal increase in the rate of synthesis of fatty acid synthetase that occurs in the presence of hormones. However, some increase in the rate of enzyme synthesis occurs during a period when no active enzyme can be detected in the tissue (Fig. 14,A,B). It is possible that this may be due to the synthesis of inactive precursor(s) of the enzyme similar to that

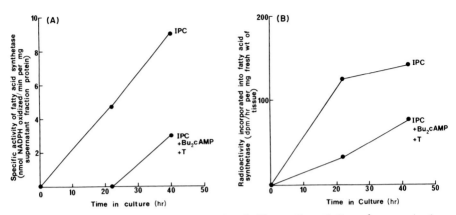

FIG. 14. Effects of dibutyryl-cAMP plus theophylline on the activity and apparent rate of synthesis of fatty acid synthetase in mammary explants cultured with insulin, prolactin, and cortisol. Explants were cultured with insulin, prolactin, and cortisol in the presence and in the absence of dibutyryl-cAMP (1 mM) plus theophylline (1 mM) for the times indicated. Groups of explants were removed and incubated with L-[U-^{14}C]leucine. The explants were homogenized, and the supernatant fractions were prepared. Fatty acid synthetase activity and the rate of incorporation of L-[U-^{14}C]leucine into fatty acid synthetase were measured in the supernatant fraction. (A) Fatty acid synthetase activity; (B) rate of incorporation of radioactivity into immunoprecipitable fatty acid synthetase. I, insulin; P, prolactin; C, cortisol; Bu$_2$cAMP, dibutyryl-cAMP; T, theophylline. Results are presented from Speake et al. (1976b) with permission of authors and publishers.

observed in liver by Yu and Burton (1974). The results with fatty acid synthetase given an insight into the mechanism by which the effects of changes in tissue content of cyclic nucleotides may be mediated in lobuloalveolar cells in mammary gland.

The tissue content of cGMP has been measured in rat mammary gland and compared with data on cAMP (Sapag-Hagar and Greenbaum, 1974b). The measurements show a coordinated change in the content of cAMP and cGMP during pregnancy and lactation. The content of cAMP is high during pregnancy and low in lactation whereas the cGMP content is low in pregnancy and high in lactation. The authors have suggested that these coordinated and opposite changes may show an antagonism between cAMP and cGMP, which may be a modulatory mechanism for the response of mammary gland to hormones. The observations on fluctuations in the cyclic nucleotide content of mammary gland during pregnancy and lactation may support the hypothesis of Goldberg et al. (1973) that there are bidirectional systems in which stimulation or inhibition of a process is achieved by a simultaneous drop in concentration of cAMP as that of cGMP is increased.

Insofar as the role of cyclic nucleotides in differentiating and developed cells is understood, it seems that cyclic nucleotides may have some type of modulatory role on mammary gland development. *In vitro,* dibutyryl-cAMP reduces the increase in the rate of synthesis of fatty acid synthetase (Speake *et al.,* 1976b) and of explant supernatant protein (B. K. Speake, R. Dils, and R. J. Mayer, unpublished observations). If this type of response is general, then increased amounts of cAMP in the mammary gland may act to suppress gene expression or translational processes required for the production of enzymes involved in the biosynthesis of milk. The fall in cAMP and rise in cGMP after parturition (Sapag-Hagar and Greenbaum, 1974b) is accompanied by a wave of mitosis in the lobuloalveolar epithelial cells in rat mammary gland so that the number of secretory cells is substantially increased. Hence the cyclic nucleotide ratio may in some way determine (or reflect) the balance in the tissue between cell proliferation and cell differentiation. Whatever the role of cyclic nucleotides, it is clear that some intracellular modulators must be involved in the harmonious response of lobuloalveolar cells to hormones during pregnancy and lactation.

V. Lipogenesis in Lactating Mammary Gland from Nonruminants

In this section it is not intended to review the large literature regarding the metabolic routes by which substrates and NADPH are provided for lipogenesis in the lactating mammary gland, but to draw attention to experimental approaches designed to study how hormones may affect these metabolic routes, or how hormones may affect the nutritional manipulation of lactating animals or *in vitro* preparations.

Two models have been presented to describe the metabolic interrelationships required to metabolize glucose and provide NADPH for lipogenesis in the lactating mammary gland of nonruminants (Bauman and Davis, 1974; Gumaa *et al.,* 1973) (Fig. 1B). The differences between the models are centered on the extent of operation of the malate transhydrogenation cycle for the generation of NADPH as well as the pentose phosphate pathway (Section II, A). The fate of cytosolic oxaloacetate, produced by the citrate cleavage enzyme, will naturally be affected by the extent of operation of the malate transhydrogenation cycle, since malate derived from cytosolic oxaloacetate is used for NADPH generation. Smith and Abraham (1975) comment that the extent of operation of the malate transhydrogenation cycle in the lactating gland is unknown. However, Katz and Wals (1972) concluded that 80–100% of the NADPH for lipogenesis could be produced by the pentose phosphate pathway and that excess production could occur. In a recent report Bartley and Abraham (1976) showed that the rate of fatty acid synthesis in lactating rat mammary gland increases linearly with the carbon flux through the pentose phosphate pathway up to a point beyond which NADPH may be produced by oxidation of malate to pyruvate. Malate would be produced by the reduction of oxaloacetate, produced during citrate cleavage, by glycolytically generated NADH. Bartley and Abraham (1976) concluded that maximal fatty acid synthesis in slices of lactating mammary gland would require the production of NADPH and NADH, a condition that was met experimentally when glucose and L-lactate were provided as substrates. The decreased rate of lipogenesis in the presence of pyruvate may support the suggested requirements for cytosolic NADH in slices of rat mammary gland.

Nonruminant mammary gland *in vivo* utilizes predominantly glucose, but also utilizes other substrates, depending on the physiological state of the animal. The concentrations of nonlipid substrates in arterial blood perfusing the mammary gland of lactating rats have been reported to be 5–6 mM glucose, 1–2 mM L-lactate, and 0.03 mM ketone bodies (Hawkins and Williamson, 1972; Elkin and Kuhn, 1975). Short-term starvation for 16 hours tends to decrease the concentrations and net uptakes of glucose and L-lactate and to increase those of β-hydroxybutyrate and acetoacetate (Hawkins and Williamson, 1972). The substrate composition of blood could have a significant influence on the rate of fatty acid synthesis in the lactating mammary gland through metabolic interactions and competitions between substrates.

Williamson *et al.* (1975) have studied the metabolic interactions of glucose and acetoacetate, and the effect of insulin on slices of mammary gland obtained from lactating rats. The utilization of glucose by the slices was decreased by 33% on adding acetoacetate to the incubation medium. This inhibition was accompanied by increases in the intracellular concentrations of citrate and glucose 6-phosphate and a doubling of the concentration of pyruvate in the culture medium. The inhibitory effect of acetoacetate on glucose utilization was completely reversed by insulin, without altering the amount of acetoacetate utilized or pyruvate formed. Similar results were obtained with slices of mammary gland from diabetic rats, except that insulin did not completely reverse the effects of acetoacetate. Acetoacetate suppressed the formation of $^{14}CO_2$ from [1-^{14}C]pyruvate. Insulin did not overcome this effect, but did increase the proportion of [3-^{14}C]acetoacetate that was converted to lipid and decrease that oxidized to CO_2. Arteriovenous difference studies on lactating mammary gland of rats have previously shown that the gland takes up ketone bodies but that their contribution to total substrate uptake is less than 3% in the fed state (Hawkins and Williamson, 1972). In short-term starvation, glucose uptake into the lactating gland declines by 50% and lactate is released. These changes are accompanied by an increase in ketone-body uptake, which may result in decreased glucose utilization and pyruvate oxidation by the gland (Hawkins and Williamson, 1972).

Williamson et al. (1975) suggested that the inhibition of glucose utilization by acetoacetate and the accumulation of intracellular citrate and glucose 6-phosphate in mammary gland slices means that the sites of inhibition of glucose utilization are at phosphofructokinase and hexokinase. The proposed inhibition of phosphofructokinase by citrate would lead to a buildup of glucose 6-phosphate, which would inhibit the hexokinase. The reversal of the inhibitory effects of acetoacetate on glucose utilization by insulin was accompanied by the highest flux of carbon (glucose and acetoacetate) to lipid. Therefore Williamson et al. (1975) proposed that the primary effect of the hormone on the system is concerned with the activation of a rate-limiting step in the lipogenic pathway. Acetyl-CoA carboxylase is proposed as the most likely candidate, since it has the lowest activity of all the enzymes involved in the conversion of glucose to lipid (McLean et al., 1972).

If the results found with slices of lactating mammary gland are applicable in vivo, then the increase in acetoacetate availability in the circulation on starvation would depress the utilization of glucose and lactate for lipid synthesis and energy supply. Ketone bodies could provide alternative substrates for both these processes which would, in short-term starvation, lead to a "sparing" of glucose for lactose synthesis (Williamson et al., 1975). When acetoacetate is administered to fed lactating rats in vivo the glucose uptake by the mammary gland is rapidly decreased. This is accompanied by an output of pyruvate from the gland, whereas lactate uptake remains the same (Robinson and Williamson, 1977a). Similar, though not identical, changes occur in starved lactating rats. In contrast to results obtained with slices of lactating mammary gland (Williamson et al., 1975) glucose 6-phosphate concentration is not increased in the gland after injection of acetoacetate into the animals. However, there is an increase in the citrate concentration in mammary slices and mammary gland in vivo after treatment with acetoacetate. The studies in vivo are not therefore completely consistent with the hypothesis that acetoacetate acts by raising the citrate concentration which then inhibits phosphofructokinase to raise the glucose 6-phosphate concentration, so inhibiting hexokinase and therefore glucose uptake into the tissue (Robinson and Williamson, 1977a). The authors suggest that the administration of acetoacetate to fed lactating rats results in changes in mammary gland that are similar to, but not identical with, those occurring after 24 hours' starvation of lactating rats. After acetoacetate administration or starvation, glucose uptake is decreased and pyruvate is released by the gland. However, in contrast with 24-hour starvation, where lactate is released by the gland, after acetoacetate administration to fed rats lactate continues to be taken up by the gland. One possible change in the mammary gland in starvation that may be associated with the observed effects is the inactivation of pyruvate dehydrogenase on starvation (Kankel and Reinauer, 1976).

Glucose metabolism in the lactating mammary gland of the rat has been compared *in vitro* and *in vivo* (Robinson and Williamson, 1977b). The authors evaluated the effects of starvation, prolactin deficiency (produced by bromocryptine injection) and insulin deficiency (produced by streptozotocin injection) on glucose metabolism *in vivo*. The results showed that there was a significant decrease in glucose uptake only in starved animals. This was accompanied by a release of lactate and pyruvate from the gland. In preparations of acini from the glands of starved, insulin-deficient, or prolactin-deficient rats, there was a greater production of lactate and pyruvate from glucose than in preparations from normal rats. This may result from a decrease in the proportion of active pyruvate dehydrogenase in these situations (Field and Coore, 1976; Kankel and Reinauer, 1976). Insulin did not increase the rate of glucose utilization in acini from normal rats but did cause a significant increase in the utilization of glucose by acini from glands of starved rats. However, insulin did not decrease the accumulation of lactate and pyruvate in any of the experiments.

The rate of lipogenesis measured from [1-^{14}C]glucose was decreased in preparations of acini obtained from mammary gland of starved, prolactin-deficient, and insulin-deficient animals. This may be related to the inactivation of pyruvate dehydrogenase, and it appears that insulin is unable to influence the interconversion of this enzyme in acini in these experiments, since accumulation of lactate and pyruvate could not be decreased (Robinson and Williamson, 1977b).

The central role of pyruvate dehydrogenase in the control of lipogenesis in nonruminant mammary gland is further suggested by studies on the enzyme in mammary gland of animals made prolactin-deficient by injection of bromocryptine. Field and Coore (1975) showed that pyruvate dehydrogenase in lactating rat mammary gland was inactivated *in vivo* by withdrawal of prolactin for 24 hours caused by injection of 2-bromo-α-ergocryptine. The inactivation was due to increased phosphorylation of the enzyme. At 12 or 21 days of lactation, but not at 4 days of lactation, the prolactin injection given at the same time as bromocryptine prevented the effect of the latter. Subsequently Field and Coore (1976) further investigated the situation at 4 days of lactation and concluded that plasma insulin may be involved, together with prolactin, in the control of enzyme activity. Prolactin may act by priming the tissue to respond directly to normal concentrations of circulating insulin, and by this means be responsible for the increased activation of the enzyme during the course of normal lactation.

Interpretation of the behavior of *in vitro* preparations obtained from lactating mammary gland must be made with caution when the observations are used to comment on the physiological behavior of the gland *in vivo*. Elkin and Kuhn (1975) have studied aerobic lactate production by mammary tissue and concluded that *in vitro* preparations (isolated cells and slices) showed extensive conversion of glucose into lactate, whereas this did not occur *in vivo*. Therefore aerobic lactate formation was considered to be not a normal feature of mammary tissue, but a consequence of some metabolic derangement of *in vitro* preparations. Studies have been made of the hormonal effects on pyruvate dehydrogenase in acini prepared by the method of Katz *et al.* (1974). The "total" activity of pyruvate dehydrogenase falls in these preparations while the degree of activation tends to rise during a 2-hour incubation period (Goheer and Coore, 1977). Similarly, it is not possible to maintain the rate of fatty acid synthesis or activity of fatty acid synthetase in explants prepared from the mammary gland of lactating rabbits (Table II).

The possible reasons for the deterioration of lactating mammary tissue *in vitro* are complex. Previously (Section II, D) the role of milk accumulation in triggering some type of feedback inhibition of biosynthetic processes and tissue response to hormones has been discussed. Whatever the reasons for the metabolic changes in mammary preparations *in vitro,* they should be borne in mind particularly when transposing results to *in vivo* systems.

It has been claimed that slices of lactating mammary gland are much better than cells (Bartley and Abraham, 1976) for metabolic studies and that acini prepared by the method of Katz *et al.* (1974) have advantages in terms of cellular homogeneity. However, responses of slices and acinar preparations to insulin have only been measured at high insulin concentrations (Williamson *et al.*, 1975; Robinson and Williamson, 1977b).

VI. LIPOGENESIS AND MAMMARY TUMORS

It has been suggested that the changes that may occur in neoplastic mammalian cells may be better understood in terms of molecular correlation (Weber, 1977). The molecular correlation concept supposes that the special gene expression in neoplastic cells could be identified from the pattern of gene expression measured by the concentration and isoenzymic distribution of key enzymes. The pattern of gene expression can be further correlated with neoplastic transformation and progression of the tumor cells. *Transformation-linked discriminants* in hepatomas have been defined as enzymes whose activities always increase or decrease on cell transformation. These changes are defined as being linked with the "reprogramming" of gene expression associated with malignant transformation. *Progression-linked discriminants* in hepatomas are defined as enzymes whose activities correlate with tumor malignancy. These changes are defined as being associated with different degrees of expression of the neoplastic program, for example in relation to tumor growth and malignancy. Irrespective of the generality of the model or applicability to the assimilated published data on enzymes in tumors, the model nevertheless provides a framework in which observations on amounts, activities, or isoenzymic patterns of enzymes can be considered. The question is whether there is sufficient data on lipogenic enzymes in mammary tumors to warrant evaluation in terms of the model.

In general, tumors seem to show abnormal lipid metabolism irrespective of the tissue of origin. The most significant metabolic derangement in several hepatomas is the lack of the normal response of lipogenesis to dietary manipulation (Sabine *et al.*, 1966, 1967; Majerus *et al.*, 1968; Elwood and Morris, 1968). Acetyl-CoA carboxylase, fatty acid synthetase (Majerus *et al.*, 1968), and a number of glycolytic and lipogenic enzymes (Sabine *et al.*, 1968) in hepatomas do not show the usual changes of activity in response to dietary manipulation. The molecular and antigenic properties of acetyl-CoA carboxylase from a hepatoma are identical to those of the enzyme from host liver (Majerus *et al.*, 1968). It seems possible therefore that the metabolic derangements may be fundamental to the neoplastic process (Sabine *et al.*, 1968) and that the enzymic changes may be transformation-linked events.

The changes in lipogenesis and the turnover of lipogenic enzymes that have been measured in mammary tumors are shown in Table V. Mouse mammary adenocarcinomas synthesize fatty acids from acetate and glucose at much lower rates than do lactating mouse mammary

TABLE V

LIPOGENESIS AND LIPOGENIC ENZYME TURNOVER IN MAMMARY TUMORS [a]

A. Lipogenesis

Parameter	Changes	References
Lipogenic rate	Reduced relative to that found in lactating mammary gland of mouse	Abraham and Bartley (1974); Bartley et al. (1971)
Fatty acid pattern	Low proportion of medium-chain fatty acids synthesized relative to the proportion in lactating mammary gland of the mouse	Abraham and Bartley (1974)

B. Enzymes

Enzyme	Species	Changes				Immunochemical properties	References
		Activity	Amount	Rate of synthesis	Rate of degradation		
Acetyl-CoA carboxylase	Rat	↓	?	?	?	Modified or much inactive enzyme	Ahmad et al. (1976)
Fatty acid synthetase	Mouse	↓	↓	?	?	Similar to enzyme in normal tissue	Lin et al. (1975)
Glucose-6-phosphate dehydrogenase	Rat	↑	↑	↑	$t_{1/2} = 17$ hr	Similar to enzyme in normal tissue	Ringler and Hilf (1975)

[a] ↑ or ↓ represents an increase or decrease, respectively, in the parameter indicated. All parameters for each enzyme are expressed relative to those for the enzyme in lactating mammary gland, except for glucose-6-phosphate dehydrogenase, where the parameters are expressed relative to those for the enzyme in virgin mammary gland.

gland, and the proportion of medium-chain fatty acids produced by preneoplastic or neoplastic mammary tissue is much lower than in normal lactating mammary gland (Bartley *et al.*, 1971; Abraham and Bartley, 1974). Thus the tumors may have a defect in production of the fatty acids characteristic of mouse milk. Since the molecular and antigenic properties of fatty acid synthetase prepared from both normal and neoplastic tissue appear to be identical, the defect may be in the factors that control fatty acid chain length (Lin *et al.*, 1975). In a recent report (Ahmad *et al.*, 1976) it was shown by immunochemical methods that either acetyl-CoA carboxylase in rat mammary tumors was antigenically distinct from the enzyme in normal tissue, or that large amounts of inactive enzyme must be present in the tumors.

It seems that defects in lipogenesis, and in the amounts and possibly the molecular properties of lipogenic enzymes, occur in mammary tumors as compared to lactating mammary gland. However, comparison of the results with those observed in lactating tissue may lead to difficulties in interpretation of the data. There is no *a priori* reason why the changes in gene expression in neoplastic mammary epithelial cells should be obvious in relation to gene expression in lactating cells. Quite the opposite might be expected if the transformation- or progression-linked discriminants concern enzymes active in cell proliferation rather than cell differentiation, since these may be mutually exclusive processes in some cell types. It is worth noting in this context that the amount and rate of synthesis of glucose-6-phosphate dehydrogenase is increased in rat mammary tumors (Table V). This change is not related to a lipogenic function, but it is probably related to the provision of substrates for mitogenic events in the cells.

Extensive studies have been carried out on the dehydrogenase enzymes of the pentose phosphate pathway, particularly glucose-6-phosphate dehydrogenase (G6PDH) in transplantable and 7,12-dimethylbenz[α]anthracene (DMBA)-induced mammary tumors. The changes in the activities of these enzymes are not necessarily related to lipogenic capacity in the tumors but deserve study because they may relate to tumor growth, regression, and hormone dependency. Glucose-6-phosphate dehydrogenase activity is increased in mammary tumors (Hershey *et al.*, 1966; Hilf *et al.*, 1970). Pharmacological doses of estradiol-17β bring about an unsustained biphasic increase in the activity of G6PDH (isoenzyme 2) in transplantable R 3230 AC mammary adenocarcinomas in Fischer rats. An unsustained larger monophasic increase was obtained in the host animal mammary gland. The hormone-induced increases in enzyme activities, expressed on a DNA basis, were considerably greater than could be attributed to cellular proliferation, which prompted the authors to suggest that estrogen was affecting the dehydrogenases both in normal tissue and in the tumor (Richards and Hilf, 1972a). It is interesting to note that the growth rate of the R 3230 AC tumor is decreased after administration of estrogen (Hilf, 1968) and a "lactation-like" response occurs, which is characterized by the appearance of a milklike fluid that contained casein, lactose, and short-chain fatty acids (Hilf, 1967; Hilf *et al.*, 1967; Zalenski and Hilf, 1974). Thus, although G6PDH activity is increased in R 3230 AC mammary tumors [approximately 4-fold (Richards and Hilf, 1972a), the further large estrogen-induced increase in G6PDH activity is associated with a lactation-like response, but in a reduced manner (Ringler and Hilf, 1975). The results indicate that the tumor can undergo some lactogenic differentiation in response to pharmacological doses of estrogen, although in more slowly proliferating cells (Hilf, 1968). It is possible, therefore, that biosynthetic processes in the tumor, including lipogenesis, may be progression-linked discriminants in the sense that the processes are related to growth and therefore to malignancy. Further studies are required to clarify the situation.

Ringler and Hilf (1975) have shown by immunochemical methods that administration of estradiol-17β results in a 2-fold increase in G6PDH activity which is preceded by a 5-fold increase in the rate of synthesis of the enzyme. Tumors induced by DMBA are hormone-dependent and require estrogens and prolactin for neoplastic growth (Meites, 1972). Many DMBA-induced mammary tumors are also insulin dependent, as shown in alloxan-induced (Hueson and Legros, 1970, 1972; Hueson *et al.*, 1972) and streptozotocin-induced (Cohen and Hilf, 1974) diabetic animals. A decrease in flux through the pentose phosphate pathway, glycolysis, and a reduced production of fatty acids occurs in regressing tumors in rats treated with streptozotocin (Cohen and Hilf, 1974). Hence DMBA-induced mammary tumors should be considered to be insulin-, prolactin-, and estrogen-dependent (Cohen and Hilf, 1974).

It is interesting that many DMBA-induced mammary tumors will regress after treatment with pharmacological doses of estrogen (Teller *et al.*, 1966). When rats were treated with estradiol, tumors regressed in 75% of the animals, but in streptozotocin-induced diabetic rats the tumors regressed in every animal. Estrogen treatment therefore appeared to enhance the effects of diabetes; this suggests that insulin deprival plus estrogen therapy may have additive effects (Cohen and Hilf, 1975). Estrogen treatment caused little change in the activities of hexokinase, phosphofructokinase, and pyruvate kinase and a slight increase in 6-phosphogluconate dehydrogenase and

G6PDH in tumors from normal rats. However, in tumors from diabetic rats estrogen treatment decreased the activities of pyruvate kinase, phosphofructokinase, and 6-phosphogluconate dehydrogenase compared to their activities in tumors of normal rats (Cohen and Hilf, 1975). These authors state that estrogen treatment did not result in the previously noted increase in G6PDH activity in DMBA tumors, but it did reverse the decrease in G6PDH activity in the tumors brought about by insulinemia.

The role of cAMP in tumor growth and regression has been studied, and it has been found that dibutyryl-cAMP treatment of rats bearing mammary tumors results in arrested growth of the tumors (Cho-Chung and Gullino, 1973a,b). Subsequently it was shown that injection of dibutyryl-cAMP into rats bearing MTW9 mammary carcinoma resulted in early disappearance of microsomal G6PDH activity, while mitochondrial and cytosol activities were not affected (Cho-Chung and Berghoffer, 1974). Prolonged treatment of rats bearing 5123 hepatoma with dibutyryl-cAMP significantly decreased G6PDH in all subcellular compartments but did not alter host liver activities. Since dibutyryl-cAMP arrested growth of these tumors the authors suggested that the loss of G6PDH may be an early event in the inhibition of tumor growth *in vivo* (Cho-Chung and Berghoffer, 1974).

It is worth considering the effect of cAMP on tumor G6PDH in relation to other known effects of cAMP on enzymes involved in lipogenesis. Rudack *et al.* (1971) have shown that cAMP could prevent the induction of G6PDH in rat liver that normally occurs in response to feeding fasted rats on a fat-free diet. These authors concluded that cAMP prevented the synthesis of lipogenic enzymes including G6PDH. Dibutyryl-cAMP prevents the increase in lipogenic enzyme activities that normally occur in mammary explants in response to hormones (Sapag-Hagar *et al.,* 1974), and, in the case of fatty acid synthetase, this effect is caused by inhibition of the increased rate of synthesis of the enzyme that normally occurs in the presence of hormones (Speake *et al.,* 1976b). Increased cAMP concentrations may therefore exert an antilipogenic effect in liver, in mammary gland, and possibly in tumors from these tissues. This effect may be part of an enhanced tissue catabolism which is known to be promoted by cAMP in regressing tumors (Cho-Chung and Gullino, 1973a); cAMP probably activates lysosomal enzymes in the early stages of tumor regression (Lanzerotti and Gullino, 1972). The decrease in the number of estrogen-binding receptors of regressing DMBA-induced tumors in ovariectomized animals (Gibson and Hilf, 1976) may be part of the enhanced tissue catabolism in regressing tumors.

At present it is difficult to decide whether lipogenic enzymes are transformation- or progression-linked discriminants in mammary tumors. However, some mammary tumors may retain the potential for lactogenic response to hormones, at least when administered in pharmacological doses.

ACKNOWLEDGMENTS

I would like to thank Miss Janice Saxton for completing the illustrations, Mr.N. Paskin for reading and correcting the manuscript, and Mrs. Jenny Paxton for typing the manuscript.

REFERENCES

Abercrombie, M. (1967). *Cell Differ., Ciba Found. Symp., 1967* pp. 3–12.

Abraham, S., and Bartley, J. C. (1974). *In* "Hormones and Cancer" (K. McKerns, ed.), p. 29. Academic Press, New York.

Abraham, S., Cady, P., and Chaikoff, I. L. (1960). *Endocrinology* **66**, 280.

Abraham, S., Matthes, K. J., and Chaikoff, I. L. (1961). *Biochim. Biophys. Acta* **49**, 268.

Agradi, E., Libertini, L., and Smith, S. (1976). *Biochem. Biophys. Res. Commun.* **68**, 894.

Ahmad, F., Ahmad, P., and Schildknecht, D. (1976). *In* "Cancer Enzymology" (J. Schultz and F. Ahmad, eds.), p. 229. Academic Press, New York.

Allred, J. B., and Roehrig, K. L. (1973). *J. Biol. Chem.* **248**, 4131.

Anderson, R. R. (1974). *In* "Lactation: A Comprehensive Treatise" (B. L. Larson and V. R. Smith, eds.), Vol. 1, p. 97. Academic Press, New York.

Baldwin, R. L., and Milligan, L. P. (1966). *J. Biol. Chem.* **241**, 2058.

Baldwin, R. L. and Yang, Y. T. (1974). *In* "Lactation: A Comprehensive Treatise" (B. L. Larson and V. R. Smith, eds.), Vol. 1, p. 349. Academic Press, New York.

Barnawell, E. B. (1965). *J. Exp. Zool.* **160**, 189.

Bartley, J. C., and Abraham, S. (1976). *J. Lipid Res.* **17**, 467.

Bartley, J. C., Abraham, S., and Chaikoff, I. L. (1967). *Biochim. Biophys. Acta* **144**, 51.

Bartley, J. C., McGrath, H., and Abraham, S. (1971). *Cancer Res.* **31**, 527.

Bauman, D. E., and Davis, C. L. (1974). *In* "Lactation, A Comprehensive Treatise" (B. L. Larson and V. R. Smith, eds.), Vol. 1, p. 31. Academic Press, New York.

Bauman, D. E., Brown, R. E., and Davis, C. L. (1970). *Arch. Biochem. Biophys.* **140**, 237.

Berlin, C. M., and Schimke, R. T. (1965). *Mol. Pharmacol.* **1**, 149.

Betts, S. A., and Mayer, R. J. (1975). *Biochem. J.* **151**, 263.

Betts, S. A., and Mayer, R. J. (1977). *Biochim. Biophys. Acta* **496**, 302.

Birkinshaw, M., and Falconer, I. R. (1972). *J. Endocrinol.* **55**, 323.

Bolton, C. E. (1971). *J. Endocrinol.* **51**, 31.

Bricker, L. A., and Levey, G. S. (1972). *J. Biol. Chem.* **247**, 4914.

Brindley, D. N. (1978). *In* "Regulation of Fatty Acid and Glycerolipid Metabolism" (R. Dils and J. Knudsen, eds.) p. 31. Pergamon, Oxford.

Butcher, R. W. (1970). *Horm. Metab. Res.* **2**, Suppl. 2, 102.

Carey, E. M. (1977). *Biochim. Biophys. Acta* **486**, 91.

Carey, E. M., and Dils, R. (1972). *Biochem. J.* **126**, 1005.

Carey, E. M., and Dils, R. (1973a). *Comp. Biochem. Physiol. B* **44**, 989.

Carey, E. M., and Dils, R. (1973b). *Biochim. Biophys. Acta* **306**, 156.

Chadwick, A. (1971). *J. Endocrinol.* **49**, 1.

Chan, L., and O'Malley, B. W. (1976). *N. Engl. J. Med.* **294**, 1322.

Chee, P. Y., and Swick, R. W. (1976). *J. Biol. Chem.* **251**, 1029.

Chivers, L., Knudsen, J., and Dils, R. (1976). *Biochim. Biophys. Acta* **487**, 361.

Cho-Chung, Y. S., and Berghoffer, B. (1974). *Biochem. Biophys. Res. Commun.* **60**, 528.

Cho-Chung, Y. S., and Gullino, P. M. (1973a). *Science* **183**, 87.

Cho-Chung, Y. S., and Gullino, P. M. (1973b). *J. Natl. Cancer Inst.* **52**, 995.

Clark, S. M. (1976). Ph.D. Thesis, University of Nottingham.

Cohen, N. D., and Hilf, R. (1974). *Cancer Res.* **34**, 3245.

Cohen, N. D., and Hilf, R. (1975). *Proc. Soc. Exp. Biol. Med.* **148**, 339.

Collier, R. J., Bauman, D. E., and Hays, R. L. (1977). *Endocrinology* **100**, 1192.

Conde, R. D., and Scornik, O. A. (1976). *Biochem. J.* **158**, 385.

Conde, R. D., and Scornik, O. A. (1977). *Biochem. J.* **166**, 115.

Cowie, A. T. (1969). *In* "Lactogenesis: The Initiation of Milk Secretion at Parturition" (M. Reynolds and S. J. Folley, eds.), p. 157. Univ. of Pennsylvania Press, Philadelphia.

Cowie, A. T., and Tindall, J. S. (1971). "The Physiology of Lactation," p. 137. Williams & Wilkins, Baltimore, Maryland.

Cowie, A. T., and Watson, S. C. (1966). *J. Endocrinol.* **35**, 213.

Cowie, A. T., Hartmann, P. E., and Turvey, A. (1969). *J. Endocrinol.* **43**, 651.

Craig, R. K., Brown, P. A., Harrison, O. S., McIlreavy, D., and Campbell, P. N. (1976). *Biochem. J.* **160**, 57.

Denamur, R. (1969a). *Prog. Endocrinol., Proc. Int. Congr., Endocrinol., 3rd, 1968* Excerpta Med. Found. Int. Congr. Ser. No. 184, p. 959.

Denamur, R. (1969b). *In* "Lactogenesis: The Initiation of Milk Secretion at Parturition" (M. Reynolds and S. J. Folley, eds.), pp. 53–64. Univ. of Pennsylvania Press, Philadelphia.

Denamur, R. (1971). *J. Dairy Res.* **38**, 237.

Dils, R. R. (1977). *In* "Lipid Metabolism in Mammals" (F. Snyder, ed.), Vol. 2, p. 131. Plenum, New York.

Djiane, J., Durand, P., and Kelly, P. A. (1977). *Endocrinology* **100**, 1348.

Durand, P., and Djiane, J. (1977). *J. Endocrinol.* **75**, 33.

Elkin, A. R., and Kuhn, N. J. (1975). *Biochem. J.* **146**, 273.

Elwood, J. C., and Morris, H. P. (1968). *J. Lipid Res.* **9**, 337.

Ephrussi, B. (1972). "Hybridization of Somatic Cells." Princeton Univ. Press, Princeton, New Jersey.

Field, B., and Coore, H. G. (1975). *Biochem. Soc. Trans.* **3**, 258.

Field, B., and Coore, H. G. (1976). *Biochem. J.* **156**, 333.

Forsyth, I. A. (1971). *J. Dairy Res.* **38**, 419.

Forsyth, I. A., Strong, C. R., and Dils, R. (1972). *Biochem. J.* **129**, 929.

Gibson, S. L., and Hilf, R. (1976). *Cancer Res.* **36**, 3736.

Goheer, M., and Coore, H. G. (1977). *Biochem. Soc. Trans.* (in press).

Goldberg, A. L., and St. John, A. C. (1976). *Annu. Rev. Biochem.* **45**, 747.

Goldberg, N. D., O'Dea, R. F., and Haddox, M. K. (1973). *Adv. Cyclic Nucleotide Res.* **3**, 155.

Green, C. D., Skarda, J., and Barry, J. M. (1971). *Biochim. Biophys. Acta* **244**, 377.

Gul, B., and Dils, R. (1969). *Biochem. J.* **111**, 263.

Gumaa, K. A., Greenbaum, L., and McLean, P. (1973). *Eur. J. Biochem.* **34**, 188.

Hallowes, R. C., Wang, D. Y., Lewis, D. J., Strong, C. R., and Dils, R. (1973). *J. Endocrinol.* **57**, 265.

Hawkins, R. A., and Williamson, D. H. (1972). *Biochem. J.* **129**, 1171.

Hers, H. G. (1976). *Annu. Rev. Biochem.* **45**, 167.

Hershey, F. B., Johnston, G., Murphy, S. M., and Schmitt, M. (1966). *Cancer Res.* **26**, 265.

Hersko, A., Mamont, P., Shields, R., and Tomkins, G. M. (1971). *Nature (London), New Biol.* **232**, 206.

Hilf, R. (1967). *Science* **155**, 826.

Hilf, R. (1968). *Cancer Res.* **28**, 1888.

Hilf, R., Michel, I., and Bell, C. (1967). *Recent Prog. Horm. Res.* **23**, 229.

Hilf, R., Goldenberg, H., Bell, C., Michel, I., Orlando, R. A., and Archer, F. L. (1970). *Enzymol. Biol. Clin.* **11**, 162.

Hill, J. M., and Malamud, M. (1974). *FEBS Lett.* **46**, 308.

Holtzer, H., and Abbot, J. (1968). *In* "The Stability of the Differentiated State" (H. Ursprüng, ed.), p. 1. Springer-Verlag, Berlin and New York.

Houdebine, L.-M. (1976). *Eur. J. Biochem.* **68**, 219.

Houdebine, L. M., and Gaye, P. (1975). *Mol. Cell. Endocrinol.* **3**, 37.

Hueson, J. C., and Legros, N. (1970). *Eur. J. Cancer* **6**, 349.

Hueson, J. C., and Legros, N. (1972). *Cancer Res.* **32**, 226.

Hueson, J. C., Legros, N., and Heimann, R. (1972). *Cancer Res.* **32**, 233.

Jones, E. A. (1967). *Biochem. J.* **103**, 403.

Jones, E. A. (1972). *Biochem. J.* **126**, 67.

Kankel, K.-F., and Reinauer, H. (1976). *Diabetologia* **12**, 149.

Katz, J., and Wals, P. A. (1972). *Biochem. J.* **128**, 879.

Katz, J. P., Wals, P. A., and Van de Velde, R. L. (1974). *J. Biol. Chem.* **249**, 7348.

Knudsen, J. (1976). *Comp. Biochem. Physiol. B* **53**, 3.

Knudsen, J., and Dils, R. (1975). *Biochem. Biophys. Res. Commun.* **63**, 780.

Knudsen, J., Clark, S., and Dils, R. (1975). *Biochem. Biophys. Res. Commun.* **65**, 921.

Knudsen, J., Clark, S., and Dils, R. (1976). *Biochem. J.* **160**, 683.

Kuhn, N. J. (1969). *J. Endocrinol.* **44**, 39.

Lanzerotti, R. H., and Gullino, P. M. (1972). *Cancer Res.* **32**, 2679.

Leader, D. P., and Barry, J. M. (1969). *Biochem. J.* **113**, 175.

Levy, H. R. (1964). *Biochim. Biophys. Acta* **84**, 229.

Libertini, L., Lin, C.-Y., and Smith, S. (1976). *Fed. Proc., Fed. Am. Soc. Exp. Biol.* **35**, 1671.

Lin, C.-Y., Smith, S., and Abraham, S. (1975). *Cancer Res.* **35**, 3094.

Mackall, J. C., and Lane, D. M. (1977). *Biochem. J.* **162**, 635.

McLean, P. (1964). *Biochem. J.* **90**, 271.

McLean, P., Greenbaum, A. L., and Gumaa, K. A. (1972). *FEBS Lett.* **20**, 277.

Majerus, P. W., Jacobs, R., Smith, M. B., and Morris, H. P. (1968). *J. Biol. Chem.* **243**, 3588.

Manning, R., Dils, R., and Mayer, R. J. (1976). *Biochem. Soc. Trans.* **4**, 241.

Mayer, R. J., and Paskin, N. (1978). *In* "Regulation of Fatty Acid and Glycerolipid Metabolism" (R. Dils and J. Knudsen, eds.), p. 53. Pergamon, Oxford.

Mayne, R., and Barry, J. M. (1970). *J. Endocrinol.* **46**, 61.

Meites, J. (1972). *J. Natl. Cancer Inst.* **48**, 1217.

Mellenberger, R. W., and Bauman, D. E. (1974). *Biochem. J.* **138**, 373.

Mellenberger, R. W., Bauman, D. E., and Nelson, D. R. (1973). *Biochem. J.* **136**, 741.

Mepham, B. (1976). "The Secretion of Milk," Inst. Biol., Stud. Biol. No. 60. Arnold, London.

Mills, E. S., and Topper, Y. J. (1970). *J. Cell Biol.* **44**, 310.

Millward, D. J., Garlick, P. J., Stewart, R. J. C., Nnanyelugo, D. O., and Waterlow, J. C. (1975). *Biochem. J.* **150**, 235.

Moretti, R. L., and Abraham, S. (1966). *Biochim. Biophys. Acta* **124**, 280.

Morkin, E., Kimata, S., and Skillman, J. J. (1972). *Circ. Res.* **30**, 690.

Morrison, W. R. (1970). *Top. Lipid Chem.* **1**, 51.

Murphy, G., and Walker, D. G. (1974). *Biochem. J.* **144**, 149.

Nakanishi, S., Tanabe, T., Horikawa, S., and Numa, S. (1976). *Proc. Natl. Acad. Sci. U.S.A.* **73**, 2304.

Oka, T., and Perry, J. W. (1974). *J. Biol. Chem.* **249**, 3586.

Paskin, N., and Mayer, R. J. (1977). *Biochim. Biophys. Acta* **474**, 1.

Paton, S., and Jensen, R. (1975). *Prog. Chem. Fats Other Lipids* **14**, 163.

Pette, D., Luh, W., and Bücher, T. (1962a). *Biochem. Biophys. Res. Commun.* **7**, 419.

Pette, D., Klingenberg, M., and Bücher, T. (1962b). *Biochem. Biophys. Res. Commun.* **7**, 425.

Philippidis, H., Hanson, R. W., Reshef, L., Hopgood, M. F., and Ballard, F. J. (1972). *Biochem. J.* **126**, 1127.

Rannels, D. E., Li, J. B., Morgan, H. E., and Jefferson, L. S. (1975). *In* "Methods in Enzymology" (B. W. O'Malley and J. G. Hardman, eds.), Vol. 37, p. 238. Academic Press, New York.

Richards, A. H., and Hilf, R. (1972a). *Cancer Res.* **32**, 611.

Richards, A. H., and Hilf, R. (1972b). *Endocrinology* **91**, 287.

Ringler, M. B., and Hilf, R. (1975). *Biochim. Biophys. Acta* **411**, 50.

Rivera, E. M., and Cummins, E. P. (1971). *Gen. Comp. Endocrinol.* **17**, 319.

Robinson, H. M., and Williamson, D. H. (1977a). *Biochem. J.* **164**, 749.

Robinson, H. M., and Williamson, D. H. (1977b). *Biochem. J.* **164**, 153.

Rosen, J. M., Woo, S. L. C., and Comstock, J. P. (1975). *Biochemistry* **14**, 2895.

Rudack, D., Davie, B., and Hotten, D. (1971). *J. Biol. Chem.* **246**, 7823.

Rutter, W. J., Ball, W. D., Bradshaw, W. S., Clark, W. R., and Sanders, T. G. (1968a). *Exp. Biol. Med.* **1**, 110.

Rutter, W. J., Clark, W. R., Kemp, J. D., Bradshaw, W. S., Sanders, T. G., and Ball, W. D. (1968b). *In* "Epithelial-Mesenchymal Interactions" (R. Fleischmajer and R. E. Billingham, eds.), p. 114. Williams & Wilkins, Baltimore, Maryland.

Rutter, W. J., Pictet, R. L., and Morris, P. W. (1973). *Annu. Rev. Biochem.* **42**, 601.

Sabine, J. R., Abraham, S., and Chaikoff, I. L. (1966). *Biochim. Biophys. Acta* **116**, 407.

Sabine, J. R., Abraham, S., Morris, H. P., and Chaikoff, I. L. (1967). *Cancer Res.* **27**, 793.

Sabine, J. R., Abraham, S., and Morris, H. P. (1968). *Cancer Res.* **28**, 46.

Sapag-Hagar, M., and Greenbaum, A. L. (1974a). *FEBS Lett.* **46**, 180.

Sapag-Hagar, M., and Greenbaum, A. L. (1974b). *Eur. J. Biochem.* **47**, 303.

Sapag-Hagar, M., Greenbaum, A. L., Lewis, D. J., and Hallowes, R. C. (1974). *Biochem. Biophys. Res. Commun.* **59**, 261.

Scornik, O. A. (1972). *Biochem. Biophys. Res. Commun.* **47**, 1063.

Scornik, O. A., and Botbol, V. (1976). *J. Biol. Chem.* **251**, 2891.

Shain, W. G., Hilfer, S. R., and Fonte, V. G. (1972). *Dev. Biol.* **28**, 202.

Smith, S., and Abraham, S. (1975). *Adv. Lipid Res.* **13**, 195.

Smith, S., and Dils, R. (1966). *Biochim. Biophys. Acta* **116**, 23.

Smith, S., Watts, R., and Dils, R. (1968). *J. Lipid Res.* **9**, 52.

Smith, S., Agradi, E., Libertini, L., and Dileepan, K. N. (1976). *Proc. Natl. Acad. Sci. U.S.A.* **73**, 1184.

Speake, B. K., Dils, R., and Mayer, R. J. (1975). *Biochem. J.* **148**, 309.

Speake, B. K., Dils, R., and Mayer, R. J. (1976a). *Biochem. Soc. Trans.* **4**, 238.

Speake, B. K., Dils, R., and Mayer, R. J. (1976b). *Biochem. J.* **154**, 359.

Stockdale, F. E., and Topper, Y. J. (1966). *Proc. Natl. Acad. Sci. U.S.A.* **56**, 1283.

Strauss, A. W., Alberts, A. W., Hennessy, S., and Vagelos, P. R. (1975). *Proc. Natl. Acad. Sci. U.S.A.* **72,** 4366.

Strong, C. R., and Dils, R. (1972). *Biochem. J.* **128,** 1303.

Strong, C. R., Forsyth, I. A., and Dils, R. (1972). *Biochem. J.* **128,** 509.

Strong, C. R., Carey, E. M., and Dils, R. (1973). *Biochem. J.* **132,** 121.

Swick, R. W., and Ip, M. M. (1974). *J. Biol. Chem.* **249,** 6836.

Tanabe, T., Horikawa, S., Nakanishi, S., and Numa, S. (1976). *FEBS Lett.* **66,** 70.

Teller, M. N., Stock, C. C., Stohr, G., Merker, P. C., Kufman, R. J., Escher, G. C., and Bowie, M. (1966). *Cancer Res.* **26,** 245.

Terry, P. M., Banerjee, M. R., and Lui, R. M. (1977). *Proc. Natl. Acad. Sci. U.S.A.* **74,** 2441.

Topper, Y. J., and Oka, T. (1974). *In* "Lactation: A Comprehensive Treatise" (B. L. Larson and V. R. Smith, eds.), Vol. 1, p. 327. Academic Press, New York.

Tucker, H. A. (1974). *In* "Lactation: A Comprehensive Treatise" (B. L. Larson and V. R. Smith, eds.), Vol. 1, p. 277. Academic Press, New York.

Turkington, R. W., and Hill, R. L. (1969). *Science* **163,** 1458.

Turkington, R. W., Brew, K., Vanaman, T. C., and Hill, R. L. (1968). *J. Biol. Chem.* **243,** 3382.

Turner, C. W. (1970). *Mo., Agric. Exp. Stan., Res. Bull.* **977.**

Volpe, J. J., and Marasa, J. C. (1975). *Biochim. Biophys. Acta* **409,** 235.

Vondehaar, B. K., Owens, I. S., and Topper, Y. J. (1973). *J. Biol. Chem.* **248,** 467.

Walker, J. H., and Mayer, R. J. (1978). *In* "Techniques in the Life Sciences, Techniques in Protein and Enzyme Biochemistry" (H. L. Kornberg *et al.*, eds.), Vol. B1/11, B119; pp. 1–32. Elsevier, Amsterdam (in press).

Walker, J. H., Betts, S. A., Manning, R., and Mayer, R. J. (1976). *Biochem. J.* **159,** 355.

Waltham, P. C., and Carey, E. M. (1976). *Biochem. Soc. Trans.* **4,** 1147.

Wang, D. Y., Hallowes, R. C., Bealing, J., Strong, C. R., and Dils, R. (1972). *J. Endocrinol.* **53,** 311.

Weber, G. (1977). *N. Engl. J. Med.* **296,** 486.

Williamson, D. H., McKeown, S. R., and Ilic, V. (1975). *Biochem. J.* **150,** 145.

Yu, H.-L., and Burton, D. N. (1974). *Arch. Biochem. Biophys.* **161,** 297.

Zalenski, D., and Hilf, R. (1974). *Cancer Biochem. Biophys.* **1,** 1.

VITAMINS AND HORMONES, VOL. 36

Biological Effects of Antibodies to Gonadal Steroids

EBERHARD NIESCHLAG AND E. JEAN WICKINGS*

Abteilung Experimentelle Endokrinologie, Universitäts-Frauenklinik, Münster, Federal Republic of Germany

I. INTRODUCTION

The neutralization of biologically active molecules is one of the basic principles of immunology. Intensive research in this field has yielded a succession of practical applications in medicine of which immunization against diphtheria and snake toxins may be mentioned as examples. However, endocrinologists have shown little interest in the ability of antibodies to neutralize the biological activity of hormones and to exploit this property as a research tool and as a means of therapy. They were confronted with these immunological problems only when a patient had developed a resistance to insulin, growth hormone, or ACTH during the course of treatment with that hormone, owing to the appearance of antibodies. Upon investigating the phenomenon of insulin resistance it could be shown for the first time that hormones are capable

* Our own investigations were supported by grants from the Deutsche Forschungsgemeinschaft.

of inducing antibody formation (Depisch and Hasenörl, 1928; Lewis, 1937; Banting et al., 1938). Indeed, it was surprising that the organism could produce antibodies against one of its own body constituents. More recently, cases of spontaneous development of antibodies against insulin have also been described, even though the patient had never received insulin (Følling and Norman, 1972; Hirata et al., 1973).

Interest in antibodies against hormones was greatly stimulated after the introduction of the principle of radioimmunoassay for hormone analysis (Yalow and Berson, 1959). These sensitive techniques could ultimately be extended to the measurement of all protein and peptide hormones. Radioimmunological methods gave great impetus to all fields of endocrinology. Whereas the production of antibodies against high-molecular-weight protein hormones provided no major problems, it proved more difficult to render the low-molecular-weight steroids antigenic. A steroid can become immunogenic only as a hapten coupled to a larger carrier molecule. Many futile attempts were made to produce stable steroid–protein conjugates for immunization. In the first experiments the steroid was coupled to the protein with an ester link, which proved to be very labile in vivo and was probably hydrolyzed before the conjugate could develop antigenic properties (Mooser and Grilliches, 1941). Not until the mid 1950s did it become possible to synthesize stable conjugates capable of inducing antibody production in experimental animals (Erlanger et al., 1957; Goodfriend and Sehon, 1958). The first application of steroid antisera was the investigation of biological activity of these hormones using passive immunization (Lieberman et al., 1959). It was only a decade later that these antisera were used in the development of radioimmunoassays for steroids (Abraham, 1969; Mikhail et al., 1970). Since that time radioimmunoassays have been established for most steroids of clinical or physiological significance; this has led to the immunization of countless experimental animals for the production of antibodies (for reviews, see Skelley et al., 1973; James and Jeffcoate, 1974; Nieschlag and Wickings, 1975). However, the interest in the biological effects resulting from immunization with steroids has remained confined to a small group of researchers.

This presentation reviews investigations of the biological effects of antibodies to gonadal steroids on male and female reproductive functions and the application of steroid antisera as tools in reproduction research. This review follows on from the first by Ferin et al. (1973), which appeared in this series 5 years ago. It serves to bring the reader up to date and, in addition, places a special emphasis on male reproductive functions.

To understand the phenomena described here it is important to bear in mind the differences between active and passive immunization. In active immunization the effects of the antibodies are investigated in the immunized animal itself, whereas in passive immunization, antibodies are transferred from actively immunized animals to recipients. The duration of the effects following passive immunization is limited by the relatively short half-life of the immunoglobulins. Repeated injections of antisera may cause serum sickness and anaphylactic reactions. High antibody concentrations can be maintained in experimental animals by active immunization without running the risk of these undesirable side effects, but other immunological problems may occur.

II. Production and Characterization of Antibodies to Steroids

A. Production of Antibodies

1. *Steroid–Protein Conjugates*

To become immunogenic, the low-molecular-weight steroid must be covalently coupled as a hapten to a larger carrier molecule, usually a protein. One prerequisite for a carrier protein is that it have sufficient lysine residues on the surface of the molecule to which the steroid can be coupled. Although several macromolecules have been investigated as suitable carriers (e.g., thyroglobulin, hemocyanin, poly-L-lysine, human serum albumin), bovine serum albumin (BSA) remains the most widely used carrier. All the studies incorporated in this review have used steroid–BSA conjugates for immunization.

The actual coupling of the steroid to the protein is brought about by either a mixed anhydride reaction (hemisuccinate or o-carboxymethyloxime) (Erlanger *et al.*, 1957, 1967) or a carbodiimide reaction (Goodfriend and Sehon, 1970). Both these methods make use of oxygen functions on the steroid skeleton. In the final conjugate the ratio of steroid molecules coupled per protein molecule is usually 8:1 to 30:1. No convincing evidence has yet been produced which demonstrates that the actual steroid:protein ratio influences the quality of the antiserum produced within these limits.

2. *Immunization*

a. Choice of Animals. Following the development of radioimmunoassay techniques, numerous methods for the production of antisera against steroids have been described in a great variety of animals. For radioimmunoassay purposes the major criterion for the choice of animal is the ability to produce suitable antibodies in large enough amounts. For biological studies, however, it is of great importance that the animal is physiologically and endocrinologically well defined. The rat is relatively unsuitable for raising antibodies for radioimmunoassay purposes because of its small blood volume and its poor immune response. It is, however, still used in biological studies since its reproductive functions have been extensively described. The rabbit is a very popular choice of animal for antibody production, as it responds well to immunization. It is, however, not suited for the study of ovarian cyclic feedback control, as it ovulates spontaneously. The rabbit is also a good source of antibodies for passive immunization (e.g., Ekre and Foote, 1972; Wuttke *et al.*, 1976), although because of their large blood volume bigger animals are preferred, such as sheep (Ferin *et al.*, 1968; Neill *et al.*, 1971; Neri *et al.*, 1964; ter Haar and MacKinnon, 1975) and goats (Furr and Smith, 1975). The possibility of using the steroid-immunized animals as a model for pathological conditions in the human, and to apply immunization with hormones in therapeutic medicine led to the use of subhuman primates, especially the rhesus monkey, as experimental animals (Sundaram *et al.*, 1973; Ferin *et al.*, 1974; Wickings and Nieschlag, 1978a). The limited availability of these animals and the difficulties of handling, however, restrict the suitability of the monkey. In addition, its similarity in respect to human reproductive functions may not be as complete as was originally assumed.

b. Immunization Schedules. The subcutaneous and the intradermal routes of administration have been applied for generating steroid antibodies for physiological studies. For primary immunization all investigators use complete Freund's adjuvant. The intradermal, multiple-site immunization technique has the advantages that only minute quantities of the antigen are required, no booster injections are necessary, and titers appear as early as 3 weeks after immunization. This method has, therefore, become the most widely used for producing antibodies for radioimmunoassay (Nieschlag and Wickings, 1975) and has also been applied successfully in physiological studies in our laboratory and in others (Nieschlag, 1975).

We have used this schedule for raising steroids in rabbits, rats, and monkeys. For this purpose, 100–300 μg of the steroid conjugate per animal are emulsified with complete Freund's adjuvant containing additional *Mycobacterium tuberculosis*. The emulsion is then injected into the back of the animal over about 20–30 sites intradermally, followed by a subcutaneous injection of 0.5 ml of pertussis vaccine.

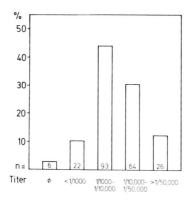

Fig. 1. Maximal antiserum titers attained in 211 rabbits after the one-time, multiple site, intradermal immunization against a testosterone-3-BSA conjugate.

Of a total of 211 rabbits only 6 (3%) did not respond or died before the third week; of the remaining, 10% showed maximal titers of up to 1/1000, 44% up to 1/10,000, and 43% of over 1/10,000 (Fig. 1). Rhesus monkeys immunized with this schedule responded well by producing titers greater than 1/10,000 (Fig. 2).

B. Characterization of Antibodies

1. *Titer*

For characterization of the antisera, the same parameters are evaluated as for radioimmunoassays (Abraham, 1974; Nieschlag and Wickings, 1975). Titer is defined as that antiserum dilution at which 50% of a given amount of labeled steroid is bound. The radioimmunological determination of titer is the easiest means of detecting the appearance and further development of specific antibodies. The specific antibody titer correlates neither with the total serum immunoglobulin concentration nor with the concentration of the individual immunoglobulins IgG and IgM (Fig. 2). The titer, however, correlates with the binding affinity as demonstrated in Fig. 3. The titer is influenced by the amount of steroid present in the serum as exemplified by the development of antiserum titers in testosterone-3-BSA immunized female, normal male, and castrated male rabbits (Fig. 4) (Wickings *et al.*, 1977).

The titer, although a useful parameter, is relatively imprecise for monitoring the immune response. It would be preferable if the actual mass of antibodies per unit volume serum or even the quotient of moles of antigen bound per mole of antibody were used as a more precise definition of antibody binding.

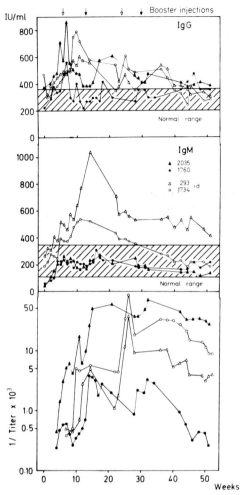

FIG. 2. Antiserum titers and serum immunoglobulin concentrations in four male rhesus monkeys actively immunized against testosterone.

2. Affinity

The binding affinity (K_a) of an antiserum for its antigen can be calculated by either a Scatchard plot (Feldman and Rodbard, 1971) or a Michaelis–Menten hyperbola (Odell *et al.*, 1971). In the second approach, the saturation data used in the calculation give an average affinity constant for the total heterogeneous population of antibody-binding sites, whereas a Scatchard plot is an indication of the number of antibody populations present. K_a is defined in the Michaelis–Menten

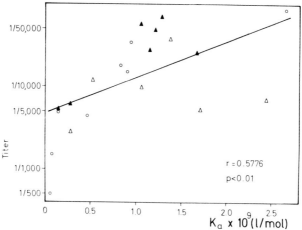

FIG. 3. Correlation between titer and binding affinity (K_a) in testosterone antisera from rhesus monkeys. $r = 0.5776$; $p < 0.01$. Sera (▲, △, ○) collected from three individual monkeys during the course of active immunization.

method as the reciprocal of the molar free (unbound) steroid concentration at half-saturation of the antibody-binding sites. Binding affinities calculated for population of steroid antibodies are of the order of 10^9 liters/mol and are thus about 100-fold higher than the affinities of the specific binding proteins, such as transcortin and testosterone-binding

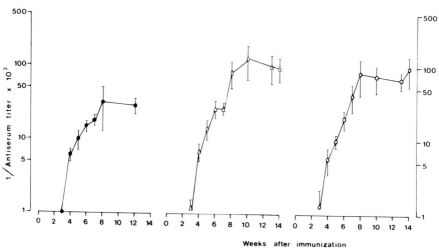

FIG. 4. Development of antiserum titers in male (●), female (△), and castrated male (○) rabbits following active immunization against testosterone. From Wickings *et al.* (1977).

globulin, but are in the same range as the binding affinities of the cellular steroid receptors.

3. Specificity

The specificity of the antibodies produced is one of the most important parameters for the interpretation of the results of physiological studies. It depends on the degree of crossreaction of the antiserum with other steroids and is established by displacement studies. The crossreaction is calculated from the ratio of the mass of immunogenic steroid required to displace 50% of the radiolabeled immunogenic steroid to the mass of crossreacting steroid required to displace the same fraction of the labeled steroid.

The factors governing specificity of antisera are not fully understood. While one cannot predict which part of the conjugate will act as the immunodeterminant site, it was soon recognized that resulting antisera were "far-sighted." That is, steroid antisera are specific for the part of the steroid moiety farthest from the site of conjugation to the carrier. Thus, if the steroid is coupled through ring D, configurations on ring A are recognized; while antisera against steroids coupled via ring A show the opposite properties and ring D is recognized. By introducing oxygen functions onto the B and C rings of the molecule, leaving the functional group on the A and D rings free, it has become possible to raise more specific antisera. For example, the use of 6-ketoestradiol as hapten has improved the specificity of the antisera for estradiol tremendously (Kuss and Goebel, 1972; Lindner et al., 1972), as has the use of 11α-hydroxyprogesterone for generating progesterone antisera (Spieler et al., 1972). For testosterone, however, the improvement in specificity using testosterone-7-BSA and testosterone-11-BSA conjugates is only moderate (Table I).

The crossreaction of the individual steroid can vary during the course of immunization. In female rabbits immunized with testosterone-3-BSA, the crossreactivity toward androstenedione increased from 3% to 12% over a 14-week period (Wickings et al., 1977). Immunization studies in male rhesus monkeys also revealed changes in antiserum specificity related to the immunization schedule (Fig. 5) (Wickings and Nieschlag, 1978b). These changes in specificity must be considered when interpreting the results from studies with active immunization.

The crossreactivity of antibodies determined in this fashion in vitro may not fully reflect the situation in vivo. In this respect it is important to differentiate between the ability of a steroid to bind to the antibody, and hence crossreact, and its ability to compete with the antigenic

TABLE I

Specificity of Antisera Raised against Different Testosterone–Bovine
Serum Albumin (T–BSA) Conjugates[a]

Steroid	Antiserum against				
	T-3-BSA	T-7-BSA	T-11-BSA	T-17-BSA	5α-DHT-3-BSA
Testosterone	100	100	100	100	100
5α-Dihydrotestosterone	60	42	15	NR	100
5β-Dihydrotestosterone	8	5	NR	NR	10
Androstenedione	0.3	1	2	31	0.5
Androstenediol	1.6	NR	0.16	0.05	NR
Progesterone	0.05	<0.1	NR	55	<0.001
Deoxycorticosterone	<0.001	<0.5	NR	55	<0.01

[a] The data on T-3-BSA and 5α-DHT–3-BSA stem from our laboratory; those on T-7-BSA from Weinstein *et al.* (1972); those on T-11-BSA from Hillier *et al.* (1973); those on T-17-BSA from Niswender and Midgley (1970). NR, not recorded.

steroid for the binding site. The first property is used in the *in vitro* assessment of crossreactivity, whereas the second may prevail *in vivo*.

4. Immunoglobulins

The actual mechanism of antibody synthesis within an immunized animal has stimulated little interest among endocrinologists. It should

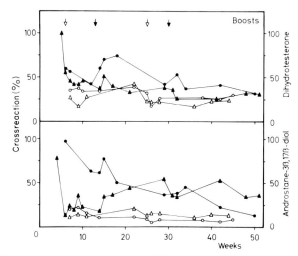

Fig. 5. Changes of crossreactivity toward dihydrotestosterone and androstanediol in testosterone antisera raised in 4 male rhesus monkeys immunized intradermally (O, △) or subcutaneously (●, ▲).

be remembered that the antibodies responsible for the endocrinological phenomena form only a small percentage of the total immune response to immunization. Immunization with antigens emulsified in complete Freund's adjuvant results in the production of antibodies to the components of the adjuvant, especially *M. tuberculosis*. Simultaneous injection of pertussis vaccine causes the production of further antibodies. In the case of steroid–protein conjugates, antibodies are also produced against the bridge and carrier moieties of the conjugate. None of these antibodies participates in the hormone-neutralizing ability of the antiserum. Hence, any immunological characterization of the antiserum, such as the measurement of the immunoglobulin fractions present, has little bearing on the endocrine properties of the antiserum.

Studies performed in the rhesus monkey demonstrate this quite clearly (Wickings and Nieschlag, 1978b). Two rhesus monkeys were immunized against testosterone-3-BSA using the multiple-site intradermal immunization technique; two further animals were immunized subcutaneously. In all 4 animals booster injections were given as indicated in the figure. Figure 2 shows the concentrations of IgG measured after immunization against testosterone. Whereas, after an initial increase, IgG levels fell to within the normal range after 40 weeks, antibody titers remained elevated for a much longer period. There was no difference in the IgG response between the two immunization schedules. Measurement of IgM levels, however, revealed significant differences between the two schemes of immunization. Whereas IgM levels in the subcutaneously immunized monkeys did not increase, there was a marked rise in IgM in the sera of the intradermally immunized monkeys. There was no correlation between antibody titer and immunoglobulin concentrations. The pattern of immunoglobulin concentrations, however, is of great importance when considering the side effects of immunization (see Section VI).

III. Effects on Male Reproductive Functions

A. Testicular Functions

1. Serum Steroid Concentrations

One of the most prominent features in the serum of male animals actively immunized with testosterone is the very high total serum testosterone concentration. These levels can be as high as 100-fold above normal. The testosterone concentrations start to rise rapidly as soon as specific steroid antibodies can be detected by radioimmunological techniques. This occurs as early as 3 weeks after immunization with the one-time, multiple-site, intradermal immunization technique. Testosterone concentrations increase parallel to the developing antibody titers for about 12 weeks after immunization in rabbits and rhesus monkeys as well as in rats (Hillier et al., 1975). After this time testosterone levels do not increase further but remain elevated as long as the animals have been observed, i.e., rabbits for 30 weeks (Thorneycroft et al., 1975) and monkeys for 1 year (Wickings and Nieschlag, 1978a).

The testes appear to be the exclusive source of these high testosterone concentrations, since castrated animals show no testosterone increase above castration levels during immunization, although they develop even higher titers than intact animals (Wickings et al., 1977).

Immunization with testosterone influences the serum concentrations of other steroids besides testosterone. For example, a 3- to 4-fold increase in Δ^4-androstenedione was observed in testosterone-immunized rabbits (Nieschlag et al., 1974). This would indicate a stimulation of the biosynthetic pathways for testosterone. In male monkeys immunized against testosterone serum dihydrotestosterone levels were 5- to 10-fold higher than control levels (Wickings and Nieschlag, 1978a). The elevated dihydrotestosterone levels reflect increased testicular secretion and increased binding to the antibodies that crossreact with dihydrotestosterone. They may also be caused by increased 5α-reduction in the enlarged tubular tissue mass, as a result of increased substrate availability in the hyperplastic testes.

2. Binding of Testosterone in Serum

The binding of testosterone in serum also increases at the same time as antibodies appear in serum and testosterone concentrations begin to increase. Using equilibrium dialysis to assess binding (Forest et al., 1968), the binding of testosterone in normal rabbits is about 90% (Nieschlag et al., 1973, 1974) and ranges from 90 to 95% in the rhesus monkey, depending on the season (Wickings and Nieschlag, 1978a). In rats, which have no specific sex hormone-binding globulin, binding of testosterone is about 65% (Hillier et al., 1975; Corvol and Bardin, 1973). With the development of antibodies, binding increases dramatically to almost 100% in all species investigated (Nieschlag et al., 1973; Hillier et al., 1975; Wickings and Nieschlag, 1978a).

It must be emphasized, however, that it is extremely difficult to generate exact results for the percentage binding using the available methodology, especially when the binding is very high. Therefore, the available data on the actual free-steroid concentration in immunized animals cannot be regarded as totally reliable. Nevertheless, when considered along with the other biological effects described in the following sections, it can be concluded that the non-protein-bound, free, biologically active fraction of serum testosterone is reduced in the immunized animals, despite the grossly elevated total testosterone concentrations.

3. Testosterone Production and Metabolism in Vivo

In order to elucidate the underlying mechanisms causing the extremely high serum testosterone levels, it was necessary to measure testosterone metabolism and production in the immunized animals. A negative correlation has been demonstrated between binding in serum and the metabolic clearance rate (Vermeulen et al., 1969), and hence a decreased metabolism of steroids in immunized animals is to be expected. Indeed, in rabbits immunized against aldosterone (Gless et al., 1974) and in female rhesus monkeys immunized against estradiol (Sundaram et al., 1973) a delayed disappearance of the respective radiolabeled steroid was observed. Longcope (1970) found that the half-life of estradiol in sheep immunized against this steroid was increased to 280 minutes, as compared to 40 minutes in normal ewes.

In male rabbits immunized against testosterone the half-life of the second component of the biphasic disappearance curve was twice as long as that in normal animals (45.4 ± 20 minutes, as compared to 22.5 ± 6.8 minutes; $p < 0.05$) (Wickings et al., 1976). The change in the gradients of the disappearance curves and of the constants α and β, as shown in Fig. 6, indicates that both the rate of transport between the inner and outer pools and the extent of metabolism in each pool are reduced. Hence, the testosterone that circulates bound to high-affinity antibodies is not readily exchangeable with the free fraction, indicating a reduction in the free fraction of testosterone. It is this free fraction that is responsible for the biological activity of the hormone (Vermeulen et al., 1971).

The decrease in the metabolic clearance rate, however, is not sufficient to maintain the extremely high circulating testosterone levels. These are also caused by an approximately 3-fold increase in plasma production of testosterone (1.20 ± 0.36 vs 0.44 ± 0.34 mg/day; $p < 0.05$) (Wickings et al., 1976). The testosterone production in 2 immunized male rhesus monkeys was also elevated to 13.7 and 62 mg/day from 1.2 ± 0.3 mg/day in normal controls (Wickings and Nieschlag, 1977). These findings indicate that the extremely high peripheral testosterone levels are caused by a decreased metabolic clearance rate as well as an increased production rate.

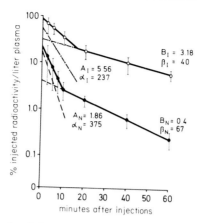

FIG. 6. Disappearance of radiolabeled testosterone from the serum of normal (●—●, ---; $n = 6$) and testosterone-immunized (○—○, -·-; $n = 4$) rabbits, used for the calculation of the metabolic clearance rate of testosterone. From Wickings et al. (1976).

4. Testosterone Production in Vitro

Parallel to the findings of an increased testosterone production in vivo, increased testicular testosterone production in vitro was also observed in immunized rabbits (Nieschlag et al., 1975a). The testosterone produced by sections of testicular tissue from testosterone-immunized rabbits incubated with hCG for 6 hours exceeded that of normal rabbits by a factor of 1.8 (see Fig. 7). The basal testosterone concentrations in the testicular tissue of testosterone-immunized rabbits were also elevated (475 ± 189 vs 180 ± 95 ng/gm wet tissue).

Hence the immunization as such would not seem to exercise any deleterious effects on testicular function, as is the case in autoimmune orchitis (Bishop, 1970; Rümke and Hekman, 1975). In fact, the testes of testosterone-immunized animals appear to have an increased endocrine capacity, paralleling the morphological signs of hypertrophy and hyperplasia.

5. Testicular Morphology

Having observed the endocrine hyperfunction of the testis, it was of interest to investigate whether the altered function was accompanied by any morphological changes. In testosterone-immunized rabbits (Nieschlag et al., 1973), rats (Hillier et al., 1975), and monkeys (Wickings and Nieschlag, 1978a) increased testicular volume and/or weight has been observed (Fig. 8). In rabbits histological examination of the testes (Figs. 9 and 10) revealed a 2- to 3-fold increase in the number of Leydig cells and a 36% increase in the nuclear volume of these cells. As

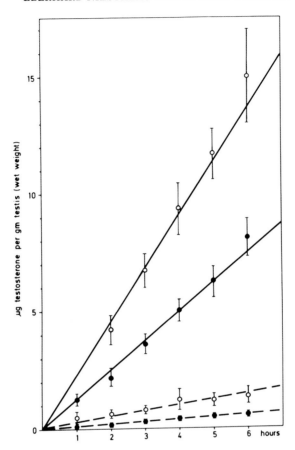

Fig. 7. Response of testicular tissue of normal (●) and testosterone-immunized (○) rabbits to incubation with hCG. - - -, Incubation without addition of hCG. From Nieschlag *et al.* (1975a).

a further sign of increased cellular activity there was augmented vascularization of the interstitial space of the testes. The tubules showed intact spermatogenesis on histological examination. Extrapolating from the testicular weight and histometry measurements, the total tubular tissue mass had increased in the same proportion as the testicular weight.

These morphological alterations in the testis can be attributed to the elevated serum gonadotropin levels reaching the testis. This type of Leydig cell hyperplasia can also be achieved by exogenous hCG application (Schoen and Samuels, 1965). It is also observed after the administration of cyproterone (Mietkiewski and Lukszyk, 1969; Heinert

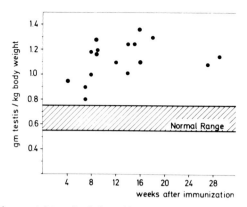

FIG. 8. Testicular weights of adult rabbits following active immunization with testosterone.

and Taubert, 1973), which is brought about by blocking of androgen-sensitive receptors in the hypothalamus and pituitary, thus resulting in increased gonadotropin secretion.

Since spermatogenesis is testosterone-dependent (Steinberger, 1971), intact spermatogenesis in the immunized animals provides evidence that testosterone reaches the tubules directly without passing through the bloodstream. Otherwise we would expect testosterone to be neutralized by the circulating antibodies and to find signs of impaired spermatogenesis.

Antibody titers could still be detected up to one year after primary immunization in rabbits. Their testicular weights also remained increased over the same period, indicating a continuing stimulation of the testis. Chronic hCG stimulation has been demonstrated to induce Leydig cell tumors in rats (Courier et al., 1964). Although Leydig cell hyperplasia is also maintained throughout immunization, no adenomas could be detected in long-term immunized animals. This absence of adenomas may be explained by the only moderate increase in gonadotropin levels, whereas high doses of hCG are required to induce Leydig cell adenomas.

In animals immunized against testicular tissue, severe morphological signs of autoimmune reaction can be observed in the testis, such as lymphatic invasion, inflammation, and destruction (Mancini, 1976). No such reactions were observed in the testosterone-immunized rabbits, suggesting that the hormone-producing tissue remains intact and that the antigen–antibody reaction occurs within the bloodstream.

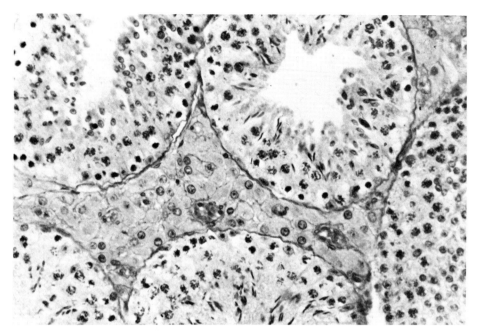

FIG. 9. Testicular histology of a normal adult rabbit. By courtesy of Dr. K.-H. Usadel, University of Frankfurt.

B. GONADAL FEEDBACK CONTROL

Active immunization of experimental animals with testosterone results in an elevation of gonadotropin levels. In general, this elevation is not as high as that seen after castration (Nieschlag *et al.*, 1974; Wickings and Nieschlag, 1978a; Thorneycroft *et al.*, 1975; Hillier *et al.*, 1975). In the first weeks after immunization there appears to be a positive correlation between antibody titers and gonadotropin levels (Nieschlag *et al.*, 1975b).

The increase in gonadotropin levels can be considered to be the result of the biological neutralization of testosterone, and hence a decrease in the biologically active free fraction of testosterone, due to antibody binding. The steroid fraction bound to antibodies in the circulation is no longer available to receptors in the hypothalamic–pituitary system, which in turn responds adequately with an increase in gonadotropin secretion. The fact that the gonadotropins do not reach castration levels indicates that the neutralization process is not complete.

The elevated LH levels in rats can be suppressed by high doses of exogenous testosterone (Table II) (Nieschlag *et al.*, 1975b). Thus, if

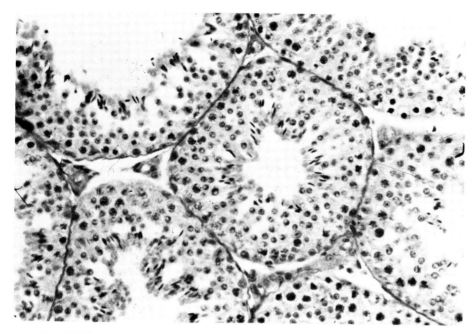

FIG. 10. Testicular histology of a testosterone-immunized adult rabbit. Same magnification as Fig. 9. Note the increase in Leydig cells. By courtesy of Dr. K.-H. Usadel, University of Frankfurt.

testosterone is administered in concentrations exceeding the binding capacity of the antibodies, it is possible to override the neutralizing effect of the antiserum by increasing the pool of unbound testosterone. Since FSH was not suppressed in these experiments, a differential hypothalamic–pituitary threshold for testosterone in regard to LH and FSH secretion can be assumed. This differential effect may also implicate the existence of separate regulatory mechanisms controlling LH

TABLE II

EFFECT OF TESTOSTERONE PROPIONATE INJECTIONS (100 μg PER ANIMAL ip) ON SERUM GONADOTROPIN LEVELS IN TESTOSTERONE-IMMUNIZED RATS (MEAN ± SEM)

Hormone	Before injection	After injection	
		60 Min	120 Min
LH (ng/ml)	124.0 ± 15.5	81.7 ± 13.7	68.4 ± 10.8
FSH (ng/ml)	338.6 ± 19.4	383.9 ± 30.9	367.4 ± 24.0

and FSH secretion, where inhibin in addition to gonadal steroids has an active role to play in the feedback mechanism.

The effect of testosterone antibodies on the pituitary gonadotropin levels in circulation provides concrete evidence that testosterone is involved in gonadal feedback control. The experiments with testosterone antibodies, however, do not rule out or confirm the possibility that feedback control is locally exerted by estradiol synthesized from testosterone in the hypothalamus. The neutralizing effect of hormonal antibodies has also been used for the study of other feedback control mechanisms. This immunological approach seems to offer certain advantages over the classical approach to the study of feedback control, which involves removal of the peripheral gland with the entire steroid spectrum and replacement of the steroid under investigation. The major difference of the immunological approach is that the animal remains intact and that a single steroid is exclusively eliminated.

However, one limitation to this immunological method is the limited specificity of most steroid antisera for one steroid. For example, the antisera produced in our studies show a high degree of crossreaction to dihydrotestosterone (Nieschlag et al., 1974). Hence, it is not possible to determine whether the pituitary response with increased gonadotropin release is due to neutralization of testosterone or dihydrotestosterone. If complete specificity cannot be achieved, the results must be considered as being effected by the group of steroids neutralized by the antibody.

All these considerations apply to studies performed in the first few weeks after immunization. There is a further phenomenon that complicates the interpretation of the feedback control studies carried out over longer periods of time as described by Thorneycroft et al. (1975) and Wickings and Nieschlag (1978a) for rabbits and rhesus monkeys, which were followed for one year after immunization with testosterone.

Antibody titers and elevated testosterone levels were found throughout this period. However, LH levels were elevated only in the first 5 months after primary immunization. In the later phases LH returned to normal levels or sank below in both species (Fig. 11). These findings are not fully understood as yet. One plausible explanation would be a change in the free fraction of testosterone, causing suppression of the pituitary. Under this assumption one would expect to see a normalization of the entire system when LH levels return to normal; this, however, is not the case. Grossly elevated testosterone levels are still found in the second half-year after immunization. A decreased clearance rate would not suffice to explain the elevated testosterone concentrations without an accompanying increase in production. The persistence of high testosterone levels in the presence of low or normal LH levels may

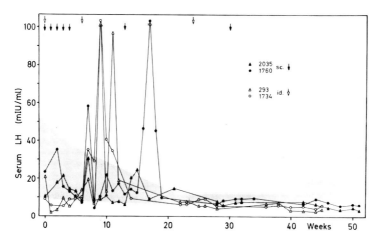

Fig. 11. Immunoreactive luteinizing hormone (LH) levels in 4 male rhesus monkeys during active immunization against testosterone. Arrows indicate booster injections. Shaded area indicates normal range from the beginning of January (week 0) to the end of December (week 52). From Wickings and Nieschlag (1978a).

reflect changes in the sensitivity of the Leydig cells. Some other (pituitary?) factor may be involved in maintaining the testicular testosterone production at the high level observed.

Other steroids are secreted in small concentrations by the testes, but their role in testicular feedback control has not been fully elucidated. Immunization with these steroids could provide further information on any possible effects in feedback mechanisms. For example, inducing antibodies to dehydroepiandrosterone in rabbits by active immunization caused a drastic increase in the percentage binding of dehydroepiandrosterone and an increase in serum levels of dehydroepiandrosterone, but not of testosterone. Testicular histology revealed no changes in the percentage of Leydig cells or other alterations. However, there were marked changes in adrenal histology, especially an increase in the nuclear volume of the zona glomerulosa cells occurred. Although these antibodies are not exclusively specific for dehydroepiandrosterone, but rather for Δ^5-3β-OH-steroids, it can be concluded that these steroids play a role in adrenal feedback, but not in testicular feedback control (Nieschlag et al., 1974).

C. ACCESSORY REPRODUCTIVE ORGANS

The first experiments using steroid antisera were designed to investigate the hormone neutralizing capacity of the antibodies. These investigations were carried out using the classical bioassay techniques for androgens. It could be demonstrated that the anabolic effect of exogenously administered testosterone on the ventral prostate, the seminal vesicles, and the levator ani muscle in castrated rats could be prevented by simultaneous administration of a testosterone antiserum (Lieberman *et al.*, 1959; Neri *et al.*, 1964). This was the first demonstration of the neutralizing capacity of a steroid antiserum.

Similarly, in actively immunized rabbits (Nieschlag *et al.*, 1975b) and rats (Hillier and Cameron, 1975) a 25–33% decrease in the weight and histological signs of atrophy of the accessory reproductive glands were found (Figs. 12 and 13). In addition, the concentration of cAMP within the prostates of testosterone-immunized rabbits was reduced by 32% compared with controls. This may indicate that cAMP is not only involved in the intracellular transmission of effects of protein hormones, but also in those of steroid hormones.

D. Sexual Differentiation

Even during fetal life testosterone exerts distinct effects on the differentiation of the reproductive tract. This role of testosterone in sex

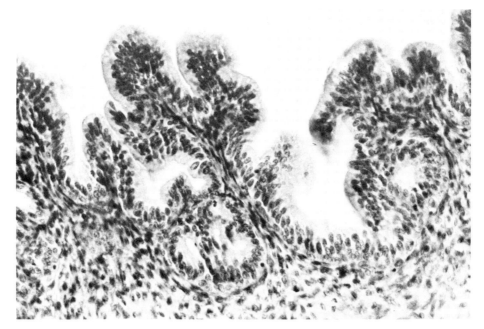

Fig. 12. Histology of the seminal vesicles from a normal adult rabbit. By courtesy of Dr. K.-H. Usadel, University of Frankfurt.

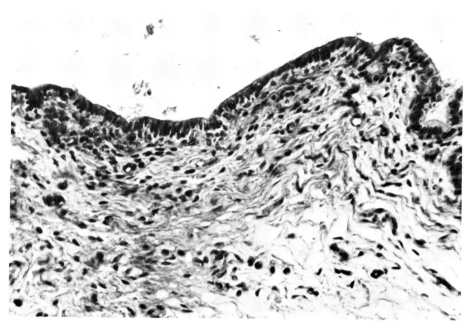

FIG. 13. Histology of the seminal vesicles from a testosterone-immunized adult rabbit. Same magnification as Fig. 12. By courtesy of Dr. K.-H. Usadel, University of Frankfurt.

differentiation has been confirmed by transplacental passive immunization of the fetus. In respect to titer, specificity, and affinity, the antibodies found in the newborn have the same characteristics as those of their mothers, who had been actively immunized with testosterone. On the day of delivery the antibody titers in the offspring are identical to those in the mothers and thereafter show a steady decline during the first days of life, indicating the maternal origin of the antibodies (Fig. 14).

In male rat fetuses from mothers to whom testosterone antibodies had been administered during pregnancy, the anogenital distance was reduced as compared to that of controls (Goldman *et al.*, 1972). A more thorough histological examination of rabbit neonates from mothers actively immunized with testosterone revealed extensive feminization of male internal and external genitalia (Bidlingmaier *et al.*, 1977). The accessory reproductive glands were underdeveloped or even absent, and the bulbo-urethral glands showed only female dimensions. The Wolffian ducts showed severe regressions. The phallus only reached female size, and hypospadias were present. As in normal males, the Müllerian ducts were completely inhibited, indicating that

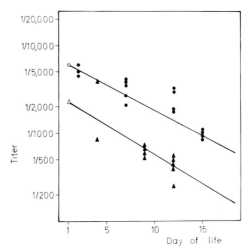

FIG. 14. Disappearance of antibody titers from the serum of offspring (●, ▲) of two female rabbits actively immunized against testosterone. ○, △, Antibody titers measured in maternal serum on the day of delivery.

the Müllerian inhibiting factor must be different from testosterone and dihydrotestosterone. There were no signs of interference with female sexual differentiation in newborns passively immunized with testosterone.

These studies show the potential applications of immunization with hormones in the elucidation of sex differentiation *in utero* and in the study of other endocrine events during fetal life.

E. SEXUAL ACTIVITY

Sexual activity was investigated as a further testosterone-dependent function in male animals. When male rabbits actively immunized with testosterone were exposed to receptive partners, they showed a lack of sexual activity. Since estrogen-immunized rabbits exhibited normal chasing, mounting, and ejaculation behavior, the lack of sexual activity in the testosterone-immunized animals can be considered to be a specific effect of the immunological neutralization of testosterone (Nieschlag and Kley, 1974). In addition to the peripheral effects already listed, this demonstrates that the antibodies also prevent testosterone from reaching central structures. Since spermatogenesis as revealed by histological examination of the testis was intact while the accessory glands were atrophied, it would have been especially interesting to evaluate ejaculates from these immunized animals. However, ejaculates could not be obtained by natural means, and artificial manipulations such as electroejaculation were not employed.

F. Pheromones

In addition to androgens, the Leydig cells of the boar testes produce a steroidal pheromone, 5α-androst-16-en-3-one, also called "boar taint." Before mating it is transmitted from the boar's saliva to the sow, where it induces the "immobilization reflex." Boar taint is also accumulated in high concentrations in the fatty tissue of the boar. Because of its unappetizing smell, boars are normally castrated before slaughtering. By elimination of the undesirable pheromone the anabolic effects of the androgens are also lost, thus diminishing the quality of the meat.

In an attempt to prevent the pheromone from entering into fat tissue, Claus (1975) actively immunized boars against this Δ^{16}-steroid. A significant reduction of the concentration in fatty tissue could be demonstrated, and after slaughtering the meat was free from distasteful odors. This preliminary experiment points to a potentially useful practical application of immunization against steroids.

IV. Effects on Female Reproductive Functions

A. Puberty

The neutralizing capacity of steroid antisera has been employed to investigate the role of estrogens in pubertal development. In immature rats (Goodfriend and Sehon, 1970), mice (Neri et al., 1964; Ferin et al., 1968), and hamsters (Ekre and Foote, 1972), the uterotrophic effect of exogenous estrogens could be prevented by simultaneous passive administration of estrogen antisera. The uptake of radiolabeled estradiol by target tissues was also inhibited by pretreatment of the animals with estradiol antibodies (Ferin et al., 1968). The immunological neutralization of endogenous estradiol could also be affected in immature hamsters, where the hCG-induced uterine weight gain was inhibited by simultaneous administration of estradiol antiserum (Ekre and Foote, 1972). The specificity of this reaction was demonstrated by the overriding effect of diethylstilbestrol, a synthetic estrogen that does not crossreact with the antibody and is thus not neutralized by the antibody (Ferin et al., 1968).

Immature female pigs actively immunized against estradiol-6-BSA did not pass through puberty and failed to ovulate (Elsaesser and

Paravizi, 1977). Ferin *et al.* (1969b) showed that pregnant mare serum (PMS)-induced ovulation in immature rats could be blocked by administration of antiestradiol serum. Ovulation could, however, still be brought about by diethylstilbestrol replacing the endogenous estradiol (see Fig. 15). This demonstrates the importance of the estrogen secretion acting as a trigger for the preovulatory LH surge. Wuttke *et al.* (1976) investigated the hypothalamic–pituitary–ovarian feedback control mechanism during puberty. In female rats pubertal development is characterized by increased estradiol levels between days 10 and 20, sporadic high LH peaks and high FSH levels (Döhler and Wuttke, 1974, 1975). The gonadostat theory (MacCann and Ramirez, 1963) attributes a positive feedback effect to estradiol on secretion of LH as well as of FSH. This role of estradiol has been reevaluated following the administration of specific estradiol antibodies to prepubertal rats (Wuttke *et al.*, 1976). In the presence of antibodies, there was a reduction of basal LH levels and the occurrence of LH peaks was prevented. Basal FSH levels, however, were increased. From this study it would seem that estradiol exerts a differential effect on LH and FSH secretion during puberty. Estradiol appears to exercise a negative feedback control effect on FSH, whereas the phasic and tonic secretion of LH would seem to be under positive estradiol feedback control.

B. OVULATION AND CYCLE

1. *Feedback Control*

Immunization with gonadal steroids has been widely used to investigate the role of steroids in the control of ovulation and cycle. Estradiol antibodies have been especially useful in confirming the positive feedback effect of estradiol on LH release in the normally cycling female animal. Either active or passive immunization against estradiol caused a blockage of the LH release normally preceding ovulation, thus suppressing ovulation (Neill *et al.*, 1971; Hillier *et al.*, 1975; Ferin *et al.*, 1969a, 1974, 1975; Sundaram *et al.*, 1973). When antibodies to estradiol were administered to normally cycling rats on the morning of the second day of diestrus, the biological activity of estrogens was neutralized, as evidenced by the absence of uterine ballooning. No LH surge and consequently no ovulation followed in these animals (Fig. 15) (Ferin *et al.*, 1969a). Antibody application was effective only when given up to approximately 15 hours prior to the expected LH surge. Later injections were not effective, suggesting that the events leading up to the LH surge did not require an estrogenic

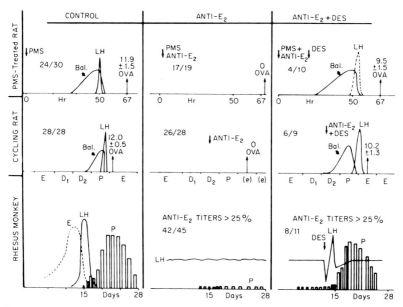

FIG. 15. Effects of antibodies to estradiol on ovulation in rats and monkeys. *Left panel:* The three biological models used to study the causal relationship between estradiol, the LH surge, and ovulation: the immature pregnant mare serum (PMS)-treated rat (10 IU) (upper section), the adult cycling rat (middle section), and the adult cycling rhesus monkey (lower section). The end points used in the experiments are outlined: Bal = ballooning of the uterus, an estrogen effect; E = plasma estrogen levels; LH = plasma LH levels; ova = mean (±SE) number of ova in fallopian tubes; P = plasma progesterone levels. *Middle panel:* The effect of passive immunization in the rat or of active immunization in the monkey. Anti-E$_2$: antibodies to estradiol. *Right panel:* Reversibility of the effects of immunization by diethylstilbestrol (DES): 10 μg in the rat; 250 μg in the monkey. From Ferin *et al.* (1975).

stimulus beyond this point. Passive immunization did not result in permanent inhibition of ovulation, but ovulation returned as soon as the antibodies had been cleared from circulation.

In contrast, when active immunization against estrogens was employed, ovulation could be suppressed for longer periods owing to the continuing production and high circulating levels of specific antibodies (Ferin *et al.*, 1974, 1975; Sundaram *et al.*, 1973). Thus the actively immunized animal is rendered chronically anovulatory and can be used as a model for the study of hypothalamic–pituitary–ovarian interrelationships (Fig. 15). This model offers distinct advantages for the investigation of feedback control mechanisms as compared to either ovariectomy or pharmacological blockage of ovulation by substances competing at the receptor sites (e.g., Clomid) (Ferin *et al.*, 1975). With ovariectomy, the organ producing the hormonal signal is removed, and at the same time the target organ is also eliminated. In the immunological approach, however, the signal from the ovary can still be mimicked by the administration of synthetic steroids, e.g., diethylstilbestrol, which are not inhibited by the antibody and can reach intact receptors. Thus ovulation can still be induced, and the effects at the target organ level can be studied as well.

This model can further serve to demonstrate the mechanism by which estrogens effect their feedback control on the hypothalamic–pituitary system. Monoamines such as L-dopa and L-epinephrine can induce LH release and ovulation when injected intraventricularly (MacCann *et al.*, 1976). This effect can be blocked by an estrogen antiserum, indicating that estrogens are necessary at the hypothalamic level to mediate the monoamine-induced pituitary stimulation (Raziano *et al.*, 1971). Using [^{35}S]methionine incorporation as an indicator of protein synthesis, ter Haar and MacKinnon (1975) demonstrated that estradiol can stimulate protein synthesis in certain brain areas, particularly in the median eminence and also in the anterior pituitary on the evening of proestrus. The specificity of this estrogenic effect could be proved by the administration of estradiol-specific antibodies, when the peak of [^{35}S]methionine incorporation usually observed in the anterior pituitary could be inhibited. Thus, ovarian steroids appear to act differently at the various central areas. There seems to be a continuous effect on the median eminence throughout the estrus cycle and a short-lived effect during proestrus on the anterior pituitary.

The immunological approach has also been used to investigate the possible role of other steroids in hypothalamic–pituitary–ovarian feedback control. In ewes actively immunized with androstenedione, effects on LH levels and its release pattern were observed that were similar to those seen following the withdrawal of estrogens (Scaramuzzi and Martensz, 1975). However, it is difficult to attribute these effects either to the neutralization of androstenedione itself acting directly at the pituitary or to the withdrawal of androstenedione as a precursor for estrogens. This could have been clarified by measuring circulating steroid levels in the immunized sheep, which was unfortunately not done during this study.

So far it has not been possible to elucidate the role of progesterone in ovulation any further using the immunological approach, since ambivalent results have been obtained. Although the biological effect of progesterone at midcycle on the uterus was blocked, the effects on the LH surge and ovulation were inconclusive in rats (Kaushansky *et al.*,

1977; Mori et al., 1977; Neill et al., 1971) and rhesus monkeys (Ferin et al., 1975). In contrast to the case in mammals, however, progesterone would seem to play a definitive role in ovulation in the hen. Passive immunization with progesterone suppressed ovulation in hens, whereas antiestradiol serum was without effect (Furr and Smith, 1975).

2. Steroid Levels and Binding in Serum

As in testosterone-immunized male rabbits, where very high levels of testosterone were found (Nieschlag et al., 1973), estradiol levels in female rats (Hillier et al., 1975) and rhesus monkeys (Ferin et al., 1974; Sundaram et al., 1973) actively immunized with estradiol were also shown to be grossly elevated. The percentage binding of estradiol was also increased (Hillier et al., 1975), indicating a decrease in the biologically active, free fraction of the steroid. However, the actual free fraction of the hormone has never been measured directly. This is also true for animals immunized against other steroids (see Section II, A, 2). A decrease in the free fraction could only be deduced from biological evidence. Although the LH levels in estrogen-immunized animals are significantly increased (Ferin et al., 1974; Hillier et al., 1975), they are not as high as in ovariectomized animals. There are also signs of continuous estrogenic effects on the vaginal epithelium and the endometrium in estradiol-immunized animals (Ferin et al., 1974; Hillier et al., 1975). These findings provide evidence that the antibodies do not completely neutralize all the circulating estrogens. Thus, in the actively immunized animals the increased ovarian estrogen production appears always to keep pace with the neutralizing capacity of the antibodies, resulting in a reduced yet still partially effective free hormone fraction.

3. Ovarian Morphology

The chronically increased LH secretion in the estradiol-immunized animals leads to certain morphological changes in the ovaries (Ferin et al., 1974; Hillier et al., 1975). They become enlarged, multiple cystic follicles develop, and a cortical fibrosis is evident. No corpora lutea are present. Active immunization with testosterone resulted in similar ovarian alterations. These changes in morphology resemble those seen in the human polycystic ovary syndrome. Thus the female animal actively immunized with estradiol or testosterone could possibly serve as a model for the study of the polycystic ovary syndrome.

C. PREGNANCY

Even though estradiol antibodies block the midcycle LH surge and ovulation in rats, animals actively immunized with estradiol can still conceive, as reported by Csapo *et al.* (1975) and by Kaushansky *et al.* (1977). Obviously mating-induced ovulation had occurred in these animals. Ensuing pregnancies were carried uneventfully to term. These results confirm that estrogens are not required for the maintenance of normal pregnancy. Indeed, it could be concluded from immunization studies that estrogens may even exert an inhibitory effect on placental growth (Csapo *et al.*, 1974).

Paradoxically, in the spontaneously ovulating rabbit immunized against estradiol, mating can obviously no longer induce ovulation, as can be concluded from the failure of these rabbits to conceive. It should be pointed out that the immunization procedure as such has no influence on conception rate and pregnancy, since all BSA-immunized controls conceived and had normal pregnancies (Table III).

The conception rate in testosterone-immunized does is also greatly reduced (Table III). In most animals conception occurred only after several matings, if at all (Bidlingmaier *et al.*, 1977; E. Nieschlag, unpublished). The ensuing pregnancies were, however, not different from normal in regard to length of gestation, but sexual differentiation of male fetuses was prevented, as discussed in Section III, B. The reduced conception rate is probably due to the ovarian hyperstimulation, which results in a polycystic ovary syndrome-like situation (Hillier *et al.*, 1975).

TABLE III

EFFECT OF ACTIVE IMMUNIZATION WITH STEROID CONJUGATES
ON CONCEPTION RATE AND PREGNANCY

Conjugate	Species	Conceptions per mating	Deliveries per mated animal	Reference[a]
Control	Rat	7/9	7/9	(1)
	Rabbit	12/12	10/12	(2)
	Rabbit	21/21	—[b]	(3)
BSA-immunized	Rabbit	6/6	6/6	(2)
control	Rabbit	33/33	—[b]	(3)
Estradiol-6-BSA	Rabbit	0/11	0/11	(2)
	Rat	5/7	5/7	(1)
Progesterone-11-BSA	Rabbit	32/41	—[b]	(3)
	Rabbit	6/6	0/6	(2)
	Rat	7/7	0/7	(1)
Testosterone-3-BSA	Rabbit	3/10	2/10	(2)
	Rabbit	—	12/25	(4)

[a] (1) Kaushansky *et al.*, 1977; (2) F. Elsaesser, unpublished results; (3) French, 1977; (4) E. Nieschlag, unpublished results.

[b] Autopsied before term.

Active immunization with progesterone does not prevent conception in rats (Kaushansky *et al.*, 1977) or rabbits (French, 1977; F. Elsaesser, unpublished) (Table III). In none of the animals, however, could pregnancy be carried to term. In some animals implantation was inhibited; in the remaining ones, resorption occurred during early or midgestation (Kaushansky *et al.*, 1977). This occurred despite progesterone levels well above the normal range (Csapo *et al.*, 1975; French, 1977; Kaushansky *et al.*, 1977; Surve *et al.*, 1976). It may be assumed that there is a reduction in the biologically active free fraction of progesterone. French (1977) provided evidence that this assumption is correct. The progesterone antibody effects on pregnancy could be prevented by the administration of medroxyprogesterone acetate, a synthetic progestin that is not neutralized by the progesterone antiserum. This experiment proves the specificity of the progesterone–antibody interaction.

The effect of passive immunization against progesterone was investigated in intact rats with normal pregnancies. Progesterone antibodies injected on day 3 of pregnancy only caused a delay in implantation and a reduction in litter size. Antibodies administered to pregnant rats on day 6, 10, or 11 provoked abortion (Csapo *et al.*, 1975; Raziano *et al.*, 1972). Csapo *et al.* (1975) demonstrated that the amount of antibodies required to terminate pregnancy during this period is directly correlated to the circulating progesterone levels. On day 6, when progesterone levels are very high, a much higher antiserum dose is required for abortion than on day 10, when progesterone levels are declining.

V. Steroid-Dependent Tumors

The original intention of Lieberman's group, who first succeeded in rendering steroids antigenic, was to investigate the biological effects of steroids using immunological neutralization (Lieberman *et al.*, 1959). In a series of experiments that demonstrated in experimental animals that steroids can be neutralized by antibodies, they also tried to employ this effect in the therapy of mammary carcinoma in humans. The patients were reported to have responded to active immunization by production of specific antibodies (Veenema *et al.*, 1959, as quoted by Ferin *et al.*, 1973), but the results were never published in full and no further reports have appeared.

In later studies, the effects of estrogen antibodies on hormone-dependent tumor development and growth was investigated in experimental animals. It had been shown that DMBA-induced mammary carcinomas in rats are estrogen dependent, since ovariectomy and hypophysectomy resulted in tumor regression (Huggins et al., 1959). Instead of regression, tumor incidence, growth rate, and size were all stimulated in rats immunized with estradiol antibodies (Dusquenoy, 1967; Hillier et al., 1975). Obviously in these animals the antibody-bound estradiol is still biologically active. This can be explained by the presence of cytoplasmic estradiol receptors, which have a higher affinity for estradiol than the circulating antibodies (Fishman and Fishman, 1974). Thus the high circulating estradiol levels resulting from immunization (see Section IV, B, 2) are fully available to the tumor receptors, in contrast to receptors in other estrogen target tissues.

In a different mammary carcinoma model—MT/W9A tumors transplanted into rats actively immunized with estradiol—the immunized animals showed inhibited tumor growth and prolonged survival times (Caldwell et al., 1971). Here it would seem that the estradiol bound to the antibodies is unavailable to the tumor receptors. However, it might be that the immunological events following immunization influence carcinogenesis and that the observed effects are unspecific. By not including BSA-immunized control animals in the study, the authors failed to demonstrate the specificity of the antibody effect.

These investigations indicate that antibodies to steroids may provide an interesting approach in the field of experimental tumor research. However, we feel that this approach has not yet been fully utilized and the data should be considered as preliminary.

VI. Immunological Side Effects

Repeated application of antisera during the course of passive immunization introduces large amounts of foreign proteins into the experimental animal. This may result in serum sickness and anaphylactic reactions and therefore limits the extent to which passive immunization can be used in experimental animals and ultimately in therapy.

Active immunization with steroid–protein conjugates may also exert deleterious effects on the immunized animals. The high concentration of circulating antibodies may result in the formation of immune complexes. If immune complexes occur, they are most likely to be deposited in the renal glomeruli. Since appropriate studies were lacking, we have examined kidneys of rabbits actively immunized with a testosterone-3-BSA conjugate for the presence of immune complex precipitation and glomerulonephritis (Wickings *et al.*, 1978; Witting *et al.*, 1978).

Immunofluorescence studies revealed the presence of varying degrees of complex precipitation in 85% of all investigated animals (Table IV; Fig. 16). The severest degrees were found at weeks 10 and 16. Exudative glomerulonephritis was also present in 10 of 20 immunized rabbits. There was a proliferation of the mesangial cells with enlargement of the mesangium area, pronounced exudation of leukocytes in the glomeruli, and vasoconstriction of the capillaries. In other experimental models, the occurrence of glomerulonephritis has been shown to lag behind the appearance of immune complexes (Dixon *et al.*, 1961). This may explain why we see evidence of glomerulonephritis in the absence of immune precipitation in 2 of the immunized rabbits (Table IV).

The occurrence of immune complex precipitation depends on the

TABLE IV

INCIDENCE OF RENAL IMMUNE COMPLEX PRECIPITATION AND GLOMERULONEPHRITIS IN RABBITS ACTIVELY IMMUNIZED AGAINST TESTOSTERONE BY THE ONE-TIME, MULTIPLE-SITE, INTRADERMAL TECHNIQUE[a]

Animal No.	Weeks	Antiserum titer	Immune complexes	Glomerulo-nephritis
1	4	1/ 7,000	+	−
2	4	1/ 9,000	+	−
3	4	1/10,000	+	−
4	10	1/14,500	+ + +	−
5	10	1/25,000	+ + +	+
6	10	1/80,000	−	+
7	16	1/10,000	+	−
8	16	1/10,000	+	−
9	16	1/ 7,000	+ + +	+
10	16	1/ 7,300	+ +	+
11	16	1/18,000	−	+
12	16	1/ 6,800	+ +	+
13	16	1/11,500	−	−
14	16	1/34,000	+ +	−
15	16	1/ 6,500	+ +	+
16	16	1/13,000	+ +	+
17	16	1/12,000	+ +	−
18	30	1/ 5,400	+	−
19	30	1/ 2,500	+	+
20	30	1/ 2,400	+	+

[a] The number of crosses signifies the severity of precipitation.

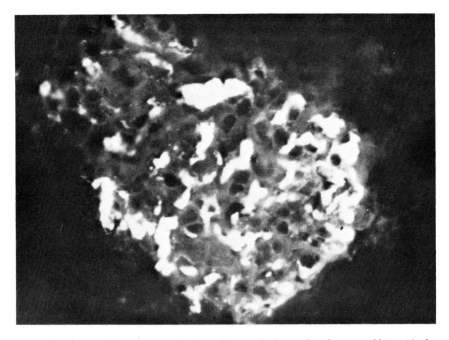

Fɪɢ. 16. Immunofluorescence staining of a renal glomerulus from a rabbit actively immunized against testosterone-3-BSA. The lighter areas indicate immune complex precipitation.

total amount of circulating immunoglobulins. From parallel studies in rhesus monkeys we know that the intradermal immunization schedule results in the production of predominantly IgM antibodies (Fig. 2), which are responsible for complement fixation and immune complex precipitation. The immunoglobulin concentrations are highest between weeks 8 and 22 after primary immunization, the period when the highest incidence and severest degree of immune complex precipitation was observed in rabbits. Despite the severe morphological renal alterations observed the immunized rabbits showed no signs of ill health during the period of observation. Neither was the mortality rate of steroid-immunized animals different from that in normal controls. To establish the clinical significance of these morphological renal findings, a careful evaluation of kidney function is mandatory.

The same renal lesions can be found in animals immunized against BSA alone (Dixon et al., 1961). Therefore we may attribute the observed effects to the use of BSA as carrier protein for the steroid hapten. Whether other carrier proteins used for active immunization also generate immune complexes remains to be investigated, but can be anticipated. Even short-term passive immunization may not circumvent this immunological side effect seen after active immunization. Kofler *et al*. (1976) demonstrated immune complex precipitation in kidneys of rats previously immunized with a rabbit anti-bLH-serum. One possible means of avoiding precipitation of immune complexes may be to use F_{AB} fragments instead of intact immunoglobulins. This approach has been used successfully in the treatment of a case of digoxin intoxication (Smith *et al*., 1976, 1977).

One unpleasant side effect of active immunization is the local reaction at the site of immunization. The intradermal immunization causes ulcerations that can last for several weeks and may leave scarring. Subcutaneous immunization in the axillary and inguinal regions may produce enlargement of the local lymph nodes, which can also ulcerate and heal only slowly. These effects are due to the use of complete Freund's adjuvant and could probably be reduced by eliminating the more virulent components of the adjuvant or by using another adjuvant (Peck *et al*., 1968).

VII. Summary and Conclusions

The studies summarized here clearly demonstrate that the biological activity of steroids can be neutralized by corresponding antibodies. Steroid-dependent developments in male sexual differentiation and in female puberty can be blocked by antibodies to testosterone or estradiol, respectively. The estradiol-induced midcycle LH peak, and thus ovulation, is prevented by estrogen antibodies. Pregnancy can be terminated by the application of progesterone antisera. In adult male animals immunization with testosterone leads to a loss of sexual activity, atrophy of accessory reproductive glands, decrease in testosterone metabolism, and increase in gonadotropin secretion. These effects are similar to those seen following castration and may therefore be characterized as "immunological castration." Paradoxically these phenomena are accompanied by hyperplasia of the Leydig cells and increased testicular testosterone production, which result from increased gonadotropin stimulation.

All these effects find a common explanation in the increased binding of the steroids to circulating antibodies. Under physiological conditions a certain proportion of gonadal steroids in blood is bound to proteins. Only the nonprotein-bound fraction is considered to be biologically active (Kawai and Yates, 1968; Slaunwhite *et al*., 1962; Vermeulen *et al.*, 1969). Gonadal steroids are bound with a low affinity relatively unspecifically to albumin and with higher affinity to the more specific sex hormone-binding globulin (SHBG) so that on average, taking into account interspecies variations, only about 10% of the total testosterone and estradiol concentration is free. The increase of the binding of steroids to high-affinity antibodies to approximately 100% is responsible for the neutralization of the hormonal activity. As discussed previously, the extent of binding is not complete, however, as evidenced by the residual hormonal activity still present in the immunized animals.

Inducing an immune reaction against steroid hormones may be considered as a form of autoimmunity in that antibodies are being produced against endogenously occurring secretions. The term "autoimmune disease" of an endocrine gland, however, is reserved for the pathological situation where antibodies are produced against tissue elements, resulting in destruction of that gland. Immunization against hormones has not been shown to induce tissue damage. The hormone-antibody interaction seems to be confined to the blood stream.

The studies reported in this review give some indications of how steroid antisera can be applied as research tools. They can be used to characterize biological effects of hormones, to investigate feedback control mechanisms, and to demonstrate hormone dependency of reproductive functions, even during fetal life. In addition the steroid-immunized animal may serve as a model for certain pathological conditions. The diverse nature of these studies illustrates that immunization against steroids is not a special field of research, but rather an investigative tool applying immunological principles to endocrinology.

Beyond the application as a research tool, immunization against steroids (as well as against other hormones) could probably be used in therapeutic medicine, when it would be necessary to inhibit hormonal activity. Although the possibility of using steroid antibodies in therapy has not been systematically investigated, immunization studies with protein hormone antigens, i.e., hCG β-subunits, have demonstrated that hormone antibodies may have a place in therapy or in fertility control (Stevens and Crystle, 1973). Therapeutic applications of antibodies to low-molecular-weight substances are also exemplified by the successful treatment of a case of severe digoxin intoxication with antibodies (Smith *et al.*, 1976, 1977).

In all experiments using antibodies against hormones, one has to be aware of the immunological side effects of active as well as passive immunization, mainly immune complex precipitation, serum sickness, and anaphylactic reactions. For the purpose of passive immunization, purification of antibodies would be desirable. It is possible to avoid the formation of complement-fixing immune complexes by removing the F_C fragment of the antibody molecule, leaving the antigenic binding site on the F_{AB} fragment intact. The use of nonimmunogenic F_{AB} fragments instead of the intact immunoglobulin molecule could open up new horizons for the application of hormone antibodies.

REFERENCES

Abraham, G. E. (1969). *J. Clin. Endocrinol. Metab.* **29**, 866.

Abraham, G. E. (1974). *Acta Endocrinol. (Copenhagen), Suppl.* **183**.

Banting, F. G., Frank, W. R., and Gairus, S. (1938). *Am. J. Psychiatry* **95**, 562.

Bidlingmaier, F., Knorr, D., and Neumann, F. (1977). *Nature (London)* **266**, 647.

Bishop, D. W. (1970). *In* "The Testis" (A. D. Johnson, W. R. Gomes, and N. L. Van-demark, eds.), Vol. 3, pp. 41–66. Academic Press, New York.

Caldwell, B. V., Tillson, S. A., Esber, H., and Thorneycroft, I. H. (1971). *Nature (London)* **231**, 118.

Claus, R. (1975). *In* "Immunization with Hormones in Reproduction Research" (E. Nieschlag, ed.), pp. 189–198. North-Holland Publ., Amsterdam.

Corvol, P., and Bardin, C. W. (1973). *Biol. Reprod.* **8**, 277.

Courier, R., Riviera, M., and Cologna, A. (1964). *C.R. Hebd. Seances Acad. Sci.* **259**, 1347.

Csapo, A., Dray, F., and Erdos, T. (1974). *Lancet* **2**, 51.

Csapo, A., Dray, F., and Erdos, T. (1975). *Endocrinology* **97**, 603.

Depisch, F., and Hasenörl, R. (1928). *Z. Gesamte Exp. Med.* **58**, 110.

Dixon, F. J., Feldman, J., and Vazquez, J. J. (1961). *J. Exp. Med.* **113**, 899.

Döhler, K. D., and Wuttke, W. (1974). *Endocrinology* **94**, 1003.

Döhler, K. D., and Wuttke, W. (1975). *Endocrinology* **97**, 898.

Dusquenoy, R. J. (1967). *Fed. Proc., Fed. Am. Soc. Exp. Biol.* **26**, 297.

Ekre, C. D., and Foote, W. C. (1972). *J. Reprod. Fertil.* **30**, 451.

Elsaesser, F., and Paravizi, N. (1977). *Acta Endocrinol. (Copenhagen), Suppl.* **208**, 107.

Erlanger, B. F., Borek, F., Beiser, S. M., and Lieberman, S. (1957). *J. Biol. Chem.* **228**, 713.

Erlanger, B. F., Beiser, S. M., Borek, F., Edel, F., and Lieberman, S. (1967). *Methods Immunol.* **1**, 144.

Feldman, H., and Rodbard, D. (1971). *In* "Principles of Competitive Protein-binding Assays" (W. D. Odell and W. H. Daughaday, eds.), pp. 158–173. Lippincott, Philadelphia, Pennsylvania.

Ferin, M., Zimmering, P. E., Lieberman, S., and Vande Wiele, R. L. (1968). *Endocrinology* **83**, 565.

Ferin, M., Tempone, A., Zimmering, P. E., and Vande Wiele, R. L. (1969b). *Endocrinology* **85**, 1070.

Ferin, M., Zimmering, P. E., and Vande Wiele, R. L. (1969a). *Endocrinology* **84**, 893.

Ferin, M., Beiser, S. M., and Vande Wiele, R. L. (1973). *Vitam. Horm. (N.Y.)* **31**, 175.

Ferin, M., Dyrenfurth, I., Cowchock, S., Warren, M., and Vande Wiele, R. L. (1974). *Endocrinology* **94**, 765.

Ferin, M., Dyrenfurth, I., Schwartz, U., and Vande Wiele, R. L. (1975). *In* "Immunization with Hormones in Reproduction Research" (E. Nieschlag, ed.), pp. 119–137. North-Holland Publ., Amsterdam.

Fishman, J., and Fishman, J. H. (1974). *J. Clin. Endocrinol. Metab.* **39**, 603.

Følling, I., and Norman, N. (1972). *Diabetes* **21**, 814.

Forest, M. G., Rivarola, M. A., and Migeon, C. J. (1968). *Steroids* **12**, 323.

French, L. R. (1977). *Biol. Reprod.* **16**, 363.

Furr, B. J. A., and Smith, K. (1975). *J. Endocrinol.* **66**, 303.

Gless, K. H., Kanka, M., Vescei, P., and Gross, F. (1974). *Acta Endocrinol. (Copenhagen)* **75**, 342.

Goldman, A. S., Baker, M. K., Chen, J. C., and Wieland, R. G. (1972). *Endocrinology* **90**, 716.

Goodfriend, L., and Sehon, A. H. (1958). *Can. J. Biochem. Physiol.* **36**, 1177.

Goodfriend, L., and Sehon, A. (1970). *In* "Immunologic Methods in Steroid Determination" (F. G. Péron and B. V. Caldwell, eds.), pp. 15–35. Appleton, New York.

Heinert, G., and Taubert, H. D. (1973). *Endocrinology* **61**, 168.

Hillier, S. G., and Cameron, E. H. D. (1975). *In* "Immunization with Hormones in Reproduction Research" (E. Nieschlag, ed.), pp. 173–184. North-Holland Publ., Amsterdam.

Hillier, S. G., Brownsey, B. C., and Cameron, E. H. D. (1973). *Steroids* **21**, 735.

Hillier, S. G., Groom, G. V., Boyns, A. R., and Cameron, E. H. D. (1975). *In* "Steroid Immunoassays" (E. H. D. Cameron, S. G. Hillier, and K. Griffiths, eds.), pp. 97–110. Alpha Omega Publ., Cardiff, Wales.

Hirata, Y., Ishizu, H., and Ito, J. (1973). *Proc. Congr. Int. Diabetes Fed., 8th, 1973* Excerpta Med. Found. Int. Congr. Ser. No. 280, Abstract No. 282.

Huggins, C., Briziarelli, G., and Sutton, H. (1959). *J. Exp. Med.* **110**, 899.

James, V. H. T., and Jeffcoate, S. L. (1974). *Br. Med. Bull.* **30**, 50.

Kaushansky, A., Bauminger, S., Koch, Y., and Lindner, H. R. (1977). *Acta Endocrinol. (Copenhagen)* **84**, 795.

Kawai, A., and Yates, F. R. (1968). *Endocrinology* **79**, 1040.

Kofler, R., Wick, G., and Loewit, K. (1976). *Lancet* **2**, 589.

Kuss, E., and Goebel, R. (1972). *In* "Hormones and Enzymes," pp. 519–523. Fortschr. Klin. Chem., Wien.

Lewis, J. H. (1937). *J. Am. Med. Assoc.* **108**, 1336.

Lieberman, S., Erlanger, B. F., Beiser, S. M., and Agate, F. J. (1959). *Recent Prog. Horm. Res.* **15**, 165.

Lindner, H. R., Perel, E., Friedlander, A., and Zeitlin, A. (1972). *Steroids* **19**, 357.

Longcope, C. (1970). *In* "Immunologic Methods in Steroid Determination" (F. G. Péron and B. V. Caldwell, eds.), p. 222. Appleton, New York.

MacCann, S. M., and Ramirez, V. D. (1963). *Recent Prog. Horm. Res.* **20**, 131.

MacCann, S. M., Harms, P. G., and Ojeda, S. R. (1976). *In* "Neuroendocrine Regulation of Fertility" (T. C. Anand Kumar, ed.), pp. 169–179. Karger, Basel.

Mancini, R. E. (1976). "Immunologic Aspects of Testicular Function." Springer-Verlag, Berlin and New York.

Mietkiewski, K., and Lukszyk A. (1969). *Acta Endocrinol. (Copenhagen)* **60**, 561.

Mikhail, G., Wu, C. H., Ferin, M., and Vande Wiele, R. L. (1970). *Steroids* **15**, 333.

Mooser, H., and Grilliches, R. K. (1941). *Z. Allg. Pathol. Bakteriol.* **4**, 375.

Mori, T., Suzuki, A., Nishimura, T., and Kambegawa, A. (1977). *J. Endocrinol.* **73**, 185.

Neill, J. D., Freeman, M. E., and Tillson, S. A. (1971). *Endocrinology* **89**, 1448.

Neri, R. O., Tolksdorf, S., Beiser, S. M., Erlanger, B. F., Agate, F. J., and Lieberman, S. (1964). *Endocrinology* **74**, 593.

Nieschlag, E., ed. (1975). "Immunization with Hormones in Reproduction Research." North-Holland Publ., Amsterdam.

Nieschlag, E., and Kley, H. K. (1974). *Experientia* **30**, 434.

Nieschlag, E., and Wickings, E. J. (1975). *Z. Klin. Chem. Klin. Biochem.* **13**, 261.

Nieschlag, E., Usadel, K.-H., Schwedes, U., Kley, H. K., Schöffling, K., and Krüskemper, H. L. (1973). *Endocrinology* **92**, 1142.

Nieschlag, E., Usadel, K.-H., Kley, H. K., Schwedes, U., Schöffling, K., and Krüskemper, H. L. (1974). *Acta Endocrinol. (Copenhagen)* **76**, 556.

Nieschlag, E., Tekook, W., Usadel, K.-H., Kley, H. K., and Krüskemper, H. L. (1975a). *Steroids* **25**, 379.

Nieschlag, E., Usadel, K.-H., Wickings, E. J., Kley, H. K., and Wuttke, W. (1975b). *In* "Immunization with Hormones in Reproduction Research" (E. Nieschlag, ed.), pp. 155–170. North-Holland Publ., Amsterdam.

Niswender, G. D., and Midgley, A. R. (1970). *In* "Immunologic Methods in Steroid Determination" (F. G. Péron and B. V. Caldwell, eds.), pp. 149–166. Appleton, New York.

Odell, W. D., Abraham, G. A., Skowsky, W. R., Hescox, M. A., and Fisher, D. A. (1971). *In* "Principles of Competitive Protein-binding Assays" (W. D. Odell and W. H. Daughaday, eds.), pp. 57–76. Lippincott, Philadelphia, Pennsylvania.

Peck, H. M., Woodhour, A. F., and Hilleman, M. R. (1968). *Proc. Soc. Exp. Biol. Med.* **128**, 699.

Raziano, J., Cowchock, S., Ferin, M., and Vande Wiele, R. L. (1971). *Endocrinology* **88**, 1516.

Raziano, J., Ferin, M., and Vande Wiele, R. L. (1972). *Endocrinology* **90**, 1133.

Rümke, P., and Hekman, A. (1975). *Clin. Endocrinol. Metab.* **4**, 496.

Scaramuzzi, R. J., and Martensz, N. D. (1975). *In* "Immunization with Hormones in Reproduction Research" (E. Nieschlag, ed.), pp. 141–152. North-Holland Publ., Amsterdam.

Schoen, E. J., and Samuels, L. T. (1965). *Acta Endocrinol. (Copenhagen)* **50**, 365.

Skelley, D. S., Brown, L. P., and Besch, P. K. (1973). *Clin. Chem.* **19**, 146.

Slaunwhite, W. R., Lockie, G. N., Black, N., and Sandberg, A. A. (1962). *Science* **135**, 1062.

Smith, T. W., Haber, E., Yeatman, L., and Butler, V. P. (1976). *N. Engl. J. Med.* **294**, 797.

Smith, T. W., Butler, V. P., and Haber, E. (1977). *In* "Antibodies in Human Diagnosis and Therapy" (E. Haber and R. M. Krause, eds.), pp. 365–389. Raven, New York.

Spieler, J. M., Webb, R. L., Saldarini, R. J., and Coppola, J. (1972). *Steroids* **19**, 751.

Steinberger, E. (1971). *Physiol. Rev.* **51**, 1.

Stevens, V. C., and Crystle, C. D. (1973). *Obstet. Gynecol.* **42**, 485.

Sundaram, K., Tsong, Y. Y., Hood, W., and Brinson, A. (1973). *Endocrinology* **93**, 843.

Surve, A. H., Bacso, I., Brinckerhoff, J. H., and Kirsch, S. J. (1976). *Biol. Reprod.* **15**, 343.

ter Haar, M. B., and MacKinnon, P. C. B. (1975). *J. Endocrinol.* **65**, 399.

Thorneycroft, I. H., Thorneycroft, N. K., Scaramuzzi, R. J., and Blake, C. A. (1975). *Endocrinology* **97**, 301.

Vermeulen, A., Verdonck, L., Van der Straeten, M., and Orie, N. (1969). *J. Clin. Endocrinol. Metab.* **29**, 1470.

Vermeulen, A., Stoica, T., and Verdonck, L. (1971). *J. Clin. Endocrinol. Metab.* **33**, 759.

Weinstein, A., Lindner, H. R., Friedlander, A., and Bauminger, S. (1972). *Steroids* **20**, 789.

Wickings, E. J., and Nieschlag, E. (1977). *Int. J. Fertil.* **22**, 56.

Wickings, E. J., and Nieschlag, E. (1978a). *Biol. Reprod.* **18**, 602.

Wickings, E. J., and Nieschlag, E. (1978b). In preparation.

Wickings, E. J., Becher, A., and Nieschlag, E. (1976). *Endocrinology* **98**, 1142.

Wickings, E. J., Tafurt, C. A., Hoogen, H., and Nieschlag, E. (1977). *J. Steroid Biochem.* **8,** 147.

Wickings, E. J., Witting, C., and Nieschlag, E. (1978). *J. Endocrinol.* **77,** 68P.

Witting, C., Wickings, E. J., and Nieschlag, E. (1978). *Acta Endocrinol. (Copenhagen)* **87,** Suppl. 215, 29.

Wuttke, W., Döhler, K. D., and Gelato, M. (1976). *J. Endocrinol.* **68,** 391.

Yalow, R. S., and Berson, S. A. (1959). *Nature (London)* **184,** 1648.

VITAMINS AND HORMONES, VOL. 36

Effects of Cannabinoids on Reproduction and Development

ERIC BLOCH, BENJAMIN THYSEN, GENE A. MORRILL,
ELIOT GARDNER, AND GEORGE FUJIMOTO

*Departments of Biochemistry, Gynecology—Obstetrics, Laboratory Medicine,
Neuroscience, Physiology, and Psychiatry, Albert Einstein College of Medicine of Yeshiva
University, Bronx, New York*

In recent years, the potential importance of the effects of marihuana on reproduction and development has been recognized. This recognition has led to an increasing number of studies and reports on the action of marihuana and its purified cannabinoid fractions on reproductive capacity and events and on embryonic and fetal development. A comprehensive, critical review of these reports, particularly from the viewpoint of reproductive biology, seems not to have been carried out. This review represents such an attempt.

203

The review encompasses the effects of cannabinoids, crude marihuana extract (CME), and of marihuana on reproduction and development. It is organized into six main topics: male reproductive system;
female reproductive system; prostaglandin synthesis; adrenal cortical
system; development; and reproductive behavior. The adrenal cortical
system is included in this review because of corticosteroid influence
on reproduction, substantial activity in this field, and a special interest
on the part of the reviewers.

Studies on sex differences in response to cannabinoids, on the influence of individual marihuana constituents on each others' biological
activities, and on activity of cannabinoids in the presence of other
drugs have not been included in this review. It is recognized that each
of these interactions between cannabis constituent and sex or drug may
profoundly affect cannabinoid activity. The interaction may occur (a) at
the genetic level, programmed during differentiation and expressed at
puberty, (b) in the induction of enzymes metabolizing cannabinoids, (c)
as competing substrates for a given enzyme, or (d) on the differential
rate of appearance of cannabinoid metabolites in a given tissue. For the
interested reader, references to these topics are included (Borgen and
Davis, 1974; Borgen et al., 1973; Burstein and Kupfer, 1971; Caldwell et
al., 1974; Cohen et al., 1971; Cohn et al., 1974; Dingell et al., 1973;
Fernandes et al., 1974; Hollister, 1974; Karniol and Carlini, 1973; Karniol et al., 1974; Lemberger and Rubin, 1976; List et al., 1975; Mitra et
al., 1976, 1977; Sofia and Barry, 1970; Thompson et al., 1973).

I. The Male Reproductive System

A. Male Reproductive Endocrine System

Marihuana and cannabinoids depress, reversibly, testicular endo-
crine function in all species studied: rats (Collu, 1976; Collu et al., 1975;
Harmon et al., 1976; Okey and Truant, 1975; Symons et al., 1976;
Thompson et al., 1973), mice (Dixit et al., 1974), rhesus monkey (Smith
et al., 1976), dogs (Dixit et al., 1977), and humans (Cohen, 1976;
Kolodny et al., 1974, 1975, 1976). This is seen in the diminished weights
of prostate (Collu, 1976; Collu et al., 1975; Okey and Truant, 1975;
Thompson et al., 1973), seminal vesicle (Dixit et al., 1974; Okey and
Truant, 1975; Solomon and Shattuck, 1974), and levator ani (Dixit et
al., 1974) and in decreased plasma testosterone levels (Cohen, 1976;
Harmon et al., 1976; R. T. Jones, 1976; Kolodny et al., 1974, 1976; Smith

et al., 1976; Symons *et al.*, 1976) following *chronic* or *acute* administration of CME, tetrahydrocannibinol (Δ^9-THC) or cannabis (Tables I–III). The involution of prostate and seminal vesicle are presumably reflections of diminished levels of circulating testosterone and testosterone synthesis (see Section I, B) rather than a direct effect of cannabinoids on these tissues (Collu, 1976) although experiments with castrated animals remain to be done. Δ^9-THC was effective whether administered by inhalation, orally, or by intraperitoneal or intramuscular injection. Gonadal activity recovers with cessation of treatment (Dixit *et al.*, 1974; Fujimoto *et al.*, 1978; Kolodny *et al.*, 1974, 1976).

A large study by Fujimoto *et al.* (1978; see also Table VIII), correlating changes in testes, androgen target systems, and sperm characteristics clearly showed the inhibitory but reversible effects of short- and long-term cannabinoid treatment on testes function. Oral administration of CME or Δ^9-THC for 5 days to adult Fischer rats led to a small but significant increase in testes weight and a pronounced decrease in plasma testosterone levels (see Table VIII). No significant changes were noted in target organ weights, cytology, or seminal vesicle fructose and citrate concentrations. Cannabidiol (CBD) was inactive. When treatment with CME was extended to 77 days (Fujimoto *et al.*, 1978), doses of 15 and 75 mg per kilogram of body weight resulted in significant reductions (27–67% at 75-mg dose) in ventral prostate, epididymal, and seminal vesicle weights, in seminal vesicle fluid volume and fructose content, and in epididymal sperm count. Histological examination indicated involution of prostate and a decrease in testicular interstitium. The effects on all these indices of male reproductive tract activity and testicular function were completely reversed by the end of a 30-day recovery period.

List *et al.* (1977) reported a significant increase in rat liver catabolism of testosterone to unidentified, "polar" metabolites after administration of Δ^9-THC or CBD. Simultaneously, cytochrome P-450 levels were reduced. These somewhat contradictory observations merit further study. If confirmed, it would suggest that cannabinoids depress plasma testosterone concentrations by increasing catabolism as well as decreasing testicular androgen synthesis. A reported effect of age on responsivity to Δ^9-THC (Collu, 1976) also needs confirmation.

In guinea pigs both Δ^8- and Δ^9-THC at low concentrations (10^{-8} M) augmented the musculotropic effects of norepinephrine and cholinergic effects of acetylcholine on the vas deferens in an *in vitro* system (Gascon and Peres, 1973). The two THCs per se exerted no action on vas deferens contractility.

TABLE I

EFFECTS OF REPEATED OR CHRONIC ADMINISTRATION OF CANNABINOIDS ON TESTES, PROSTATE, AND SEMINAL VESICLE WEIGHTS[a]

Species	Strain	Age or body weight	Cannabinoid	Dose[b] (mg/kg/day)	Duration (days)	Route	Effect on weight/kg body weight — Testes	Prostate	Seminal vesicle	References[f]
Rat	Fischer	100 gm	Δ8-, Δ9-THC	50	28–119	Po	↑±[c]	→	—	1
			CME	150	28–119	Po	↑±[c]	→	—	1
	Fischer	100 gm	Δ9-THC	50	28	Po	↑	→[j]	—	2
					90, 180	Po	↑	0[j]	—	2
	Fischer	100 gm	Δ9-THC	10	28–180	Po	↑	0	—	3
				50	28–180	Po	↑±[e]	↓±[e]	—	3
				4	28, 57	Inhalation	→	→	—	3
					87, 180	Inhalation	0	0	↓[j]	3
	Fischer	Adult	CME	15, 75	77	Po	→	→	0	4
	Sprague–Dawley	21 days	Δ9-THC	10 (3/wk)	28	Ip	0	→	→	5
	Sprague–Dawley	25 days	Δ9-THC	20	70	Not stated	—	—	→	6
	Wistar	20 days	CME	90 ppm[f]	37	Diet	→	→	→	7
	Wistar	Adult	Δ9-THC	16	4	Ip	0	0	0	8
	Sprague–Dawley	23 days	Δ9-THC	20 μg[g]	7	Intraventricular	0	→	0	9
	Sprague–Dawley	50 days	Δ9-THC	50 μg[g]	7	Intraventricular	0	0	0	9
	Walter Reed	20 days	Δ9-THC	8	40	Po	→	—	—	10

Mouse	Swiss–Albino	Adult	CME	70	45	Ip	↓	—	↓[i,k]	11
	Swiss–Albino	Adult[h]	CME	200	?	Ip	—	→	↓[k]	12

[a] Effect expressed as increase (↑), no change (0), decrease (↓), or questionable effect (±).

[b] Minimum dose giving consistent results in relation to higher dose(s) or over a period of time.

[c] After 5 and 28 days: (↑); after 91 and 119 days: (0).

[d] After 180 days: 0.

[e] After 28 and 57 days: (↓); after 87 and 180 days: (0).

[f] 50 ppm Δ^9-THC or ca. 5 mg of Δ^9-THC/kg per day po; for testes, effective dose ~270 ppm of CME (Okey and Truant, 1975).

[g] Equal to ca. 10 mg/kg per day injected peripherally (Collu, 1976).

[h] Castrated with end point of testosterone stimulation of accessory reproductive organ weights.

[i] Effects reversible after cessation of treatment.

[j] Epididymal weight, seminal fluid volume, and fructose content (↓), reversibly.

[k] Levator ani weight (↓).

[l] References: (1) Thompson et al., 1973; (2) Rosenkrantz et al., 1975; (3) Rosenkrantz and Braude, 1976; (4) Fujimoto et al., 1978; (5) Collu et al., 1975; (6) Solomon and Shattuck, 1974; (7) Okey and Truant, 1975; (8) Ling et al., 1973; (9) Collu, 1976; (10) Harmon et al., 1976; (11) Dixit et al., 1974; (12) Dixit and Lohiya, 1975.

TABLE II

EFFECTS OF REPEATED OR CHRONIC ADMINISTRATION OF Δ^9-THC OR MARIHUANA ON PLASMA TESTOSTERONE AND LH CONCENTRATIONS[a]

Species	Strain	Dose[b] (mg/kg/day)	Duration (days)	Route	Effect on Testosterone	Effect on LH	References[e]
Rat	Wistar	5 (2/wk)	42	Im	↓	↓	1
	Fischer[c]	4	14	Inhalation	↓	—	2
		10	14	Po	↓	—	2
	Sprague–Dawley	10 (3/wk)	28	Ip	—	↓	3
	Sprague–Dawley	20 μg[d]	7	Intraventricular	—	0	4
		50 μg[d]	7	Intraventricular	—	0	4
	Walter Reed	8	40	Po	↓	—	5
Rhesus		2.4	1 Year	Diet	0	—	6
Human		6 Cigarettes	21	Smoking	0	—	7
		5–> 10 Cigarettes (4/wk)	>6 Months	Smoking	↓	0	8, 9
		1 Cigarette	3	Smoking	0	—	10
		1–3 Cigarettes	63	Smoking	↓	↓	11
		>3 Cigarettes/wk	10–28 Years	Smoking	0	—	12

[a] Rats were 21–23 days old; rhesus monkey and human subjects were adults. Rats and rhesus were administered Δ^9-THC; humans smoked marihuana. Effect expressed as increase (↑), no change (0), or decrease (↓), not determined (—). Plasma FSH levels determined and found unchanged (Collu, 1976; Kolodny et al., 1974, 1975, 1976); plasma prolactin increased in 23- but not in 50-day-old rats after intraventricular Δ^9-THC administration (Collu, 1976).

[b] Minimum dose giving consistent results in relation to higher dose(s) or over a period of time.

[c] Age not specified; designation based on other work by author's group (Rosenkrantz et al., 1975; Rosenkrantz and Braude, 1976).

[d] Equal to ca. 10 mg/kg per day injected peripherally (Collu, 1976); 50-μg dose given to 50-day-old rats.

[e] References: (1) Symons et al., 1976; (2) Esber et al., 1976; (3) Collu et al., 1975; (4) Collu, 1976; (5) Harmon et al., 1976; (6) Sassenrath and Chapman, 1975; (7) Mendelson et al., 1974; (8, 9) Kolodny et al., 1974, 1975; (10) Schaefer et al., 1975; (11) Kolodny et al., 1976; (12) Coggins et al., 1976.

TABLE III
Effect of Single Administration of Δ^9-THC on Plasma Testosterone, LH, and Prolactin Levels[a]

Species	Strain	Dose[b] (mg/kg/day)	Duration (days)	Effect on Testosterone	Effect on LH	Effect on Prolactin	References[e]
Rat	Wistar	16	S + 24[d]	—	—	↕	1
	Hebrew U. Sabra	2	S + 0.5	—	—	→	2
	Not stated	5[c]	S + 2	→	→	→	3
	Wistar	5	S + 2	→	—	—	4
Human		1 cig.	S + 2, 3	→	—	—	5
Rhesus		2.5	S + 6, 12 ...	→	→	—	6

[a] Δ^9-THC was administered to adult rhesus monkeys and rats, except for 36-day-old rats used by Daley et al. (1974). Humans smoked marihuana. Animal administration was intraperitoneal or intramuscular. Effect expressed as increase (↑), decrease (↓), not determined (—).

[b] Minimum dose giving consistent results in relation to higher dose(s) or over a period of time.

[c] Doses of 30, 60 mg ineffective.

[d] Single injection of Δ^9-THC (S) with blood removal n hours (+n) later (e.g., S + 0.5 = blood collection 0.5 hour after THC injection; S + 2, 3 = collection at 2 and 3 hours post-THC).

[e] References: (1) Daley et al., 1974; (2) Kramer and Ben-David, 1974; (3) Bromley and Zimmerman, 1976; (4) Symons et al., 1976; (5) Kolodny et al., 1976; (6) Smith et al., 1976.

B. TESTES

Chronic administration of Δ^9-THC or CME to rats or mice results in testicular weight changes characterized by limited magnitude (0–30%) and considerable variability and scatter (Table I). Δ^9-THC dissolved in oil and given orally at a cumulative dose greater than 1 gm over a 1-month period led initially to modest increases in testicular weight (Rosenkrantz and Braude, 1976; Rosenkrantz et al., 1975; Thompson et al., 1975). Some tolerance or escape also developed with longer administration. At lower cumulative dosages in these studies, or in investigations in which lower dosages of Δ^9-THC were administered in diverse vehicles via different routes (Coggins, 1976; Collu, 1976; Collu et al., 1975; Goldstein et al., 1977; Harmon et al., 1976; Okey and Truant, 1975), testes weight was the same or somewhat less than those of the vehicle-injected controls. It should be recognized that relatively few studies have been made on cannabinoid effects on adult testes weight. Most have dealt with initially immature rats, thereby studying the influence of cannabinoid on testes maturation.

Cannabinoids exert a direct inhibitory action on testicular androgen synthesis and cell metabolism (Table IV). This is in contrast to the variable weight changes but explains in part the drop in plasma testosterone levels following cannabinoid intake. The addition of Δ^9-THC or cannabinol (CBN) to mouse testes minces in incubation medium inhibited endogenous testosterone production by more than 50% (Dalterio et al., 1977). Inhibition was obtained with testes from both immature and adult mice, although the specificity of cannabinoid activity in this interesting study remains to be established. Similarly, a single or a 10-day regime of daily intraperitoneal administration of Δ^9-THC or CBD decreased the capacity of rat testicular microsomes to convert progesterone to testosterone (List et al., 1977).

Cannabinoids added to testes slice preparations in vitro depress protein, nucleic acid, and lipid synthesis and ATP concentrations (Jakubović and McGeer, 1976, 1977). Some of the metabolic derivatives of Δ^9-THC (e.g., 11-hydroxy-Δ^9-THC, 8β-hydroxy-Δ^9-THC) were more active in suppressing protein, lipid, and nucleic acid synthesis than their parent compound. However, the doses required (10^{-5} to 10^{-4} M) to achieve a 30–60% inhibition of synthetic activity seem high. Limited solubility may be involved since the highest activity was shown by 1-[4-(morpholino)butyryloxy]-3-n-pentyl-6,6,9-trimethyl-10a,6a,7,8-tetrahydrodibenzo[b,d]pyran hydrobromide, a water-soluble derivative of Δ^9-THC (Jakubović and McGeer, 1977). Mice treated in vivo with 90 mg of CME over a 45-day period showed decreased testes weight and

RNA content, and smaller seminal tubule diameters (Dixit *et al.*, 1974). Dogs given CME subcutaneously for 30 days (12.5 mg/kg per day) exhibited a moderate decrease in testicular weight, protein, RNA, and sialic acid content. Seminiferous tubules and Leydig cell nuclei were shrunk (Dixit *et al.*, 1977). Chronic intraperitoneal THC or CBD injections significantly reduced testicular esterase activity in rats, indicating Leydig cell involution (Goldstein *et al.*, 1977). The reduction in metabolic activity and macromolecular synthesis following exposure to cannabinoids correlates with and may be the basis for the diminished spermatogenesis and testosterone synthesis found after Δ^9-THC administration.

C. Effect on Gonadotropin and Prolactin Production

Cannabinoids exert a direct action on testicular activity and metabolism. However, at least part of the diminution of gonadal function caused by cannabinoids is mediated via the hypothalamic–pituitary axis, and pituitary gonadotropin production responds to marihuana (Tables II and III). Whether this response is solely or only partially responsible for the decrease in testes endocrine activity remains to be resolved; work with hypophysectomized animals has not yet been carried out.

Symons *et al.* (1976) elegantly demonstrated a depression of pituitary *gonadotropic* and gonadal activity following the intramuscular administration of 5 mg of Δ^9-THC, either (a) into 21-day-old rats, twice weekly, for 6 weeks, or (b) into adult male rats, acutely, with sampling 2 hours later at time of maximum blood Δ^9-THC concentrations. In both groups, plasma testosterone (T) and luteinizing hormone (LH), levels decreased markedly, as shown in the accompanying tabulation.

	Acute (adult)		Chronic (immature)	
	Vehicle	Δ^9-THC	Vehicle	Δ^9-THC
Plasma testosterone (ng/ml)	1.43 ± 0.11	1.09 ± 0.14	2.15 ± 0.26	1.12 ± 0.14
Plasma LH (ng/ml)	82 ± 10	<15	99 ± 8	75 ± 8

Furthermore, there was less increase in plasma LH levels after exogenous LH-releasing hormone (LH-RH) in Δ^9-THC-treated rats than in animals injected with vehicle only. Plasma LH levels respond acutely to marihuana in humans, as will be discussed below.

TABLE IV

EFFECT OF CANNABINOIDS ON SPERMATOGENESIS AND OTHER PARAMETERS OF MALE REPRODUCTIVE PHYSIOLOGY

Species	Strain	Cannabinoid	Dose (mg/kg/day)	Duration (days)	Route	Effects[a]		References[d]
Effects on spermatozoa								
Rat	Fischer	CME	750	28	Po	Spermatogonia	↓	1
Rat	Fischer	Δ⁸-, Δ⁹-THC	500	28	Po	Spermatogonia	0	1
Rat	Fischer	CME	15, 75	77	Po	Spermatogonia	↓	2
Mouse	Swiss	CME	70	45	Ip	Spermatogenesis	↓	3
Human	—	Marihuana	5->10 Cigarettes, 4×/wk	>6 months	Smoking	Spermatogenesis	↓	4
			10–31 Cigarettes	21	Smoking	Spermatogenesis	0	5
				14–21	Smoking	Spermatogenesis	↓	6
Dog	—	CME	12.5	30	Sc	Spermatogenesis	↓	7
Miscellaneous effects in vivo								
Rat	Wistar	Δ⁹-THC	4, 16	S + 20	Ip	[³H]Testosterone uptake	0	8
Mouse	Swiss	CME	70	45	Ip	Testes RNA content	↓	9
Rat	Long–Evans	Δ⁹-THC	1	21	Sc	Mammary development	↑	10
Human	—	CME	"Heavy"	—	Smoking	Breast development	↑	11
Dog		CME	12.5	30	Sc	Testes RNA, protein, sialic acid synthesis; Leydig cell nucleus	↓	7
Rat	Wistar	Δ⁹-THC	2, 10	S + 6	Ip }	Testes testosterone (↓); liver testosterone hydroxyl (↑)		12
		CBD	2	10ᶜ	Ip }			

212

Miscellaneous effects in vitro

Rat	Wistar	$2\text{--}100 \times 10^{-5}$ M Δ^8-, Δ^9-THC. 6 metabolites	Testes RNA, DNA, protein, lipid synthesis	$\rightarrow$	13, 14
Guinea pig		$10^{-8} M$ Δ^8-, Δ^9-THC	Vas deferens NE and ACH effects[b]	$\uparrow$	9
Bovine		$3\text{--}30 \times 10^{-4} M$ Δ^9-THC	Sperm motility, respiration, ATP	$\rightarrow$	4
Mouse		34–37-day-old testes} incubated with $8\text{--}800 \times 10^{-7} M$ 2–3-month-old testes} Δ^9-THC or CBN	Testosterone production	$\rightarrow$	15

[a] Effect expressed as increase ($\uparrow$), no change (0) or decrease ($\downarrow$).

[b] Potentiation of tropic and contractile effects of norepinephrine (NE) and acetylcholine (ACH), respectively.

[c] CBD, 2 mg dose × 10 days ineffective in testosterone production.

[d] References: (1) Thompson *et al.*, 1973; (2) Fujomoto *et al.*, 1978; (3) Dixit *et al.*, 1974; (4) Kolodny *et al.*, 1974; (5) Smith *et al.*, 1976; (6) Hembree *et al.*, 1976; (7) Dixit *et al.*, 1977; (8) Ling *et al.*, 1973; (9) Gascon and Peres, 1973; (10) Harmon and Aliapoulios, 1974; (11) Harmon and Aliapoulios, 1972; (12) List *et al.*, 1977; (13) Jakubović and McGeer, 1976; (14) Jakubović and McGeer, 1977; (15) Dalterio *et al.*, 1977.

Cannabinoids influence circulating *prolactin* levels in male rats; an age-dependent reactivity may exist. A single intraperitoneal administration of 2, 5, or 10 mg of Δ^9-THC to *adult* rats resulted in an immediate drop in serum prolactin (65% at the 5-mg dose) with a minimum reached in 30 minutes; a return to near-normal values occurred 4 hours later (Kramer and Ben-David, 1974). Similar activity was reported by Bromley and Zimmerman (1976). In contrast, *36-day-old* rats had a 2-fold rise in serum prolactin levels 24 hours after the intraperitoneal injection of 16 mg of Δ^9-THC, a dose equal in activity to that of 40 μg of estradiol benzoate (Daley *et al.*, 1974). Further support for an age dependency is found in the work of Collu (1976), where the intraventricular administration of Δ^9-THC to 23-day-old rats led to increased pituitary prolactin levels. No change was observed in 50-day-old rats. Kramer and Ben-David (1974) suggested prolactin suppression to be a consequence of TRH inhibition, a known effect of Δ^9-THC.

D. SPERMATOGENESIS

Cannabis extracts depress sperm maturation (Table IV). Daily intraperitoneal injection of mice with 2 mg of CME for 45 days resulted in complete arrest of spermatogenesis (Dixit *et al.*, 1974). Exposure of sperm to Δ^9-THC *in vitro* has been reported to decrease sperm motility, respiration, and ATP content and to cause morphological changes (Shahar and Bino, 1973). Rats treated orally with 750 or 1500 mg of CME per kilogram per day for 28 days (but not after longer intervals) showed spermatogonial degeneration (Thompson *et al.*, 1973). The effect was moderate and may have been caused by noncannabinoid constituents in CME; Δ^8- and Δ^9-THC at equivalent dosages were inactive. In Fischer rats, CME at 75 mg/kg per day orally for 77 days reduced epididymal sperm content, which returned to basal levels at the end of a 30-day recovery period (Fujimoto *et al.*, 1978). Daily administration of CME (12.5 mg/kg body weight) for 30 days produced complete arrest of spermatogenesis in dogs (Dixit *et al.*, 1977).

E. HUMANS

The *acute* administration of marihuana by smoking usually leads to a decrease in circulating testosterone and LH levels (Cohen, 1976; Kolodny *et al.*, 1975, 1976; R. Jones, 1977). For example, Kolodny *et al.* (1976) reported that marihuana inhalation (20 mg of Δ^9-THC per cigarette) resulted 3 hours later in a marked decrease in plasma testosterone and LH concentrations in both naive and experienced smokers (see tabulation). Plasma FSH levels remained unchanged.

Tested at	Before smoking	After smoking	
		Naive	Experienced
	Testosterone (ng/ml)		
0 Hour	7.33 ± 0.63	7.79 ± 0.56	6.39 ± 0.53
3 Hours	7.16 ± 0.47	5.05 ± 0.37	4.32 ± 0.31
	LH (mU/ml)		
0 Hour	8.6 ± 1.0	8.0 ± 1.2	8.4 ± 1.1
3 Hours	8.0 ± 0.9	4.9 ± 0.5	4.6 ± 0.5

This is in contrast to the *chronic* effects of marihuana. In the earliest study on this subject, Kolodny *et al.* (1974) found blood testosterone levels, but not those of LH, FSH, or prolactin, depressed in chronic marihuana cigarette smokers. This study suffered from inadequate controls. Cohen (1976) confirmed this observation, but others found plasma testosterone concentration in chronic smokers to be the same as those in nonsmokers (Coggins *et al.*, 1976; Mendelson *et al.*, 1974, 1976; Nahas, 1976; Schaefer *et al.*, 1975).

In an extensive study, Coggins *et al.* (1976) saw no difference in testosterone levels in paired male nonsmokers and smokers who had smoked at least 3 times a week for 10 years or more. A subgroup of 13 males consuming at least 10 cigarettes per day (26–74 mg of Δ^9-THC per day) had 5.22 ± 1.76 ng of testosterone per milliliter of plasma compared to 5.50 ± 1.18 among paired, nonsmoking controls. Subgroups with high β-globulin (sex steroid-binding globulin) levels or unilateral testicular atrophy also showed no differences. Both nonsmokers and heavy smokers fathered an average of 2.6 children. Coggins concluded that "these findings cast serious doubt on a cause and effect relationship between marihuana smoking and plasma testosterone levels in long-term users" (Coggins *et al.*, 1976, p. 160).

The differences in findings may reflect variations in dose and length of administration, and in the time of sampling relative to episodic secretion and a diurnal rhythm pattern. The time interval between smoking and plasma sampling is of importance; blood levels return to presmoking levels 12 hours after marihuana intake (R. Jones, 1977).

Among the suppressive effects of cannabinoids reported on male reproductive organs and their functions has been one on lowering sperm output in young men smoking marihuana cigarettes for 6 months (Kolodny *et al.*, 1974). Oligospermia was observed in 35% of the patients, with reversal after cessation of smoking. Mendelson *et al.* (1974), however, reported no change in sperm counts in young men smoking for a 3-week period. The relatively shorter time period in the latter study may have been a factor in explaining these discrepant results. In a third study, smoking 10–31 cigarettes (200–600 mg of Δ^9-THC equivalent) per day for 2–3 weeks led to a 25–50% drop in sperm count (Hembree *et al.*, 1976). The temporal relationship between initiation of marihuana smoking, spermatogenesis, and the reduction in sperm counts has been interpreted as a perturbation of spermiogenesis, although altered epididymal transit or failure to complete meiosis are not excluded by the data (Hembree *et al.*, 1976).

II. The Female Reproductive System

One of the earliest reports on any productive effect of marihuana dealt with female reproduction. It described the relaxation of rat uterine strips by CME and the antioxytoxic activity of CME (Bose *et al.*, 1963, 1964). Since 1963, further work has been done, although less than in males. Cannabinoid effects on female reproduction have been studied largely in rats and mice; investigations with other species are increasing.

A. The Reproductive System in Nonpregnant Females

CME administration to rats and mice over periods of 8–64 days resulted generally in reduced uterine metabolism (Table V). Uterine weight (Dixit *et al.*, 1975; Okey and Truant, 1975), glycogen content (Chakravarty *et al.*, 1975a), and RNA and sialic acid levels (Dixit *et al.*, 1975) declined during cannabis administration. CME antagonizes the effects of estrogens in some systems. Chakravarty *et al.* (1976) reported the counteraction of CME on the inhibition of monoamine oxidase activity by estradiol in 11-day-old rats. The uterotropic effect of estradiol in suckling rats was delayed, although not abolished, by the prior subcutaneous injection of CME (~20 mg of Δ^9-THC equivalent per kilogram) over a 10-day period (Chakravarty *et al.*, 1975a). Δ^9-THC restored the estradiol-suppressed plasma LH concentrations to their uninhibited levels (Marks, 1972).

The long-term studies by Dixit *et al.* (1975) showed atrophy of ovarian function by CME. Cessation of the ovarian cycle as judged by vaginal smear occurred after 30 days of treatment, and by 64 days the ovaries were significantly reduced in size and number of primordial ova. Many atretic follicles were seen in the 64-day ovaries, and luteinization was inhibited. In contrast, A/J mice on an oral regime of CME or Δ^9-THC continued with normal estrous cycles (Kostellow et al., 1978). In a single study with primates, 2 macaca monkeys retained a normal menstrual cycle while ingesting 2.4 mg of Δ^9-THC per kilogram per day for one year (Sassenrath and Chapman, 1975).

Δ^9-THC did not produce significant weight or morphological change in uteri and ovaries of intact, adult rats which had received oral doses of up to 50 mg/kg per day for 28–180 days (Rosenkrantz et al., 1975). On the other hand, Solomon described a uterine weight gain in adult rats ovariectomized 1 day prior to the beginning of intraperitoneal injection of 2.5 mg of Δ^9-THC per kilogram for 14 days (Solomon et al., 1976). The magnitude of response was about two-thirds that obtained from inject-ing 2 μg of estradiol. Doses of both 1 and 10 mg/kg gave a smaller response. Cytologically, the uterus showed hyperplasia and hyper-trophy of the surface epithelium, endometrial stroma and glands, and myometrium. Δ^9-THC produced vaginal stratification (Solomon et al., 1977). Conflicting claims for Δ^9-THC as a weak competitor with estradiol-17β for uterine cytoplasmic estrogen receptors have been made. This is discussed in Section II, C.

Nir et al. (1973) found that intraperitoneal injections of Δ^9-THC on the afternoon of proestrus effectively delayed ovulation in rats for 24 hours, although many of the oocytes entrapped in the follicles had matured. The preovulatory surge in LH concentration was completely suppressed. A dose of 10 mg/kg was required to block ovulation. Since the concurrent administration of 2.5 μg of LH was not as effective in restoring ovulation as when given together with a blocking dose of Nembutal, the investigators do not exclude a direct effect of Δ^9-THC on the ovary.

Δ^9-THC causes a striking depression in serum LH concentrations (Table V). This was first described by Marks (1972) in ovariectomized rats and later confirmed in cycling rats (Chakravarty et al., 1975b; Nir et al., 1973). A brief report (Esber et al., 1975) described increased LH and FSH levels in rat serum after gavage of 50 mg of THC per kilogram for 14 days but not longer. This stands rather in contrast to the depress-ing effects of acute Δ^9-THC administration seen in both sexes. In a report by Chakravarty et al. (1975b), a dramatic decrease from 172 to 23 ng/ml was observed in serum prolactin levels after the in-traperitoneal injection of 50 mg of THC per kilogram.

In rhesus monkeys, Besch and co-workers (1977) showed that a single dose of Δ^9-THC administered intramuscularly 3–5 weeks after ovariec-tomy resulted in a precipitous drop in plasma LH and FSH levels. These reached minimum concentrations 6–12 hours after Δ^9-THC injec-

TABLE V
Effects of Cannabinoids on Endocrine and Reproductive System of the Nonpregnant Female[a]

Species	Strain	Age	Canna-binoid	Dose[b] (mg/kg/dose)	Duration (days)	Route	Effect on Uterus	Effect on Ovary (weight/kg/body wt)	Effect on Cycle	References[i]
Rat	Fischer	100 gm	Δ9-THC	2–50	28–180	Po	0	0	—	1
	CD	75 Days	Δ9-THC	1	14	Ip	←→	—	—	2, 3
	Wistar	20 Days	CME	360 ppm	8	Diet	→	—	—	4
		20 Days	CME	200	8	Ip	0/↓[d]	—	—	4
		Adult[c]	CME	360 ppm	15	Diet	↓[e]	—	—	4
	Not stated	11 Days	CME	120	10	Sc	↓[e]	—	—	5
	Not stated	Adult	CME	25	64	Ip	0[f]	→	Absent	6
Mouse	Swiss–Albino	Adult	CME	40	64	Ip	↓[f]	→	Absent	6
Macaca	—	Adult	Δ9-THC	2.4	1 year	Diet	—	—	Present	7

218

							LH	Other (weight/ml plasma)	Cycle	
Rat	Fischer	100 gm	Δ⁹-THC	50	14	Po	↑±[a]	FSH: ↑±	—	8
	Not stated	120 gm	Δ⁹-THC	5	2S + 2	Ip	→	—	→	9
		Adult[h]	Δ⁹-THC	50	S + 6	Ip	→	Prolactin: ↓	—	10
		Adult[h]	Δ⁹-THC	1–5	S + 1	Iv	→	—	—	11
Rhesus	—	Adult[h]	Δ⁹-THC	0.625	5 + 6, 12	Im	→	FSH: ↓	—	12

[a] Effect expressed as increase (↑), no change (0), decrease (↓), or questionable effect (±).

[b] Minimum dose giving consistent results in relation to higher dose(s) or over a period of time.

[c] Ovariectomized 6 weeks prior to cannabinoid administration.

[d] See Table I, footnote f.

[e] Antagonistic effect to estradiol-induced increase in uterine weight, glycogen and water content.

[f] Decrease in uterine glycogen and in uterine and vaginal RNA and sialic acid.

[g] After 14 days: ↑; after 23–180 days: 0.

[h] Ovariectomized 3–5 weeks prior to cannabinoid administration.

[i] References: (1) Rosenkrantz et al., 1975; (2) Solomon et al., 1976; (3) Solomon et al., 1977; (4) Okey and Truant, 1975; (5) Chakravarty et al., 1975a; (6) Dixit et al., 1975; (7) Sassenrath and Chapman, 1975; (8) Esber et al., 1975; (9) Nir et al., 1973; (10) Chakravarty et al., 1975b; (11) Marks, 1972; (12) Besch et al., 1977.

tion, and then rapidly returned to basal levels. Duration of effect, but not magnitude, was related to dosage. Acute marihuana smoking by human females depressed plasma FSH and LH levels, while chronic smoking increased the number of anovulatory cycles and lowered both LH peaks and luteal progesterone levels, according to Johnson, citing work by Kolodny (in Besch *et al.*, 1977).

Except for the inhibition of LH release, no general conclusions on the effects of marihuana or its components on the female reproductive system seem possible. The number of studies to date have been few, and the experimental designs from study to study quite varied. The activity of Δ^9-THC on the female reproductive tract is not identical to that of CME. The activity of noncannabinoid constituents in CME on reproductive processes and structures requires investigation. More work should be carried out with other species, particularly suitable primates.

B. Effect of Cannabinoids on Maternal Physiology during Pregnancy and on Lactation

The changes in maternal physiology during pregnancy in response to cannabinoids have been the subject of a small number of investigations. Few cannabinoid effects have been described, and most of these are not restricted to the pregnant state.

In *rats,* cumulative doses of 1–4 gm of Δ^9-THC (!) resulted in prolongation of gestation by 2–3 days (Borgen *et al.*, 1971). Since birth weights were normal, the extended gestation suggested to Pace and co-workers (1971) delayed nidation rather than delayed parturition. A brief report by the Rosenkrantz group (Esber *et al.*, 1975) indicated a Δ^9-THC effect on plasma gonadotropin and estradiol concentrations in pregnant rats.

The maternal weight gain normally seen in pregnancy is abolished or reversed after intake of a sufficient dose of Δ^9-THC. Long–Evans rats injected with Δ^9-THC subcutaneously throughout pregnancy lost weight when the dose exceeded 75 mg of THC (Borgen *et al.*, 1971; Pace *et al.*, 1971). Very similar results were obtained by Banerjee *et al.* (1975) working with Sprague–Dawley rats. This decreased rate of growth has also been reported after long-term administration of higher doses of CME or Δ^9-THC to nonpregnant rats (Bartova and Birmingham, 1976; Manning *et al.*, 1971; Rosenkrantz and Braude, 1976; Rosenkrantz *et al.*, 1975; Thompson *et al.*, 1973) and has been ascribed to decreased food consumption, THC being anorexigenic (Manning et al., 1971; Rosenkrantz and Braude, 1976). However, the reduction in food intake is small (10–30%).

Reduced gain in body weight is not shared equally by all organ systems. In the work by Borgen et al. (1971), cumulative doses of 1–4 gm of THC resulted in increased maternal adrenal, thyroid, and heart weights and decreased liver weights. As in the nonpregnant rat, adrenal and thyroid weight increments were substantial (40–75%).

Moderate or low doses of cannabinoids did not influence length of gestation, maternal viability, or maternal weight gain (Borgen et al., 1971; Keplinger et al., 1973; Pace et al., 1971).

Other effects of potential importance to the pregnant rat and fetuses include hemoconcentration, rise in erythocyte count (Rosenkrantz and Braude, 1976; Thompson et al., 1973), a questionable hyperglycemia (Rosenkrantz and Braude, 1976; Rosenkrantz et al., 1975; Sprague et al., 1973), and, at very high doses of THC or CME, severe depletion of fat depots (Thompson et al., 1973).

Pregnancy and fertility in *mice*, unlike rats, were not influenced by Δ^9-THC consumption (Legator et al., 1976; Maker et al., 1974; Mantilla-Plata et al., 1975). Following an extensive protocol, in which cumulatively 100–900 mg of Δ^9-THC were injected intraperitoneally in single or multiple doses into Swiss–Webster mice between day 8 and day 16 of gestation, maternal weight gains were unaffected (Mantilla-Plata et al., 1975). Pregnant CFI-S mice did not respond to 5 mg of Δ^9-THC per kilogram body weight added to their diet (Maker et al., 1974). Inhalation of 500 mg of CME "near term" increased the heart rate and caused electrocardiogram changes in *guinea pigs* (Singer et al., 1973).

Potentially significant is the report that corpora lutea of pregnant mice very effectively concentrated [^{14}C]Δ^9-THC administered intravenously and as determined by radioautography (Freudenthal et al., 1972; Kennedy and Waddell, 1972). In contrast, ovarian follicles and stroma of pregnant and nonpregnant mice (Freudenthal et al., 1972; Kennedy and Waddell, 1972), dogs (Martin et al., 1976), and rabbits (Agurell et al., 1970) did not seem to localize Δ^9-THC in concentrations greater than those found in plasma. The localization in luteal tissue may indicate protein binding, with its physiological implications, or more simply reflect the lipophilic solubility of Δ^9-THC.

In one study using *chimpanzees*, male and female smokers who had consumed 50–150 doses of Δ^9-THC, 1–2 mg/kg, were mated with nonsmoking partners as well as with each other. The interval between smoking and mating in these 9 chimpanzees was 48 to 535 days. Pregnancy and fertility among smokers did not differ from animals in the colony who had never smoked marihuana (Grilly et al., 1974).

Lactation

Lactation appears to be reduced by Δ^9-THC. Pups of rats which had been injected subcutaneously with a cumulative dose of 1.2 gm of Δ^9-THC during Day 10–16 of pregnancy showed a high neonatal mortality (Pace et al., 1971). This significant rise in the mortality of rat pups 1–3 days old was ascribed to diminished milk reaching the newborn; no milk was visible in the pups' stomachs (Borgen et al., 1971; Pace et al., 1971). Cross-fostering confirmed that Δ^9-THC-treated rats were not successfully lactating. The mechanism or locus of action is unknown. It may involve inhibition of prolactin production or be a direct effect on mammary gland metabolism; mammary glands accumulate [^{14}C]Δ^9-THC in 15-day pregnant mice (Freudenthal et al., 1972).

Δ^9-THC can be retained by the mother and transmitted to her young, as shown in the radioactivity present in rat pups whose mothers had received 20 μCi (53 mg/kg) of 2[^{14}C]Δ^9-THC 3 days earlier (Jakubović et al., 1973). Δ^9-THC was presumably retained in mammary tissue and transmitted via milk, although both skin and salivary secretions are alternative possibilities. No effects on lactation were noted with low doses of Δ^9-THC or CME (Keplinger et al., 1973; Maker et al., 1974). [^{14}C]Δ^9-THC, administered on marshmallows to lactating squirrel monkeys, was found in low concentrations in both milk and suckling infants (Chao et al., 1976). Of the injected dose, 43% appeared in maternal urine and feces, within 24 hours, 0.2% in milk, and 0.13% in infants' excreta.

C. CANNABINOIDS AS ESTROGENS

Neto et al. (1975), Solomon et al. (1976), and Rawitch et al. (1977) point out the similarity between the biological activity of Δ^9-THC (or CME) and estrogens in females and males. Indeed, there is an impressive list of organs, cells, and processes responding qualitatively similarly to both estradiol (Emmens and Parkes, 1947; Greep and Jones, 1950; Pantanelli, 1975; Price and Williams-Ashman, 1961) and cannabinoids: increased adrenal and pituitary weights, stimulation of ACTH secretion, altered prolactin production, follicular atresia, depression of weight of testes, seminal vesicle, and prostate, suppression of pituitary LH release and of spermatogenesis, and stimulation of mammary gland development. [One of the earliest "alerts" of cannabis as an estrogen came from the observation by Harmon and Aliapoulios

(1972) of gynecomastia in 3 heavy marihuana users. Harmon and Aliapoulios (1974) also demonstrated in rats that Δ^9-THC administration stimulated mammary tissue development.]

Arguments have been raised against considering Δ^9-THC as an estrogen. (a) A uterotrophic effect with a dose-response relationship is one of the primary criteria for assigning estrogenicity to a compound. In general, Δ^9-THC decreases rather than increases uterine weight and metabolism. The report by Solomon et al. (1976) of uterotrophic activity by Δ^9-THC lacked such a dose-response relationship. More extensive experiments with lower doses, such as those used by Solomon and Cocchia (1977) in later work, might reveal a dose-dependent uterotrophic response to Δ^9-THC. (b) The "estrogenic" dosage of Δ^9-THC is 10^3 to 10^5 orders higher than that of estradiol-17β for all criteria. (c) In our laboratories, preliminary studies using the chick oviduct system did not indicate estrogenic activity by Δ^9-THC. (d) Δ^9-THC suppresses or antagonizes estradiol-stimulated processes in several systems.

Cannabinoids have been studied for their ability to compete with estradiol for uterine cytosol binding (Okey and Truant, 1975; Okey and Bondy, 1977; Rawitch et al., 1977, Shoemaker and Harmon, 1977). The competition, at best, is weak, and its specificity has not been adequately documented. Cannabis resin, Δ^9-THC, or 11-hydroxy-Δ^9-THC at concentrations equal to 10^{-5} M Δ^9-THC either did not compete with estradiol (Okey and Truant, 1975; Okey and Bondy, 1977) or only weakly (Shoemaker and Harmon, 1977). Shoemaker and Harmon (1977) claimed [³H]Δ^9-THC and [³H]11-hydroxy-Δ^9-THC to bind with high affinity to uterine and mammary cytosol, a binding that was inhibited by estradiol pretreatment. Sucrose gradient sedimentation characteristics and tissue-binding specificities were the same as those of estradiol-17β (Shoemaker and Harmon, 1977) or showed a new, 10.4 S peak (Rawitch et al., 1977).

Δ^9-THC may act by reducing the availability of specific receptors to estradiol. Δ^9-THC may bind weakly to estrogen receptors at the receptor site. This would either diminish nuclear translocation of estrogen receptors or have the translocated receptor bound weakly to Δ^9-THC. Under conditions of high and sustained Δ^9-THC tissue concentrations, such binding would explain both the estradiol-like effects of Δ^9-THC and its antagonistic actions to estradiol. Alternatively, a change in conformation of the estrogen receptor (10.4 S form?) or an increased rate of destruction of receptor induced by Δ^9-THC would also explain the antiestrogenic action of this cannabinoid. On the whole, the "estrogen–antiestrogen" aspects of Δ^9-THC and CME activity remain to be clarified.

III. Prostaglandin Synthesis

Cannabinoids exert an inhibitory action on prostaglandin synthesis in diverse tissues and organs. Howes and Osgood (1976) have postulated that some of the effects of cannabinoids can be explained by their inhibition of prostaglandin synthesis.

Prostaglandins influence or regulate gonadotropic stimulation of ovarian function, degeneration of the corpus luteum, parturition, the contractility and motility of uterus, oviducts, vas deferens, and epididymis, and the tonus of associated circulatory systems. Burstein and Raz (1972) and Burstein *et al.* (1973) demonstrated that several crystalline cannabinoids, including Δ^9- and Δ^8-THC, CBD, and CBN inhibited prostaglandin synthesis from [^{14}C]8,11,14-epicosatrienoic acid in microsomal preparations from bovine seminal vesicles. The order of inhibitory activity correlated fairly well with that shown as antiinflammatory agents (Burstein *et al.*, 1973; Howes and Osgood, 1976). However, the inhibitory effect required rather large concentrations of cannabinoids, about 100-fold that of indomethacin, a sensitive inhibitor of the conversion of arachidonic acid to prostaglandins (Burstein *et al.*, 1973). Inhibition of synthesis was restricted to the prostaglandin E series; prostaglandin F synthesis was unaffected. The major activity in CME resided not with cannabinoids, but with the aromatic alcohols eugenol (Burstein *et al.*, 1975) and *p*-vinyl phenol (Burstein *et al.*, 1976). This finding emphasizes the potential importance of other constituents in marihuana, including alkaloids, terpene derivatives, and aromatic alcohols and acids.

Several reproductive processes seem to be inhibited or depressed by cannabinoids, e.g., LH secretion, uterine contractility, sperm counts, ovarian follicular maturation. Reduced tissue prostaglandin concentrations have similar effects. If cannabinoids or other marihuana constituents do exert a major inhibitory effect on prostaglandin synthesis, some of their effects on reproductive processes may be reflections of reduced prostaglandin synthesis.

IV. Adrenal Cortical System

A. Cannabinoid Effects on Pituitary–Adrenal Axis

CME, Δ^9-THC, and other cannabinoids stimulate adrenal cortical activity, probably by increasing ACTH output (Barry *et al.*, 1972; Biswas *et al.*, 1976; Bromley and Zimmerman, 1976; Dewey *et al.*, 1970; Drew and Slagel, 1973; Dixit *et al.*, 1974; Kokka and Garcia, 1974;

Kubena et al., 1971; Maier and Maitre, 1975; Warner et al., 1977). The acute response to cannabinoids is usually a prompt rise in plasma corticosteroid levels and decreased adrenal ascorbic acid levels (see Tables VI and VII; note also exceptions to generalization). Doses of 2–20 mg of Δ^9-THC to rats, usually administered intraperitoneally, are effective as acute stimulants. Since these acute effects can be abolished by hypophysectomy (Kubena et al., 1971; Maier and Maitre, 1975), or by pentobarbital (Barry et al., 1972; Dewey et al., 1970; Mitra et al., 1977) or dexamethasone (Kokka and Garcia, 1974) administration, a primary locus of action appears to be at the hypothalamus and pituitary, with cannabinoids acting as stressors (Barry et al., 1972). Drew and Slagel (1973) had reported acute stimulation of ACTH release by Δ^9-THC. They postulated that cannabinoids exert their stressor effect by blocking the negative feedback activity of circulating corticosterone. Whether cannabinoids also reduce corticosteroid metabolism or renal clearance has not been determined.

The acute action of cannabinoids on the pituitary–adrenal axis is well illustrated by the study of Maier and Maitre (1975). Intraperitoneal injection of Δ^9-THC into adult male rats resulted in a 5- to 6-fold elevation of plasma corticosterone concentration, a decrease in adrenal ascorbic acid and cholesterol ester content, and a 2-fold rise in plasma free fatty acids. The same effects were obtained with Δ^8-THC, dimethylheptyl-Δ^{6a-10a}-THC and ACTH, but with differing dose-response curves and decay in plasma corticosterone and free fatty acid concentrations with time. Hypophysectomy abolished the adrenal effects; adrenalectomy did not prevent the plasma free fatty acid increase. The results clearly suggest stimulation of ACTH production.

Cannabinoids and corticosteroids interact at the brain and pituitary level. The amygdala, preoptic area, hypothalamus, and pituitary localize labeled Δ^9-THC, but not in a manner strikingly different from other brain structures (Erdmann et al., 1976; Just et al., 1975; Kennedy and Waddell, 1972; Layman and Milton, 1971; Martin et al., 1976; McIsaac et al., 1971; Shannon and Fried, 1972). Hypothalamic and thalamic uptake of [^{3}H]corticosterone in adult male rats was reduced after the intraperitoneal injection of 9 mg of Δ^9-THC, but increased with a 3-mg dose (Drew and Slagel, 1973). Daily intraventricular injections of 50 μg of Δ^9-THC for 7 days into 50-day-old rats led to adrenal and pituitary hypertrophy and increased corticosterone secretion (Collu, 1976). An age dependence may exist (Hattmeyer et al., 1966; Milković and Milković, 1963); 23-day-old rats did not respond to intraventricular or intraperitoneal injection of Δ^9-THC (Collu, 1976; Collu et al., 1975).

TABLE VI

Effects of Cannabinoids on Adrenal, Thymus, and Pituitary Weights and Adrenal Ascorbic Acid Content[a]

Species	Strain	Age	Sex	Cannabinoid	Dose[b] (mg/kg/day)	Duration (days)	Route	Adrenal (wt/kg)	Thymus (body wt)	Adrenal ascorbic acid	Pituitary (wt/body wt)	References[j]
Rat	Fischer	100 gm	M, F	Δ⁸,Δ⁹-THC	10	28–119	Po	↑	—	—	↑[c]	1
	Fischer	100 gm	M, F	CME	30	28–119	Po	↑	—	—	↑	1
	Fischer	100 gm	M, F	Δ⁹-THC	10	28–180	Po	↑	0	—	↑±[d]	2
	Fischer	100 gm	M	Δ⁹-THC	4	13–180	Inhalation	↑	—	—	—	3
	S.D.	21 Days	M	Δ⁹-THC	10 (3/wk)	28	Ip	↑	0	—	0	4
	Wistar	Adult	M	Δ⁹-THC	16	4	Ip	0	↓	—	—	5
	Not stated	Adult	—[e]	CME	25	64	Ip	↑	↓	—	↑	6
	Wistar	70 Days	F	CME	20	25	Ip	↑	—	↓	—	7
	Albino	100 gm	M	Δ⁹-THC	18	15	Ip	↑	—	0	↑	8
	Sprague–Dawley		M	Δ⁹-THC	5	5	Ip	↑	—	↓[i]	—	9
	Wistar	Adult	M	Δ⁹-THC	20	8	Ip	0	0	—	0	10
	Sprague–Dawley	23 Days	M	Δ⁹-THC	20 µg[g]	7	Intraventricular	0	—	—	0	11
	Sprague–Dawley	50 Days	M	Δ⁹-THC	50 µg[g]	7	Intraventricular	↑	—	—	—	11
Mouse	Tuck No. 1	21 Days	F	CME	100	5	Sc	—	↓	—	—	12
	Swiss–Albino	Adult	M	CME	100	5	Sc	—	↓	—	—	12
	Swiss–Albino	Adult	M	CME	70	45	Ip	↑[f]	↓	↑	—	13
	Swiss–Albino	Adult	F	CME	40	64	Ip	0	—	—	—	6
Guinea pig	English short hair	Adult	M	Δ⁹-THC	3	180	Ip	0	↓	↑	—	14[h]
Rhesus		Adult	M, F	Δ⁹-THC	15	28	Iv	—	0	—	—	15
				Δ⁹-THC			Po	—	—	—	—	15

[a] Effects expressed as increase (↑), no change (0), or decrease (↓).
[b] Minimum dose giving consistent results in relation to higher dose(s) or over a period of time.
[c] Increase at 50 mg dose after 91 days administration.
[d] Increase after 180 days administration of 10 mg to females only.
[e] Ovariectomized at 60 days of age.
[f] Neutral lipid content, Δ⁵-3β-hydroxysteroid dehydrogenase and glucose-6-phosphate dehydrogenase activities increased.
[g] Equal to ca. 10 mg/kg per day injected peripherally (Collu, 1976).
[h] Plasma free fatty acid concentrations declined.
[i] Depletion of adrenal ascorbic acid after single, acute Δ⁹-THC administration.
[j] (1) Thompson et al., 1973; (2) Rosenkrantz et al., 1975; (3) Rosenkrantz and Braude, 1976; (4) Collu et al., 1975; (5) Ling et al., 1973; (6) Dixit et al., 1975; (7) Neto et al., 1975; (8) Biswas et al., 1976; (9) Dewey et al., 1970; (10) Birmingham and Bartova, 1976; (11) Collu, 1976; (12) Pertwee, 1974; (13) Dixit et al., 1974; (14) Huy et al., 1975; (15) Thompson et al., 1974.

Chronic Δ^9-THC or CME administration to rats or mice, usually orally or by intraperitoneal injection, has been carried out for 4–8 days or 25–180 days (see Tables VI–VIII). Such chronic treatments led to increased adrenal (Dixit et al., 1975; Neto et al., 1975; Rosenkrantz et al., 1975; Thompson et al., 1973) and decreased thymus weights (Dixit et al., 1974, 1975; Ling et al., 1973; Smith et al., 1976). These effects appear to be reversible (Dixit et al., 1974). The capacity to respond acutely to Δ^9-THC by a prompt rise in plasma corticosterone levels (Barry et al., 1972; Neto et al., 1975 Pertwee, 1974) and a rapid depletion of adrenal ascorbic acid (Dewey et al., 1970; Dixit et al., 1975) was unimpaired after 2 months of cannabinoid administration. Similarly, in vitro corticosteroidogenesis and ACTH responsivity were not affected by chronic Δ^9-THC administration (Birmingham and Bartova, 1976; Ling et al., 1973). Birmingham and Bartova (1976) reported that 20 mg of Δ^9-THC injected daily intraperitoneally for 8 days into rats did not result in adrenal enlargement or thymic regression; the reason for this exception is not apparent. Neto et al. (1975) found CME to potentiate estradiol stimulation of adrenal and pituitary weight gain and of corticosteroidogenesis. Progesterone abolished both the primary estradiol activity and its CME potentiation.

The reports on the appearance of tolerance to cannabinoids conflict. The 5- to 8-day schedules of intraperitoneal injections of 2–20 mg of Δ^9-THC per day to rats did not impair the depletion in ascorbic acid (Dewey et al., 1970) or the rise in plasma corticosterone (Barry et al., 1972) in response to an acute test-dose of Δ^9-THC. However, in a third study with rats (Birmingham and Bartova, 1976), an acute 8-fold rise in plasma corticosterone on day 1 of treatment decreased to 2-fold on day 8. Tolerance was also observed in mice after a 5-day treatment schedule (Pertwee, 1974). However, the "protection" against the stress of acute CME or Δ^9-THC injection did not extend to the stress of immobilization (Pertwee, 1974).

Rabbits, Guinea Pigs, Monkeys

In contrast to studies with rats and mice, isolated publications of work with rabbits (Maier and Maitre, 1975; Thompson et al., 1975), guinea pigs (Huy et al., 1975), monkeys (Sassenrath and Chapman, 1975; Thompson et al., 1974), and man (Hollister, 1969; Hollister et al., 1970; Kolodny et al., 1974) reported no change in adrenocortical activity following CME or Δ^9-THC administration. In the case of rabbits and guinea pigs, the stress of handling alone may have maximally stimulated the hypothalamic–pituitary axis. Additionally, a low dose (3 mg of Δ^9-THC per kilogram) was administered to the guinea pigs. Oral

TABLE VII
EFFECTS OF CANNABINOIDS ON CORTICOSTEROID PRODUCTION

Species	Strain[a]	Cannabinoid	Dose (mg/kg/day)	Duration (days)	Route	Plasma corticosteroid response[b]	References[b]
Long-term administration							
Rat	Wistar	CME	20	25	Ip	↑	1
	Sprague–Dawley	Δ⁹-THC	20 μg[c]	7	Intraventricular	0	2
			50 μg[c]	7	Intraventricular	↑	2
	"Albino"	Δ⁹-THC	8	8	Ip	↓	3
	Wistar	Δ⁹-THC	2	8	Ip	↓	4
	Charles River	Δ⁹-THC	20[d]	8	Ip	↓	5
	Charles River	Δ⁹-THC	10	21	Ip	↓	6
			10	Single	Ip	↑	6
Mouse	Tuck No. 1	CME	500	5	Sc	0	7
		Δ⁹-THC	10	5	Sc	0	7
Human	—	Marihuana	5–>10 cigarettes (4/wk)	>6 Months	Smoking	0	8
			2–21 cigarettes	1–12 Years	Smoking	±[e]	9
			1–24 cigarettes	7–37 Years	Smoking	0	10
Single-dose administration							
Rat	"Albino"	Δ⁹-THC	1	Single	Ip	↓	3
	Sprague–Dawley	Δ⁸-,Δ⁹-THC	1	Single	Ip	↓	4
		DMPH	30	Single	Ip	↑	11[f]
		DMPH	30	Single	Ip		
	Sprague–Dawley	Δ⁹-THC	10	Single	Ip	↓	12
	Wistar	Δ⁹-THC	3	Single	Ip	↓	5
	Not stated	Δ⁹-THC	30	Single	Ip	↑	13

Mouse	Tuck No. 1	Δ^9-THC	20	Single	Ip	↑	14
Human	—	Δ^9-THC	<0.2–1[g]	Single	Po	0	15
		Δ^9-THC	<0.35–1[g]	Single	Po	0	
			In vitro incubation				
Rat	Wistar	Δ^9-THC	4, 16	4	Ip	0	16
			10^{-5} M	—	*In vitro*	0	5
Mouse	(adrenal tumor in culture)	Δ^9-THC, CBD	10^{-5} M			(inhibited ACTH; stimulated ↑ in B[i])	17, 18

[a] All subjects were adult males except those reported by Neto *et al.* (1975) (70-day male and female rats) and Collu (1976) (see footnote *c*).

[b] Plasma corticosteroid response expressed as increase (↑), no change (0) or questionable (±). Corticosteroid determined is usually corticosterone (rats, mice) or cortisol (human). *Plasma sample for corticosteroid determination obtained usually within 2 hours after "challenge" or single dose of cannabinoid.* Elevation of plasma corticosteroid level by cannabinoid inhibited or abolished by hypophysectomy (Kubena *et al.*, 1971; Maier and Maitre, 1975; dexamethasone (Kokka and Garcia, 1974), pentobarbital (Barry *et al.*, 1972; Dewey *et al.*, 1970), pentobarbital + morphine (Kubena *et al.*, 1971).

[c] Injected intraventricularly: 20 μg to 23-day-old males, 50 μg to 50-day-old males. Both doses approximated about 10 mg/kg per day injected peripherally (Collu, 1976).

[d] Increase at 3-mg dose injected ip for 2 days; no response after 8-day regime.

[e] Significant decrease from control group only at 1 hour after insulin administration (see text).

[f] Adrenal cholesterol ester and ascorbic acid content decreased; plasma free fatty acid levels increased; dose-response curves and effective doses were not identical between Δ^8-THC, Δ^9-THC, and DMPH.

[g] Δ^9-THC equivalents, administered as Δ^9-THC, synhexyl or, by Hollister *et al.* (1970) only, CME. Dose given is maximum; possible loss from aqueous diluting medium not stated.

[h] References: (1) Neto *et al.*, 1975; (2) Collu, 1976; (3) Kubena *et al.*, 1971; (4) Barry *et al.*, 1972; (5) Birmingham and Bartova, 1976; (6) Mitra *et al.*, 1977; (7) Pertwee, 1974; (8) Kolodny *et al.*, 1974; (9) Benowitz *et al.*, 1976; (10) Cruickshank, 1976; (11) Maier and Maitre, 1975; (12) Kokka and Garcia, 1974; (13) Bromley and Zimmerman, 1976; (14) Hollister *et al.*, 1970; (15) Hollister, 1969; (16) Ling *et al.*, 1973; (17) Carchman *et al.*, 1976; (18) Warner *et al.*, 1977.

[i] B = corticosterone.

TABLE VIII

EFFECT OF SHORT-TERM, ORAL ADMINISTRATION OF CRUDE MARIHUANA EXTRACT (CME), Δ^9-TETRAHYDROCANNABINOL (THC), AND CANNABIDIOL (CBD) ON PARAMETERS OF THE REPRODUCTIVE AND ADRENOCORTICAL SYSTEM IN ADULT (200 gm) MALE FISCHER RATS[a]

Parameter	CME		THC		CBD	
	0	75 mg	0	25 mg	0	25 mg
Adrenals, pair (mg/100 gm)	21.3 ± 1.9	24.0 ± 2.8*	21.3 ± 1.4	25.5 ± 2.7*	18.8 ± 0.80	18.5 ± 1.1
Testes, pair (mg/100 gm)	1160 ± 66	1230 ± 48*	1170 ± 67	1260 ± 24*	1250 ± 57	1200 ± 35
Ventral prostate (mg/100 gm)	88 ± 9.2	96 ± 16.9	107 ± 9.8	100 ± 18	84 ± 13.2	82 ± 7.6
Epididymis (mg/100 gm)	203 ± 13.7	209 ± 20.0	160 ± 19.2	168 ± 9.8	134 ± 25.6	128 ± 14
Seminal vesicle (SV) (mg/100 gm)	154 ± 11.0	152 ± 14.8	147 ± 19.3	134 ± 24.4	125 ± 19.8	135 ± 46
SV fructose (μg/100 gm)	68 ± 13.9	69 ± 26.5	63.3 ± 21.4	60.8 ± 36.4	—	—
SV citrate (μg/100 gm)	42 ± 6.0	29.7 ± 5.2	—	—	—	—
Serum corticosterone (ng/ml)	110 ± 40	170 ± 8.3*	68 ± 47	35.4 ± 16.3	118 ± 78	95 ± 85
Serum corticosterone-24 hr[b]	116 ± 98	247 ± 84*	—	—	—	—
Serum testosterone (ng/ml)	6.4 ± 3.1	5.4 ± 1.58	5.7 ± 1.94	1.7 ± 0.81**	4.7 ± 0.72	5.2 ± 2.2

[a] Groups of 10 rats were administered by intubation 0, 3, 15, or 75 mg of CME or 0, 1, 5, or 25 mg of THC or CBD per kilogram body weight per day for 5 days. Cannabinoids were dissolved in Tween 80:sesame oil:0.012 M saline (1:1:130). Rats were sacrificed 2 hours after last cannabinoid administration. Data were analyzed by analysis of variance for independent measures and individual mean comparison using Dunnett's t statistic. Values differ significantly from those of control group: *, $P = 0.01$ to <0.05; **, $P < 0.01$. Table shows only control and maximum dose data; tissue weights are wet weights per 100 gm body weight.

[b] Rats were sacrificed 24 hours after last intubation.

administration of 2.4 mg of THC daily to macaques for 1 year affected neither excretion of urinary cortisol, epinephrine, or norepinephrine nor responsivity to ACTH (Sassenrath and Chapman, 1975). An exception was thymus involution following the *intravenous* injection of 15 mg of Δ^9-THC per kilogram per day for 28 days into adult rhesus monkeys (Thompson *et al.*, 1974).

B. DIRECT EFFECTS ON ADRENAL CORTEX

Cannabinoids exert a direct and apparently inhibitory action on adrenocortical activity. The variations in the time-course of the steroidogenic and lipolytic responses to different cannabinoids and to ACTH (Maier and Maitre, 1975) have been mentioned above. Δ^9-THC, CBN, or CBD added to cultured mouse adrenal tumor cells largely abolished cellular responsivity to subsequent ACTH stimulation (Carchman *et al.*, 1976; Warner *et al.*, 1977). CBD was most active with half-maximal stimulation of $3 \times 10^{-7}M$ compared to 1×10^{-4} M for THC and 2×10^{-5} M for CBN (Warner *et al.*, 1977). Further, CBD depressed basal levels of corticosteroid production in this *in vitro* system. The inhibition of steroidogenesis was not the result of a generalized diminution of cell function or viability. The site of cannabinoid action on steroidogenesis seemed to be between cAMP and pregnenolone production (Warner *et al.*, 1977).

The adrenal cortex of mice (Freudenthal *et al.*, 1972; Kennedy and Waddell, 1972) rats (Ho *et al.*, 1970), rabbits (Agurell *et al.*, 1970), and dogs (Martin *et al.*, 1976, 1977) takes up ^{14}C- or ^{3}H-labeled Δ^9-THC to achieve tissue : plasma ratios of 2 to 6 within 20 minutes to 3 hours after administration. In rabbits, Agurell *et al.* (1970) noted a tissue :plasma ratio > 1 as late as 3 days after THC administration. These data suggest selective Δ^9-THC retention in the adrenal cortex, as in the corpus luteum (see Section II, B), with its implication of localized action. Entry of the highly lipophilic Δ^9-THC into adrenocortical mitochondrial lipids with subsequent inhibition of steroidogenesis may be visualized. Indeed, Δ^9-THC has been shown to be an effective inhibitor *in vitro* of NADH-oxidase activity of rat brain and heart mitochondria (Bartova and Birmingham, 1976; Birmingham and Bartova, 1976). However, alternative explanations for adrenocortical localization of Δ^9-THC are its solubility in lipid droplets and deposition as Δ^9-THC-plasma proteins.

C. HUMANS

In humans, cannabinoid intake did not alter adrenocortical activity or function (Hollister, 1969; Hollister *et al.*, 1970; Kolodny *et al.*, 1974).

Hollister (1969) and Hollister *et al.* (1970) emphasized the contrast between the responsivity of rat adrenal corticosteroid secretion and the lack of response of human adrenals to comparable cannabinoid doses. Benowitz *et al.* (1976) reported diminished plasma cortisol in Δ^9-THC-treated males after insulin-induced hypoglycemia. A group of 30 adult males, having smoked for 7–37 years, 1–24 cigarettes per day (Δ^9-THC content varied from 0.7 to 10.3%), did not differ from nonsmokers in their excretion of the major urinary metabolites of cortisol (Cruickshank, 1976). Similarly, smoking marihuana did not impair adrenocortical reactivity to ACTH (Perez-Reyes, 1976).

V. Development

A. Placental Transfer of Cannabinoids

Δ^9-THC is transferred to a limited extent across the placenta to the fetus. Pace *et al.* (1971) studied the transfer of [^{14}C]Δ^9-THC across the placenta after intravenous injection into rats. At least 80% of the injected dose remained in the mother rat. On a wet-weight basis, placental cotyledons contained 50–60% as much activity as that found in maternal tissues and 2- to 3-fold as much as in the fetus, thereby suggesting a partial restriction of placental transfer by these structures. More radioactivity per unit weight was found 1 hour after injection in the fetuses plus placentas at 18 or 20 days than at 13 or 15 days of pregnancy. Similar transfer gradients have been described in rats by Vardaris *et al.* (1976), mice (see next paragraph), and dogs (Martin *et al.*, 1977).

The loss of Δ^9-THC from fetus and placenta may be slower than from the maternal animal. When [^{14}C]Δ^9-THC was injected intraperitoneally (Harbison and Mantilla-Plata, 1972) or intravenously (Mantilla-Plata and Harbison, 1974, 1976a,b) into pregnant Swiss–Webster *mice,* at least 80% of the injected radioactivity remained in the mother. Of the total recovered radioactivity during the first 24-hour postinjection period, maximally 2% resided in the combination of placenta, fetus plus amniotic fluid. However, at 48 hours postinjection, 10% of the recoverable radioactivity was found in these fetal–placental compartments. The activity ratio in placenta:fetus was about 3:1, with an exponential decay in ^{14}C concentrations with time.

Much of the maternal Δ^9-THC is found in adipose tissue. Peak concentrations of Δ^9-THC in maternal fat and in mouse fetuses are reached at 1–4 hours after injection; 40% of peak values are found in adipose tissue after 24 hours and 3% after 48 hours (Harbison and Mantilla-

Plata, 1972). Maternal adipose tissue may be viewed as a potential THC reservoir vis-à-vis the fetus (Mantilla-Plata and Harbison, 1976a). Another organ that concentrates Δ^9-THC is the adrenal of both the mother (see Section IV) and fetus (Martin *et al.*, 1977).

In *hamsters* (Geber and Schramm, 1969b; Wilson, 1965), labeled THC crosses the placenta when administered either intraperitoneally or subcutaneously on day 6 or 15 of pregnancy. Placental uptake was 2- to 3-fold that by fetuses, and release was slow; i.e., whereas a fetal peak was noted at 30 minutes after injection, radioactivity was still present in fetal hamsters 24 hours postinjection.

From the foregoing discussion, the similarities in the disposition of injected [^{14}C] THC in pregnant rats and mice, and probably also in the pregnant hamster, are seen to be rather striking. There appears to be a concentration gradient of radioactivity of mother > placenta > fetus. Placental uptake of Δ^9-THC is severalfold that of the fetus, and release is slow. This may be viewed effectively as a restriction in Δ^9-THC transfer into the fetus. On the other hand, slow release into the fetal compartment makes the placenta another potential reservoir of Δ^9-THC for the fetus.

B. DEVELOPMENTAL TOXICITY

"The general principle is now well accepted that any agent which is capable of producing embryonic death may also, if the dosage and timing are appropriate, cause derangement of specific tissues and result in congenital deformity" (Rennert, 1972). The nature of deformity depends on the site of action of the noxious agent and the stage of development of the target organ, i.e., on the temporal coexistence between active concentrations of the agent and a susceptible molecular or metabolic process of differentiation. The teratogenic expression of a noxious agent is usually largely dependent on the agent reaching the embryo during organogenesis. During earlier stages of development or at higher concentrations, drugs tend to be lethal; later, to be growth-retarding. The activity of any exogenous drug will also be influenced by metabolic and physiologic changes in the embryo, fetus, and placenta during gestation.

The effects of marihuana on embryonic and fetal survival and prenatal growth and development are summarized in Table IX. The details of Table IX are considered in the following sections.

1. Embryonic and Fetal Survival

The administration of Δ^9-THC or CME to rats, mice, or rabbits, by different routes, in doses of 30–50 mg per kilogram body weight per day

TABLE IX

EFFECTS OF MARIHUANA DERIVATIVES ON PREGNANCY AND FETAL DEVELOPMENT IN LABORATORY ANIMALS

Species	Strain	Cannabinoid	Dose (mg/kg/day)	Vehicle[v]	Duration (days of gestation)	Route	Effects on Litter size[a]	Effects on Fetal growth[a]	Effects on Teratogenicity[a]	Effective dose; remarks	References[m]
Rat	Not stated	CME	0.2%	?	"Months"	Po	Reduced	?	None	—	M[r]
	Inbred albino	CME	4.2	1%T	1–6	Ip	Reduced	Reduced	Yes	—	1
	Long–Evans	Δ⁹-THC	0.01–200	O.o.	1–20	Sc	Reduced	None	None[b]	100, 200 mg	2
	Wistar	Δ⁸-, Δ⁹-THC	20, 40[c]	O.o.	1–20	Sc	None	None	None	—	3
	Wistar	Δ⁹-THC	100–250	O.o.	9–16	Sc	NS	Reduced	None	—	3
	Wistar	Δ⁹-THC	10	O.o.	10–12	Sc	NS	None	None	—	B[r]
	Wistar	Δ⁹-THC	5, 20	PG	9–21	Po	NS	NS	Yes	—	4
	Wistar	Δ⁹-THC	3.3	Cig.	—	Smoke	NS	Reduced	Yes	—	5
	Charles River	CME	30–300	NS	6–15	Po	None	NS	None	—	6
		Δ⁹-THC	5–50	NS	6–15	Po	None	NS	None	—	6
	Charles River	CME	3–30	NS	15–wean	Po	None	NS	None	—[d]	7
		Δ⁹-THC	0.5–5.0	NS	15–wean	Po	Reduced	NS	None	5 mg[d]	7
	Sprague–Dawley	Δ⁹-THC	25–100	PG	6–15	Sc	None	None	None	—	8
	Wistar	Δ⁹-THC	30–120	?	10–12	Sc	Reduced	?	None	—	U[v]
	Wistar	Δ⁹-THC	30–120	ETOH	4	Sc	Reduced	NS	None	—	9
	A/Jax	Δ⁹-THC	120, 240	1%T	12–13	Po	Reduced	NS	Yes	—	10
Mouse	Not stated	CME	16	1%T	1–6	Ip	Complete	Resorption	—	—	11
	Not stated	CME	16	1%T	6	Ip	Reduced	Reduced	None	—[v]	P[x]
	Not stated	Δ⁹-THC	200	?	8–9	Ip	Reduced	?	None	—	12
	Swiss–Webster	Δ⁹-THC	200	10%T	8–13[b]	Ip	Reduced	Reduced	ND	Growth ↓: 10–13 days	12
	Swiss–Webster	Δ⁹-THC	40–100	10%T	6–15	Ip	Reduced	Reduced	Yes	100 mg	13,14,15
	Swiss–Webster	Δ⁹-THC	50, 200	10%T	8–13[b]	Ip	Reduced	Reduced	Yes	Resorption max.: 8–9 days	13,14,15
	Swiss–Webster	Δ⁹-THC	25, 50, 75	10%T	8–10/12–14	Ip	Reduced	Reduced	Yes	ter.: 75 mg, days 12–14	13,14,15
	Swiss–Webster	Δ⁹-THC	300	10%T	12 or 14	Ip	Reduced	Reduced	Yes	—[t]	13,14,15
	Swiss–Webster	Δ⁹-THC	100–400	O.o.	7–11 (1×)	Po	None	Reduced	Yes	200, 400 mg.;	16
	DBA/2J	Δ⁹-THC	100–400	O.o.	7–11 (1×)	Po	Reduced	Reduced	Yes	days 8, 9, 10	16
	CFI-S	Δ⁹-THC	5	Food	1–20	Po	None	None	ND	—[j]	17
	Charles River CD-1	Δ⁹-THC	5–150	S.o.	6–15	Po	None	None	None	Skeletal malformations?	18

			Dose (mg/kg)	Vehicle	Days	Route					Ref.
Rabbit	New Zealand	CME	130–500	Oil	7–10	Sc	Reduced	Reduced	?	250, 500 mg; edema	19
	New Zealand White	CME	3–90	NS	6–18	Po	Reduced	Reduced	None	90 mg	6
	New Zealand White	Δ^9-THC	0.5–15	NS	6–18	Po	NS	None	None	90 mg	6
	Fauve de Bourgogne	CME	15, 30	Tablet	5–12	Po	Reduced	Reduced	Yes	Few abnormals	20
Hamster	Golden	CME	25–300	Oil	6–8	Sc	Reduced	None	Yes	200, 300 mg; edema	21
	Golden	CME	200, 300	O.o.	6–8	Sc	None	NS	None	—	3
	Golden	Δ^9-THC	125–500	O.o.	7–12 (1×)	Po	Reduced	Reduced	—[i]	—	10
	Golden	Δ^9-THC	25–100	O.o.	7–12	Po	Reduced	Reduced	—[i]	—	10
Chimpanzee	—	Δ^9-THC	1.0–2.1	NS	—[k]	Po	—	None	None	—	22
Rhesus monkey	—	Δ^9-THC	2.4	Food	1 Year	Po	2 Births	Reduced	—	1 with hydrocephalia	23

[a] NS = not stated; ND = not determined; 1%T = 1% Tween 80 in saline; 10%T = 10% Tween 80 in saline; O.o. = olive oil; S.o. = sesame oil; PG = propylene glycol; ETOH = anhydrous ethanol.

[b] Gross examination of external appearance only.

[c] Injected every other day for 30 days prior to conception plus every day until day 20 of gestation.

[d] No effects were obtained when rats were subjected to same protocol beginning 14 (females) and 60 days (males) prior to mating and continued into pregnancy (14 or 21 days).

[e] As cited by Fleischman et al. (1975); B = Borgen (1973), P = Phillips (1971), M = Miras (1962).

[f] As cited by Uyeno (1975): U = Uyeno (1973).

[g] Effects of treatment not expressed quantitatively.

[h] Dose given for 2-day periods; i.e., days 8–9, 10–11, and 12–13.

[i] Not teratogenic when administered on day 8, 10, or 16; little or no growth retardation on days 8, 10, or 12.

[j] "Not teratogenic . . . before and during gestation and lactation" (Maker et al. (1974).

[k] Gave THC.

[l] Males and females received 50–150 doses prior to mating; time between last dose and mating was 48–535 days. Eight offspring from 3 females, including one fetal death.

[m] Statistically significant increase in bent tails at 100 mg/day, days 7–10, and in gyropodin at 500 mg on day 10. However, Joneja 1977 attaches little meaning to these findings.

References: (1) Persaud and Ellington, 1968; (2) Borgen et al., 1971; (3) Pace et al., 1971; (4) Siegel et al., 1977; (5) Fried, 1977; (6) Haley et al., 1973; (7) Keplinger et al., 1973; (8) Banerjee et al., 1975; (9) Uyeno, 1975; (10) Joneja, 1977; (11) Persaud and Ellington, 1967; (12) Harbison and Mantilla-Plata, 1972; (13) Mantilla-Plata et al., 1975; (14) Mantilla-Plata and Harbison, 1976b; (15) Harbison et al., 1977; (16) Joneja, 1976; (17) Maker et al., 1974; (18) Fleischman et al., 1975; (19) Geber and Schramm, 1969b; (20) Fournier et al., 1976; (21) Geber and Schramm, 1969a; (22) Grilly et al., 1974; (23) Sassenrath and Chapman, 1975.

or greater, during the first half of gestation is associated with increased fetal and embryonic mortality, i.e., increased resorption and decreased litter size (Banerjee *et al.*, 1975; Borgen *et al.*, 1971; Fleischman *et al.*, 1975; Fournier *et al.*, 1976; Geber and Schramm, 1969b; Haley *et al.*, 1973; Harbison and Mantilla-Plata, 1972; Joneja, 1976; Mantilla-Plata *et al.*, 1973; Persaud and Ellington, 1968; Uyeno, 1975). In general, administration for one or more days through day 15 of gestation reduced fetal survival. There are reports to the contrary (Joneja, 1976; Mantilla-Plata *et al.*, 1973; Pace *et al.*, 1971). Later administration appears either not to be lethal or to have been insufficiently studied (Fleischman *et al.*, 1975; Haley *et al.*, 1973; Joneja, 1976; Keplinger *et al.*, 1973).

Fetal survival in small groups of mice (6–34 mice per group) given Δ^9-THC intraperitoneally was reduced by 40–70% if the cumulative dose was 150 mg/kg or more and injected during days 8, 9, and 10 of gestation (Harbison and Mantilla-Plata, 1972; Mantilla-Plata *et al.*, 1973, 1975; Mantilla-Plata and Harbison, 1976a). Δ^9-THC administered over days 12, 13, and 14 of gestation resulted in only 25% resorption. Intragastric administration of 120 mg and 240 mg of Δ^9-THC per kilogram body weight per day to A/Jax mice during days 11.5 and 12.5 of gestation led to a small but significant increase in the incidence of resorption (Kostellow *et al.*, 1978).

In another study, Fournier *et al.* (1976) found that the ingestion of CME at 30 mg/kg body weight per day by pregnant rabbits during days 5 through 12 of pregnancy resulted in increased resorptions (from 6.8% in controls to 10.0% in the treated group), number of macerated fetuses (from 4.1 to 8.3%), and stillbirths (from 4.4 to 10.2%). A reference group of 1850 births with 14,430 fetuses was available. Litter size in hamsters was not affected by the subcutaneous administration of CME (Geber and Schramm, 1969a). Based on total implants rather than implants per litter, Joneja (1977) reported increased resorption of Syrian hamster fetuses when given intragastric Δ^9-THC during a period including days 8 and 9 of gestation.

2. *Growth Retardation*

Fetal or neonatal growth retardation and "stunting" were frequently reported after the administration of larger amounts of CME or THC to mice, rats, rabbits, and hamsters (Banerjee *et al.*, 1975; Borgen *et al.*, 1971; Fournier *et al.*, 1976; Geber and Schramm, 1969a,b; Harbison and Mantilla-Plata, 1972; Harbison *et al.*, 1977; Joneja, 1976, 1977; Mantilla-Plata *et al.*, 1973, 1975; Mantilla-Plata and Harbison, 1976a; Pace *et al.*, 1971; Persaud and Ellington, 1967, 1968). In general, schedules of administration leading to increased resorption also resulted in growth retardation in the surviving fetuses or neonates. Growth retardation here was the product of drug administration during the embryonic and organogenic, rather than fetal, phases of development.

3. Congenital Defects

Persaud and Ellington (1968) reported congenital defects in *rat* fetuses of mothers administered 4.2 mg of marihuana resin intraperitoneally per kilogram per day on days 1–6 of gestation. In 93 fetuses from 13 experimental rats, 57% were malformed as compared to no malformations in 49 fetuses from 7 control rats. Syndactyly (76% of affected fetuses), encephalocele (57%), phocomelia (15%), and eventration of abdominal viscera (30%) were the most common malformations. Unfortunately, any evaluation of the vehicle as a teratogen and the frequency of malformation per litter were not reported. In other studies with rats, a teratogenic action of CME or Δ^9-THC could not be established (Banerjee *et al.*, 1975; Borgen *et al.*, 1971; Haley *et al.*, 1973; Keplinger *et al.*, 1973; Pace *et al.*, 1971; Uyeno, 1975). However, these studies are not easily compared to that of Persaud and Ellington in that route of administration, vehicle, gestational age, or developmental criteria differed.

Recent reports describe a cannabis effect on dental development in rats. Wistar albino rats exposed to cannabis smoke delivered and reared pups with retarded weight gain, eye opening, and incisor eruption (Fried, 1976). Mandibular and maxillary asymmetry was seen in rat offspring given Δ^9-THC (Siegel *et al.*, 1977).

Intraperitoneal injection of 300 mg of Δ^9-THC led to cleft-palate formation in fetal Swiss–Webster *mice*. A 50% and 27% frequency, respectively, was observed when single maternal injections were carried out on days 12 or 14 of pregnancy. Treatment with lesser amounts, later in gestation, or 300 mg/kg on day 8, 10, or 16 was essentially without effect. On the other hand, phenobarbital and SKF-525 A increased the incidence of cleft palate to 76% and 36%, respectively (Harbison *et al.*, 1977). Harbison *et al.* (1977) explain the increased incidence by drug facilitation of Δ^9-THC transfer to the fetus, where it is rapidly metabolized. Skeletal abnormalities were looked for but not found. A/Jax mice given doses of up to 240 mg of Δ^9-THC per kilogram per day administered intragastrically on days 11.5–12.5 (but not when given on days 10.5–11.5) had increased incidence of cleft palate, about double that seen with vehicle alone (Kostellow *et al.*, 1978).

Joneja (1976) also reported some structural abnormalities in Swiss–Webster and DBA/2J mice, given a single 100, 200, or 400 mg dose intragastrically of Δ^9-THC per kilogram on gestational day 7, 8, 9, 10, *or* 11. The total number of abnormalities after 400 mg of Δ^9-THC given to DBA mice on day 8, to either strain on day 9, and 200 mg to DBA mice on day 10, was significantly higher than in the corresponding control groups. Exencephaly and, of less certain significance, fused ribs and cleft palate, where the malformations seen. Joneja's extensive study employed adequate numbers of mice. However, a clear dose-response pattern for the frequency of malformations was not found. The frequency of other soft-tissue or skeletal abnormalities did not exceed control values; administration by other routes was ineffective.

In contrast to Harbison's and Joneja's findings, Fleischman *et al.* (1975) observed no malformations in fetuses from CD-1 mouse mothers who had received up to 150 mg of Δ^9-THC in oil per kilogram body weight per day during days 6–15 of gestation.

CME administered as oil subcutaneously to *hamsters* on days 6, 7, and 8 of pregnancy produced fetal congenital defects and edema (Geber and Schramm, 1969a). Doses of 200 and 300 mg/kg per day were clearly effective; malformations consisted of phocomelia, omphalocele, spina bifida, exencephaly, myelocele, and multiple malformations (no data on frequency). In their study, Geber and Schramm compared two CME preparations, one derived from marihuana grown in Mexico and rich in marihuana seed oils (preparation A), the other grown in New Jersey and devoid of seed oils (preparation B). The effect of uncontrolled variables, e.g., natural oils, vehicle, growth and metabolic characteristics of cannabis due to soil, climate, is clearly reflected in the difference in the frequency of edema and perhaps of abnormalities found with the two preparations:

CME	Percent abnormalities		Percent edema	
	A	B	A	B
100 mg/kg	3	0	12	0
200 mg/kg	7	4	18	8
300 mg/kg	9	8	31	8

A seasonal difference was also noted; at any given dose of CME, experiments performed during November, December, and January resulted in 2- to 3-fold the number of abnormal fetuses as when these studies were carried out during the remainder of the year.

Up to 500 mg of Δ^9-THC per kilogram per day, administered by gavage during gestational days 7–12, produced only a small increase in the incidence of external anomalies and none in internal anomalies (Joneja, 1977).

Geber and Schramm (1969b) extended their work in hamsters to *rabbits*. Deformity and edema formation were seen when 250 or 500 mg of CME was given daily on gestation days 7 through 10, with sacrifice and examination on day 16 or 17. Administration of preparation B was associated with a greater incidence of fetal abnormalities (33% at 500-mg dose) than that of A, but lesser incidence of edema (35% at 500 mg of A vs. 17% at 500 mg of B). The edema effect is opposite to that seen with hamsters. The types of malformation are reported to be identical to those observed in hamster fetuses. Fournier *et al.* (1976) claimed a teratologic effect of CME administered orally to rabbits during days 5–12 of pregnancy (see Table VI). The very low incidence of total malformations found (control = 0/68, 1/74; experimental = 1/60, 1/49, 3/60, 4/73) requires confirmation and extension before the significance of these data can be evaluated. Haley *et al.* (1973), giving orally Δ^9-THC or CME for 13 days during pregnancy (days 6–18), found no evidence of maldevelopment in 794 30-day-old rabbit fetuses.

Two reports deal with primates. Oral intake of 2.4 mg of Δ^9-THC per kilogram by two macaque females for 1 year was associated with 2 babies; one was a hyperactive but otherwise normal male, the other a hydrocephalic female who died shortly after birth (Sassenrath and Chapman, 1975). Eight offspring from chimpanzees who had smoked Δ^9-THC prior to mating were normal (Grilly *et al.*, 1974).

4. Summary

In the studies with mice by Mantilla-Plata *et al.* (1973, 1975), Mantilla-Plata and Harbison (1976a), Harbison *et al.* (1977), Joneja (1976), and Kostellow *et al.* (1978), a teratogenic response was clearly observed: (a) the frequency of two specific developmental lesions, cleft palate and exencephaly, was quite high and showed some relationship to dose; (b) the susceptible period for the induction of cleft palate and exencephaly coincided with the critical period of plate and brain development (Burdi *et al.*, 1972; Wilson, 1965) and that found after the administration of other teratogens (Burdi *et al.*, 1972; Fraser and Fainstat, 1951; Saxén, 1976; Wilson, 1965); (c) agents that affected Δ^9-THC metabolism enhanced its activity in interfering with palate closure (Harbison *et al.*, 1977; Mantilla-Plata and Harbison, 1976a); and (d) sufficient control and experimental groups with enough litters per group were used (Palmer, 1972). In three other studies with rats (Persaud and Ellington, 1968), hamsters (Geber and Schramm, 1969a), and rabbits (Geber and Schramm, 1969b), treatment probably caused the observed malformations, although a definite judgment cannot be made in the absence of data on the frequency and litter-distribution of each malformation.

It is of unknown significance but interesting that most dosages of CME and δ^9-THC eliciting a teratogenic response in mice, rabbits, hamsters, and rats were of the same order of magnitude, i.e., several hundred milligrams per kilogram body weight. The data also illustrate the difference between CME and Δ^9-THC. Except in mice, teratogenic effects tended to be seen more often after CME administration than after intake of purified Δ^9-THC. This difference again calls attention to the role of other cannabinoids and of noncannabinoids in the activities of marihuana.

C. Conclusions and Summary

In mice, rats, and rabbits, marihuana extracts and Δ^9-tetrahydrocannabinol, in sufficient dosage, produce resorption, growth retardation, and malformations. Their lethal action is perhaps more pronounced during the embryonic stages of development, although this requires more study. The locus (or loci) of action of marihuana resulting in resorption is unknown.

Growth retardation as manifest in reduced fetal or neonatal weight was frequently observed. A clear-cut maldevelopmental effect was seen less often. Whether growth retardation and teratogenecity are a direct consequence of cannabinoid administration or are a result of diminished food consumption remains to be resolved. Δ^9-THC diminishes food intake in rats (Banerjee et al., 1975; Pace et al., 1971) and may interfere with gastrointestinal absorption (Joneja, 1976). Reduced food consumption (Kalter, 1965) or starvation (Runner, 1959) has been shown to be teratogenic in mice. The incidence of cleft palate rose from 1.4 to 5.6% when food intake was restricted to 40% of normal during the day 12 through day 16 of gestation (Kalter, 1965). In the studies by Mantilla-Plata et al. (1975) the high incidence of cleft palate after injection of 300 mg of THC was associated with a significant decrease in fetal weight gain.

Retardation in growth and development in rodents as a consequence of marihuana intake is an important and significant finding. It emphasizes the relationship between marihuana consumption, nutritional status, and embryonic and fetal development. The direct effects of cannabinoids on growth and development should be separated from indirect effects via malnutrition in future research. Appropriate human populations should be carefully monitored for analogous trends and correlations.

VI. REPRODUCTIVE BEHAVIOR

A. CANNABINOID UPTAKE AND LOCALIZATION IN BRAIN AREAS SUBSERVING REPRODUCTIVE BEHAVIOR

Speculation has appeared in the scientific literature that cannabinoid compounds may affect reproductive processes and behavior by acting directly upon brain systems subserving these processes (e.g., Kolodny, 1975; Erdman et al., 1976; Besch et al., 1977). Many of these speculations appear to be based upon reported findings of cannabinoid-induced depression of circulating sex hormone levels [e.g., in male monkeys (Smith et al., 1976), female monkeys (Besch et al., 1977), and humans (Kolodny et al., 1974)] and the assumption that such effects are due to direct cannabinoid action on brain. However, insufficient data currently exist either to confirm or refute such speculations of direct cannabinoid action on brain systems subserving reproductive behavior.

That the preoptic and hypothalamic areas are the principal brain regions subserving the elicitation and regulation of reproductive behavior is well established (see reviews by Malsbury and Pfaff, 1974; Pfaff et al., 1974; Myers, 1974). Evidence in this regard consists of (a) the concentration of steroid sex hormones by cells in these brain regions (e.g., McEwen et al., 1972; Pfaff and Keiner, 1973), (b) the elicitation of reproductive behavior by direct intracranial hormonal stimulation of these regions (e.g., Lisk, 1966; Michael, 1966), (c) the abolition of reproductive behavior by discrete lesions in these brain regions (e.g., Singer, 1968), (d) the direct elicitation of reproductive behavior by discretely delimited electrical stimulation in these regions (e.g., Caggiula and Hoebel, 1966; Pfaff et al., 1973; Vaughan and Fisher, 1962). Additional evidence also exists for the implication of portions of the amygdala and associated limbic circuitry in reproductive behavior and in the feedback inhibition of reproductive behavior (Schreiner and Kling, 1953; Shealy and Peele, 1957; Kling, 1968; Pfaff and Keiner, 1973) and selective uptake of circulating sex hormones (Pfaff et al., 1974).

Unfortunately, considerably less work has been devoted to the question of cannabinoid uptake, localization, and action in these brain areas (cf. Drew and Miller, 1974).

Aside from a number of studies demonstrating the penetration into the whole brain of cannabinoid compounds administered systemically [e.g., by injection (Miras, 1965); by inhalation (Ho et al., 1970)], only limited information is available, to date, on finer cannabinoid brain distribution patterns. And, furthermore, the available information is contradictory, both with respect to the presence or absence of regional differences in distribution and with respect to the specific patterns of distribution. Thus, Layman and Milton (1971) reported finding no differences in [³H]Δ⁹-THC concentration in different brain regions of rat following intraperitoneal administration, whereas Shannon and Fried (1972) reported highly significant uptake and distribution differences between rat brain regions in a methodologically similar study. Using intravenous administrations, Martin *et al.* (1976) reported significant regional differences in dog brain [³H]Δ⁹-THC distribution, and McIsaac *et al.* (1971) and Erdmann *et al.* (1976) both reported significant regional brain differences in infrahuman primates for [³H]Δ⁹-THC and [¹⁴C]Δ⁹-THC, respectively. Dewey *et al.* (1973) reported uptake and gross localization differences for [³H]Δ⁹-THC in the pigeon brain, but made no attempt to study fine brain distribution patterns.

Of the brain regions implicated in the elicitation and regulation of reproductive behavior (see above), no autoradiographic evidence was found for cannabinoid uptake or distribution in either preoptic or anterior hypothalamic areas (McIsaac *et al.*, 1971; Shannon and Fried, 1972; Erdmann *et al.*, 1976). Evidence for selective cannabinoid uptake or binding in other hypothalamic nuclei involved in reproduction is problematic. Thus, Shannon and Fried (1972) and Erdmann *et al.* (1976) reported heavy radiolabeling of, respectively, the lateral hypothalamic nucleus and the supraoptic and paraventricular hypothalamic nuclei following administration of radioactive Δ⁹-THC. On the other hand, McIsaac *et al.* (1971) and Martin *et al.* (1976) reported hypothalamus to have lower levels of radiolabel than almost any other brain area following administration of [³H]Δ⁹-THC. Although such differences are perplexing, they may be at least partially attributable to differences in method, since McIsaac *et al.* (1971) and Martin *et al.* (1976) used microdissection combined with liquid scintillation spectrometry, whereas Shannon and Fried (1972) and Erdmann *et al.* (1976) used autoradiographic techniques. (However, McIsaac *et al.* (1971) used autoradiography in addition, and reported no hypothalamic labeling.)

Of the three hypothalamic areas implicated in Δ⁹-THC uptake by Shannon and Fried (1972) and Erdmann *et al.* (1976), there is reasonable evidence for lateral hypothalamic involvement in reproductive behavior (Fisher, 1956; Porter *et al.*, 1957; Vaughan and Fisher, 1962; Barraclough and Cross, 1963; Singer, 1968; Malsbury and Pfaff, 1974; Myers, 1974), but only very slight evidence for involvement of the supraoptic and paraventricular nuclei (Lisk, 1966; Michael, 1966; Malsbury and Pfaff, 1974; Myers, 1974; Pfaff *et al.*, 1974).

With respect to the amygdala and associated limbic circuitry involved in reproductive behavior (see above), the situation seems somewhat clearer. McIsaac *et al.* (1971), Shannon and Fried (1972), and Martin *et al.* (1976) all reported heavy radiolabeling of amygdala following administration of [³H]Δ⁹-THC. However, the specific amygdaloid nuclei showing the label are not specified, an important omission since not all portions of the amygdala seem equally involved in the regulation of reproductive behavior (Pfaff and Keiner, 1972; Pfaff *et al.*, 1974).

In addition, Hockman *et al.* (1971) and Miller and Drew (1974) both reported significantly altered electrographic activity in amygdala following cannabinoid administration to cats with chronic indwelling subcortical recording electrodes. Similarly, Heath (1976) reported altered amygdaloid electrographic activity in monkeys given Δ⁹-THC or chronically exposed to marihuana smoke.

Shannon and Fried (1972) reported abrupt and major alterations in amygdaloid electrographic activity in rats given Δ⁹-THC intraperitoneally. However, the portion of amygdala affected in the study by Shannon and Fried (1972) was the lateral nucleus, a portion of the amygdala not as clearly involved in reproductive processes as the cortical and medial nuclei (Pfaff *et al.*, 1974).

The work of Miller and Drew (1974) and Hockman *et al.* (1971) implicates another hypothalamic area involved in reproductive behavior, the ventromedial nucleus (Myers, 1974; Pfaff *et al.*, 1974). They reported significantly altered electrographic activity, following systemic cannabinoid administration, in cat ventromedial hypothalamus.

Summary

Selective cannabinoid action on brain areas regulating reproductive behavior is not established. The two brain regions most important for the regulation of reproductive behavior, the preoptic and anterior hypothalamic areas, seem not to be sites of direct cannabinoid action. However, some (tenuous) evidence does exist for cannabinoid action on other brain systems involved in reproductive behavior, especially portions of the amygdala and, perhaps, portions of the lateral, ventromedial, and supraoptic nuclei of the hypothalamus.

B. Cannabinoid Effects on Reproductive Behavior of Infrahuman Species

The research literature on cannabinoid effects on animal reproductive behavior is sparse.

With respect to acute cannabinoid administration, Merari *et al.* (1973) found that male rats given intraperitoneal Δ⁹-THC, 30 minutes before being placed with estrous females, showed significantly lengthened first-mount latencies, ejaculation latencies, and postejaculation intervals. Corcoran *et al.* (1974), also working with rats, reported that intraperitoneal administration of hashish resin (doses containing Δ^9-THC at 8.3 mg/kg and 16.6 mg/kg) significantly impaired male copulation (defined as number of animals achieving intromission). Cutler *et al.* (1975a,b), working with mice, reported that intraperitoneal administration of a tincture of cannabis significantly decreased the frequency and duration of mounts and attempted mounts, and also inhibited other forms of male sexual investigation. Of special interest is their report (Cutler *et al.*, 1975b) that alcohol administration in a similar situation increased male sexual behavior.

With respect to chronic cannabinoid administration, Miras (1965) reported that reproductive activity of rats fed 0.2% resin in the diet was significantly lower than that of controls. On the other hand, Keplinger *et al.* (1973) and Wright *et al.* (1976) reported finding no differences in mating behavior of male or female rats given oral doses of either Δ^9-THC or crude marihuana extract every day for 60 and 14 days (males and females, respectively) prior to mating. Corcoran *et al.* (1974) found that chronic administration of hashish resin for 5 days impaired male rat copulation, but that the impairment was indistinguishable from that caused by acute administration.

Methodologically, several of these studies are problematic. In none of them was there adequate experimental control for the general depressant effects of cannabinoids on motor activity (Masur *et al.*, 1971; Brown, 1972; Gill and Jones, 1972; Fernandes *et al.*, 1974; Fried, 1977; Meyer, 1978) and on appetitive and consummatory behaviors (Abel and Schiff, 1969; Orsingher and Fulginiti, 1970; Cutler *et al.*, 1975a; Fried, 1977; Meyer, 1978). Nor were there experimental controls for the possibility of behavioral stimulation at low Δ^9-THC dose levels (e.g., Luthra *et al.*, 1976) or from chronic administration (e.g., Luthra *et al.*, 1975). In most of the studies (excepting that of Merari *et al.*, 1973), the quantification and analysis of the reproductive behavior seems crude (cf. Beach *et al.*, 1969; Wilhelmsson and Larsson, 1973; Diakow, 1974, 1975). In most of the studies (again excepting that of Merari *et al.*, 1973), no attempt was made to control the degree of estrous or stimulus female receptivity. In several studies, crude hashish or cannabis preparations were used, and the relative contributions of Δ^9-THC or other constituents to the reported effects on reproductive behavior are thus unknown. In only one study (Keplinger *et al.*, 1973) was an attempt made to study the mating behavior of the female animal, and this one attempt was apparently not very detailed. Finally, as pointed out by numerous authorities (e.g., Lehrman, 1961), reproductive behavior in the female (and, depending on the species, often in the male as well) extends far beyond the mating act. In fact, totally separate categories of reproductive behavior other than the mating act, all under the control of reproductive brain systems and sex hormones, have been identified (Lehrman, 1961; Milner, 1970). To date, the effects of cannabinoids on these aspects of reproductive behavior are unknown, with the exception of the observation by Sassernath and Chapman (1975) that a single female macaque treated chronically with Δ^9-THC exhibited irritable rejection behavior toward its infant.

Summary

The few studies in the literature of cannabinoid effects on male animal reproductive behavior are suggestive of an inhibitory effect on mounting, intromission, and ejaculation. Owing to methodological problems, none of these studies can be considered definitive. The effects of cannabinoids on female mating behavior and on reproductive behavior other than the mating act are unknown.

C. CANNABINOID EFFECTS ON HUMAN REPRODUCTIVE BEHAVIOR

Reports of cannabinoid-induced sexual stimulation in humans are common (Chopra and Chopra, 1957; Robinson, 1966; Hollister *et al.,* 1968; Tart, 1970; R. Jones, 1977), and purely anecdotal reports in this regard are especially common (e.g., Mendelson *et al.,* 1975). Bouquet (1951) and Chopra (1969; Chopra and Chopra, 1957) reported the widespread belief in North Africa and India, respectively, that cannabis preparations stimulate sexual desire and improve and prolong sexual performance, and the widespread use of such preparations as aphrodisiacs. In apparent contradiction, cannabis is often used in India as a sexual depressant (Chopra and Chopra, 1957; Chopra, 1969).

In one of the earliest experiments with cannabis administration in humans (Mayor's Committee on Marihuana, 1944), it was found that, out of 150 experimental marihuana administrations, sexual stimulation was subjectively reported in 10%. In a somewhat better-controlled experiment, Hollister *et al.* (1968) reported stimulation of sexual thoughts following cannabinoid administration, but not following administration of lysergic acid diethylamide.

In two fairly extensive surveys of experienced marihuana users, a large majority of cannabis users, male and female, reported sexual stimulation and heightened and prolonged sexual performance following marihuana use (Tart, 1971; Berke and Hernton, 1974). Similarly,

Traub (1977) found that 94% of experienced marihuana users report heightened sexual pleasure during marihuana use. Other surveys of cannabis users have found similar reports of increased sexual desire and enjoyment following acute marihuana exposure (Halikas *et al.*, 1971; Goode, 1972b; Fisher and Steckler, 1974; Koff, 1974). Roth *et al.* (1976) found that, among experienced marihuana and alcohol users, subjective impression of enhanced sexual sensation was significantly more common following marihuana than following alcohol.

On the other hand, sexually assaultive behavior is reported to be much lower following cannabinoid use than following alcohol use (Tinklenberg *et al.*, 1974).

With respect to chronic, rather than acute, cannabinoid administration, Chopra and Jandu (1976), in a study of 275 Indian chronic cannabis users, reported that 25% experienced increased sex drive and enjoyment with controlled daily cannabis doses, but that chronic use of high doses produced lack of sexual desire and impotence. There are additional quasi-anecdotal reports from both India and North Africa of sexual impotence resulting from prolonged use of high doses of cannabis (Bouquet, 1951; Benabud, 1957; Chopra and Chopra, 1957). Also, Kolodny *et al.* (1974) reported finding decreased plasma testosterone levels and a suggestion of decreased sexual drive following chronic intensive cannabinoid use. On the other hand, sexual promiscuity is reported to be higher among chronic Indian users of high doses of cannabis than among control subjects (Mehndiratta and Wig, 1975), and regular American users of marihuana report a higher incidence of sexual activity than do nonusers (Goode, 1972a; Brill and Christie, 1974).

Unfortunately, all the above-cited reports and studies are based upon subjective self-reports of the effects of cannabinoid administration. Such approaches to the study of behavior are notoriously inaccurate (Hebb, 1972), and, with specific respect to the study of cannabinoid action, Peters *et al.* (1976) have demonstrated a clear dissociation between objectively measured behavioral effects following Δ^9-THC administration and subjectively reported effects.

In addition, reports of increased sexual activity being associated with marihuana use, even if correct, may have nothing to do with direct pharmacological action of cannabis. For instance, personality and life-style are strongly associated with sexual and drug-taking behavior (Brill and Christie, 1974). Thus, both sexual activity and marihuana use may reflect a general sensation-seeking, risk-taking set, rather than one following from the other (Brill *et al.*, 1971; Brill and Christie, 1974). Also, since those who expect to be sexually aroused by cannabis are more likely to be so aroused than those who do not (Grinspoon, 1977), a significant percentage of the subjective reports of enhanced arousal following marihuana may merely represent placebo reaction.

Furthermore, it seems possible that at least some of the above-cited subjectively reported cannabinoid effects on human sexual behavior may, if correct, actually be secondary to cannabinoid effects on other bodily systems (Paton and Pertwee, 1973b). Thus, cannabinoids cause a reduction in sympathetic tone (Paton and Pertwee, 1973a), which may in turn produce a genital vasodilation. In addition, time perception is altered by Δ^9-THC (see, e.g., Paton and Pertwee, 1973b; Miller, 1974; Karniol et al., 1975), and, thus, sexual behavior may seem subjectively prolonged when, in actual fact, it is not. Also, ejaculation in the male may be genuinely delayed, but by a sympathetic action rather than a direct effect on brain systems organizing and regulating reproductive behavior. Moreover, the documented effects of cannabinoids on sensory perception (Paton and Pertwee, 1973b) may, in turn, cause the tactile stimulation of the sex act to be more intensely perceived, without there being any objectively measurable behavioral changes in the act itself (Zinberg, 1974).

For all the foregoing reasons, and as pointed out by many workers (e.g., Kolodny, 1975; Kolodny et al., 1976; R. Jones, 1977), it is unfortunate that no controlled objective experimental studies, as opposed to subjective self-reports, of cannabinoid effects on human sexual or reproductive behavior have yet appeared in the scientific literature. Plans for such studies were blocked by a special act of the U.S. Congress for reasons apparently having little to do with scientific merit (Rubin, 1976; Meyer, 1978).

Summary

Tenuous evidence (based exclusively on subjective self-reports) exists for a stimulation and prolongation of sexual behavior by acute administration of cannabinoid compounds. Equally tenuous evidence has been reported for an inhibitory effect on sexual behavior of chronic high doses of cannabinoid. None of these purported effects have been confirmed by objective study, and, even if genuine, they may be secondary to cannabinoid effects on other bodily systems.

VII. Conclusions and Summary

Relatively few definitive findings or generalizations have emerged from the studies on the effects of marihuana and its derivatives on reproduction and development. To the contrary, the variability in experimental design, with widely differing dosages, schedules, routes, and vehicles of cannabinoid administration, document the need for standardized and well-designed studies. Most work has been done with rats, except in developmental studies, where rats, mice, and rabbits have been used. Studies in subhuman primates should be encouraged. Most studies have concentrated on the effects of crude extract of marihuana (CME) or of Δ^9-tetrahydrocannabinol (Δ^9-THC). Both other cannabinoids and noncannabinoid constituents in marihuana deserve far more intensive study. Their role in marihuana action and the general question of specificity of observed marihuana effects require clarification. The relationship between cannabinoid effect and age (e.g., prepuberal vs. adult), and interaction with sex hormones and glucocorticoids should be more closely examined.

To conclude and in summary:

1. Cannabinoids inhibit *testicular* function in all species studied. Testicular metabolic activity and *in vitro* testosterone synthesis are decreased; plasma testosterone levels fall; and prostate, seminal vesicles, and epididymis show varying degrees of functional and morphological involution. Effects on testes weight are small and inconsistent. Prolonged cannabinoid intake leads to diminished spermatogenesis. The effects of marihuana and cannabinoids on male reproductive physiology are reversible, and no permanent changes have been described following cessation of cannabinoid intake. The reduction in metabolic activity and macromolecular synthesis following exposure to cannabinoids correlates with and may be the basis for the diminished spermatogenesis and testosterone synthesis found after Δ^9-THC administration.

In humans, marihuana smoking decreases plasma testosterone levels. The effect is acute and rapidly reversible. Oligospermia and gynecomastia have been reported. Hence, in man, as in rats, consumption of marihuana can lead to transiently diminished testicular function.

2. Prolonged administration of CME leads to impaired reproductive function in *female* rats and mice. Estrous cycles become irregular and anovulatory or are abolished; follicular atresia increases, and uteri and vaginae show signs of morphological and functional involution. These actions are reversible. The effects of Δ^9-THC are conflicting. Δ^9-THC seems to replace CME only partially in its activity. It must be remembered that CME contains noncannabinoid constituents, some of which may be active, as has been shown for CME action on prostaglandin synthesis (see Section III).

Very few studies have been carried out with primates, including man. Δ^9-THC rapidly and transiently depressed plasma LH levels in rhesus monkeys, suggesting the potential of impaired ovarian function with heavy and chronic intake of marihuana.

Cannabinoids antagonize the action of estradiol in several systems. But there is also evidence for "estrogenicity" of Δ^9-THC. Cannabinoids may exert some of their effects at the estradiol receptor site, cannabinoids decreasing the availability of cytosol receptors for estradiol binding.

3. Reduced gonadal function may be a secondary effect of diminished *pituitary gonadotropin* formation. Δ^9-THC markedly and acutely reduced serum LH concentrations in both male and female rats. The preovulatory LH surge is suppressed in rats and mice. An effect on FSH has yet to be unequivocally demonstrated. The data suggest suppression or reduction of pituitary LH production in rats by CME and Δ^9-THC, secondarily leading to reduced gonadal function. However, some evidence for a direct effect of marihuana constituents on gonadal morphology and function also exists; more such studies need be done (e.g., in hypophysectomized animals). This duality of action, i.e., on the pituitary and its target gland, is also encountered with the pituitary–adrenal cortical axis. The relative importance of the direct and indirect effects of cannabinoids on gonad activity needs be assessed and any direct effects of cannabinoids on androgen and estrogen target sites explored.

4. In *pregnant* rats and mice, Δ^9-THC exerted few maternal effects unique to pregnancy. High doses of Δ^9-THC abolished the weight gain of pregnant rats and exerted a variable effect on maternal body organ weights. The reduction in weight gain was partially independent of reduced food intake. Prolonged gestation with normal birth weights suggests delayed nidation. Corpora lutea of mice very effectively concentrated THC, indicating specific protein binding or, more simply, the lipophilic solubility of Δ^9-THC.

5. *Lactation* is markedly reduced. Δ^9-THC decreased *prolactin* levels in adults of both sexes. This diminution may explain the reduced and inadequate lactation seen in the postpartum rat. Ingested Δ^9-THC appears in *mammary* tissue and *milk* and is transferred to suckling pups. This was also shown in lactating squirrel monkeys.

6. Several cannabinoids at high dosages inhibit *prostaglandin* synthesis. Some of the cannabinoid effects on reproductive processes are similar to those observed after reduced tissue prostaglandin concentrations. Hence, some of the cannabinoid effects on reproductive processes may be via reduced prostaglandin levels.

7. Little firm evidence exists for cannabinoids or marihuana modifying *reproductive behavior*. In male rats and mice, an inhibiting effect on mounting, intromission, and ejaculation is suggested. The effects on male reproductive behavior other than the mating act, on female reproductive behavior, and on reproductive behavior independent of depressed generalized motor activity are unknown.

In humans, acute administration of marihuana may stimulate and prolong sexual behavior, while chronic high doses may inhibit sexual behavior. These tenuous conclusions are based on subjective self-reports. Objective studies are lacking, as are studies differentiating between direct effects of cannabinoids on sexual behavior and effects secondary to cannabinoid action on other physiological systems.

8. Cannabinoids and CME stimulate *adrenal cortical* function in rats and mice. *Acute* administration results in increased plasma corticosterone concentrations. Administration of CME, Δ^9-THC, and other cannabinoids has resulted in increased plasma corticosterone levels and adrenal cortical changes consistent with those seen after *acute* or *chronic* stimulation by ACTH. Since the cannabinoid effects can be abolished by agents and procedures that block ACTH production, a primary locus of cannabinoid action must be the hypothalamic–pituitary area. This anatomic region localizes Δ^9-THC, but not remarkably more than other brain regions.

The adrenal cortex of several species concentrates Δ^9-THC, suggesting a direct action on adrenal cortical metabolism. Abolution of responsivity to ACTH by adrenal tumor cells and depression of local corticosteroid production *in vitro* support this suggestion. Conflicting reports on an acquired adrenal tolerance to cannabinoids have appeared.

In contrast to studies with rats and mice, isolated publications of work with rabbits, guinea pigs, monkeys, and humans reported little or no change in adrenocortical activity following administration of CME or Δ^9-THC. The absence of such effects may reflect differing thresholds of responsivity to cannabis or a pituitary adrenal cortical system functioning already under maximum stimulation.

9. ^{14}C-Labeled Δ^9-tetrahydrocannabinol injected into pregnant rodents results in a concentration gradient of radioactivity of mother $>$ placenta $>$ fetus. *Placental* uptake of THC is severalfold that of the fetus, with only slow release. This makes the placenta potentially both a barrier against and a reservoir for THC transfer into the fetus.

10. Marihuana preparations, CME, and Δ^9-THC variably affected reproductive *efficiency* and *development* in mice, rats, and rabbits. Litter size was reduced; resorption frequency increased and birth weights decreased; and the incidence of malformation increased. These effects

were seen primarily when larger amounts of cannabinoids were administered during the first half of gestation.

Malformations consisted of cleft palate and exencephaly in mice in response to high doses of Δ^9-THC given during the critical periods of palate and brain development, respectively. Other reports on associations between cannabinoid intake and teratogenicity were less well supported by the experimental data.

Growth retardation and developmental malformations may be a direct consequence of cannabinoid intake by the pregnant mother or an indirect result of diminished food intake, the latter a consequence of marihuana ingestion. These findings emphasize the relationship between marihuana consumption, nutritional status, and developmental processes—relationships that merit further analysis, study, and clarification.

ACKNOWLEDGMENTS

Preparation of this review was supported by contract No. 271-76-3318 from the National Institute of Drug Abuse. The excellent and devoted assistance of Ms. Genevieve Cohen in the preparation of this manuscript is gratefully acknowledged.

REFERENCES

Abel, E. L., and Schiff, B. B. (1969). *Psychon Sci.* **16**, 38.

Agurell, S., Nilsson, I. M., Ohlsson, A., and Sandberg, F. (1970). *Biochem. Pharmacol.* **19**, 1333.

Banerjee, B. N., Galbreath, C., and Sofia, R. D. (1975). *Teratology* **11**, 99.

Barraclough, C. A., and Cross, B. A. (1963). *J. Endocrinol.* **26**, 339.

Barry, H., III, Kubena, R. K., and Perhach, J. L., Jr. (1972). *Prog. Brain Res.* **39**, 323.

Bartova, A., and Birmingham, M. K. (1976). *J. Biol. Chem.* **251**, 5002.

Beach, F. A., Noble, R. G., and Orndoff, R. K. (1969). *J. Comp. Physiol. Psychol.* **68**, 490.

Benabud, A. (1957). *Bull. Narc.* **9**, 1.

Benowitz, N. L., Jones, R. T., and Lerner, C. B. (1976). *J. Clin. Endocrinol. Metab.* **42**, 938.

Berke, J., and Hernton, C. (1974). "The Cannabis Experience." Peter Owen, London.

Besch, N. F., Smith, C. G., Besch, P. K., and Kaufman, R. H. (1977). *Am. J. Obstet. Gynecol.* **128**, 635.

Birmingham, M. K., and Bartova, A. (1976). *In* "Marihuana: Chemistry, Biochemistry, and Cellular Effects" (G. G. Nahas and G. Gabriel, eds.), p. 425. Springer-Verlag, Berlin and New York.

Biswas, B., Dey, S. K., and Ghosh, J. J. (1976). *Endocrinol. Exp.* **10**, 139.

Borgen, L. A., and Davis, W. M. (1974). *Res. Commun. Chem. Pathol. Pharmacol.* **7**, 613.

Borgen, L. A., Davis, W. M., and Pace, H. B. (1971). *Toxicol. Appl. Pharmacol.* **20**, 480.

Borgen, L. A., Lott, G. C., and Davis, W. M. (1973). *Res. Commun. Chem. Pathol. Pharmacol.* **5**, 621.

Bose, B. C., Vijayvargiya, R., Saifi, A. Q., and Bhagwat, A. W. (1963). *Arch. Int. Pharmacodyn. Ther.* **146**, 99.

Bose, B. C., Vijaybargiya, R., Saifi, A. Q., and Bhagwat, A. W. (1964). *Arch. Int. Pharmacodyn. Ther.* **147**, 291.

Bouquet, J. (1951). *Bull. Narc.* **3**, 22.

Brill, N. Q., and Christie, R. L. (1974). *Arch. Gen. Psychiatry* **31**, 713.

Brill, N. Q., Crumpton, E., and Grayson, H. M. (1971). *Arch. Gen. Psychiatry* **24**, 163.

Bromley, B., and Zimmerman, E. (1976). *Fed. Proc., Fed. Am. Soc. Exp. Biol.* **35**, 220.

Brown, H. (1972). *Psychopharmacologia* **27**, 111.

Burdi, A., Feingold, M., Larsson, K. S., Leck, I., Zimmerman, E. F., and Fraser, F. C. (1972). *Teratology* **6**, 255.

Burstein, S., and Kupfer, D. (1971). *Ann. N.Y. Acad. Sci.* **191**, 61.

Burstein, S., and Raz, A. (1972). *Prostaglandins* **2**, 369.

Burstein, S., Levin, E., and Varanelli, C. (1973). *Biochem. Pharmacol.* **22**, 2905.

Burstein, S., Varanelli, C., and Slade, L. T. (1975). *Biochem. Pharmacol.* **24**, 1053.

Burstein, S., Taylor, P., El-Feraly, F. S., and Turner, C. (1976). *Biochem. Pharmacol.* **25**, 2003.

Caggiula, A. R., and Hoebel, B. G. (1966). *Science* **153**, 1284.

Caldwell, B. B., Bailey, K., Paul, C. J., and Anderson, G. (1974). *Toxicol. Appl. Pharmacol.* **29**, 59.

Carchman, R. A., Warner, W., White, A. C., and Harris, L. S. (1976). *In* "Marihuana: Chemistry, Biochemistry and Cellular Effects"(G. C. Nahas and G. Gabriel, eds.), p. 329. Springer-Verlag, Berlin and New York.

Chakravarty, I., Sengupta, D., Bhattacharya, P., and Ghosh, J. J. (1975a). *Toxicol. Appl. Pharmacol.* **34**, 513.

Chakravarty, I., Sheth, A. R., and Ghosh, J. J. (1975b). *Fertil. Steril.* **26**, 947.

Chakravarty, I., Sengupta, D., Bhattacharya, P., and Ghosh, J. J. (1976). *Biochem. Pharmacol.* **25**, 377.

Chao, F. C., Green, D. E., Forrest, I. S., Kaplan, J. N., Winship-Ball, A., and Braude, M. (1976). *Res. Commun. Pathol. Chem. Pharmacol.* **15**, 303.

Chopra, G. S. (1969). *Int. J. Addict.* **4**, 215.

Chopra, G. S., and Jandu, B. S. (1976). *Ann. N.Y. Acad. Sci.* **282**, 95.

Chopra, I. C., and Chopra, R. N. (1957). *Bull. Narc.* **9**, 4.

Coggins, W. J. (1976). *In* "Pharmacology of Marihuana" (M. C. Braude and J. Szara, eds.), Vol. 2, p. 667. Raven, New York.

Coggins, W. J., Swenson, E. W., Dawson, W. W., Fernandez-Salas, A., Hernandez-Bolanus, J., Jiminez-Antillon, C. F., Solano, J. R., Vinocour, R., and Faerron-Valdez, F. (1976). *Ann. N.Y. Acad. Sci.* **282**, 148.

Cohen, G. M., Peterson, D. W., and Mannering, G. J. (1971). *Life Sci.* **10**, Part 1, 1207.

Cohen, S. (1976). *Ann. N.Y. Acad. Sci.* **282**, 211.

Cohn, R. A., Barratt, E. S., and Pirch, J. H. (1974). *Proc. Soc. Exp. Biol. Med.* **146**, 109.

Collu, R. (1976). *Life Sci.* **18**, 223.

Collu, R., Letarte, J., Leboeuf, G., and Ducharme, J. R. (1975). *Life Sci.* **16**, 533.

Corcoran, M. E., Amit, Z., Malsbury, C. W., and Daykin, S. (1974). *Res. Commun. Chem. Pathol. Pharmacol.* **7**, 779.

Cruickshank, E. K. (1976). *Ann. N.Y. Acad. Sci.* **282**, 162.

Cutler, M. G., MacKintosh, J. H., and Chance, M. R. A. (1975a). *Psychopharmacologia* **41**, 271.

Cutler, M. G., MacKintosh, J. H., and Chance, M. R. A. (1975b). *Psychopharmacologia* **45**, 129.

Daley, J. D., Branda, L. A., Rosenfeld, J., and Younglai, E. V. (1974). *J. Endocrinol.* **63**, 415.

Dalterio, S., Bartke, A., and Burstein, S. (1977). *Science* **196**, 1472.

Dewey, W. L., Peng, T.-C., and Harris, L. S. (1970). *Eur. J. Pharmacol.* **12**, 382.

Dewey, W. L., McMillan, D. E., Harris, L. S., and Turk, R. F. (1973). *Biochem. Pharmacol.* **22**, 399.

Diakow, C. (1974). *Adv. Study Behav.* **5**, 227.

Diakow, C. (1975). *J. Comp. Physiol. Psychol.* **88**, 704.

Dingell, J. V., Miller, K. W., Heath, E. C., and Klausner, H. A. (1973). *Biochem. Pharmacol.* **22**, 949.

Drew, W. G., and Miller, L. L. (1974). *Pharmacology* **11**, 12.

Drew, W. G., and Slagel, D. E. (1973). *Neuropharmacology* **12**, 909.

Dixit, V. P., and Lohiya, N. K. (1975). *Indian J. Physiol. Pharmacol.* **19**, 98.

Dixit, V. P., Sharma, V. N., and Lohiya, N. K. (1974). *Eur. J. Pharmacol.* **26**, 111.

Dixit, V. P., Arya, M., and Lohiya, N. K. (1975). *Endokrinologie* **66**, 365.

Dixit, V. P., Gupta, C. L., and Agrawal, M. (1977). *Endokrinologie* **69**, 299.

Emmens, C. W., and Parkes, A. S. (1947). *Vitam. Horm. (N.Y.)* **5**, 233.

Erdmann, G., Just, W. W., Thel, S., Werner, G., and Wiechmann, M. (1976). *Psychopharmacology* **47**, 53.

Esber, H. J., Kuo, E. H., Rosenkrantz, H., and Braude, M. C. (1975). *Fed. Proc., Fed. Am. Soc. Exp. Biol.* **34**, 783.

Esber, H. J., Rosenkrantz, H., and Bogden, A. E. (1976). *Fed. Proc., Fed. Am. Soc. Exp. Biol.* **35**, 727.

Fernandes, M., Schabarek, A., Coper, H., and Hill, R. (1974). *Psychopharmacologia* **38**, 329.

Fisher, A. E. (1956). *Science* **124**, 228.

Fisher, G., and Steckler, A. (1974). *Int. J. Addict.* **9**, 101.

Fleischman, R. W., Hayden, D. W., Rosenkrantz, H., and Braude, M. C. (1975). *Teratology* **12**, 47.

Fournier, E., Rosenberg, E., Hardy, N., and Nahas, G. (1976). *In* "Marihuana: Chemistry, Biochemistry and Cellular Effects" (G. G. Nahas and G. Gabriel, eds.), p. 457. Springer-Verlag, Berlin and New York.

Fraser, F. C., and Fainstat, T. D. (1951). *Pediatrics* **8**, 527.

Freudenthal, R. I., Martin, J., and Wall, M. E. (1972). *Br. J. Pharmacol.* **44**, 244.

Fried, P. A. (1976). *Psychopharmacologia* **50**, 285.

Fried, P. A. (1977). *Behav. Biol.* **21**, 163.

Friedman, M. A., and Wrenn, J. M. (1977). *Toxicol. Appl. Pharmacol.* **41**, 345.

Fujimoto, G. I., Rosenbaum, R. M., Ziegler, D., Rettura, G., and Morrill, G. A. (1978). *Proc. 60th Annu. Meet. Endocr. Soc.* (in press).

Gascon, A. L., and Peres, M. T. (1973). *Can. J. Physiol. Pharmacol.* **51**, 12.

Geber, W. F., and Schramm, L. C. (1969a). *Arch. Int. Pharmacodyn. Ther.* **177**, 224.

Geber, W. F., and Schramm, L. C. (1969b). *Toxicol. Appl. Pharmacol.* **14**, 276.

Gill, E. W., and Jones, G. (1972). *Biochem. Pharmacol.* **21**, 2237.

Goldstein, H., Harclerode, J., and Nyquist, S. E. (1977). *Life Sci.* **20**, 951.

Goode, E. (1972a). *Am. J. Psychiatry* **128**, 1272.

Goode, E. (1972b). *Sex Behav.* **2**, 45.

Greep, R. O., and Jones, I. C. (1950). *Recent Prog. Horm. Res.* **5**, 197.

Grilly, D. M., Ferraro, D. P., and Braude, M. C. (1974). *Pharmacology* **11**, 304.

Grinspoon, L. (1977). "Marihuana Reconsidered," 2nd ed. Harvard Univ. Press, Cambridge, Massachusetts.

Haley, S. L., Wright, P. L., Plank, J. B., Keplinger, M. L., Braude, M. C., and Calandra, J. C. (1973). *Toxicol. Appl. Pharmacol.* **25**, 450.

Halikas, J. A., Goodwin, D. W., and Guze, S. B. (1971). *J. Am. Med. Assoc.* **217**, 692.

Harbison, R. D., and Mantilla-Plata, B. (1972). *J. Pharmacol. Exp. Ther.* **180**, 446.

Harbison, R. D., Mantilla-Plata, B., and Lubin, D. J. (1977). *J. Pharmacol. Exp. Ther.* **202**, 455.

Harmon, J. W., and Aliapoulios, M. A. (1972). *N. Engl. J. Med.* **287**, 936.

Harmon, J. W., and Aliapoulios, M. A. (1974). *Surg. Forum* **25**, 423.

Harmon, J. W., Locke, D., Aliapoulios, M. A., and MacIndoe, J. H. (1976). *Surg. Forum* **27**, 350.

Hattmeyer, G. C., Denenberg, V. H., Thatcher, J., and Zarrow, M. X. (1966). *Nature (London)* **212**, 1371.

Heath, R. G. (1976). *In* "Pharmacology of Marihuana" (M. C. Braude and S. Szara, eds.), Vol. 1, p. 345. Raven, New York.

Hebb, D. O. (1972). "Textbook of Psychology," 3rd ed. Saunders, Philadelphia, Pennsylvania.

Hembree, W. C., III, Zeidenberg, P., and Nahas, G. G. (1976). *In* "Marihuana: Chemistry, Biochemistry and Cellular Effects" (G. G. Nahas and G. Gabriel, eds.), p. 521. Springer-Verlag, Berlin and New York.

Ho, B. T., Fritchie, G. E., Kralik, P. M., Englart, L. F., McIsaac, W. M., and Idanpaan-Heikkila, J. E. (1970). *J. Pharm. Pharmacol.* **22**, 538.

Hockman, C. H., Perrin, R. G., and Kalant, H. (1971). *Science* **172**, 968.

Hollister, L. E. (1969). *J. Clin. Pharmacol.* **9**, 24.

Hollister, L. E. (1974). *Pharmacology* **11**, 3.

Hollister, L. E., Richards, R. K., and Gillespie, H. K. (1968). *Clin. Pharmacol. Ther.* **9**, 783.

Hollister, L. E., Moore, F., Kanter, S., and Noble, E. (1970). *Psychopharmacologia* **17**, 354.

Howes, J. F., and Osgood, P. F. (1976). *In* "Marihuana: Chemistry, Biochemistry, and Cellular Effects" (G. G. Nahas and G. Gabriel, eds.), p. 416. Springer-Verlag, Berlin and New York.

Huy, N. D., Gailis, L., Cote, G., and Roy, P. E. (1975). *Int. J. Clin. Pharmacol.* **12**, 284.

Jakubović, A., and McGeer, P. L. (1976). *In* "Marihuana: Chemistry, Biochemistry, and Cellular Effects" (G. G. Nahas and G. Gabriel, eds.) p. 223. Springer-Verlag, Berlin and New York.

Jakubović, A., and McGeer, P. L. (1977). *Toxicol. Appl. Pharmacol.* **41**, 473.

Jakubović, A., Hattori, T., and McGeer, P. L. (1973). *Eur. J. Pharmacol.* **22**, 221.

Joneja, M. G. (1976). *Toxicol. Appl. Pharmacol.* **36**, 151.

Joneja, M. G. (1977). *J. Toxicol. Environ. Health* **2**, 1031.

Jones, R. T. (1977). *In* "Marihuana Research Findings: 1976" (R. C. Petersen, ed.), Natl. Inst. Drug Abuse Res. Monogr. No. 14, p. 128. US Govt. Printing Office, Washington, D.C.

Jones, R. T. (1976). *Ann. N.Y. Acad. Sci.* **282**, 182.

Just, W. W., Erdmann, G., Thel, S., Werner, G., and Wiechmann, M. (1975). *Naunyn-Schmiedeberg's Arch. Pharmacol.* **287**, 219.

Kalter, H. (1965). *In* "Teratology" (J. G. Wilson and J. Warkany, eds.). p. 57. Univ. of Chicago Press, Chicago, Illinois.

Karniol, I. G., and Carlini, E. A. (1973). *Psychopharmacologia* **33**, 53.

Karniol, I. G., Shirakawa, I., Kasinski, N., Pfefferman, A., and Carlini, E. A. (1974). *Eur. J. Pharmacol.* **28**, 172.

Karniol, I. G., Shirakawa, I., Takahashi, R. N., Knobel, E., and Musty, R. E. (1975). *Pharmacology* **13**, 502.

Kennedy, J. S., and Waddell, W. J. (1972). *Toxicol. Appl. Pharmacol.* **22**, 252.

Keplinger, M. L., Wright, P. L., Haley, S. L., Plank, J. B., Braude, M. C., and Calandra, J. C. (1973). *Toxicol. Appl. Pharmacol.* **25**, 449.

Kling, A. (1968). *J. Comp. Physiol. Psychol.* **65**, 466.

Koff, W. C. (1974). *J. Sex Res.* **10**, 194.

Kokka, N., and Garcia, J. F. (1974). *Life Sci.* **15**, 329.

Kolodny, R. C. (1975). *In* "Marihuana and Health Hazards: Methodological Issues in Current Research" (J. R. Tinklenberg, ed.), p. 71. Academic Press, New York.

Kolodny, R. C., Masters, W. H., Kolodner, R. M., and Toro, G. (1974). *N. Engl. J. Med.* **290**, 872.

Kolodny, R. C., Toro, G., and Masters, W. H. (1975). *N. Engl. J. Med.* **292**, 868.

Kolodny, R. C., Lessin, P. J., Toro, G., Masters, W. H., and Cohen, S. (1976). *In* "Pharmacology of Marihuana" (M. C. Braude and S. Szara, eds.), Vol. I, p. 217. Raven, New York.

Kostellow, A. B., Bloch, E., Morrill, G. A., and Fujimoto, G. I. (1978). *Fed. Proc., Fed. Am. Soc. Exp. Biol.* **37**, 858.

Kramer, J., and Ben-David, M. (1974). *Proc. Soc. Exp. Biol. Med.* **147**, 482.

Kubena, R. K., Perhach, J. L., Jr., and Barry, H., III. (1971). *Eur. J. Pharmacol.* **14**, 89.

Layman, J. M., and Milton, A. S. (1971). *Br. J. Pharmacol.* **42**, 308.

Legator, M. S., Weber, E., Connor, T., and Stoeckel, M. (1976). *In* "Pharmacology of Marihuana" (M. C. Braude and S. Szara, eds.), Vol. 2, p. 699. Raven, New York.

Lehrman, D. S. (1961). *In* "Sex and Internal Secretions" (W. C. Young, ed.), 3rd ed., Vol. 2, p. 1268. Williams & Wilkins, Baltimore, Maryland.

Lemberger, L., and Rubin, A. (1976). *Life Sci.* **17**, 1637.

Ling, G. M., Thomas, J. A., Usher, D. R., and Singhal, R. L. (1973). *Int. J. Clin. Pharmacol., Ther. Toxicol.* **7**, 1.

Lisk, R. D. (1966). *In* "Brain and Behavior" (R. A. Gorski and R. E. Whalen, eds.), Vol. 3, p. 98. Univ. of California Press, Los Angeles.

List, A., Burtram, S. F., Nazar, B., and Harclerode, J. (1975). *J. Pharm. Pharmacol.* **27**, 606.

List, A., Nazar, B., Nyquist, S., and Harclerode, J. (1977). *Drug Metab. Dispos.* **5**, 268.

Luthra, Y. K., Rosenkrantz, H., Heyman, I. A., and Braude, M. C. (1975). *Toxicol. Appl. Pharmacol.* **32**, 418.

Luthra, Y. K., Rosenkrantz, H., and Braude, M. C. (1976). *Toxicol. Appl. Pharmacol.* **35**, 455.

McEwen, B. S., Zigmond, R. E., and Gerlach, J. (1972). *Struct. Funct. Nerv. Tissue* **5**, 206.

McIsaac, W. M., Fritchie, G. E., Idanpaan-Heikkila, J. E., Ho, B. T., and Englert, L. F. (1971). *Nature (London)* **230**, 593.

Maier, R., and Maitre, L. (1975). *Biochem. Pharmacol.* **24**, 1695.

Maker, B. S., Khan, M. A., and Lehrer, G. M. (1974). *Fed. Proc., Fed. Am. Soc. Exp. Biol.* **33**, 540.

Malsbury, C., and Pfaff, D. W. (1974). *In* "Limbic and Autonomic Nervous Systems Research" (L. V. DiCara, ed.), p. 86. Plenum, New York.

Manning, F. J., McDonough, J. H., Jr., Elsmore, T. F., Saller, C., and Sudetz, F. J. (1971). *Science* **174**, 424.

Mantilla-Plata, B., and Harbison, R. D. (1974). *Toxicol. Appl. Pharmacol.* **29**, 78.

Mantilla-Plata, B., and Harbison, R. D. (1976a). *In* "Pharmacology of Marihuana" (M. C. Braude and S. Szara, eds.), Vol. 2, p. 733. Raven, New York.

Mantilla-Plata, B., and Harbison, R. D. (1976b). *In* "Marihuana: Chemistry, Biochemistry and Cellular Effects" (G. G. Nahas and G. Gabriel, eds.), p. 469. Springer-Verlag, Berlin and New York.

Mantilla-Plata, B., Clewe, G. L., and Harbison, R. D. (1973). *Fed. Proc., Fed. Am. Soc. Exp. Biol.* **32**, 476.

Mantilla-Plata, B., Clewe, G. L., and Harbison, R. D. (1975). *Toxicol. Appl. Pharmacol.* **33**, 333.

Marks, B. H. (1972). *Prog. Brain Res.* **39**, 331.

Martin, B. R., Dewey, W. L., Harris, L. S., and Beckner, J. S. (1976). *J. Pharmacol. Exp. Ther.* **196**, 128.

Martin, B. R., Dewey, W. L., Harris, L. S., and Beckner, J. S. (1977). *Res. Commun. Chem. Pathol. Pharmacol.* **17**, 457.

Masur, J., Martz, R. M., and Carlini, E. A. (1971). *Psychopharmacologia* **19**, 388.

Mayor's Committee on Marihuana. (1944). "The Marihuana Problem in the City of New York: Sociological, Medical, Psychological and Pharmacological Studies." Jaques Cattell Press, Lancaster, Pennsylvania.

Mehndiratta, S. S., and Wig, N. N. (1975). *Drug. Alc. Depend.* **1**, 71.

Mendelson, J. H., Kuehnle, J., Ellingboe, J., and Babor, T. F. (1974). *N. Engl. J. Med.* **291**, 1051.

Mendelson, J. H., Kuehnle, J., Ellingboe, J., and Babor, T. F. (1975). *In* "Marihuana and Health Hazards: Methodological Issues in Current Research" (J. R. Tinklenberg, ed.), p. 83. Academic Press, New York.

Mendelson, J. H., Barbor, T. F., Kuehnle, J. C., Rossi, A. M., Bernstein, J. G., Mello, N. K., and Greenberg, I. (1976). *Ann. N.Y. Acad. Sci.* **282**, 186.

Merari, A., Barak, A., and Plaves, M. (1973). *Psychopharmacologia* **28**, 243.

Meyer, R. E. (1978). *In* "Psychopharmacology: A Generation of Progress" (M. A. Lipton, A. DiMascio, and K. F. Killam, eds.), p. 1639. Raven, New York.

Michael, R. P. (1966). *In* "Brain and Behavior" (R. A. Gorski and R. E. Whalen, eds.), Vol. 3, p. 82. Univ. of California Press, Los Angeles.

Milković, K., and Milković, S. (1963). *Endocrinology* **73**, 535.

Miller, L. L. (1974). *In* "Marihuana: Effects on Human Behavior" (L. L. Miller, ed.), p. 189. Academic Press, New York.

Miller, L. L., and Drew, W. G. (1974). *In* "Marihuana: Effects on Human Behavior" (L. L. Miller, ed.), p. 158. Academic Press, New York.

Milner, P. M. (1970). "Physiological Psychology." Holt, New York.

Miras, C. J. (1965). *Ciba Found. Study Group* **21**, 37.

Mitra, G., Poddar, M. K., and Ghosh, J. J. (1976). *Toxicol. Appl. Pharmacol.* **35**, 523.

Mitra, G., Poddar, M. K., and Ghosh, J. J. (1977). *Toxicol. Appl. Pharmacol.* **42**, 505.

Myers, R. D. (1974). "Handbook of Drug and Chemical Stimulation of the Brain." Van Nostrand-Reinhold, New York.

Nahas, G. G. (1976). *Ann. N.Y. Acad. Sci.* **282**, 181.

Neto, J. P., Nunes, J. F., and Carvalho, F. V. (1975). *Psychopharmacologia* **42**, 195.

Nir, I., Ayalon, D., Tsafriri, A., Cordova, T., and Lindner, H. R. (1973). *Nature (London)* **243**, 470.

Okey, A. B., and Bondy, C. P. (1977). *Science* **195**, 904.

Okey, A. B., and Truant, G. S. (1975). *Life Sci.* **17**, 1113.

Orsingher, O. A., and Fulginiti, S. (1970). *Pharmacology* **3**, 337.

Pace, H. B., Davis, W. M., and Borgen, L. A. (1971). *Ann. N.Y. Acad. Sci.* **191**, 123.

Palmer, A. K. (1972). *Adv. Exp. Biol. Med.* **27**, 45.

Patanelli, D. J. (1975). *Handb. Physiol., Sect. 7: Endocrinol.* **5**, 245.

Paton, W. D. M., and Pertwee, R. G. (1973a). *In* "Marihuana: Chemistry, Pharmacology, Metabolism and Clinical Effects" (R. Mechoulam, ed.), p. 192. Academic Press, New York.

Paton, W. D. M., and Pertwee, R. G. (1973b). *In* "Marihuana: Chemistry, Pharmacology, Metabolism and Clinical Effects" (R. Mechoulam, ed.), p. 288. Academic Press, New York.

Perez-Reyes, M. (1976). *Ann. N.Y. Acad. Sci.* **282**, 168.

Persaud, T. V. N., and Ellington, A. C. (1967). *Lancet* **2**, 1306.

Persaud, T. V. N., and Ellington, A. C. (1968). *Lancet* **2**, 406.
Pertwee, R. G. (1974). *Br. J. Pharmacol.* **51**, 391.
Peters, B. A., Lewis, E. G., Dustman, R. E., Straight, R. C., and Beck, E. C. (1976). *Psychopharmacologia* **47**, 141.
Pfaff, D. W., and Keiner, M. (1972). *Adv. Behav. Biol.* **2**, 775.
Pfaff, D. W., and Keiner, M. (1973). *J. Comp. Neurol.* **151**, 121.
Pfaff, D. W., Lewis, C., Diakow, C., and Keiner, M. (1973). *Prog. Physiol. Psychol.* **5**, 253.
Pfaff, D. W., Diakow, C., Zigmond, R. E., and Kow, L.-M. (1974). *In* "The Neurosciences: Third Study Program" (F. O. Schmitt and F. G. Worden, eds.), p. 621. MIT Press, Cambridge, Massachusetts.
Porter, R. W., Cavanaugh, E. B., Critchlow, B. V., and Sawyer, C. H. (1957). *Am. J. Physiol.* **189**, 145.
Price, D., and Williams-Ashman, H. G. (1961). *In* "Sex and Internal Secretions" (W. C. Young, ed.), 3rd ed., Vol. 1, p. 421. Williams & Wilkins, Baltimore, Maryland.
Rawitch, A. B., Schultz, G. S., Ebner, K. E., and Vardaris, R. M. (1977). *Science* **197**, 1189.
Rennert, O. M. (1972). *Adv. Exp. Biol. Med.* **27**, 97.
Roberts, W. W., Steinberg, M. L., and Means, L. W. (1967). *J. Comp. Physiol. Psychol.* **64**, 1.
Robinson, V. (1966). *In* "The Marihuana Papers" (D. Solomon, ed.), p. 201. Bobbs-Merrill, Indianapolis, Indiana.
Rosenkrantz, H., and Braude, M. C. (1976). *In* "Pharmacology of Marihuana" (M. C. Braude and S. Szara, eds.), Vol. 2, p. 571. Raven, New York.
Rosenkrantz, H., Sprague, R. A., Fleischman, R. W., and Braude, M. C. (1975). *Toxicol. Appl. Pharmacol.* **32**, 399.
Roth, W. T., Tinklenberg, J. R., and Kopell, B. S. (1976). *In* "The Therapeutic Potential of Marihuana" (S. Cohen and R. C. Stillman, eds.), p. 255. Plenum, New York.
Rubin, H. (1976). *Pap., Meet. Am. Psychol. Assoc.* Oral presentation.
Runner, M. N. (1959). *Pediatrics* **23**, 245.
Sassenrath, E. N., and Chapman, L. F. (1975). *Fed. Proc., Fed. Am. Soc.* **34**, 1666.
Saxén, L. (1976). *J. Embryol. Exp. Morphol.* **36**, 1.
Schaefer, C. F., Gunn, C. G., and Dubowski, K. M. (1975). *N. Engl. J. Med.* **292**, 867.
Schreiner, L., and Kling, A. (1953). *J. Neurophysiol.* **16**, 643.
Shahar, A., and Bino, T. (1973). *Biochem. Pharmacol.* **23**, 1341.
Shannon, M. E., and Fried, P. A. (1972). *Psychopharmacologia* **27**, 141.
Shealy, C. N., and Peele, T. L. (1957). *J. Neurophysiol.* **20**, 125.
Shoemaker, R. H., and Harmon, J. W. (1977). *Fed. Proc., Fed. Am. Soc. Exp. Biol.* **36**, 345.
Siegel, P., Siegel, M. I., Krimmer, E. C., Doyle, W. J., and Barry, H., III. (1977). *Toxicol. Appl. Pharmacol.* **42**, 339.
Singer, J. J. (1968). *J. Comp. Physiol. Psychol.* **66**, 738.
Singer, P. R., Seibetta, J. J., and Rosen, M. G. (1973). *Am. J. Obstet. Gynecol.* **117**, 331.
Smith, C. G., Moore, C. E., Besch, N. F., and Besch, P. K. (1976). *Pharmacologist* **18**, 248.
Sofia, R. D., and Barry, H., III. (1970). *Eur. J. Pharmacol.* **13**, 134.
Solomon, J., and Cocchia, M. A. (1977). *Science* **195**, 905.
Solomon, J., and Shattuck, D. X. (1974). *N. Engl. J. Med.* **291**, 309.
Solomon, J., Cocchia, M. A., Gray, R., Shattuck, D., and Vossmer, A. (1976). *Science* **192**, 559.
Solomon, J., Cocchia, M. A., and DiMartino, R. (1977). *Science* **195**, 875.
Sprague, R. A., Rosenkrantz, H., and Braude, M. C. (1973). *Life Sci.* **12**, Part 2, 409.
Symons, A. M., Teale, J. D., and Marks, V. (1976). *J. Endocrinol.* **68**, 43P.
Tart, C. T. (1970). *Nature (London)* **226**, 701.

Tart, C. T. (1971). *In* "On Being Stoned: A Psychological Study of Marihuana Intoxication," p. 141. Science and Behavior Books, Palo Alto, California.

Thompson, G. R., Mason, M. M., Rosenkrantz, H., and Braude, M. C. (1973). *Toxicol. Appl. Pharmacol.* **25,** 373.

Thompson, G. R., Fleischman, R. W., Rosenkrantz, H., and Braude, M. C. (1974). *Toxicol. Appl. Pharmacol.* **27,** 648.

Thompson, G. R., Fleischman, R. W., Rosenkrantz, H., and Braude, M. C. (1975). *Toxicology* **4,** 41.

Tinklenberg, J. R., Murphy, P. L. Murphy, P., Darley, C. F., Roth, W. T., and Kopell, B. S. (1974). *Arch. Gen. Psychiatry* **30,** 685.

Traub, S. H. (1977). *Br. J. Addict.* **72,** 67.

Uyeno, E. T. (1975). *Pharmacologist* **17,** 181.

Vardaris, R. M., Weiss, D. J., Fazel, A., and Rawitch, A. B. (1976). *Pharmacol., Biochem. Behavior* **4,** 249.

Vaughan, E., and Fisher, A. E. (1962). *Science* **137,** 758.

Warner, W., Harris, L. S., and Carchman, R. A. (1977). *Endocrinology* **101,** 1815.

Wilhelmsson, M., and Larsson, K. (1973). *Physiol. Behav.* **11,** 227.

Wilson, J. G. (1965). *In* "Teratology" (J. G. Wilson and J. Warkaray, eds.), p. 251. Univ. of Chicago Press, Chicago, Illinois.

Wright, P. L., Smith, S. H., Keplinger, M. L., Calandra, J. C., and Braude, M. C. (1976). *Toxicol. Appl. Pharmacol.* **38,** 223.

Zinberg, N. E. (1974). *N. Engl. J. Med.* **291,** 309.

VITAMINS AND HORMONES, VOL. 36

Steroid Hormone Regulation of Specific Gene Expression

LAWRENCE CHAN, ANTHONY R. MEANS, AND
BERT W. O'MALLEY

Departments of Cell Biology and Medicine, Baylor College of Medicine, Houston, Texas

I. Introduction

The regulation of specific gene expression is undoubtedly a major mechanism of action of the steroid hormones. Much of our present knowledge in this area has been derived from studies on a limited number of systems. The topic has been recently reviewed by a number of authors (Gorski and Gannon, 1976; Yamamoto and Alberts, 1976; Liao, 1977; Jensen and DeSombre, 1974; Vedeckis et al., 1978) and by ourselves (O'Malley and Means, 1974; Chan and O'Malley, 1976a,b,c). In the present review we will discuss some of the individual systems used by investigators in the field of hormone action. Most of the advances over the last three years were in the area of steroid hormone regulation of specific mRNA production and translation. We will attempt to update the current status of steroid hormone regulation of transcription *in vivo* and *in vitro*. Taken together, the experimental evidence currently available strongly supports the idea that steroid hormones act primarily at the level of transcription.

II. INDUCTION OF SPECIFIC PROTEIN SYNTHESIS BY STEROID HORMONES

A large number of proteins have been reported to increase in concentration or activity after steroid hormone treatment (Pitot and Yatvin, 1973; Gelehrter, 1973). However, the exact level of regulation of most of these proteins is unclear. There are indirect studies involving drugs like actinomycin D, from which conclusions have been drawn. However, such studies are fraught with dangers of over- or misinterpretation because of the multiplicity of action of most drugs. It is evident that major conceptual advances will occur primarily through use of reconstituted cell-free systems for transcription and translation and through cell culture systems amenable to genetic manipulations. To assess the level of regulation and differentiate translational from pretranslational events, the mRNAs of a handful of such proteins have been partially purified and their activities assayed *in vitro* (Table I). In a few instances, the mRNAs have been purified to homogeneity and their complementary DNAs (cDNAs) have been synthesized *in vitro*. Studies using the radiolabeled cDNAs as hybridization probes have generally confirmed the results obtained via the translation experiments. We will confine our survey specifically to those proteins the mRNA of which has been studied either by *in vitro* translation or by nucleic acid hybridization.

III. PROTEINS REGULATED BY ESTROGEN

A. EGG WHITE PROTEINS

One of the systems used most extensively in the study of steroid hormone regulation of gene expression is the chick oviduct system

(O'Malley et al., 1969; Palmiter, 1975). In the chick, the administration of estrogen (primary stimulation) induces growth and differentiation and the synthesis of a number of egg white proteins, the major one of which is ovalbumin. The weight of the oviduct increases several hundredfold, and there is a massive proliferation of tubular gland cells. If estrogen treatment is interrupted, the oviduct atrophies and ovalbumin synthesis gradually becomes undetectable. However, some tubular gland cells persist, so that the readministration of either estrogen or progesterone (secondary stimulation) results in the rapid induction of ovalbumin synthesis (Palmiter, 1972; Chan et al., 1973). Secondary stimulation lends itself to a simpler analysis, since cell division is unnecessary for the ovalbumin response. When ovalbumin mRNA levels were measured by in vitro translation, there was a close correlation between the mRNA activity and the rate of ovalbumin synthesis following estrogen (Chan et al., 1973). Similarly, when ovalbumin mRNA sequences were quantified by cDNA hybridization, the number of mRNA molecules was also found to increase rapidly after estrogen treatment (Cox et al., 1974; Harris et al., 1975; McKnight et al., 1975). Ovalbumin mRNA sequences decreased to barely detectable levels after withdrawal of the hormone. One interesting observation was that ovalbumin mRNA activity as measured by translation in vitro disappeared more rapidly after acute withdrawal of estrogen than predicted by the biological half-life of the mRNA in the presence of the hormone (Palmiter and Carey, 1974). This phenomenon was further studied by Cox (1977) in some detail by nucleic acid hybridization. It appears that the concentration of ovalbumin mRNA, as well as of other high-abundance, low-complexity mRNAs, is selectively and rapidly reduced in polysomes after estrogen withdrawal. The exact mechanism of this apparent change in biological half-life of the different mRNAs is, however, unclear.

An apparent discrepancy has been reported in different laboratories in the kinetics of induction of ovalbumin mRNA by estrogen in the hormone-withdrawn oviduct. McKnight et al. (1975), Palmiter (1975, and Palmiter et al., 1976) observed a 3-hour lag period between the injection of estradiol and the increase in ovalbumin mRNA as quantified by translation or cDNA hybridization. The lag was shorter (2 hours) when progesterone was administered, and a much shorter lag (30 minutes) was observed also for the estrogen-induced conalbumin mRNA accumulation. Based on these observations, Palmiter et al. (1976) proposed a model of estrogen action involving a rate-limiting translocation of the estrogen receptor from initial nonproductive chromatin-binding sites to productive sites. In contrast to these findings, Harris et al. (1975) observed no appreciable lag between hormone

TABLE I

SPECIFIC PROTEINS INDUCED BY STEROID HORMONES[a]

Hormone	Tissue	Protein	Reference
I. Estrogen	Chick oviduct	Ovalbumin	Chan et al. (1973); Cox et al. (1974); Harris et al. (1975); McKnight et al. (1975)
	Chick oviduct	Conalbumin	Palmiter et al. (1976)
	Chick liver	ApoVLDL-II	Chan et al. (1976)
	Chick liver	Vitellogenin	Mullinix et al. (1976); Deeley et al. (1977b)
	Xenopus liver	Vitellogenin	Shapiro et al. (1976); Baker and Shapiro (1977); Ryffel et al. (1977)
	Rat pituitary	Prolactin	Stone et al. (1977)
II. Progesterone	Chick oviduct	Avidin	Chan et al. (1973)
	Rabbit uterus	Uteroglobin	Beato and Rungger (1975); Levey and Daniel (1976); Bullock et al. (1976)
III. Androgen	Rat liver	α_{2u}-Globulin	Sippel et al. (1975); Kurtz and Feigelson (1977)
	Mouse liver	Major urinary protein complex	Osawa and Tomino (1977)
	Rat prostate	Aldolase	Mainwaring et al. (1974)

IV. Glucocorticoids	Rat liver	Tyrosine aminotransferase	Roewekamp et al. (1976); Nickol et al. (1976); Diesterhaft et al. (1977)
	Rat liver	Tryptophan oxygenase	Schultz et al. (1975)
	Rat kidney	Phosphoenolpyruvate carboxykinase	Iynedjian and Hanson (1977b)
	Mouse mammary cells	Mammary tumor virus RNA	Parks et al. (1974); Ringold et al. (1975); Young et al. (1977)
	Embryonic chicken retina	Glutamine synthetase	Sarkar and Griffith (1976)
	Rat pituitary cell culture	Growth hormone	Tushinski et al. (1977); Martial et al. (1977a)
	Rat pituitary	Corticotropin[b]	Nakanishi et al. (1977)

[a] Includes those proteins the mRNAs of which have been demonstrated by translation or nucleic acid hybridization. The level of regulation can be evaluated only in these instances.

[b] Corticotropin mRNA is "turned off" rather than induced by glucocorticoids.

administration and mRNA accumulation as measured by hybridization. A noteworthy increase in ovalbumin mRNA was observed by 60 minutes of estrogen treatment. The discrepancy in observations in the different laboratories is more apparent than real. Harris et al. (1975) were studying the induction process in chicks withdrawn from estrogen for only 11 days, whereas McKnight et al. (1975) and Palmiter et al. (1976) studied animals withdrawn from the hormone for 26 and more days. This could account for a shorter lag in the former study. Furthermore, if the data of McKnight et al. are examined carefully, a definite but slow increase in the number of ovalbumin mRNA molecules was observed at 1 and 2 hours after hormone. The rate of this increase trebled after 3 hours. So the 3-hour lag is only relative, not absolute. Similarly, if Harris' data are carefully analyzed, one finds a slow initial phase of response for 60 minutes, followed by a much more rapid response. These studies support the conclusion that ovalbumin mRNA starts to accumulate within a short time after estrogen administration. Such changes do not support the unmodified "receptor translocation" hypothesis of Palmiter et al. (1976). The much more rapid increase in response after 3 hours observed by all the laboratories can be explained either by a purely transcriptional model, in which induction requires 90 minutes to reach a maximum rate with respect to the whole organ, or perhaps by a combination of transcriptional and post-transcriptional events.

Other oviduct proteins regulated by estrogen include conalbumin, ovomucoid, and lysozyme. The synthesis of these proteins, however, is not strictly coordinated, and each is synthesized more or less independently in response to estrogen (Palmiter, 1972).

B. Apo-Very Low Density Lipoprotein-II (ApoVLDL-II)

Women taking oral contraceptives containing estrogen often develop hypertriglyceridemia and hyperlipoproteinemia (Wynn et al., 1969; Hazzard et al., 1977). The exact mechanism for this observation is unclear. In the chick, a similar response to estrogen was first observed by Hillyard et al. (1956). Luskey et al. (1974) demonstrated that the hyperlipoproteinemia involved mainly the very low density lipoproteins (VLDL) and the hepatic synthesis of VLDL was increased. Progesterone, a component in many contraceptives, was found to be without significant effect on the VLDL response to estrogen (Chan et al., 1977b).

To localize the level of regulation of VLDL by estrogen, Chan et al. (1976) purified a major VLDL apoprotein, apoVLDL-II. The mRNA for apoVLDL-II was partially purified and translated in vitro. When apoVLDL-II mRNA levels were compared to the actual rate of VLDL synthesis, an excellent correlation was observed, suggesting that estrogen regulates VLDL synthesis predominantly at the transcriptional level. Unlike the massive effect of estrogen in the chick oviduct, where every protein examined was found to be stimulated, apoVLDL synthesis appeared to be selectively stimulated by the hormone in the cockerel liver. The rates of synthesis of apoA-I, a major avian high density apolipoprotein (Jackson *et al.*, 1976), and of albumin were not affected by estrogen. The mRNA levels for these two proteins were similarly unaffected by the hormone (Chan *et al.*, 1978).

An interesting observation (Chan *et al.*, 1978) in the VLDL system was that when apoVLDL-II mRNA was translated in a wheat germ system *in vitro*, the product, preapoVLDL-II, had a molecular weight of 12,000, compared to 9400 for plasma apoVLDL-II. Sequence determination revealed the extra stretch of 23 amino acid residues on preapoVLDL-II to be located at the amino terminal of apoVLDL-II and to be rich in hydrophobic residues. The presence of a putative precursor to apoVLDL-II is compatible with Blobel's signal hypothesis that secretory proteins are initially synthesized as higher molecular weight precursors (Blobel and Dobberstein, 1975).

Apo VLDL-II mRNA has been purified to apparent homogeneity. A cDNA synthesized on the purified mRNA as template was used to quantify the number of structural apoVLDL-II genes in total avian DNA. Only a limited number (probably one) of such genes was found per haploid genome, both in control and in estrogen-treated animals. This suggests that estrogen stimulates apoVLDL-II gene expression at the transcriptional, or possibly posttranscriptional, level rather than at the DNA level.

C. Vitellogenin

The estrogen induction of vitellogenin synthesis in the *Xenopus laevis* and in the rooster represents promising systems for investigating the regulation of specific gene expression in the eukaryotes (Tata, 1976). Vitellogenin is the precursor to the major yolk proteins phosvitin and lipovitellin. It is a phosphoprotein rich in serine residues. The exact molecular weight of the protein is unknown, but, on denaturing gel electrophoresis, its apparent molecular weight is over 2×10^6 in both the amphibian and the avian species (Bergink and Wallace, 1974; Deeley *et al.*, 1975). In the avian species, each vitellogenin monomer molecule contains two phosvitin molecules and one lipovitellin molecule (Deeley *et al.*, 1975).

In both the male *Xenopus* and the rooster, vitellogenin is normally undetectable. The protein appears in the liver and blood within about 12 hours after estrogen treatment in the frog (Wittliff and Kenney, 1972) and within 4 hours after similar treatment in the cockerel (Jackson et al., 1977). Different authors have commented on the apparent lag in hormone induction. However, since the reported lag varies considerably among various investigators [from several days (Berridge et al., 1976) to less than an hour in an in vitro system (Waugh and Knowland, 1975)], it is likely that the discrepancy is explained at least partially by the sensitivity of the detection methods (Jackson et al., 1977). An interesting observation on the effects of estrogen on vitellogenin synthesis is that repeated exposure of the animal to the hormone ("secondary stimulation") results in a much more rapid accumulation of the protein in both the liver and in blood than the initial hormonal treatment ("primary stimulation") (Bergink et al., 1973; Talwar et al., 1973; Berridge et al., 1976). This difference in the kinetics of vitellogenin induction by estrogen has been termed the "memory effect." It cannot be attributed to a requirement for cell division in the primary induction as in the case of ovalbumin, since in this instance DNA synthesis is not prerequisite to the response to hormone (Jost et al., 1973; Green and Tata, 1976).

The mRNAs for vitellogenin from both the frog (Shapiro et al., 1976; Berridge et al., 1976; Berridge and Lane, 1976) and the chick (Wetekam et al., 1975; Jost and Pehling, 1976) have been translated in vitro. For Xenopus, an excellent correlation between mRNA activity in vitro and rate of vitellogenin synthesis in liver slices was observed (Shapiro et al., 1976). In the rooster, comparison was made only of the hepatic mRNA levels and the hepatic and plasma concentrations of vitellogenin (rather than its rate of synthesis). Whereas the induction was accomplished by an accumulation of the mRNA in the liver and the protein in the blood, the hormone withdrawal pattern was more complex. When the protein was no longer detectable in the liver or plasma, appreciable quantities of vitellogenin mRNA activity were still present. These mRNA molecules were free and unassociated with polysomes (Mullinix et al., 1976). Whether this observation is related to the more rapid secondary stimulation by estrogen is entirely speculative, since significant amounts of vitellogenin mRNA as measured by cDNA hybridization were not detected in postwithdrawal rooster liver in a subsequent study (Deeley et al., 1977a). However, the exact time of estrogen withdrawal was not given in the translation studies. In the Xenopus system, Baker and Shapiro (1977) found significant amounts of vitellogenin mRNA even 50 days after hormone withdrawal. Furthermore, the failure to detect vitellogenin in the plasma or liver could be related to the sensitivity of the assay used (Jackson et al., 1977).

To further understand the mechanism of vitellogenin induction, the mRNA for this protein has been purified to apparent homogeneity in both the *Xenopus* and the chick (Shapiro and Baker, 1977; Ryffel *et al.,* 1977; Deeley *et al.,* 1977b). A complementary DNA to the RNA has been used in both instances to study the kinetics of induction of vitellogenin under conditions of primary as well as of secondary stimulation (Baker and Shapiro, 1977; Ryffel *et al.,* 1977; Deeley *et al.,* 1977a). In the *Xenopus,* considerable variance in the induction kinetics was reported by different investigators. Baker and Shapiro (1977) found that after primary stimulation, vitellogenin mRNA accumulation was first detected 4.5 hours after hormone. In secondarily stimulated animals, the mRNA increased at a much more rapid rate, such that the number of sequences present 6 hours after restimulation with estrogen was more than 10 times greater than that observed 6 hours after primary stimulation. Unfortunately, since the early time points (less than 6 hours) after estrogen restimulation were not studied, they presented no data on the absolute lag periods before mRNA sequences were observed to accumulate. Ryffel *et al.* (1977), on the other hand, observed a 12-hour lag before vitellogenin mRNA was detected after primary stimulation, and a 6–12-hour lag (depending on the animals) in secondary stimulated animals. The reason for the difference in observations between the two groups of investigators is unclear. However, Baker and Shapiro (1977) used a slightly higher dose of estrogen, which could at least partly explain this apparent discrepancy.

In the rooster, Deeley *et al.* (1977a) also carried out similar studies with a vitellogenin cDNA. They observed an accumulation of vitellogenin mRNA as early as 30 minutes after either primary or secondary stimulation. However, there was a 6- to 7-fold difference in the rates of accumulation between the two types of manipulation. Furthermore, in the primary response, there was a 5- to 6-fold increase in accumulation rate between 5 and 12 hours as compared to the first 4 hours after hormonal stimulation, whereas in the secondary response, no significant change in the accumulation rate was observed and the maximal rate of mRNA accumulation was achieved almost immediately after hormone treatment. The rate at which the mRNA sequences disappeared was the same in both primary and secondary responses.

The rapidity of the vitellogenin response and the absence of any detectable vitellogenin mRNA in the untreated liver in both the *Xenopus* and the rooster suggests a primary effect at the transcriptional level. The anamnestic response, on the other hand, is an observation that could be explained by (a) a persistent change in the conformation of the vitellogenin gene; (b) a permanent change in the estrogen-receptor generation or response; or (c) some other unknown "commitment" mechanism brought about by primary stimulation with estrogen. Future work in this area will likely shed some light on this interesting phenomenon.

D. PROLACTIN

Prolactin secretion and synthesis in the anterior pituitary is regulated by a number of factors (Thorner, 1977). The hormone is under tonic inhibitory control by the hypothalamus by a prolactin release inhibiting factor (PIF). Apart from PIF, other factors known to modulate prolactin secretion include dopamine (which may or may not be identical to PIF), thyrotropin-releasing hormone (TRH) (Tashjian *et al.*, 1971), possibly a prolactin-releasing factor distinct from TRH (Boyd *et al.*, 1976; Szabo and Frohman, 1976), and serotonin (MacLeod, 1977). Apart from PIF and dopamine, these other factors all stimulate prolactin secretion. In addition, estrogen also appears to have a stimulatory effect on prolactin secretion.

In the rat the administration of estrogen resulted in increased synthesis of prolactin (MacLeod *et al.*, 1969; Yamamoto *et al.*, 1975; Maurer and Gorski, 1977) as demonstrated by incorporation of radiolabeled amino acids into the peptide. The effect of estrogen was quite specific in that other pituitary proteins did not seem to be affected by it and incorporation of radioactivity into growth hormone actually declined (Maurer and Gorski, 1977). When daily estrogen injections were given to ovariectomized female and intact male rats, the rate of synthesis of prolactin increased by 50% on day 1 and reached maximum levels at 3–7 days. In intact rats estrogen could exert its effect by influencing PIF production by the hypothalamus (Ratner and Meites, 1964) or by directly acting on the pituitary. Studies *in vitro*, however, indicate that the hormone has a direct effect on the gland (Nicoll and Meites, 1962, 1964).

To investigate the level of regulation of prolactin synthesis, prolactin mRNA was isolated from rat anterior pituitaries and prolactin-secreting pituitary tumors. Translation of the mRNA *in vitro* showed that prolactin is synthesized initially as a larger precursor, preprolactin (Evans and Rosenfeld, 1976; Dannies and Tashjian, 1976; Maurer *et al.*, 1976, 1977). The precursor has 29 amino acid residues at the N terminus of the prolactin sequence, and is another example of a signal sequence on a precursor of a secretory protein (Maurer *et al.*, 1977; Blobel and Dobberstein, 1975).

When preprolactin mRNA activity from male rat pituitary was assayed *in vitro*, estrogen was found to stimulate the mRNA activity. On daily treatment with estrogen, preprolactin mRNA increased daily to a maximum of 300% of controls after 7 days of treatment. After estrogen treatment was discontinued, the mRNA activity declined to 50% of the maximum stimulation after 2 days. The stimulating effects of estrogen on preprolactin mRNA activity were also observed in ovariectomized female rats (Stone *et al.*, 1977). It thus appears that estrogen regulates prolactin synthesis at a pretranslational level. Whether this is a direct effect of estrogen, or whether some intermediate steps (e.g., changes in dopamine and/or other factors) are involved cannot be determined from these studies in intact animals. It has been shown that TRH stimulates prolactin mRNA activity directly in an *in vitro* system (Evans and Rosenfeld, 1976; Dannies and Tashjian, 1976).

IV. PROTEINS REGULATED BY PROGESTERONE

A. AVIDIN

Avidin was one of the first hormone-regulated proteins studied. Hertz *et al.* (1943) first reported its induction in the chick oviduct by estrogen plus progesterone. The observation was later extended, and the protein was induced *de novo* by progesterone both *in vivo* and in minced oviduct tissue and monolayer cultures *in vitro* (O'Malley, 1967; O'Malley and Kohler, 1967a,b; Korenman and O'Malley, 1968). The induction was inhibited by both actinomycin D and cycloheximide. When avidin mRNA was extracted and translated *in vitro*, its activity was found to increase after progesterone treatment (Chan *et al.*, 1973). Avidin mRNA has been purified about 1000-fold by Sperry *et al.* (1976), who also confirmed its absence in immature oviduct and induction by a single injection of progesterone.

B. UTEROGLOBIN

One important function of the hormone progesterone is the preparation of the uterine environment for proper implantation and maintenance of pregnancy. Progesterone appears to accomplish such a function through direct influence on the properties of the uterine musculature, the endometrium, and most important, the uterine secretions (Beier, 1975). The effects of pregnancy or progesterone on the secretory proteins of the uterus have been studied extensively in the rabbit as well as the human (Beier, 1975, 1976a,b; Beier and Beier-Hellwig, 1973). A specific protein, uteroglobin, was found to be the predominant protein in rabbit uterine secretion and in endometrial tissue extracts during the normal cycle, during pregnancy before implantation, and during pseudopregnancy (Beier, 1967, 1976a; Krishnan and Daniel, 1967). It was also found in blastocyst fluid. Krishnan and Daniel (1967) named the protein blastokinin and suggested that it might be important in supporting blastocyst development. Such a function, however, has not been confirmed by other workers (Mauer and Beier, 1976).

Progesterone has been shown to induce uteroglobin synthesis (Beier, 1970, 1976b; Arthur and Daniel, 1972). This probably explains the appearance of the protein in uterine secretions in large amounts between day 3 and day 8 of pregnancy or pseudopregnancy. One interesting observation was that the protein was no longer detectable by day 10 of pregnancy (Krishnan and Daniel, 1967). This observation was initially quite puzzling because the protein apparently disappeared while plasma progesterone was still rising (Hilliard *et al.*, 1968). An explanation was readily apparent when Bullock and Willen (1974) demonstrated that concomitant administration of estradiol suppressed the progesterone-induced synthesis of uteroglobin, and plasma estradiol was noted to be rising at the time of disappearance of uteroglobin in the rabbit (Hilliard and Eaton, 1971).

Uteroglobin mRNA isolation was first reported by Beato and Rungger (1975). The authors extracted the RNA from progesterone-primed rabbits and translated it in *Xenopus* oocytes. Subsequently, the *in vitro* translation of uteroglobin mRNA in wheat germ extracts has been reported by a number of workers (Beato and Nieto, 1976; Levey and Daniel, 1976; Bullock *et al.*, 1976; Atger and Milgrom, 1977). An interesting observation was the presence of a "preuteroglobin" as the translation product. Preuteroglobin has a molecular weight of 11,000 whereas uteroglobin monomer has a molecular weight of about 8000 (Beato and Nieto, 1976; Bullock *et al.*, 1976; Atger and Milgrom, 1977). The proportion of uteroglobin mRNA was found to be markedly increased in the endometrium either by administration of progesterone or during pregnancy. Such observations suggest that progesterone stimulates uteroglobin synthesis at the level of transcription.

One additional piece of observation was presented by Bullock (1977): mRNA isolated from the rabbit lung directed the synthesis *in vitro* of a product indistinguishable from authentic uteroglobin immunologically. The product was also identical in size to preuteroglobin. The concentration of the pulmonary uteroglobin-like protein mRNA was the same in nonpregnant and the pregnant state. If this RNA is indeed identical to the endometrial uteroglobin mRNA, the action of progesterone on the same protein appears to be totally different in the uterus and in the lung. Future studies on this interesting phenomenon will likely shed some light on the molecular mechanism of progesterone action.

V. Proteins Regulated by Androgen

A. α_{2u}-Globulin

α_{2u}-Globulin is a protein found by Roy and Neuhaus (1966) in the urine of mature male rats and absent from the urine of female rats. The protein is synthesized in the liver and is rapidly filtered and excreted through the kidneys. The regulation of the biosynthesis of this protein was reviewed in our previous review on steroid hormone action (Chan and O'Malley, 1976b); suffice it to say that pituitary growth hormone, thyroid hormones, insulin, and glucocorcorticoids all seem to act synergistically with androgens to stimulate synthesis of α_{2u}-globulin. That androgen works predominantly at the nuclear level was first demonstrated by Sippel et al. (1975). They isolated α_{2u}-globulin mRNA from rat liver and translated it in vitro. Message activity was demonstrated only in male livers and was absent from female livers. Furthermore, androgen treatment of spayed female rats or castrated male rats was found to induce the parallel appearance of both α_{2u}-globulin and its corresponding mRNA (Sippel et al., 1975; Kurtz et al., 1976b). The importance of other hormones in the regulation of this protein was further established by a series of experiments (Sippel et al., 1975; Kurtz et al., 1976a; Roy et al., 1977; Roy and Dowbenko, 1977). Thyroidectomy resulted in a complete disappearance of α_{2u}-globulin and its mRNA in the male rat. Both the protein and its mRNA could be restored by administration of L-thyroxine or triiodo-L-thyronine to the animals. Androgens were ineffective in inducing the protein or its mRNA in thyroidectomized animals. Hypophysectomy and adrenalectomy both reduced the level of α_{2u}-globulin and its mRNA (Sippel et al., 1975; Roy and Dowbenko, 1977). Reversal of the effect of hypophysectomy on the synthesis of the protein requires simultaneous treatment with androgen, glucocorticoid, thyroxine, and growth hormone. The multihormonal regulation appears to be exerted at the level of transcription, since similar effects on α_{2u}-globulin mRNA were observed.

Recently Kurtz and Feigelson (1977) succeeded in preparing a complementary DNA (cDNA) specific for α_{2u}-globulin mRNA. Using the cDNA as a hybridization probe, they confirmed the previous results with translation assays on the hormonal regulation of α_{2u}-globulin mRNA accumulation by androgens, estrogens, and thyroid hormones.

B. MAJOR URINARY PROTEIN COMPLEX

Quite analogous to the α_{2u}-globulin in the rat, the major urinary protein (MUP) complex in the mouse is synthesized in the liver and excreted in the urine. Its excretion is also under sex-hormone control. Urine from male mice contains a greater amount of the MUP complex than that from females (Finlayson et al., 1963). Its level in the female can be stimulated by testosterone administration. When mRNA extracted from mouse livers was assayed in vitro, males and androgen-treated females were shown to contain higher MUP complex mRNA activities than control females. In contrast to the α_{2u}-globulin mRNA, however, small amounts of MUP complex mRNA activity were detectable in the female (Osawa and Tomino, 1977). Hence, in the mouse, androgen appears to control the synthesis of MUP at a pretranslational level.

C. FRUCTOSE DIPHOSPHATE ALDOLASE

In the prostate of the castrated rat, androgen administration stimulates the activity of the enzyme fructose diphosphate aldolase (Butler and Schade, 1958). Mainwaring et al. (1974) took advantage of this observation and studied the regulation of aldolase mRNA by testosterone. Message activity was measured in a Krebs II ascites-tumor cell extract in vitro at various times after hormone treatment. Testosterone was found to stimulate prostatic aldolase mRNA activity and was without significant effect on hepatic aldolase mRNA activities. These findings support the view that androgen stimulates the transcription of aldolase mRNA in the prostate. However, from the published data, it is not clear whether or not transcription control is a primary event in this system. Aldolase is an extremely minor component of total prostatic protein, and aldolase mRNA activity accounts for less than 1% of the total mRNA activity. The changes following androgen are relatively slow, taking 4 hours or more, whereas the total protein biosynthetic response to testosterone occurred within 45 minutes. Furthermore, there is some discrepancy between the time course of isolated mRNA activity and rate of aldolase synthesis on whole tissue and polyribosomes. These observations suggest that the authors might be studying some secondary effects of testosterone and that the prostatic aldolase system may not be an ideal model to investigate the *primary* action of androgens.

VI. Proteins Regulated by Glucocorticoids

A. Tyrosine Aminotransferase

Tyrosine aminotransferase is probably the best-studied of the glucocorticoid-induced proteins. The protein was induced by glucagon, glucocorticoids, insulin, and a serum factor (Lin and Knox, 1957; Tomkins *et al.*, 1972; Kenney *et al.*, 1968, 1973; Gelehrter and Tomkins, 1970). Based on the observation of superinduction by the administration of actinomycin D after glucocorticoid induction, Tomkins *et al.* (1969) proposed a model of gene regulation involving labile posttranscriptional "repressors" that inhibit the utilization of tyrosine aminotransferase mRNA. In the last few years, the translation of the mRNA in heterologous systems has been examined in a number of laboratories (Roewekamp *et al.*, 1976; Nickol *et al.*, 1976; Diesterhaft *et al.*, 1977). It is now apparent that tyrosine aminotransferase induction can be simply explained by the hormone-induced accumulation of its specific mRNA. The phenomenon of superinduction can be explained by the differential stability of mRNAs and competition of these RNAs for rate-limiting factors involved in the translation process (D. Granner *et al.*, personal communication). Thus the mechanism of superinduction appears to be the same for the glucocorticoid induction of hepatic tyrosine aminotransferase and the estrogenic induction of ovalbumin mRNA (Palmiter and Schimke, 1973).

B. Tryptophan Oxygenase

Hepatic tryptophan 2,3-dioxygenase is an enzyme that appears at the end of the second postnatal week in the rat. It increases to the adult level by 22 days after birth (Nemeth, 1959; Franz and Knox, 1967; Greengard and Dewey, 1971; Roper and Franz, 1977). The factors that control this process were studied by various workers using techniques involving adrenalectomy and administration of glucocorticoids. It is apparent that the developmental pattern probably results from increased glucocorticoid release between the second and third weeks postnatally. Administration of the hormone leads to induction of the enzyme (Schimke *et al.*, 1965). This process results from an increased synthetic rate of the enzyme, as well as an accumulation of its specific mRNA (Schultz *et al.*, 1975). Similarly, the developmental pattern of the enzyme also parallels that of the specific mRNA activity (Killewich and Feigelson, 1977). Interestingly, tryptophan oxygenase activity can also be induced by administration of tryptophan (Knox and Mehler,

1951). When its mRNA activity was measured by *in vitro* translation, Schultz *et al.* (1975) found that the profound elevation of enzyme activity after tryptophan treatment was unaccompanied by any significant change in the mRNA coding for the protein. This observation is in agreement with the finding of Schimke *et al.* (1965) that whereas glucocorticoids increase enzyme levels by increasing its synthesis, tryptophan does so by stabilizing and thereby decreasing the rate of degradation of the enzyme.

C. PHOSPHOENOLPYRUVATE CARBOXYKINASE

The activity of the gluconeogenic enzyme phosphoenolpyruvate (PEP) carboxykinase is regulated by various hormones and the nutritional state of the animal. The enzyme can be demonstrated in the liver (Wicks *et al.*, 1973; Gunn *et al.*, 1975a) and in the kidney (Gunn *et al.*, 1975b; Iynedjian *et al.*, 1975) and its activity is increased following glucocorticoid treatment. The hormone appears to stimulate the synthesis of the enzyme in hepatoma cells *in vitro* (Gunn *et al.*, 1975a) or in the kidney *in vivo* (Gunn *et al.*, 1975b; Iynedjian *et al.*, 1975). The effect of glucocorticoids on this enzyme can be blocked by actinomycin D.

In an attempt to elucidate the mechanism of action of glucocorticoid, Iynedjian and Hanson (1977a) extracted mRNA from rat kidney and translated PEP carboxykinase in a wheat germ system *in vitro*. They studied the mRNA activity for the enzyme at various times after glucocorticoid treatment. PEP carboxykinase activity was assayed in the tissue, and the rate of enzyme synthesis was monitored by a pulse label and specific immunoprecipitation of radioactivity incorporated into the PEP carboxykinase (Iynedjian and Hanson, 1977b). Glucocorticoid treatment was found to result in a simultaneous stimulation of all three parameters: PEP carboxykinase mRNA activity, its rate of synthesis, and its total enzymic activity. It thus appears that a gluconeogenic enzyme is induced at the pretranslational level by glucocorticoids.

D. MOUSE MAMMARY TUMOR VIRUS RNA

In establishing virus infection of cell lines *in vitro,* it was observed by a number of virologists that glucocorticoids stimulate the production of various tumor viruses in tissue culture cells (McGrath, 1971; Paran *et al.*, 1973; Morhenn *et al.*, 1973; Parks *et al.*, 1974; Dickson *et al.*, 1972; Fine *et al.*, 1974). The best studied of these systems was the effect of glucocorticoids on mouse mammary tumor virus (MMTV) production in tissue culture cells. In short-term cultures of mammary adenocarcinoma cells of BALB/cf C3H mice, McGrath (1971) showed that hydrocortisone added *in vitro* induced the production and release of MMTV, which was quantified by actual isolation of the viral particles and RNA. Subsequently this observation was confirmed in mammary tumor cell lines by others, and increased MMTV production under the influence of the synthetic glucocorticoid, dexamethasone, could be detected by molecular hybridization to MMTV [³H]cDNA (Parks *et al.*, 1974, 1975). Concomitantly, viral DNA polymerase activity (Dickson *et al.*, 1972; Parks *et al.*, 1975) and MMTV antigens (Parks *et al.*, 1974, 1975) were increased by the hormone. These changes were accompanied by electron microscopic evidence of increased production of type B particles morphologically typical of MMTV particles (Parks *et al.*, 1974). Concentrations of dexamethasone as low as $1 \times 10^{-10} M$ were effective, and actinomycin D, but not inhibitors of DNA or protein synthesis, blocked MMTV RNA induction (Ringold *et al.*, 1975; Scolnick *et al.*, 1976).

It is likely that the dexamethasone induction of MMTV is receptor-mediated. In the cell lines studied, typical glucocorticoid receptors could be demonstrated. The receptor was steroid specific and similar in size, hormone affinity, and DNA-binding properties to the glucocorticoid receptors previously demonstrated in another hormone-responsive mouse cell line (Young *et al.*, 1975; Ringold *et al.*, 1975). It also undergoes a temperature-sensitive nuclear translocation similar to other steroid hormone receptor systems (Young *et al.*, 1975; Chan and O'Malley, 1976a). Furthermore, an excess of progesterone, a competitive inhibitor of glucocorticoid receptor binding (Rousseau *et al.*, 1972), completely abolished the dexamethasone induction of MMTV RNA (Ringold *et al.*, 1975).

The dexamethasone-induced increase in MMTV RNA concentration could be explained either by an increase in synthesis or a decrease in degradation of the RNA. Because of the limitation of the assay systems in the initial studies, changes in the RNA concentration were demonstrated only after prolonged periods of time, e.g., hours or days after hormone treatment. Recently Ringold *et al.* (1975) presented evidence that RNA accumulation was stimulated within 15 minutes. Furthermore, Young *et al.* (1977) were able to demonstrate with short-term labeling experiments that within 10 minutes of dexamethasone treatment there was a 3-fold increase in newly synthesized MMTV RNA. The stimulation reached 5- to 10-fold within 30 to 60 minutes. They also observed that MMTV RNA had a half-life greater than 8 hours, and dexamethasone probably accelerated the rate of decay of the RNA.

Thus, the magnitude and rapidity of dexamethasone action on MMTV RNA synthesis strongly suggested a primary action at the level of transcription.

E. GLUTAMINE SYNTHETASE

The embryonic chick retina is another defined system used for the study of developmental patterns of the enzyme glutamine synthetase (Moscona and Hubby, 1963). The enzyme was inducible by the administration of glucocorticoids, and nascent enzyme synthesis appeared to be involved (Alescio and Moscona, 1969). Sarkar and Moscona (1973) also found the amount of immunoprecipitable nascent enzyme in retinal polysomes to be increased by the hormone. Furthermore, Sarkar and Griffith (1976) extracted total mRNA from embryonic retinal cells and translated it in a wheat germ system. Amount of enzyme synthesized *in vitro* was quantified by incorporation of radioactive amino acids into immunoprecipitable glutamine synthetase. Comparison of the amount of mRNA activity from control and glucocorticoid-treated embryos indicated that the hormone stimulated the accumulation of glutamine synthetase mRNA. In this system, glucocorticoid regulates specific protein synthesis at least partially at a pretranslational level.

F. GROWTH HORMONE

A tissue-culture system used extensively in investigations on the mechanism of action of glucocorticoids and thyroid hormones is a rat pituitary cell line that secretes growth hormone (Samuels *et al.*, 1973; Kohler and Bridson, 1973). In this system both glucocorticoid and thyroid hormones stimulate production of growth hormone. Messenger RNA from this system directs the synthesis of growth hormone *in vitro*. When Krebs II ascites tumor cell extracts were used as the translation assay, the size of the product was shown to be similar to that of growth hormone (Bancroft *et al.*, 1973). However, when wheat germ extracts were used, the major translation product, designated pregrowth hormone, was about 20% larger than native growth hormone (Sussman *et al.*, 1976).

Tushinski *et al.* (1977) examined the effect of glucocorticoid on growth hormone synthesis in the rat pituitary cell line. Growth hormone synthesis was measured by immunoprecipitable radioactivity incorporated into the hormone following a pulse label with a radiolabeled amino acid. They observed good agreement between the enhancement of growth hormone synthesis and the stimulation of cytoplasmic levels of pregrowth hormone mRNA as assayed by translation *in vitro*. The pregrowth hormone mRNA was also demonstrated on polyacrylamide gel as a band that was detectable only after glucocorticoid treatment. Martial *et al.* (1977a) independently investigated the level of control of glucocorticoids and thyroid hormones on growth hormone in a similar rat pituitary cell line (GC). Growth hormone mRNA activity was quantified by translation *in vitro* as well as by cDNA hybridization. They found a good correlation of degree of stimulation of growth hormone production and the changes in pregrowth hormone mRNA activity after glucocorticoid or triiodothyronine treatment. Furthermore, these investigators (Martial *et al.,* 1977b) observed a synergistic effect of thyroid and glucocorticoid hormones on growth hormone production, and that this synergistic effect was also mediated at the level of the mRNA for growth hormone.

G. CORTICOTROPIN

All the steroid hormone-regulatable proteins discussed so far involve the induction of a specific protein by a steroid, or the modulation of the steroid-mediated response by another hormone. The only situation in which a specific mRNA concentration is decreased is upon the withdrawal of the inducing hormone or by the addition of a second hormone that interferes with the action of the first one. In our studies of gene regulation, it would be of interest to have a system where a specific protein or mRNA is "turned off" upon treatment with a single hormone. Such a system is found in the negative regulation of corticotropin by glucocorticoids.

In investigating the level of glucocorticoid regulation of corticotropin production by the pituitary, Nakanishi *et al.* (1976) and Jones *et al.* (1977) identified a corticotropin-like product resulting from the *in vitro* translation of mRNA extracted from the bovine pituitary and mouse pituitary cell line. Corticotropin is a single polypeptide consisting of 39 amino acid residues (Li *et al.,* 1961). The product that Nakanishi *et al.* (1976) synthesized *in vitro* had a molecular weight of approximately 33,000–35,000. It is thus some seven times larger than plasma corticotropin. This putative precursor is larger than the common precursor of secretory proteins, which usually contains in addition a signal sequence of only about 20–30 amino acid residues (Blobel and Dobberstein, 1975). The apparent discrepancy in size of the *in vitro* product is readily explained by some recent observations on the high-molecular-weight forms of corticotropin in the pituitary. Mains and Eipper (1976) and Eipper *et al.* (1976) studied corticotropin biosynthesis in a mouse pituitary tumor cell line. They found that the tumor cells, as well as normal pituitary tissue, contained several high-molecular-weight glycoprotein forms of corticotropin with molecular weights of 31,000, 23,000, and 13,000 in addition to the "normal size" of 4500. Kinetics of labeling suggest that the 31 K corticotropin is the biosynthetic precursor of the smaller forms of corticotropin and 23 K corticotropin a biosynthetic intermediate. Moreover, by tryptic peptide map analysis and specific immunoprecipitation studies, Mains et al. (1977) showed that the 31 K peptide was actually a common precursor to corticotropin and β-lipotropin (and hence β-endorphin). The large product of cell-free translation of bovine pituitary mRNA that Nakanishi et al. (1976) observed was probably equivalent to the 31 K precursor that Mains et al. (1977) found in the mouse pituitary tumor cell line. Indeed, Roberts and Herbert (1977a,b) repeated the experiment of Nakanishi et al. (1976) using mRNA from the mouse tumor cells, and identified corticotropin and β-lipotropin peptide sequences in a 31 K product. They also showed that β-lipotropin sequence was located on the carboxyl-terminal side of the corticotropin molecule.

The demonstration of a common precursor to corticotropin and β-lipotropin (and β-endorphin) explains some earlier observations that these three peptides all change in a parallel fashion in response to various stimuli (Abe et al., 1967, 1969; Gilkes et al., 1975) and that these molecules are all demonstrated within the same pituitary cells (Moriarty, 1973; Dubois et al., 1973) and within the same secretory granules (Moriarty, 1973).

The role of glucocorticoid in the regulation of the mRNA for this 31 K common precursor was studied by Nakanishi et al. (1977). They measured the specific mRNA activity of RNA isolated from the rat pituitary after various hormonal manipulations. The activity was found to be increased 3- to 6-fold by adrenalectomy. Glucocorticoid administration to adrenalectomized rats resulted in a marked suppression of the mRNA activity, whereas other steroid hormones, such as progesterone and aldosterone, were without effect. These observations indicate that glucocorticoids regulate the levels of corticotropin precursor mRNA. The glucocorticoid–corticotropin negative feedback system will be an exciting system in which to study how a specific gene is "turned off" by a specific ligand.

VII. REGULATION OF SPECIFIC GENE EXPRESSION BY NONSTEROID HORMONES

While there are a number of different systems involving steroid hormone regulation of gene expression, relatively few studies of a similar nature have been reported involving nonsteroid hormones. As we have discussed in the sections on the individual steroid-induced proteins, nonsteroidal hormones frequently modulate the response of the target cell to the steroid. Nonsteroids as primary regulators of specific protein synthesis have been studied at the mRNA level in only three systems: the induction of tyrosine aminotransferase mRNA by adenosine 3',5'-monophosphate (cyclic AMP; cAMP) and glucagon (Ernest and Feigelson, 1978), the induction of phosphoenolpyruvate carboxykinase by cAMP (Iynedjian and Hanson, 1977a), and the induction of casein mRNA by prolactin (Matusik and Rosen, 1978).

As discussed in the section on glucocorticoids, hepatic tyrosine aminotransferase mRNA and PEP carboxykinase in hepatoma cells are readily induced by this steroid hormone. It has been known for a long time, however, that both of these enzymes can be induced by cAMP administration (Wicks, 1974). Until recently the mechanism of action of this cyclic nucleotide in the stimulation of the synthesis of these two enzymes was unclear, and it has been proposed that this action of cAMP could be mediated at the translational level (Wicks, 1974). However, Iynedjian and Hanson (1977a) demonstrated that the functional level of hepatic mRNA coding for PEP carboxykinase rapidly increased in concert with the enzyme activity during induction by dibutyryl cAMP administration *in vivo*. Similarly, Ernest and Feigelson (1978) demonstrated that a single injection of dibutyryl cAMP and theophylline stimulated both the hepatic tyrosine aminotransferase enzymic activity as well as the functional activity of its mRNA as assayed in the wheat germ system. This effect of cAMP was completely inhibited by α-amanitin. They further demonstrated that glucagon given *in vivo* also stimulated hepatic tyrosine aminotransferase at the level of its mRNA.

These studies on hepatic enzyme regulation by cAMP and glucagon are interesting and raise the possibility that these two hormones regulate specific gene expression at a pretranslational level. However, since the studies were carried out in intact animals and mRNA activities were examined hours after hormone administration, some indirect effects of these hormones on mRNA activity could not be excluded. Undoubtedly similar studies will soon be carried out in tissue-culture systems involving the same enzymes, since all the techniques are presently available. Only then can one conclude whether cAMP and glucagon exert direct effects on the mRNA activity of PEP carboxykinase or tyrosine aminotransferase.

The only system in which studies *in vitro* were performed is the rodent mammary gland organ culture, where casein mRNA is induced by prolactin (Matusik and Rosen, 1978). Terry *et al.* (1977) first demonstrated the induction of casein mRNA in a mouse mammary gland culture. The mRNA activity was assayed in a cell-free protein system, and the induction was carried out over a 6-day period by a combination of insulin + prolactin + cortisol. Matusik and Rosen (1978) studied the induction process in a rat mammary gland explant. They detected casein mRNA sequences by molecular hybridization with a specific cDNA probe, and observed induction of the mRNA within 1 hour of addition of prolactin to the culture medium. They further demonstrated that hydrocortisone was not necessary for casein mRNA induction by prolactin, but the steroid was required for maximal accumulation of casein mRNA. Furthermore, the induction of the mRNA by prolactin was inhibited in a dose-dependent manner by the simultaneous addition of progesterone to the organ culture. The study of Matusik and Rosen (1978) appears to be the first demonstration of the rapid induction of a specific mRNA by a peptide hormone, and their system will serve as a valuable model for further studies on the peptide hormone regulation of specific gene expression.

VIII. Effects of Steroid Hormones on Specific Gene Transcription *in Vitro*

The availability of pure mRNAs for a number of proteins has allowed the synthesis of specific radiolabeled cDNAs. Such cDNA probes have been used to quantify mRNA sequences synthesized *in vitro* from isolated chromatin in the presence of added *Escherichia coli* RNA polymerase (Gilmour and Paul, 1973; Axel *et al.*, 1973). Such an approach was taken by Harris *et al.* (1976). They found that RNA isolated from such preparations contained significant amounts of ovalbumin mRNA when estrogen-stimulated chick oviduct chromatin was used. However, such sequences were extremely low in the RNA synthesized from estrogen-withdrawn oviduct chromatin.

Since this original observation, a number of advances have been made. First, Dale and Ward (1975) reported that, using mercurated nucleotides as substrate for *in vitro* RNA synthesis, the newly synthesized mercurated RNA could be separated from contaminating nonmercurated RNA sequences by means of affinity chromatography on sulfhydryl–Sepharose columns. Using this technique, Towle *et al.* (1977) were able to confirm the earlier studies by Harris *et al.* (1976). However, since these studies, a number of investigators (Crouse *et al.*, 1976; Konkel and Ingram, 1977; Zasloff and Felsenfeld, 1977a,b) demonstrated that there are certain problems inherent to the mercury-substitution method, and if used indiscriminately the method could lead to erroneous conclusions about the extent of transcription from DNA templates on chromatin. The possible sources of error are as follows: (1) inability of the sulfhydryl–Sepharose column to separate the newly synthesized mercurated RNA due to aggregation; (2) mercurated polyuridylate formation which hybridizes to the polyadenylate tail of contaminating mRNA sequences, thus preventing a clean separation of the latter from newly synthesized RNA; and (iii) anti-mRNA synthesis by an RNA-dependent RNA polymerase activity inherent in *E. coli* RNA polymerase. Tsai *et al.* (1978b) systematically investigated each of these possibilities in the chick oviduct system. They found that if application of the RNA mixture on the sulfhydryl-Sepharose column was immediately preceded by heating the sample to disaggregate the mercurated RNA from contaminating mRNA sequences, over 90% of the latter could be removed by one passage through the column. They also found that mercurated polyuridylate formation did not account for retention of contaminating ovalbumin mRNA sequences on the affinity column since, if the chromatography was performed on the *in vitro* mercurated RNA under renaturation conditions (allowing RNA aggregates to reform), the presence of excess polyuridylate did not affect the binding of added ovalbumin mRNA to the column. Finally, by substituting $MgCl_2$ for $MnCl_2$, they completely eliminated the RNA-dependent RNA synthesis activity of the *E. coli* RNA polymerase and excluded such a process as a source of newly synthesized mercurated RNA.

The use of the stringent conditions for assaying the *in vitro* transcripts has allowed Tsai *et al.* (1978b) to demonstrate that *de novo* synthesis of ovalbumin mRNA occurs on estrogen-stimulated chick oviduct chromatin *in vitro* in the presence of *E. coli* RNA polymerase. Such sequences were essentially undetectable in similar studies employing estrogen-withdrawn chromatin. The studies of Tsai *et al.* strongly favor primary gene derepression as the most important mechanism for the estrogenic induction of ovalbumin synthesis.

IX. Role of Receptors in Steroid Hormone Action

Upon entering the cell, steroid hormones are initially bound to specific cytoplasmic protein receptors. The hormone–receptor complex undergoes "activation" and translocates from the cytoplasm into the nucleus. In the nuclear compartment, the hormone–receptor complex binds to "acceptor sites" on the target cell chromatin. This is followed by the activation (and in some cases inactivation) of specific genes resulting in the appearance of a new species of RNA. This general model seems to hold for all the major steroid hormones examined including estrogens, progesterone, androgens, glucocorticoids, and aldosterone (Chan and O'Malley, 1976a).

There are important recent developments in the area of steroid hormone receptor biology. Greene *et al.* (1977) succeeded in immunizing rabbits with a purified preparation of estrogen–receptor complex from calf uterine nuclei. The specific estrogen–receptor complex antibodies were shown to crossreact with the nuclear receptor of rat uterus, as well as with the extranuclear receptors of calf, rat, mouse, and guinea pig uterus and of human breast cancer. The antibodies did not react with either the nuclear or extranuclear dihydrotestosterone–receptor complex of rat prostate or with the extranuclear progesterone–receptor complex of chick oviduct. The availability of a monospecific receptor antibody should be useful in future studies, such as the development of radioimmunoassays for receptor content of different cell types, especially of human breast cancer as a guide to therapy (McGuire *et al.*, 1975; Jensen *et al.*, 1976); the efficient purification of specific hormone receptors by affinity chromatography; and the ultrastructural localization of nuclear and cytoplasmic receptors by electron microscopy.

Another aspect of receptor biology that might have some direct bearing on steroid hormone action resides in the subunit structure of the progesterone receptor in the chick oviduct (Vedeckis *et al.*, 1978). This receptor is a dimer composed of A and B subunits. This subunit structure has been confirmed recently by use of a reversible crosslinking reagent that will crosslink the native dimer. After extraction and partial purification the dimer can be dissociated, releasing equimolar amounts of the A and B proteins. Both the two subunits have been purified. The A protein has a molecular weight of 79,000, and that of the B protein is 117,000. The hormone-binding specificity and kinetics for the two receptor proteins are virtually identical (Schrader and O'Malley, 1972), suggesting that their hormone-binding sites may be very similar. The intact 6 S dimer containing 1 mol each of A and B is located in the cytoplasm of the target cell in the absence of hormone stimulation and translocates to the nuclear compartment on administration of progesterone. The B subunit binds to the nonhistone protein–DNA complexes of oviduct chromatin but not to pure DNA, whereas the A subunit binds to pure DNA but poorly to chromatin (Schrader *et al.*, 1972). These observations on the properties of the A and B subunits have led to a hypothesis of their mechanism of interaction with the target cell genome (O'Malley and Schrader, 1976). It is believed that the A subunit could be the actual gene regulatory protein. In the absence of the B protein, the A subunit would encounter difficulty in locating the specific chromosomal regions it is to regulate, while the B subunit, the "specifier" protein, should be totally inactive as the sole transcriptional regulator. Consistent with this concept was the observation that purified A subunit protein was capable of stimulating transcription on withdrawn chromatin but only at much higher concentrations (approximately 10- to 50-fold) than that required for the intact dimer (Buller *et al.*, 1976). The isolated B subunit was totally ineffective in stimulating transcription from oviduct chromatin at any concentration tested. These observations are consistent with a model in which the B subunit acts as a site-specific binder to localize the dimer in certain regions of chromatin, whereas the A subunit may alter the local structure or conformation of a portion of the chromatin DNA so that initiation of new RNA synthesis can occur (O'Malley and Schrader, 1976).

X. Implications of Recent Concepts of Gene Structure on Steroid Hormone Action

In this review, we have attempted to present recent studies bearing on the regulation of specific protein synthesis by steroid hormones. The pattern of all the systems examined is quite similar: steroid hormones appear to regulate the concentration of specific proteins predominantly at the level of their mRNAs. The conclusion is inescapable that, in general, steroid hormones regulate specific gene expression mainly at a pretranslational level.

Until a few years ago, the concept of pretranslational control would have been compatible with only a few fairly straightforward alternatives. It was generally held that in certain eukaryote cells transcription could result in the production of high-molecular-weight nuclear RNAs (HnRNA). Subsequent processing of the HnRNAs was thought to involve simple scission with conservation of specific mRNA sequences that were exported into the cytoplasm, where they were translated into the corresponding proteins. Over the past few years, processing was found to be much more complicated. The first good evidence for a pre-mRNA was found in the globin mRNA system where, by means of cDNA-cellulose chromatography, a radioactive pre-mRNA has been identified (Ross, 1976; Curtis and Weismann, 1976; Kwan *et al.*, 1977; Bastos and Aviv, 1977). As yet definite evidence for pre-mRNA has not been presented for any of the hormone-regulatable proteins. The "processing" step is complicated by at least two processes, polyadenylation at the 3' end (Darnell *et al.,* 1973; Brawerman, 1974) and "capping" at the 5' end (Shatkin and Both, 1976; Chan *et al.,* 1977a). The polyadenylation and capping appear also to be potential sites of regulation in the eukaryote. There is, however, no definitive evidence for this effect.

Recently a much more amazing observation has completely changed our concept of the basic transcriptional unit in eukaryotes. It was previously assumed that mRNA was directly copied from a gene sequence. It turns out that such is not the case for at least (at the time of writing) three eukaryotic genes: the rabbit β-globin (Jeffreys and Flavell, 1977), mouse immunoglobulin light chain (Tonegawa *et al.,* 1978), and ovalbumin (Doel *et al.,* 1977; Breathnach *et al.,* 1977; Lai *et al.,* 1978; Weinstock *et al.,* 1978) genes. In each of these instances, inserts of DNA sequences were found that appeared in the middle of the protein coding region of the genome.

The structure of the ovalbumin gene, a steroid hormone-regulated gene, was studied in the following fashion. Full-length cDNA synthesized from ovalbumin mRNA was inserted into plasmid DNA and amplified by molecular cloning. The resultant chimeric plasmid (pOV230) was cleaved with restriction enzymes (*Hae* III and *Hind* III) to yield two distinct DNA fragments containing the left (OV_L) and right (OV_R) halves of the ovalbumin DNA insert. The two fragments were labeled with ^{32}P and were used as specific hybridization probes to study the organization of the ovalbumin gene in native chick DNA. Total chick DNA was digested with a variety of restriction endonucleases, and the fragments were hybridized with the OV_R and OV_L halves of the structural ovalbumin gene. While *Hae* III generated only one hybridizable fragment with OV_R as expected, it generated two DNA fragments with OV_L, indicating the presence of a *Hae* III site in native chick DNA that is absent in structural ovalbumin cDNA. Furthermore, *Eco* RI, another restriction endonuclease, produced 3 discrete fragments although it does not cleave the structural cDNA. While the two smaller fragments (2.4 and 1.8 kilobases, respectively) hybridized only with OV_L, the larger (9.5 kilobase) fragment formed a hybrid only with OV_R. These results are consistent with the interpretation that at least two nonstructural sequences may exist in the native ovalbumin structural gene that were cleaved by *Hae* III and *Eco* RI. The probable location of these inserted sequences within the native ovalbumin gene is shown in Fig. 1.

It is too early yet to speculate on the function(s) of these "insert" sequences within the natural ovalbumin structural gene. Using DNA isolated from hen liver and oviduct cells, identical restriction banding

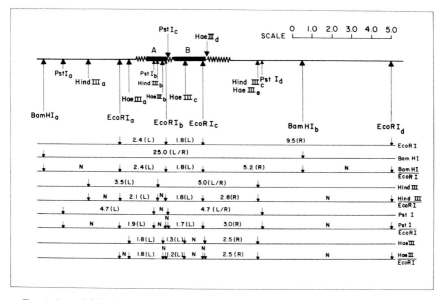

FIG. 1. A model for the organization of the natural ovalbumin gene in chick DNA. DNA sequences present in ovalbumin complementary DNA (cDNA$_{ov}$) are represented by ∿∿∿∿∿ and "insert" sequences are represented by ▬▬, while flanking DNA sequences are represented by ──. Various restriction sites on the DNA are shown by arrows. Those above the line are restriction sites present in double-stranded cDNA$_{ov}$, and those below are predicted by data summarized elsewhere (Lai *et al.*, 1978). A scale is also shown in the upper right-hand corner. An exception to the scale is the *Bam* HI$_a$ site, which should be 25 kilobases to the left of the *Bam* HI$_b$ site. The generation of DNA fragments of different sizes by various restriction digestions of this DNA is shown beneath the model: numbers represent the sizes of DNA fragments in kilobases; (L), (R), and (L/R) indicate that the DNA fragments was detected either by hybridization with OV$_L$, OV$_R$, or both OV$_L$ and OV$_R$, respectively. N represents DNA fragments that should have resulted from various restriction digests but were not detected in the radioautograms because either there was no DNA sequence complementary to the probes employed, or lengths of the complementary sequences were insufficient to form stable hybrids under the conditions employed.

patterns were obtained. Since ovalbumin is not synthesized in hen liver but is produced in great abundance in mature oviduct tubular gland cells, it may be concluded that a function of these "inserts" is not to directly inhibit the expression of the ovalbumin gene in the liver. Finally, the definitive sequence organization map of the natural ovalbumin gene must be derived from characterizing each of the fragments after amplification by molecular cloning. Only then can specific hybridization probes be generated so that such important questions as whether these "inserts" are repeating or unique sequences within the chick genome or whether they are transcribed into RNA during gene expression can be answered.

The presence of these DNA inserts presents a few additional possibilities concerning the regulation of gene expression (Williamson, 1977): First, the primary transcripts might include both the inserts and the mRNA sequences, and the inserts are specifically nicked out during processing and the mRNA sequences ligated. The conservation of both the 3' polyadenylate and the 5' cap during processing is then easily explained. Second, it is possible that the DNA inserts are never transcribed. Finally, it is possible that different regions of the mRNA are synthesized separately and then ligated together during processing. Currently available evidence favors the first alternative. It should be noted that hormone-mediated accumulation of mRNA-containing sequences from each of the three coding regions (separated by inserts) in nuclei of target cells occurs coordinately. In each of these instances, however, there is ample room for new potential loci of regulation by steroid hormones. For example, whether transcribed or not, the excision sites for the inserts could be binding sites for various enzymes and regulatory proteins and could interact directly or indirectly with hormone receptors. In both the β-globin and ovalbumin systems, inserts were found both in tissues that were active and in those that were inactive in the synthesis of the corresponding mRNAs. Active investigations are currently in progress in a number of laboratories on the significance of the DNA inserts, and by the time this review is published we will undoubtedly have partial answers to some of our questions.

XI. Summary and Prospects for the Future

While there is little doubt that steroid hormonal regulation occurs at the nuclear transcriptional and perhaps the posttranscriptional (in certain instances) level, much information is yet to be obtained concerning the exact mechanism by which the hormones carry out their regulatory functions. Steroid hormones are initially bound to specific cytoplasmic protein receptors. The hormone–receptor complex then translocates from the cytoplasm into the nucleus, where it apparently binds to chromatin. This is followed by accumulation of the product of specific genes. The mechanism by which the hormone–receptor complex induces the transcription of specific genes will be an area of active research in the immediate future. A number of synthetic eukaryotic genes have now been made and sequenced. With respect to a hormone-regulatable gene, the structural ovalbumin gene has been synthesized *in vitro* and cloned in plasmids. Recently, we have purified and cloned the natural ovalbumin gene so that it retains its flanking and possibly regulatory sequences. With the availability of this hormone-inducible gene in quantity, microchromosomes can be constructed and reconstitution experiments can be carried out with purified hormone receptors. Other hormone-regulatable genes will surely be available within the near future. Details of the hormone-receptor–gene interaction will probably engage the imagination and efforts of numerous investigators in the next decade, during which one can hope to see the unraveling of many of the mysteries of eukaryotic gene expression and regulation.

XII. UPDATE ON STEROID HORMONE REGULATION OF SPECIFIC GENE EXPRESSION

Since the original manuscript went to press, a number of significant advances have been made. In the following section, we will attempt to provide an up-to-date account of some of these advances.

A. PROTEINS REGULATED BY ESTROGEN—EGG WHITE PROTEINS: OVOMUCOID

Since the original study by Palmiter (Palmiter, 1972), the regulation of the transcription of the ovomucoid gene has been further investigated by Tsai *et al.* (Tsai *et al.*, 1978a).

A fragment of ovomucoid cDNA was purified by cloning of the DNA in plasmids (Stein *et al.*, 1978). The cloned fragment was radioactively labeled to high specific activity and used as a hybridization probe to quantify the number of ovomucoid mRNA sequences in the chick oviduct under various hormonal conditions. About 1900 copies of the ovomucoid mRNA sequences were found in each tubular gland cell nucleus of the chick oviduct after 14 days of diethylstilbestrol treatment. Only very low levels of ovomucoid mRNA sequences were detected in nuclear RNA isolated from chick liver or chick spleen tissues. After 14 days of withdrawal of diethylstilbestrol from the chick, the concentration of ovomucoid mRNA in the chick oviduct decreased to 3 molecules per tubular gland cell nucleus. Readministration of a single dose of diethylstilbestrol to these chicks resulted in a gradual increase in the concentration of ovomucoid mRNA within the first four hours (from 3 to 38 molecules per tubular gland cell nucleus). By 16 hours, the nuclear concentration of ovomucoid mRNA was 120 molecules per tubular gland cell nucleus. However, with a second injection of estrogen at 48 hours, the amount of ovomucoid mRNA sharply increased to a level (620 molecules per tubular gland cell nucleus) approximately one-third of that observed for chicks stimulated chronically with estrogen.

In vitro synthesis of ovomucoid mRNA in isolated nuclei was measured by hybridization to nitrocellulose filters containing cloned ovomucoid DNA and compared with the synthesis of ovalbumin mRNA under the same conditions. In oviduct nuclei isolated from chronically stimulated chicks, the rate of transcription of the ovomucoid gene was almost 5-fold slower than that determined for the ovalbumin gene.

These studies on ovomucoid gene expression are interesting. They illustrate the usefulness of molecular cloning in the purification of specific gene products, and the value of adoption of such a technique in the investigation of steroid-hormone mediated regulation of gene expression.

B. Recent Concepts of Gene Structure and Steroid Hormone Action—Update

Since the initial discovery that there were intervening inserts in the natural ovalbumin gene, much more detailed studies have been performed on the structure of the natural gene.

Successful cloning of a major fragment of the natural ovalbumin gene (Woo *et al.*, 1978) has permitted Dugaiczyk *et al.* (Dugaiczyk *et al.*, 1978) to construct a detailed map of the gene and compare it to the mature ovalbumin mRNA sequence. Somewhat surprisingly, it was found that the left half of the structural gene is interrupted by a total of at least seven intervening DNA sequences (Fig. 2). Using DNA-hybridization probes specific to the intervening sequences, it was possible to study the transcription of these regions of the ovalbumin gene (Roop *et al.*, 1978).

By these techniques, the intervening sequences were found to be transcribed. However, the amount of nuclear RNA corresponding to these sequences was approximately 10-fold less than that observed for structural sequences. The accumulation of RNA corresponding to structural and intervening sequences was also determined during acute estrogen stimulation and the results suggest that there were either different rates of transcription for these regions of the ovalbumin gene or that RNA sequences corresponding to the intervening sequences were preferentially processed and degraded. The *in vitro* expression of the ovalbumin gene was also studied in nuclei isolated from

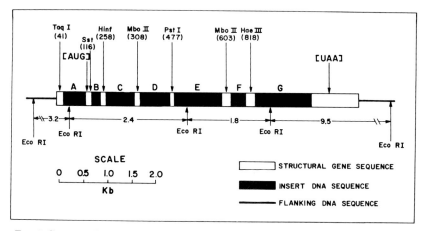

FIG. 2. Structural organization of the natural ovalbumin gene. A map of the organization of structural and intervening DNA sequences comprising the chick ovalbumin gene. Each of the noncontiguous structural segments is identified by one restriction endonuclease site.

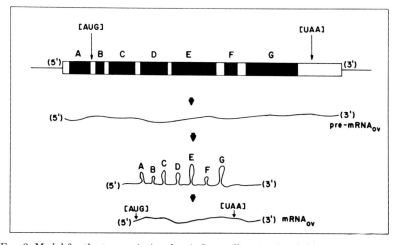

FIG. 3. Model for the transcriptional unit for ovalbumin. Available data indicate that the intervening sequences within the ovalbumin gene are unique chick DNA sequences and are transcribed in their entirety during gene expression. Furthermore, the expression of the intervening sequences is inducible by steroid hormones in a coordinate manner with the structural gene sequences. Hence the ovalbumin gene appears to be transcribed into a precursor RNA which is at least 3 times the size of the mature mRNA and the intervening sequences are subsequently enzymatically processed away from the mature mRNA by precise excision and proper ligation.

chronically stimulated oviducts. Structural and intervening sequences of the ovalbumin gene were preferentially transcribed *in vitro* with similar rates, approximately 500-fold greater than would be expected for random transcription of the haploid chick genome.

Recently, nuclear RNA from stimulated chick oviduct has been fractionated by electrophoresis under denaturing conditions to reveal multiple species of RNA that are high in molecular weight and hybridize to structural and intervening sequences of the ovalbumin gene. One of the species of RNA (approximately 40 S) may be large enough to be a transcript of the entire natural ovalbumin gene.

Taken together, the recent studies in ovalbumin gene structure are compatible with a model for expression of the ovalbumin gene shown in Fig. 3. The ovalbumin gene appears to be transcribed in its entirety in response to estrogen treatment. The initial transcript undergoes fairly extensive modification and is processed into the mature ovalbumin mRNA. The role of estrogen in the post-transcriptional steps, if any, is still unclear.

ACKNOWLEDGMENTS

The work described in the review in the authors' laboratories were supported by grants HD-7857 and HD-8188, and HL-16512 from the National Institutes of Health, and grant-in-aid 75-914 of the American Heart Association. L. Chan is an Established Investigator of the American Heart Association. A. R. Means is the recipient of a Faculty Research Award from the American Cancer Society.

REFERENCES

Abe, K., Nicholson, W. E., Liddle, G. W., and Orth, D. N. (1967). *J. Clin. Invest.* **46,** 1609.
Abe, K., Nicholson, W. E., Liddle, G. W., Orth, D. N., and Island, D. P. (1969). *J. Clin. Invest.* **48,** 1580.
Alescio, T., and Moscona, A. A. (1969). *Biochem. Biophys. Res. Commun.* **34,** 176.
Arthur, A. T., and Daniel, J. C., Jr. (1972). *Fertil. Steril.* **23,** 115.
Atger, M., and Milgrom, E. (1977). *J. Biol. Chem.* **252,** 5412.
Axel, R., Cedar, H., and Felsenfeld, G. (1973). *Proc. Natl. Acad. Sci. U.S.A.* **70,** 2029.
Baker, H. J., and Shapiro, D. J. (1977). *J. Biol. Chem.* **252,** 8428.
Bancroft, F. C., Wu, G., and Zubay, G. (1973). *Proc. Natl. Acad. Sci. U.S.A.* **70,** 3646.
Bastos, R. N., and Aviv, H. (1977). *Cell* **11,** 641.
Beato, M., and Nieto, A. (1976). *Eur. J. Biochem.* **64,** 15.
Beato, M., and Rungger, D. (1975). *FEBS Lett.* **59,** 305.
Beier, H. M. (1967). *Verh. Zool. Ges. Heidelberg* **31,** 139.
Beier, H. M. (1970). *In* "Ovo-Implantation, Human Gonadotropins and Prolactin" (P. O. Hubinot *et al.*, eds.), pp. 157–163. Karger, Basel.
Beier, H. M. (1975). *J. Reprod. Fertil.* **37,** 221.
Beier, H. M. (1976a). *J. Reprod. Fertil., Suppl.* **25,** 53.
Beier, H. M. (1976b). *Curr. Top. Pathol.* **62,** 105.
Beier, H. M., and Beier-Hellwig, K. (1973). *Acta Endocrinol. (Copenhagen), Suppl.* **180,** 404.

Bergink, E. W., and Wallace, R. A. (1974). *J. Biol. Chem.* **249,** 2897.

Bergink, E. W., Korsterboer, H. J., Gruber, M., and Ab, G. (1973). *Biochim. Biophys. Acta* **294,** 497.

Berridge, M. V., and Lane, C. D. (1976). *Cell* **8,** 283.

Berridge, M. V., Farmer, S. R., Green, C. D., Henshaw, E. C., and Tata, J. R. (1976). *Eur. J. Biochem.* **62,** 161.

Blobel, G., and Dobberstein, B. (1975). *J. Cell Biol.* **67,** 835.

Boyd, A. E., III, Spencer, E., Jackson, I. M. D., and Reichlin, S. (1976). *Endocrinology* **99,** 861.

Brawerman, G. (1974). *Annu. Rev. Biochem.* **43,** 621.

Breathnach, R., Mandel, J. L., and Chambon, P. (1977). *Nature (London)* **270,** 314.

Buller, R. E., Schwartz, R. J., Schrader, W. T., and O'Malley, B. W. (1976). *J. Biol. Chem.* **251,** 5178.

Bullock, D. W. (1977). *Biol. Reprod.* **17,** 104.

Bullock, D. W., and Willen, G. F. (1974). *Proc. Soc. Exp. Biol. Med.* **146,** 294.

Bullock, D. W., Woo, S. L. C., and O'Malley, B. W. (1976). *Biol. Reprod.* **15,** 435.

Butler, W. W., and Schade, A. L. (1958). *Endocrinology* **63,** 271.

Chan, L., and O'Malley, B. W. (1976a). *N. Engl. J. Med.* **294,** 1322.

Chan, L., and O'Malley, B. W. (1976b). *N. Engl. J. Med.* **294,** 1372.

Chan, L., and O'Malley, B. W. (1976c). *N. Engl. J. Med.* **294,** 1430.

Chan, L., Means, A. R., and O'Malley, B. W. (1973). *Proc. Natl. Acad. Sci. U.S.A.* **70,** 1870.

Chan, L., Jackson, R. L., O'Malley, B. W., and Means, A. R. (1976). *J. Clin. Invest.* **58,** 368.

Chan, L., Harris, S. E., Rosen, J. M., Means, A. R., and O'Malley, B. W. (1977a). *Life Sci.* **20,** 1.

Chan, L., Jackson, R. L., and Means, A. R. (1977b). *Endocrinology* **100,** 1636.

Chan, L., Jackson, R. L., and Means, A. R. (1978). *Circ. Res.* **43,** 209.

Cox, R. F. (1977). *Biochemistry* **16,** 3433.

Cox, R. F., Haines, M. E., and Emtage, S. (1974). *Eur. J. Biochem.* **49,** 225.

Crouse, G. F., Fodor, E. J., and Doty, P. (1976). *Proc. Natl. Acad. Sci. U.S.A.* **70,** 1594.

Curtis, P. J., and Weismann, C. (1976). *J. Mol. Biol.* **106,** 1061.

Dale, R. M. R., and Ward, D. C. (1975). *Biochemistry* **14,** 2458.

Dannies, P. S., and Tashjian, A. H., Jr. (1976). *Biochem. Biophys. Res. Commun.* **70,** 1180.

Darnell, J. E., Jelenek, W. R., and Molloy, G. R. (1973). *Science* **181,** 1215.

Deeley, R. G., Mullinex, K. P., Wetekam, W., Kronenberg, H. M., Meyers, M., Eldridge, J. D., and Goldberger, R. F. (1975). *J. Biol. Chem.* **250,** 9060.

Deeley, R. G., Udell, D. S., Burns, A. T. H., Gordon, J. I., and Goldberg, R. F. (1977a). *J. Biol. Chem.* **252,** 7913.

Deeley, R. G., Gordon, J. L., Burns, A. T. H., Mullinix, K. P., Bina-Stein, M., and Goldberger, R. F. (1977b). *J. Biol. Chem.* **252,** 8310.

Dickson, C., Haslam, S., and Nandi, S. (1972). *Virology* **62,** 242.

Diesterhaft, M., Noguchi, T., Hargrove, J., Thornton, C., and Granner, D. (1977). *Biochem. Biophys. Res. Commun.* **79,** 1015.

Doel, M. T., Houghton, M., Cook, E. A., and Carey, N. H. (1977). *Nucleic Acids Res.* **4,** 3701.

Dubois, P., Vargues-Regairaz, H., and Dubois, M. P. (1973). *Z. Zellforsch. Mikrosk. Anat.* **145,** 131.

Dugaiczyk, A., Woo, S. L. C., Lai, E. C., Mace, M. L., Jr., McReynolds, L., and O'Malley, B. W. (1978). *Nature* **274,** 328.

Eipper, B. A., Mains, R. E., and Guenzi, D. (1976). *J. Biol. Chem.* **251,** 4121.

Ernest, M. J., and Feigelson, P. (1978). *J. Biol. Chem.* **253**, 319.

Evans, G. A., and Rosenfeld, M. G. (1976). *J. Biol. Chem.* **251**, 2842.

Fine, D. L., Plowman, J. K., Kelley, S. P., Arthur, L. O., and Hillman, E. A. (1974). *J. Natl. Cancer Inst.* **52**, 1881.

Finlayson, J. S., Potter, M., and Runner, C. C. (1963). *J. Natl. Cancer Inst.* **31**, 91.

Franz, J. M., and Knox, W. E. (1967). *Biochemistry* **6**, 3464.

Gelehrter, T. D. (1973). *Metab., Clin. Exp.* **22**, 85.

Gelehrter, T. D., and Tomkins, G. M. (1970). *Proc. Natl. Acad. Sci. U.S.A.* **66**, 390.

Gilkes, J. J. H., Bloomfield, G. A., Scott, A. P., Lowry, P. J., Ratcliffe, J. G., Landon, J., and Rees, L. H. (1975). *J. Clin. Endocrinol. Metab.* **40**, 450.

Gilmour, R. S., and Paul, J. (1973). *Proc. Natl. Acad. Sci. U.S.A.* **70**, 3440.

Gorski, J., and Gannon, F. (1976). *Annu. Rev. Physiol.* **38**, 425.

Green, C. D., and Tata, J. R. (1976). *Cell* **7**, 131.

Greene, G. L., Closs, L. E., Fleming, H., DeSombre, E. R., and Jensen, E. V. (1977). *Proc. Natl. Acad. Sci. U.S.A.* **74**, 3681.

Greengard, O., and Dewey, H. K. (1971). *Proc. Natl. Acad. Sci. U.S.A.* **68**, 1698.

Gunn, J. M., Tilghman, S. M., Hanson, R. W., Reshef, L., and Ballard, F. J. (1975a). *Biochemistry* **14**, 2350.

Gunn, J. M., Hanson, R. W., Meyuhas, O., Reshef, L., and Ballard, R. J. (1975b). *Biochem. J.* **150**, 195.

Harris, S. E., Rosen, J. M., Means, A. R., and O'Malley, B. W. (1975). *Biochemistry* **14**, 2072.

Harris, S. E., Schwartz, R. J., Tsai, M.-J., O'Malley, B. W., and Roy, A. K. (1976). *J. Biol. Chem.* **251**, 524.

Hazzard, W. R., Brunzell, J. D., Appelbaum, D. M., Goldberg, A. P., Gague, C., Albers, J. J., Wahl, P. W., and Hoover, J. J. (1977). *In* "Pharmacology of Steroid Contraceptive Drugs" (S. Garattini and H. W. Berendes, eds.), p. 251. Raven, New York.

Hertz, R., Fraps, R. M., and Sebrell, W. H. (1943). *Proc. Soc. Exp. Biol. Med.* **52**, 142.

Hilliard, J., and Eaton, L. W., Jr. (1971). *Endocrinology* **89**, 522.

Hilliard, J., Spies, H. G., and Sawyer, C. H. (1968). *Endocrinology* **82**, 157.

Hillyard, L. A., Entenman, C., and Chaikoff, I. L. (1956). *J. Biol. Chem.* **223**, 359.

Iynedjian, P. B., and Hanson, R. W. (1977a). *J. Biol. Chem.* **252**, 655.

Iynedjian, P. B., and Hanson, R. W. (1977b). *J. Biol. Chem.* **252**, 8398.

Iynedjian, P. B., Ballard, F. J., and Hanson, R. W. (1975). *J. Biol. Chem.* **250**, 5596.

Jackson, R. L., Lin, H.-Y., Chan, L., and Means, A. R. (1976). *Biochim. Biophys. Acta* **420**, 342.

Jackson, R. L., Lin, H.-Y., Mao, J. T. S., Chan, L., and Means, A. R. (1977). *Endocrinology* **101**, 849.

Jeffreys, A. J., and Flavell, R. A. (1977). *Cell* **12**, 429.

Jensen, E. V., and DeSombre, E. R. (1974). *Vitam. Horm. (N.Y.)* **32**, 89.

Jensen, E. V., Smith, S., and DeSombre, E. R. (1976). *J. Steroid Biochem.* **7**, 911.

Jones, R. E., Pulbrabek, P., and Grunberger, D. (1977). *Biochem. Biophys. Res. Commun.* **74**, 1490.

Jost, J.-P., and Pehling, G. (1976). *Eur. J. Biochem.* **66**, 339.

Jost, J.-P., Keller, R., and Dierks-Ventling, C. (1973). *J. Biol. Chem.* **248**, 5262.

Kenney, F. T., Red, J. R., Hager, C. B., and Wittliff, J. L. (1968). *In* "Regulatory Mechanisms for Protein Synthesis in Mammalian Cells" (A. San Pietro, M. R. Lamborg, and F. T. Kenney, eds.), p. 119. Academic Press, New York.

Kenney, F. T., Lee, K.-L., Stiles, C. D., and Fritz, J. E. (1973). *Nature (London), New Biol.* **246**, 208.

Killewich, L. A., and Feigelson, P. (1977). *Proc. Natl. Acad. Sci. U.S.A.* **74**, 5392.

Knox, W. E., and Mehler, A. H. (1951). *Science* **113**, 237.

Kohler, P. O., and Bridson, W. E. (1973). *In* "Tissue Culture: Methods and Applications" (P. F. Kruse, Jr. and M. K. Patterson, Jr., eds.), p. 570. Academic Press, New York.

Konkel, D. A., and Ingram, V. (1977). *Nucleic Acids Res.* **4**, 1979.

Korenman, S. E., and O'Malley, B. W. (1968). *Endocrinology* **83**, 11.

Krishnan, R. S., and Daniel, J. C., Jr. (1967). *Science* **158**, 490.

Kurtz, D. T., and Feigelson, P. (1977). *Proc. Natl. Acad. Sci. U.S.A.* **74**, 4791.

Kurtz, D. T., Sipple, A. E., and Feigelson, P. (1976a). *Biochemistry* **15**, 1031.

Kurtz, D. T., Sippel, A. E., Ansah-Yiadom, R., and Feigelson, P. (1976b). *J. Biol. Chem.* **251**, 3594.

Kwan, S., Wood, T. G., and Lingrel, J. B. (1977). *Proc. Natl. Acad. Sci. U.S.A.* **74**, 178.

Lai, E. C., Woo, S. L. C., Dugaiczyk, A., Catterall, J. F., and O'Malley, B. W. (1978). *Proc. Natl. Acad. Sci. U.S.A.* **75**, 2205.

Levey, I. L., and Daniel, J. C., Jr. (1976). *Biol. Reprod.* **14**, 194.

Li, C. H., Dixon, J. S., and Chung, D. (1961). *Biochim. Biophys. Acta* **46**, 324.

Liao, S. (1977). *Biochem. Actions Horm.* **4**, 351.

Lin, E. C. C., and Knox, W. E. (1957). *Biochim. Biophys. Acta* **26**, 85.

Luskey, K. L., Brown, M. W., and Goldstein, J. L. (1974). *J. Biol. Chem.* **249**, 5939.

McGrath, C. M. (1971). *J. Natl. Cancer Inst.* **47**, 455.

McGuire, W. L., Carbone, P. P., and Vollmer, E. P., eds. (1975). "Estrogen Receptors in Human Breast Cancer." Raven, New York.

McKnight, G. S., Pennequin, P., and Schimke, R. T. (1975). *J. Biol. Chem.* **250**, 8105.

MacLeod, R. M. (1977). *In* "Reproductive Physiology and Sexual Endocrinology" (P. Hubinot, ed.), p. 54. Karger, Basel.

MacLeod, R. M., Abad, A., and Eidson, L. L. (1969). *Endocrinology* **84**, 1475.

Mains, R. E., and Eipper, B. A. (1976). *J. Biol. Chem.* **251**, 4115.

Mains, R. E., Eipper, B. A., and Ling, N. (1977). *Proc. Natl. Acad. Sci. U.S.A.* **74**, 3014.

Mainwaring, W. I. P., Mangan, F. R., Irving, R. A., and Jones, D. A. (1974). *Biochem. J.* **144**, 413.

Martial, J. A., Baxter, J. D., Goodman, H. M., and Seeburg, P. H. (1977a). *Proc. Natl. Acad. Sci. U.S.A.* **74**, 1816.

Martial, J. A., Seeburg, P. H., Guenzi, D., Goodman, H. M., and Baxter, J. D. (1977b). *Proc. Natl. Acad. Sci. U.S.A.* **74**, 4293.

Matusik, R. J., and Rosen, J. M. (1978). *J. Biol. Chem.* **253**, 2343.

Maurer, R. A., and Gorski, J. (1977). *Endocrinology* **101**, 76.

Maurer, R. A., Stone, R., and Gorski, J. (1976). *J. Biol. Chem.* **251**, 2801.

Maurer, R. A., Gorski, J., and McKean, D. J. (1977). *Biochem. J.* **161**, 189.

Maurer, R. R., and Beier, H. M. (1976). *J. Reprod. Fertil.* **48**, 33.

Morhenn, V., Rabinowitz, Z., and Tomkins, G. M. (1973). *Proc. Natl. Acad. Sci. U.S.A.* **70**, 1088.

Moriarty, G. C. (1973). *J. Histochem. Cytochem.* **21**, 855.

Moscona, A. A., and Hubby, J. L. (1963). *Dev. Biol.* **7**, 192.

Mullinix, K. P., Wetekam, W., Deeley, R. G., Gordon, J. I., Meyers, M., Kent, K. A., and Goldberger, R. F. (1976). *Proc. Natl. Acad. Sci. U.S.A.* **73**, 1442.

Nakanishi, S., Taii, S., Hirata, Y., Matsukura, S., Imura, H., and Numa, S. (1976). *Proc. Natl. Acad. Sci. U.S.A.* **73**, 4319.

Nakanishi, S., Kita, T., Taii, S., Imura, H., and Numa, S. (1977). *Proc. Natl. Acad. Sci. U.S.A.* **74**, 3283.

Nemeth, A. M. (1959). *J. Biol. Chem.* **234**, 2921.

Nickol, J. M., Lee, K.-L., Hollinger, T. G., and Kenney, F. T. (1976). *Biochem. Biophys. Res. Commun.* **72**, 687.

Nicoll, C. S., and Meites, J. (1962). *Endocrinology* **70**, 272.

Nicoll, C. S., and Meites, J. (1964). *Proc. Soc. Exp. Biol. Med.* **117**, 579.

O'Malley, B. W. (1967). *Biochemistry* **6**, 2546.

O'Malley, B. W., and Kohler, P. O. (1967a). *Proc. Natl. Acad. Sci. U.S.A.* **58**, 2359.

O'Malley, B. W., and Kohler, P. O. (1967b). *Biochem. Biophys. Res. Commun.* **28**, 1.

O'Malley, B. W., and Means, A. R. (1974). *Science* **183**, 610.

O'Malley, B. W., and Schrader, W. T. (1976). *Sci. Am.* **234**, 232.

O'Malley, B. W., McGuire, W. L., Kohler, P. O., and Korenman, S. G. (1969). *Recent Prog. Horm. Res.* **25**, 105.

Osawa, S., and Tomino, S. (1977). *Biochem. Biophys. Res. Commun.* **77**, 628.

Palmiter, R. D. (1972). *J. Biol. Chem.* **247**, 6450.

Palmiter, R. D. (1975). *Cell* **4**, 189.

Palmiter, R. D., and Carey, N. H. (1974). *Proc. Natl. Acad. Sci. U.S.A.* **70**, 2367.

Palmiter, R. D., and Schimke, R. T. (1973). *J. Biol. Chem.* **248**, 1502.

Palmiter, R. D., Moore, P. B., Mulvihill, E. R., and Emtage, S. (1976). *Cell* **8**, 557.

Paran, M., Gallo, R. C., Richardson, L. S., and Wu, A. M. (1973). *Proc. Natl. Acad. Sci. U.S.A.* **70**, 2391.

Parks, W. P., Scolnick, E. M., and Kozikowski, E. H. (1974). *Science* **184**, 158.

Parks, W. P., Ransom, J. C., Young, H. A., and Scolnick, E. M. (1975). *J. Biol. Chem.* **250**, 3330.

Pitot, H. C., and Yatvin, M. B. (1973). *Physiol. Rev.* **53**, 228.

Ratner, A., and Meites, J. (1964). *Endocrinology* **75**, 377.

Ringold, G., Yamamoto, K. R., Tomkins, G. M., Bishop, J. M., and Varmus, H. E. (1975). *Cell* **6**, 299.

Roberts, J. L., and Herbert, E. (1977a). *Proc. Natl. Acad. Sci. U.S.A.* **74**, 4826.

Roberts, J. L., and Herbert, E. (1977b). *Proc. Natl. Acad. Sci. U.S.A.* **74**, 5300.

Roewekamp, W. G., Hofer, E., and Sekeris, C. E. (1976). *Eur. J. Biochem.* **70**, 259.

Roop, D. R., Tsai, S. Y., Tsai, M-J., and O'Malley, B. W. (1978). *Cell.* Submitted for publication.

Roper, J. D., and Franz, J. M. (1977). *J. Biol. Chem.* **252**, 4354.

Ross, J. (1976). *J. Mol. Biol.* **106**, 403.

Rousseau, G. G., Baxter, J. D., and Tomkins, G. M. (1972). *J. Mol. Biol.* **67**, 99.

Roy, A. K., and Dowbenko, D. J. (1977). *Biochemistry* **16**, 3918.

Roy, A. K., and Neuhaus, O. W. (1966). *Proc. Soc. Exp. Biol. Med.* **121**, 894.

Roy, A. K., Dowbenko, D. J., and Schiop, M. J. (1977). *Biochem. J.* **164**, 91.

Ryffel, G. U., Wahli, W., and Weber, R. (1977). *Cell* **11**, 213.

Samuels, H. H., Tsai, J. S., and Cintron, R. (1973). *Science* **181**, 1253.

Sarkar, P. K., and Griffith, B. (1976). *Biochem. Biophys. Res. Commun.* **68**, 675.

Sarkar, P. K., and Moscona, A. A. (1973). *Proc. Natl. Acad. Sci. U.S.A.* **70**, 1667.

Schimke, R. T., Sweeney, E. W., and Berlin, C. M. (1965). *J. Biol. Chem.* **240**, 322.

Schrader, W. T., and O'Malley, B. W. (1972). *J. Biol. Chem.* **247**, 51.

Schrader, W. T., Toft, D. O., and O'Malley, B. W. (1972). *J. Biol. Chem.* **247**, 2401.

Schultz, G., Killewich, L., Chen, G., and Feigelson, P. (1975). *Proc. Natl. Acad. Sci. U.S.A.* **72**, 1017.

Scolnick, E. M., Young, H. A., and Parks, W. P. (1976). *Virology* **69**, 148.

Shapiro, D. J., and Baker, H. J. (1977). *J. Biol. Chem.* **253**, 5244.

Shapiro, D. J., Baker, H. J., and Stitt, D. T. (1976). *J. Biol. Chem.* **251**, 3105.

Shatkin, A. J., and Both, G. W. (1976). *Cell* **7**, 305.

Sippel, A. E., Feigelson, P., and Roy, A. K. (1975). *Biochemistry* **14**, 825.

Sperry, P. J., Woo, S. L. C., Means, A. R., and O'Malley, B. W. (1976). *Endocrinology* **99**, 315.

Stein, J. S., Catterall, J. F., Woo, S. L. C., Means, A. R., and O'Malley, B. W. (1978). *Biochemistry* (in press).

Stone, R. T., Maurer, R. A., and Gorski, J. (1977). *Biochemistry* **16**, 4915.

Sussman, P. M., Tashinski, R. J., and Bancroft, F. C. (1976). *Proc. Natl. Acad. Sci. U.S.A.* **73**, 29.

Szabo, M., and Frohman, L. A. (1976). *Endocrinology* **98**, 1451.

Talwar, G. P., Jailkhani, B. L., Narayanan, P. R., and Narasimhan, C. (1973). *In* "Endocrinology: Protein Synthesis in Reproductive Tissue" (E. Diczfalusy, ed.), p. 341. Karolinska Institutet, Stockholm.

Tashjian, A. H., Baroski, N. J., and Jensen, D. J. (1971). *Biochem. Biophys. Res. Commun.* **43**, 516.

Tata, J. R. (1976). *Cell* **9**, 1.

Terry, P. M., Banerjee, M. R., and Lui, R. M. (1977). *Proc. Natl. Acad. Sci. U.S.A.* **74**, 2441.

Thorner, M. O. (1977). *Clin. Endocrinol. Metab.* **6**, 201.

Tomkins, G. M., Gelehrter, T. D., Granner, D., Martin, D., Samuel, H. H., and Thompson, E. B. (1969). *Science* **166**, 1474.

Tomkins, G. M., Levinson, B. B., Baxter, J. D., and Dethlefsen, L. (1972). *Nature (London), New Biol.* **239**, 9.

Tonewaga, S., Maxam, A. M., Tezaid, R., Bernard, O., and Gilbert, W. (1978). *Proc. Natl. Acad. Sci. U.S.A.* **75**, 1485.

Towle, H. C., Tsai, M.-J., Tsai, S. Y., and O'Malley, B. W. (1977). *J. Biol. Chem.* **252**, 2396.

Tsai, S. Y., Roop, D. R., Tsai, M-J., Stein, J. P., Means, A. R., and O'Malley, B. W. (1978a). *Biochemistry* (in press).

Tsai, M.-J., Tsai, S. Y., Chang, C., and O'Malley, B. W. (1978b). *Biochim. Biophys. Acta* (in press).

Tushinski, R. J., Sussman, P. M., Yu, L.-Y., and Bancroft, F. C. (1977). *Proc. Natl. Acad. Sci. U.S.A.* **74**, 2357.

Vedeckis, W. V., Schrader, W. T., and O'Malley, B. W. (1978). *Biochem. Actions Horm.* **5**, 321.

Waugh, L. J., and Knowland, J. (1975). *Proc. Natl. Acad. Sci. U.S.A.* **72**, 3172.

Wetekam, W., Mullinix, K. P., Deeley, R. G., Kronenberg, H. M., Eldridge, J. D., Meyers, M., and Goldberg, R. F. (1975). *Proc. Natl. Acad. Sci. U.S.A.* **72**, 3364.

Weinstock, R., Swelt, R., Weiss, M., Cedar, H., and Axel R. (1978). *Proc. Natl. Acad. Sci. U.S.A.* **75**, 1299.

Wicks, W. D. (1974). *Adv. Cyclic Nucleotide Res.* **4**, 335.

Wicks, W. D., van Wijk, R., and McKibbin, J. B. (1973). *Adv. Enzyme Regul.* **11**, 117.

Williamson, B. (1977). *Nature (London)* **270**, 295.

Wittliff, J. L., and Kenney, F. T. (1972). *Biochim. Biophys. Acta* **269**, 485.

Woo, S. L. C., Dugaiczyk, A., Tsai, M-J., Lai, E. C., Caterall, J. F., and O'Malley, B. W. (1978). *Proc. Natl. Acad. Sci. U.S.A.* **75**, 3688.

Wynn, V., Doar, J. W. H., Mills, G. L., and Stokes, T. (1969). *Lancet* **2**, 756.

Yamamoto, K., Kawai, K., and Ieiri, T. (1975). *Jpn. J. Physiol.* **25**, 645.

Yamamoto, K. R., and Alberts, B. M. (1976). *Annu. Rev. Biochem.* **45**, 721.

Young, H. A., Scolnick, E. M., and Parks, W. P. (1975). *J. Biol. Chem.* **250**, 3337.

Young, H. A., Shih, T. Y., Scolnick, E. M., and Parks, W. P. (1977). *J. Virol.* **21**, 139.

Zasloff, M., and Felsenfeld, G. (1977a). *Biochem. Biophys. Res. Commun.* **75**, 598.

Zasloff, M., and Felsenfeld, G. (1977b). *Biochemistry* **16**, 5135.

Enkephalins and Endorphins

RICHARD J. MILLER AND PEDRO CUATRECASAS

Department of Pharmacological and Physiological Sciences, The University of Chicago, Chicago, Illinois, and Wellcome Research Laboratories, Research Triangle Park, North Carolina

I. INTRODUCTION

Reports of the effects of opioids in animals and man stretch back for hundreds of years. The subjective effects of these drugs have been documented by many writers. Individuals in many countries and in every age have used them either for their pharmacological and therapeutic properties or else to savor the delights of these drugs in relation to personal aesthetic goals. Unfortunately, as many have found to their dismay, the misuse of morphine is fraught with dangers and problems.

Consideration of the therapeutic side of morphine use shows that the drug has many roles to play in medical treatment. As analgesics, morphine and related compounds are clearly the most effective drugs available when it comes to dealing with really severe pain. Other well known uses of opioid drugs include the treatment of diarrhea and coughing. Morphine also has effects on respiration, the endocrine system, and mood (Martin, 1967). The latter effect, that is, the "high"

297

associated with the use of these drugs, is undoubtedly one of the main reasons people find them pleasurable to take. The use of narcotics is also typified by so-called tolerance and addiction phenomena and the associated withdrawal syndrome (Snyder and Matthysse, 1975). These behavioral effects are responsible for much of the misery associated with the misuse of narcotics. It has long been the aim of researchers to produce a morphinelike compound that is free of such side effects.

In the last decade considerable advances have been made at the molecular level in understanding the mechanism of action of narcotics. The fundamental concept in understanding this work is that of the opioid receptor, which may be defined as that entity which recognizes and binds opioid drugs, with binding transduced into various biochemical and physiological sequelae. The concept of the opiate receptor arose from the development of various pharmacological assay systems that were sensitive to the effects of narcotics. For example, it was found that electrical stimulation of the guinea pig ileum or of the mouse vas deferens would cause the tissue to contract (Schaumann, 1955; Paton, 1957; Kosterlitz and Waterfield, 1975). This was a result of acetylcholine in the case of the ileum and norepinephrine in the case of the vas deferens being released by the electrical stimulation. It was found that narcotic agonists, such as morphine, could inhibit the electrically stimulated output of transmitter in these tissues and consequently inhibit the electrically stimulated contraction. This action of morphine and related natural and synthetic drugs was shown to have high specificity in the pharmacological sense. Thus structural requirements for agonist activity were stringent, the action of agonists were stereospecific, and certain structural modifications produced molecules that acted as partial agonists or antagonists (Kosterlitz and Watt, 1968). In addition, there was shown to be an exceedingly good correlation between the potency of a drug in these bioassays and its potency as an analgesic *in vivo* (Kosterlitz and Waterfield, 1975). This suggested that these analgesic effects were mediated by a receptor that was extremely similar, if not identical to, that mediating the effects of narcotics on transmitter release.

In the early 1970s a further breakthrough occurred. Molecular endocrinologists had previously devised assay systems for looking at the binding of radioactive hormones, e.g., insulin, to their receptors (Cuatrecasas, 1971). Taking a leaf from this book, neuropharmacologists applied these techniques to the presumed opioid receptor. Utilizing opioid agonists and antagonists of high specific activity several groups of workers were able to demonstrate a stereospecific interaction of labeled ligand with some entity in brain synaptic membranes

(Terenius, 1973; Pert and Synder, 1973a,b; Simon *et al.*, 1973), and guinea pig ileal homogenates (Creese and Snyder, 1975). Subsequent investigations showed that the entity that bound the labeled drugs appeared to have all the properties of the opioid receptor as previously defined from bioassay and analgesic effects. Intensive investigation of the biochemical properties of the opioid receptor has revealed a wealth of interesting data that are outside the scope of this review. One particular observation, however, is extremely important. It was found that only opioidlike drugs interacted selectively with the receptor (Snyder, 1975). Thus, drugs related to cholinergic, adrenergic, serotonergic, and histaminergic systems were all ineffective. So were such substances as steroid and peptide hormones. Apart from illustrating the necessary specificity of the opioid receptor, such observations raised a question in the mind of many investigators: "Why should specific receptors exist in mammals for recognizing morphine—a plant alkaloid?" One exciting possibility was that these receptors were in fact receptors for some previously unknown morphinelike substance normally found in the central nervous system (CNS) and possibly elsewhere. Clearly such a compound might be involved in the control of pain and mood. Other observations also supported the notion of an endogenous morphinelike factor. In particular it was demonstrated that electrical stimulation of certain areas by the brain, such as the periaqueductal gray could produce analgesia in animals and man (Tsou and Janq, 1964; Reynolds, 1969; Mayer and Price, 1976). This could signify that the electrical stimulation was causing the release of some morphinelike material *"in situ."* The observation that the electrically produced analgesic effects could be reversed, at least partially, by naloxone, an opioid antagonist, further implicated the opioid nature of the phenomenon (Mayer and Price, 1976; Akil *et al.*, 1976).

In the light of the above discussion it is reasonable that several groups set out to look for the possible morphinelike factor. Initially workers made extracts of brain and tried to identify opioidlike material in such extracts by means of bioassay and opioid receptor-binding assay. Several reports were published showing that in fact such brain extracts did contain some activity that would depress the contraction of the electrically stimulated guinea pig ileum and mouse vas deferens in a naloxone-reversible fashion (Hughes, 1975; Terenius and Wahlström, 1975a; Hughes *et al.*, 1975a; Pasternak *et al.*, 1975). Moreover, these extracts would compete with [^{3}H]naloxone for the opioid receptor in brain homogenates (Pasternak *et al.*, 1976). Extracts and incubation fluids of pituitary (Cox *et al.*, 1975, 1976a; Ross *et al.*, 1977; Teschemacher *et al.*, 1975) and gut (Puig *et al.*, 1977; Schulz *et al.*, 1977a,b) were also found to contain these opioidlike materials. In addition, these crude morphinelike factor preparations produced analgesia after intraventricular injection (A. Pert *et al.*, 1977) in rats. One study examined the distribution in detail of the morphinelike factor in monkey brain (*Macaca mulata*) (Simantov *et al.*, 1976a). In this case the areas with the highest concentrations were found to be the head of the caudate nucleus, the globus pallidus, the body of the caudate nucleus, and the anterior hypothalamus. Moderate concentrations were found in the amygdala, posterior hypothalamus, tail of the caudate nucleus, periaqueductal gray, raphe area, and floor of the fourth ventricle. Other regions contained lower concentrations, but in no area was morphinelike activity completely absent.

It was also realized even at this early stage that several features of the morphinelike factor were in fact not at all like morphine. First, the molecular weight of the factor was rather high. Estimates in the brain hovered around 800–1000 (Hughes, 1975; Pasternak *et al.*, 1975). In the pituitary, however, activity obtained on gel filtration had molecular weights in the range of 1500–3000 (Cox *et al.*, 1975). Second, some work was performed in which the morphinelike factor was treated in various ways to try to gain some insight into its chemical composition. Surprisingly, both leucine aminopeptidase and carboxypeptidases were found to destroy the activity, in some brain extracts at any rate (Hughes, 1975; Pasternak *et al.*, 1975). It thus became clear that the morphinelike factor was, in fact, a peptide.

Certain other interesting observations were made on the nature of the morphinelike factor even before its structure had been resolved. For example, the opioid activity in brain extracts was found to be localized in the synaptosomal fraction after subcellular fractionation (Queen *et al.*, 1976; Simantov *et al.*, 1976b). One phylogenetic study investigated the presence of opioidlike material in a wide variety of species (Simantov *et al.*, 1976c). It was found that vertebrates ranging from humans to the hagfish all had some morphinelike factor extractable from their brains and in addition appeared to possess opioid receptors as measured in binding assays. The highest concentration was found in the toad. This perhaps is not surprising, as toads and frogs have been reported to be particularly rich in all sorts of bioactive peptides. Invertebrates such as tarantulas and cockroaches, however, contained neither morphinelike factors nor opioid receptors.

Apart from the pituitary, brain, and gut, morphinelike factors have been described in the cerebrospinal fluid and blood of humans and animals. These factors also seem likely to be peptides (Terenius and Wahlström, 1975b; Pert *et al.*, 1976a). One factor, however, is almost certainly not a peptide and was isolated from the brain by means of immunoprecipitation with antimorphine antibodies. This factor is therefore immunochemically very similar to morphine and may resemble it chemically (Gintzler et al., 1976). As things stand at the moment not all the structures of the morphinelike factors originally described have been completely elucidated. We shall therefore concentrate here on those factors whose structure seems fairly certain. It is our belief that many of the others that have been described will ultimately prove to be related to those whose structures are now known.

The first success in elucidating the structure of a morphinelike factor was reported by Hughes and colleagues in 1975. These workers elucidated the structure of the morphinelike factor from brain, which they had previously named "enkephalin." Here again there was another surprise. Enkephalin proved to be a mixture of two pentapeptides. These had the sequences H_2N-Tyr-Gly-Gly-Phe-Met-OH ([Met^5]-enkephalin) and H_2N-Tyr-Gly-Gly-Phe-Leu-H ([Leu^5]-enkephalin). In the brains of most species the former peptide was found to predominate (Smith et al., 1976). The existence of these peptides was rapidly confirmed by Simantov and Snyder (1976a), who found that in the calf brain [Leu^5]-enkephalin was the major component. It was shown that synthetic [Met^5]- and [Leu^5]-enkephalins produced the full spectrum of opioidlike effects (see below).

One other surprising and subsequently extremely important observation was made in the original paper in Nature (Hughes et al., 1975b). This was that the structure of [Met^5]-enkephalin was contained within the sequence of a previously isolated peptide of 91 amino acids known as β-lipotropin. This hormone had been previously isolated by Li and co-workers (1965; Li, 1964, 1977), originally from ovine pituitaries but subsequently from bovine, porcine, and human sources as well. It was known previously that the N-terminal 58 amino acids of β-lipotropin, known as γ-lipotropin, could also be isolated from the pituitary and that this portion of the molecule contained the entire sequence of the hormone β-MSH (β-lipotropin, 41–58). It was therefore thought that β-lipotropin might function as a biosynthetic precursor to β-MSH via γ-lipotropin. In addition, β- and γ-lipotropins themselves had some lipolytic activity in the fat pads of certain species (Lohmar and Li, 1967). No particular role had been assigned to the piece of β-lipotropin which remained after cleavage to form γ-lipotropin. This fact was reflected by its name, C-fragment, i.e., β-lipotropin residues 61–91 (Bradbury et al., 1976a). The realization, however, that the first five amino acids of C-fragment were identical to [Met^5]-enkephalin was a revelation. Workers now rushed to investigate the opioid activity of this entire 31-amino acid C-fragment portion of β-lipotropin and found it to be at least as potent as [Met⁵]-enkephalin by several criteria (Bradbury *et al.*, 1976b; Cox *et al.*, 1976b). C-fragment has now been isolated from the pituitaries of several species including man, pig, sheep, and camel (Li, 1977). It probably exists also in the central nervous system (see below).

A word should be mentioned concerning the nomenclature in this field. It is generally accepted that the overall name for opioid peptides related to β-lipotropin is endorphin. The enkephalins are considered to be the two pentapeptides described by Hughes and colleagues, and are thus a particular case of endorphin. Other endorphins, intermediate in length between [Met⁵]-enkephalin and β-endorphin, have also been isolated from the pituitary, and these are known as α-, β-, and γ-endorphins (Ling and Guillemin, 1976; Guillemin *et al.*, 1976). These are therefore all fragments of the C terminus of β-lipotropin. In addition, the fragment β-lipotropin 61–87 has also been isolated from pituitary and is known as C'-fragment. The relationship between all these fragments is illustrated in Fig. 1.

The above discussion provides a basic historical background to the discovery and nature of the opioid peptides. During the last 2 years the subject cannot be said to have suffered from a lack of attention. In fact, over one thousand publications covering every aspect of the area have appeared. We shall try to summarize the field primarily by using our own results where relevant as a starting point for discussion. Some aspects of this research have been briefly reviewed elsewhere (Snyder, 1977).

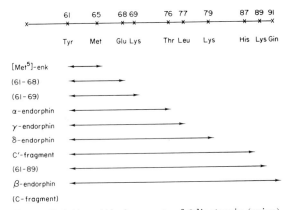

FIG. 1. Opioid peptide fragments of β-lipotropin (ovine).

II. Identification of the Opioid Peptides

The two main methods of detecting and quantitating enkephalins and endorphins used so far are radioimmunoassay and bioassay. In addition, opioid receptor binding assays were originally utilized a great deal to detect general opioid activity. While this latter method is still extremely useful for some purposes, it lacks the potential specificity associated with radioimmunoassay. Clearly radioimmunoassay is the method of choice for detection of opioid peptides in terms of its convenience and potential sensitivity. In addition the antisera obtained are useful for immunohistochemical localization of the relevant peptides (see below). However, when carrying out radioimmunoassay, certain precautions and controls must be run. If these are performed, then the method is certainly invaluable. To date several laboratories have developed antisera to the enkephalins, and a few papers have reported antisera for endorphins and β-lipotropin. We shall consider the radioimmunoassay for enkephalins first of all.

Most antisera prepared against [Met^5]- or [Leu^5]-enkephalins show some crossreactivity to both peptides (Simantov and Snyder, 1976b; Miller et al., 1978a; Simantov et al., 1977a; Rossier et al., 1977a; Weissman et al., 1976; Yang et al., 1977). Although this is not surprising, it does make the interpretation of results rather complicated. The average crossreactivity between peptides reported has been in the range of 0.1% to 10%. As the concentrations of [Leu^5]-enkephalin in rat brain have been reported to be about one-tenth those of [Met^5]-enkephalin, when using antibodies to [Leu^5]-enkephalin it is often hard to say without reservation that [Met^5]-enkephalin is not also being detected. One way to overcome this problem is to perform some preliminary separation of the two peptides. This may be done by high-pressure liquid chromatography (J. Meek, personal communication) or by affinity chromatography (Miller et al., 1978a). Another useful method is to treat extracts with cyanogen bromide to destroy the [Met^5]-enkephalin immunoreactivity, theoretically just leaving the [Leu^5]-enkephalin (Smith et al., 1976). Although the problems of crossreactivity have been recognized by most investigators, it is worth keeping in mind when considering the absolute reliability of published data.

A second problem relates to the best procedure for extraction of the various peptides. Originally several groups used a technique of sucrose homogenization followed by boiling, centrifugation, and lyophilization (Simantov and Snyder, 1976b). However, it was subsequently found that this process leads to a very low recovery of enkephalin. It appears, however, that the use of 1 N acetic acid or 0.1 N HCl is satisfactory for extraction of enkephalins in high yield. Both 1 N acetic acid and 0.1 N HCl also appear to be satisfactory for extraction of the large endorphins from brain in high yield and are generally useful (Miller *et al.*, 1978a). In the case of β-endorphin it has been suggested that boiling the tissue before homogenization in acid is also a prerequisite for obtaining the peptide in high yield, although enkephalins were found to be efficiently extracted even without boiling (Rossier *et al.*, 1977a). It is important to note that it is essential to monitor the recovery of peptides during extraction in order to make accurate quantitative estimates of tissue concentrations. In some reports such controls have not been performed, making the absolute value of the data somewhat questionable except in a qualitative sense. An example of the size distribution of brain opioid activity and enkephalin immunoreactivity is illustrated in Fig. 2.

Hughes and colleagues have generally used the mouse vas deferens bioassay in order to quantitate enkephalins. The peptides are isolated

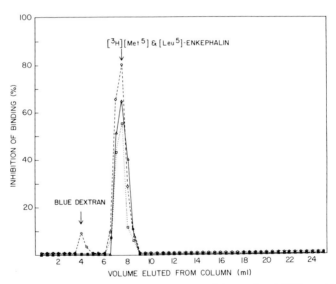

FIG. 2. Distribution of enkephalinlike immunoreactivity and opioidlike activity in whole rat brain extract determined by chromatography of 0.1 N HCl extract on BioGel P2. $\triangle$—$\triangle$, [Met⁵]-enkephalin immunoreactivity. Inhibition of binding of [¹²⁵I][Met⁵]-enkephalin to anti-[Met⁵]-enkephalin antibody. $\square$··$\square$, [Leu⁵]-enkephalin immunoreactivity. Inhibition of binding of [¹²⁵I][Leu⁵]-enkephalin to anti-[Leu⁵]-enkephalin antibody. $\bigcirc$---$\bigcirc$, Opioidlike activity. Inhibition of binding of [¹²⁵I][DAla²,DLeu⁵]-enkephalin to opioid receptors in N4TG1 neuroblastoma cells. From Miller *et al.* (1978a).

by extracting tissue in 0.1 N HCl followed by chromatography on XAD-2 hydrophobic resin from which peptides are eluted by 90% methanol. Differential measurements of [Met[5]]- or [Leu[5]]-enkephalins are achieved by treatment of part of the extract with cyanogen bromide as mentioned above (Smith et al., 1976).

Recently, several reports have appeared giving details of radioimmunoassays for the endorphins, especially for β-endorphin (Guillemin et al., 1977a; LaBella et al., 1977; Li et al., 1977; Snell et al., 1977). From these reports, one problem seems to be the difficulty in producing an antibody to β-endorphin that does not have very substantial crossreactivity to β-lipotropin. However, as it should be quite possible to separate β-lipotropin and β-endorphin easily on the basis of their molecular weights, such antisera should still be suitable for radioimmunoassay provided that they have the required sensitivity. This cannot be said, however for immunohistochemistry, where results must be interpreted with due caution.

One other question relating to methodology which has turned up in the literature to date is that of the use of microwave irradiation for fixing tissue before extraction. Potentially, this method is useful as it should provide the most rapid and direct method for preserving the levels of peptides in the animal. Three groups have reported that animals sacrificed in this way have concentrations of opioid peptides in the brain, which are somewhat higher than in those sacrificed by conventional means (Cheung et al., 1977; Simantov et al., 1977a; Yang et al., 1977). However, another group has reported that the method is technically demanding and difficult to reproduce (Rossier et al., 1977a). In addition, one cannot be completely sure as to the effects of the microwaves themselves in elevating peptide levels. Therefore, at present this method remains potentially useful, but not as yet generally accepted.

One particularly powerful technique for the extraction and microsequencing of peptides developed by Udenfriend and colleagues has recently been applied to the problem of the opioid peptides (Rubinstein et al., 1977a,b). This technique includes the use of fluorescent derivatives and high-pressure liquid chromatography for the "ultramicroanalytical" sequencing of peptides. Rubinstein et al. have so far managed to isolate and sequence both β-lipotropin and β-endorphin from rat pituitaries. β-Endorphin in the rat is identical to that in camel and sheep. These workers have also confirmed the existence of [Met[5]]-enkephalin in pituitary and brain. No [Leu[5]]-enkephalin was found in the pituitary, but one peak running in the correct position for [Leu[5]]-enkephalin was found in the brain. However, the material in this peak has not yet been completely identified. In addition, this group has also identified the high molecular weight precursor to ACTH and β-endorphin reported by others (see below). The reader is referred to the original articles for further details of these powerful and important analytical techniques.

III. Distribution of Opioid Peptides by Radioimmunoassay

Considering the different variables that have been described above there is a fairly good agreement between the various reports that have presented data on the distribution of enkephalins in the central nervous system. One early paper reported concentrations that were substantially lower than those of more recent reports (Simantov and Snyder, 1976b). However, these authors subsequently found this to be due to a relatively poor extraction procedure and in later reports have demonstrated concentrations closer to those reported by others (Hong *et al.*, 1977a; Kobayashi *et al.*, 1978; Rossier *et al.*, 1977b; Yang *et al.*, 1977). A representative set of data is shown in Table I and Fig. 3. In these

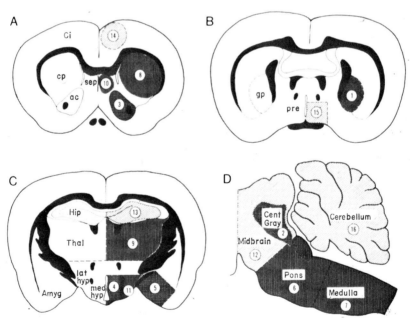

FIG. 3. Distribution of enkephalin-like immunoreactivity in rat brain. Areas are ranked for enkephalin content from 1 (highest) to 16 (lowest). Data are taken from Table I (Kobayashi *et al.*, 1978).

TABLE I

REGIONAL DISTRIBUTION OF BRAIN ENKEPHALIN AND EFFECTS OF HYPOPHYSECTOMY (PMOL/MG PROTEIN)[a]

Rank order	Region	Normal				Hypophysectomized			
		Total	Met	Leu	M:L	Total	Met	Leu	M:L
1	Globus pallidus	35.0	29.5 ± 3.5	5.5 ± 0.10	5.4	36.5	31.5 ± 2.8	5.0 ± 0.35	6.3
2	Central gray	6.5	4.8 ± 0.2	1.7 ± 0.09	2.8	6.6	5.1 ± 0.4	1.5 ± 0.07	3.4
3	Nucleus accumbens	6.3	5.2 ± 0.4	1.1 ± 0.09	4.7	6.5	5.6 ± 0.4	0.91 ± 0.06	6.2
4	Medial hypothalamus	5.0	4.4 ± 0.3	0.60 ± 0.07	7.3	4.2	3.7 ± 0.3	0.53 ± 0.01	7.0
5	Amygdala	4.5	3.3 ± 0.3	1.2 ± 0.07	2.8	5.1	3.3 ± 0.2	1.8 ± 0.1	1.8
6	Pons	3.4	2.8 ± 0.4	0.55 ± 0.04	5.1	2.7	2.2 ± 0.4	0.51 ± 0.02	4.3
7	Medulla	3.3	2.6 ± 0.6	0.70 ± 0.06	3.7	2.9	2.2 ± 0.3	0.66 ± 0.08	3.3
8	Caudate-putamen	3.1	2.6 ± 0.4	0.53 ± 0.06	4.9	3.3	2.5 ± 0.2	0.75 ± 0.06	3.3
9	Thalamus	2.6	2.0 ± 0.1	0.64 ± 0.03	3.1	3.0	2.3 ± 0.2	0.66 ± 0.02	3.5
10	Septal area	2.3	2.0 ± 0.3	0.40 ± 0.02	5.0	2.2	1.8 ± 0.2	0.37 ± 0.03	4.9
11	Lateral hypothalamus	2.1	1.9 ± 0.3	0.22 ± 0.02	8.6	1.6	1.4 ± 0.1	0.18 ± 0.01	7.8
12	Midbrain	1.5	1.2 ± 0.1	0.31 ± 0.04	3.9	1.3	1.0 ± 0.1	0.28 ± 0.03	3.6
13	Hippocampus	1.3	1.1 ± 0.08	0.17 ± 0.02	6.5	1.5	1.3 ± 0.10	0.17 ± 0.04	7.7
14	Cerebral cortex	1.3	0.81 ± 0.09	0.44 ± 0.04	1.8	1.4	1.0 ± 0.05	0.37 ± 0.04	2.7
15	Preoptic area	1.1	0.95 ± 0.10	0.11 ± 0.01	8.6	0.9	0.79 ± 0.06	0.10 ± 0.02	7.9
16	Cerebellum	—	0.2 ± 0.03	<0.1	—	—	0.1 ± 0.1	<0.1	—

[a] From Kobayashi et al. (1978).

studies detailed localization was obtained by measuring enkephalins in nuclei punched out of frozen sections of rat brain with a hollow needle. Such methods have been used elsewhere to obtain detailed localization of other bioactive substances in the nervous system. It is quite clear from these data that in the rat at any rate the concentrations of [Met^5]-enkephalin are considerably higher than those of [Leu^5]-enkephalin. This also appears to be true of mouse, guinea pig, and rabbit (Smith *et al.*, 1976). One study, however, reported that in calf brain there was about twice as much [Leu^5]-enkephalin as [Met^5]-enkephalin (Simantov and Snyder, 1976a). A second point to note is that the ratio of [Met^5]- to [Leu^5]-enkephalin differs considerably in different brain areas. This observation is hard to interpret at the moment, as little is known about the relative cellular and subcellular distributions of the two enkephalins or their biosynthesis and degradation. It might perhaps be expected that if both peptides were always found in the same cells their relative concentrations would remain the same, other factors being constant. It is, however, possible that selective biosynthetic or degradative processes may occur at the subcellular level and these may alter depending on the area in question. Such mechanisms would result in differing ratios of the two peptides in different brain regions.

There are some particularly interesting facts to note concerning the distribution of enkephalins in the central nervous system. One of the most striking features is the localization of the peptides in the globus pallidus. The concentrations of enkephalins in this area are 5–10 times higher than any other area in the brain. Exactly what function is served by these vast quantities of enkephalin is not really clear at this point. Certainly it is a reasonable starting hypothesis that it may be involved in the extrapyramidal control of motor activity. It is well known that many narcotics and synthetic or natural opioid peptides can produce both hypermotility or cataleptic effects, depending on dosage and other factors (see below). In addition it may also be that such effects are mediated in certain cases by interaction with dopaminergic systems in the basal ganglia. This evidence is discussed below. With respect to the origin of the enkephalin within the globus pallidus, some immunohistochemical evidence, also discussed below, suggests that there may be a pathway originating from cell bodies within the caudate nucleus that gives rise to enkephalinergic fibers within the globus pallidus (Cuello and Paxinos, 1978).

Parts of the limbic system also contain high concentrations of enkephalin. For example, the nucleus accumbens and amygdala are rich in both peptides. It is tempting to suppose that enkephalinergic systems in this part of the brain may be involved in the control of mood and other subjective effects usually associated with morphine use. In addition, such a role would also certainly increase the likelihood of enkephalinergic systems playing a role in mental illness, as some workers have suggested (Bloom *et al.*, 1977b).

In the midbrain, concentrations of enkephalin are moderate to low with the notable exception of the periaqueductal gray and raphe nuclei. It is interesting to note that these areas are known to be important in the transmission of pain signals. For example, electrical stimulation of the periaqueductal gray produces analgesia in both animals and man, and in addition microinjection of narcotics into this region also produces analgesia (Reynolds, 1967). Similar experiments have illustrated the importance of the raphe nuclei and associated serotoninergic systems in the mediation of pain sensations (Mayer and Price, 1976). Histological data in this area support and complement the radioimmunoassay data (see below).

Another area of the brain in which the localization of enkephalin seems to tie in well with certain effects of narcotics is the hypothalamus. Immunohistochemistry reveals that both enkephalin-containing terminals and cell bodies are localized within the hypothalamus. In particular, enkephalinergic terminals are localized in the external layer of the median eminence. This is most interesting in view of the fact that morphine is able to release several pituitary hormones including prolactin, growth hormone, and vasopressin after systemic administration (see below). The observation that the opioid peptides and their synthetic analogs are also able to release these hormones together with their localization in the median eminence suggests that they may play a role as neuroendocrine modulators.

Other areas of the brain generally contain lower concentrations of enkephalins, although in no areas is it completely absent. This is reminiscent of the data on the distribution of morphinelike factor in monkey brain discussed previously. Even in areas such as the cortex, where concentrations are low, some staining can be seen in immunohistochemical studies (see below).

Table I also illustrates the fact that enkephalin concentrations in the central nervous system are not changed following hypophysectomy. Thus it appears that if β-endorphin is the biosynthetic precursor of [Met^5]-enkephalin, as many have suggested, then the source of such β-endorphin cannot be the pituitary but an independent source of β-endorphin must exist in the brain. This as we shall see appears to be the case. This observation has been repeated by other workers (e.g., Cheung and Goldstein, 1976).

In contrast to the enkephalins, few data are available so far on the distribution of β-endorphin or β-lipotropin in the central nervous system by radioimmunoassay. It is at least fairly certain that these peptides do exist in the brain. The evidence is predominantly immunochemical. Owing to the relatively low concentrations of such peptides in the brain compared to the pituitary, they have not as yet been isolated from nervous tissue and sequenced. However, other criteria such as crossreactivity to antisera and chromatographic properties suggest that these peptides in the brain are probably identical to those previously identified in the pituitary (Bloom et al., 1978; Krieger et al., 1977a; LaBella et al., 1977; Rossier et al., 1977b).

Quantitative radioimmunoassay data have been reported by two groups for β-endorphin, both using the same antibody. One group investigated rat brain (Rossier et al., 1977b), and the other used bovine brain (Krieger et al., 1977a). Table II illustrates a representative sample of the data obtained. In addition, another group has reported the presence of β-endorphin and β-lipotropin in the brain, but not their distribution (LaBella et al., 1977). Although the data are scanty, certain facts are already obvious. For example, it is clear that the concentrations of β-lipotropin and β-endorphin in the basal ganglia are not nearly as high as those of the enkephalins. Moreover, it is also apparent that concentrations of β-endorphin in the spinal cord are low whereas they are high for enkephalin. The assay of β-endorphin in brain is found to be somewhat complicated by several crossreacting species that are also picked up by the radioimmunoassay. As these are all of higher molecular weight that β-endorphin, a simple column sep-

TABLE II
DISTRIBUTION OF IMMUNOASSAYABLE β-ENDORPHIN IN RAT BRAIN[a]

Brain area	β-Endorphin (ng/gm tissue)[b]
Whole	108 ± 8 (10)
Hypothalamus	490 ± 30 (5)
Septum	234 ± 34 (3)
Midbrain	207 ± 15 (5)
Medulla and pons	179 ± 5 (5)
Striatum	None (5)
Hippocampus	None (5)
Cortex	None (5)
Cerebellum	None (5)

[a] Adapted from Rossier et al. (1977b).
[b] Data are means $\pm$SEM; number of animals shown in parentheses.

aration prior to radioimmunoassay helps to produce reliable data. The potential crossreacting species are β-lipotropin, "Big ACTH," and also myelin basic protein, which has been found to have some crossreactivity to anti-β-endorphin antisera (Bloom et al., 1978; Rossier et al., 1977b). In crude extracts of some areas of the brain, in particular cortical areas or the striatum, all the immunoreactivity is due to these high-molecular-weight species, and no β-endorphin is detectable. One paper reporting on the distribution of β-lipotropin by radioimmunoassay in bovine brain demonstrated the presence of β-lipotropin in the striatum and cortex, and so this may make up part of the high-molecular-weight crossreactivity (Krieger et al., 1977a). Clearly, however, myelin basic protein may also be involved owing to the high concentrations of this substance found in the central nervous system. The status of "Big ACTH" in the central nervous system is not yet certain. However, as both β-lipotropin and ACTH in the brain appear to be contained in the same nerve cell bodies from immunohistochemical studies (see below) it may well be that such a molecule is present and that the synthesis of β-lipotropin and ACTH is linked as it appears to be in the pituitary (see below).

Concentrations of β-endorphin and β-lipotropin in the pituitary are extremely high (Rossier et al., 1977a,b). The main localization of this peptide by radioimmunoassay appears to be the neurohypophysis/pars intermedia area rather than in the adenohypophysis. In fact, immunohistochemical work shows that this localization is actually in the intermediate lobe rather than in both the neural and intermediate lobes (Bloom et al., 1977a). Kobayashi et al. (1978) reported that enkephalin concentrations in the pituitary were low. However, Rubinstein et al. (1977a) and Rossier et al. (1977b) reported appreciable pituitary enkephalin concentrations. It appears, however, that the pituitary contains only [Met^5]-enkephalin, as Rubinstein et al. (1977a,b), using their microanalytical fluorescent technique, found no evidence of [Leu^5]-enkephalin. [Met^5]-enkephalin also appears to be primarily localized in the pars intermedia/neurohypophysis area as opposed to the anterior lobe, as is β-endorphin (Rossier et al., 1977b). However, the immunohistochemical staining patterns for [Met^5]-enkephalin differ somewhat from those for β-endorphin in that some fiberlike staining for [Met^5]-enkephalin is found in the neurohypophysis in addition to staining of the intermediate lobe (Bloom et al., 1978). This, again, would represent a difference in the distribution of enkephalin and β-endorphin, as has been mentioned above for some areas of the brain, such as the basal ganglia. More data concerning the relative distributions of the enkephalins and β-endorphins are discussed below when immunohistochemical experiments are considered.

Apart from the nervous system and pituitary, the main localization of enkephalin is in the gastrointestinal tract. In the small intestine of several species investigated, appreciable concentrations of enkephalin have been found (Linnoilla et al., 1978; Polak et al., 1977; Smith et al., 1976). These species include the guinea pig, rat, hamster, monkey, and human (Table III). Enkephalins have also been localized in the gut by immunohistochemistry, where they appear to be present both in neurons and endocrine cells in the human and in neurons in the guinea pig and rat. In the case of the human, the endocrine cells that stained for enkephalin also stained for gastrin (Polak et al., 1977). The presence of enkephalin in the gastrointestinal tract again fits in well with what is known of the pharmacology of narcotics. Such drugs are known to affect the guinea pig ileum, and this is the basis of a classical bioassay for narcotic agonist activity (Kosterlitz and Waterfield, 1975). Moreover, one of the main effects of morphine is to produce constipation. Thus, one other function for enkephalinergic systems "in vivo" may be in the control of gastrointestinal motility. This aspect will be further discussed below.

It should be noted that the enkephalins are one of a large group of peptides now known to be localized both in the gut and the brain (Pearse, 1976). Other peptides in this category include somatostatin,

TABLE III
CONCENTRATIONS OF ENKEPHALIN IN THE GASTROINTESTINAL TRACT[a,b]

Area	Guinea pig	Rat
	[Met^5]-enkephalin	
Duodenum	6.2 ± 0.7	1.6 ± 0.2
Jejunum	4.4 ± 0.2	1.1 ± 0.1
Ileum	4.1 ± 0.3	0.81 ± 0.05
Colon	3.3 ± 0.3	0.33 ± 0.01
Cecum	0.7 ± 0.1	0.3 ± 0.01
	[Leu^5]-enkephalin[b]	
Duodenum	0.55 ± 0.04	0.08 ± 0.01
Jejunum	0.57 ± 0.02	0.09 ± 0.01
Ileum	0.38 ± 0.02	0.10 ± 0.02
Colon	0.67 ± 0.04	0.05 ± 0.01
Cecum	0.10 ± 0.01	0.02 ± 0.003

[a] Unpublished observations of I. Linoilla, R. Di Augustine, R. J. Miller, K.-J. Chang, and P. Cuatrecasas.

[b] Results are the mean for 3 animals expressed as picomoles per gram wet weight.

neurotensin, substance P, gastrin, cholecystokinin, and vasoactive intestinal polypeptide. Moreover, in the gut such peptides are often found both in neurons and endocrine cells, although the distribution alters considerably from species to species (Hakanson et al., 1970). It is also worth noting that one report has also localized some enkephalin-containing endocrine cells within the human pancreas (Polak et al., 1977). However, there are no reports as yet of any metabolic effects of the opioid peptides that might be related to alterations of pancreatic function.

Only one report has been published so far on the radioimmunoassay of α- and β-endorphin in the gut. These peptides were not detected although high concentrations of enkephalin were detectable in the same samples (Polak et al., 1977). Unfortunately, the authors did not present any data on the recovery of enkephalin or β-endorphin in their experiments.

IV. BIOSYNTHESIS AND DEGRADATION

One of the most fascinating pieces of data as yet reported concerning the opioid peptides relates to the biosynthesis of β-endorphin by the pituitary gland and possibly by the brain. In order to understand these data, it is first necessary to give some background information concerning the biosynthesis of corticotropin.

It has been known for some time that some size heterogeneity exists in immunoreactive ACTH found either in normal pituitaries or secreted by some lung or pituitary tumors (Eipper and Mains, 1976; Yalow and Berson, 1971, 1973; Scott and Lowry, 1974; Orth et al., 1973). The largest form of ACTH reported has a molecular weight in the range of 31,000. This peptide is a glycoprotein known as "Big ACTH" (Mains and Eipper, 1976; Eipper et al., 1976). Some patients have lung tumors that secrete predominantly "Big ACTH," and because this molecule has low bioactivity such patients do not have Cushing's syndrome (Rees, 1975). It was postulated previously that "Big ACTH" might be a biosynthetic precursor to ACTH (1–39). Mains and Eipper (1976) performed pulse-chase labeling experiments utilizing a mouse pituitary tumor line (AtT-20) that synthesizes ACTH. They were able to show that label initially appearing in a high-molecular-weight fraction of immunoreactive ACTH could be chased through several species of lower molecular weight until the ACTH (1–39) stage was reached. These experiments, therefore, demonstrated directly the precursor relationship between "Big ACTH" and ACTH (1–39). Other experiments have shown that mRNA isolated from bovine pituitaries can be translated in a cell-free system to produce "Big ACTH" (Roberts and Herbert, 1977; Nakanishi *et al.*, 1976). Moreover, administration of dexamethasone to animals, which reduces the pituitary of ACTH, also reduces the content of mRNA in the pituitary that can be translated to give "Big ACTH" (Nakanishi *et al.* (1976).

Recent experiments have shown that after pulse-labeling of the pituitary cell line described above in the synthesis of "Big ACTH," β-endorphin antisera can also be used to immunoprecipitate various labeled peptides (Mains *et al.*, 1977). The largest of these peptides is the same as one that can be precipitated by anti-ACTH antisera, i.e., the MW 31,000 form—"Big ACTH." Thus, the "Big ACTH" molecule appears to contain the antigenic determinants for both ACTH and β-endorphin. Smaller peptides immunoprecipitable with β-endorphin antisera do not correspond to smaller peptides immunoprecipitable with anti-ACTH antisera. Thus, the two antigenic determinants are found separately in the largest molecular species obtained. All this has led to considerable speculation that "Big ACTH" may function as a biosynthetic precursor to both ACTH and related peptides, on the one hand, and β-lipotropin and related peptides on the other. This contention is also supported by several other pieces of evidence. For example, one report has demonstrated that the pituitary tumor line AtT-20 used in the above pulse-chase experiments produces peptides with opioid agonist activity (Giagnoni *et al.*, 1977). In these experiments the peptides were not characterized beyond their opioid agonist properties. Second, it appears that the two classes of peptides are found in the same cells in the pituitary. Thus, staining the pituitary with antibodies to both ACTH or β-endorphin shows staining in the same cells of the pars intermedia and adenohypophysis (F. Bloom, personal communication). It is not known as yet whether the antisera stain the same population of secretory vesicles. Third, the release of the two peptides appears to be orchestrated in an identical fashion *in vivo* (Guillemin *et al.*, 1977b). For example, it has been recently demonstrated that circulating concentrations of β-endorphin and ACTH in the rat respond in a parallel fashion to various physiological manipulations. During stress β-endorphin levels increased, as did ACTH levels. On the other hand, dexamethasone depressed both circulating ACTH and β-endorphin but adrenalectomy increased levels of both peptides in the circulation. In one human patient with Nelson's syndrome, who had very high circulating levels of ACTH, very high circulating levels of β-endorphin were also detected. Another piece of evidence comes from the work of Rubinstein *et al.* (1977a), who reported that during their investigations into the sequence of rat pituitary β-lipotropin they also observed a large (MW $>$ 30,000) molecule that yielded opioid peptides after trypsinization. This again indicates that a molecule of the "Big ACTH" type is found in normal as well as neoplastic tissue. A final and most compelling piece of evidence in support of the hypothesis that "Big ACTH" is the biosynthetic precursor to ACTH and β-lipotropin/β-endorphin comes from very recent work by Herbert and colleagues. This group has translated mRNA from the AtT-20 pituitary tumor line in a cell-free system. They find that the main product is a nonglycosylated peptide of molecular weight about 28,500. Peptide mapping of this protein shows that it contains the sequences of both ACTH and β-lipotropin, probably only one copy of each (Roberts and Herbert, 1977).

It is well known that there is an amino acid sequence common to both ACTH and the γ-lipotropin portion of β-lipotropin. This sequence is ACTH (4–10). It seems likely from consideration of the above evidence that both ACTH and β-lipotropin are synthesized on the same precursor molecule. The common sequence suggests that possibly this may be the result of a partial gene duplication event. Certainly, clarification of the biosynthetic routes in the pituitary involved in the production of the opioid peptides is one of the most interesting problems in this field at the moment.

It is also known that ACTH, β-lipotropin, and β-endorphin all occur in the central nervous system (Krieger et al., 1977b; LaBella et al., 1977; Rossier et al., 1977b). However, it is not known whether their biosynthesis is linked in this tissue. Certainly, this question is considerably harder to study in the central nervous system than in the pituitary. However, some evidence from immunohistochemical studies discussed below suggests that ACTH and β-endorphin synthesis may be linked in the brain as well.

In addition to the above data, other workers have shown that by pulse labeling of bovine pituitary slices or dissociated cells from the pars intermedia, radiolabeled β- or γ-lipotropin or β-endorphin can be obtained. However, little if any β-MSH was obtained, indicating that turnover of γ-lipotropin is rather slow. It was also found that very little β-lipotropin was formed in comparison to γ-lipotropin or β-endorphin. The authors suggest, therefore, that β-lipotropin may be a transient form that is readily cleaved to produce γ-lipotropin and β-endorphin (Crine et al., 1977a,b).

Very little is known at present about the biosynthesis of [Met^5]- and [Leu^5]-enkephalins. Attempts to label enkephalins in situ by pulsing brain slices with radioactive amino acid have met with only limited success (Yang et al., 1978). It has been hypothesized that [Met⁵]-enkephalin is derived from β-endorphin, and indeed this seems to be a reasonable starting hypothesis. However, there is rather little evidence to date supporting this contention, and some data actually tends to argue against it (see below). However, if [Met⁵]-enkephalin is not derived from β-endorphin, it is not at all clear where it does come from. It is very unlikely that it is synthesized as [Met⁵]-enkephalin on the ribosome, because synthesis of such small peptides has not been demonstrated in eukaryotes. Also it is unlikely to be synthesized by some template mechanism, because biosynthesis of small peptides by this method is known to occur with certainty only in prokaryotes (Kurhashi, 1974). Thus, it must be assumed that it does derive from some biosynthetic precursor. Whether this ultimately proves to be β-endorphin or not remains to be seen.

All that has been said above about [Met⁵]-enkephalin can also be said for [Leu⁵]-enkephalin. In this case, however, no potential biosynthetic precursor has surfaced at all. For example no [Leu⁶⁵]-β-lipotropin or [Leu⁵]-β-endorphin has been found, although some workers have looked for such a molecule. The biosynthetic origins of [Leu⁵]-enkephalin are therefore considered to be mysterious at this time.

Some investigations have been carried out on the metabolism of the various opioid peptides, although it is hard in general to know quite what to make of most of them. Certain features, however, are quite clear. For example, it has been shown that the enkephalins are extremely rapidly degraded by enzymes in various tissue homogenates or in blood, whereas β-endorphin is considerably more stable (Dupont et al., 1977a; Hambrook et al., 1976; Miller et al., 1977). This observation serves to explain, at least partly, the greatly increased antinociceptive potency of β-endorphin over [Met⁵]-enkephalin following intraventricular injection, as their opioid receptor affinities are similar (see below). In homogenates of guinea pig ileum or in the brain, enkephalin appears to be degraded mainly by removal of the N-terminal tyrosine residue, although other minor modes of degradation may also exist (Hambrook et al., 1976). It is therefore not surprising that enkephalin analogs containing a D-amino acid in the second position instead of a glycine are considerably more stable than the naturally occurring enkephalins (Hambrook et al., 1976). The subcellular distribution of the enkephalin-degrading activity in the brain has been examined (Lane et al., 1977). Significant "enkephalin-hydrolyzing activity" (EHA) was found to be associated with all subcellular fractions. In synaptosomes high activity was found associated with soluble, synaptosomal membrane and mitochondrial fractions, whereas that associated with vesicles was low. In addition EHA was detected in plasma, but was rather low in cerebrospinal fluid. Both bacitracin (Miller *et al.*, 1977) and *o*-phenanthroline (Meek *et al.*, 1977) will effectively protect enkephalin from degradation by enzymes in brain homogenates. It is well known that bacitracin can also protect other peptides from metabolism in a similar fashion (Desbuquois *et al.*, 1974).

β-Endorphin can also be degraded by an enzyme in synaptosomal membranes (Austen *et al.*, 1977). The products formed depend on the pH at which the experiment is performed and also on whether or not bacitracin is present. However, depending on the conditions, α-endorphin, γ-endorphin, or [Met^5]-enkephalin can be formed. Little is known about the nature of the various enzymes involved in these cleavages. Apparently bacitracin can protect γ-endorphin from further breakdown by striatal slices, indicating that the enzyme involved in this case is probably an aminopeptidase. On the other hand, bacitracin does not protect β-endorphin from breakdown, indicating that the first step in the proteolysis of this peptide involves attack by an endopeptidase.

The trouble with all the data on the metabolism of opioid peptides is that one does not know whether the reactions involved are really "relevant" in the functional sense, i.e., whether these reactions are actually those that are concerned with the metabolism of the opioid peptides *in vivo*. This problem will be quite difficult to resolve. It might be tackled by the development of specific inhibitors of the enzymes that metabolize the opioid peptides *in situ*, as has been done with the catecholamines, for example. It seems likely that the main method of termination of action of opioid peptides *in vivo* will prove to be by degradation, as with acetylcholine, rather than by presynaptic reuptake, as with biogenic amines.

V. Immunohistochemistry

In addition to radioimmunoassay the technique of immunohistochemistry is ideally suited for investigation of the distribution of the opioid peptides and other neuropeptides for that matter. When proper care is taken over the interpretation of results this method is certainly the most powerful available for precisely localizing these substances. Several groups have used immunohistochemistry to try to localize the enkephalins and endorphins and to examine the various relationships between them (Elde *et al.*, 1976; Hökfelt *et al.*, 1977a,b; Simantov *et al.*, 1977b; Uhl *et al.*, 1977, 1978; Watson *et al.*, 1977a,b). The following discussion is based on results obtained by our colleagues and ourselves but with reference to other data where appropriate.

A. CENTRAL NERVOUS SYSTEM

1. *Enkephalins*

Elde *et al.* (1976) were the first to report on the distribution of enkephalin in the central nervous system (CNS) using anti-[Leu⁵]-enkephalin antisera and fluorescent immunohistochemical method. In this study no nerve cell bodies were found to stain with antibody, but many terminals were detected. In a later study the same workers reported that neuronal perikarya could also be stained if animals were first treated with colchicine (Hökfelt *et al.*, 1977a). Such treatment has been utilized successfully to enhance the staining of neuronal perikarya with antisera to various peptides and enzymes. The rationale here is that the colchicine inhibits axonal transport allowing a buildup of the antigen in the cell body, thus facilitating the staining procedure. Two points should be made with respect to these early studies. First, staining using anti-[Met⁵]-enkephalin antibodies in subsequent studies has revealed virtually identical patterns of staining to those found with anti-[Leu⁵]-enkephalin antibody, in the central nervous system at any rate. Thus, staining for both peptides is widely distributed in confirmation of the radioimmunoassay data, and both are found in the same areas. It is not possible to tell as yet with certainty whether both peptides are localized in the same cells. Moreover, because of the crossreactivity of the enkephalins to the various antisera available, it may not be possible to obtain an answer to this question very easily. Second, it is true to say that in the main all studies, whether using the fluorescent method or the Sternberger peroxidase technique, have revealed a distribution of the enkephalins very similar to that originally reported. However, the detail of the descriptions has increased considerably.

We have studied the distribution of enkephalin-like immunoreactivity in the CNS in collaboration with Drs. M. Sar and W. Stumpf of the University of North Carolina at Chapel Hill, using a modification of the Sternberger method. The staining obtained may be summarized as follows.

Immunoreactive [Leu⁵]-enkephalin and [Met⁵]-enkephalin fibers, terminals, and cell bodies are distributed throughout the CNS. The intensity of staining varies markedly among different brain structures and may be classified as weak, intermediate, and heavy. The distribution of [Leu⁵]-enkephalin-positive staining appears to be similar to that of [Met⁵]-enkephalin staining. The staining is specific for enkephalins since [Met⁵]- or [Leu⁵]-enkephalin antisera, previously adsorbed either with [Met⁵]- or [Leu⁵]-enkephalin, when incubated with the sections does not show any peroxidase staining in terminals, fibers, or cell bodies. Enkephalin-positive perikarya are found in brains of colchicine-treated rats and also in hypophysectomized rats.

a. *Telencephalon*. In the tuberculum olfactorium some immunoreactive enkephalin fibers appear to exist. In the CNS the globus pallidus shows the heaviest staining of fibers resembling a reticulum. In the caudate-putamen, staining of weak to medium intensity is observed. The staining is not uniform throughout, and the areas adjacent to the lateral ventricle and to the globus pallidus are of medium intensity whereas the lateral part of the nucleus is weakly stained. The nucleus accumbens around the anterior commissure shows staining of medium intensity. The nucleus (n.) septi lateralis does not show positive staining throughout its extension. Only a small portion of this nucleus at its middle part close to the lateral ventricle shows staining of fibers and terminals with a medium to heavy intensity. These cells are densely surrounded by enkephalin fibers and terminals, giving a beaded appearance. In contrast, the medial nucleus of the septum does not reveal any staining. Dense immunoreactive enkephalin fibers and terminals are observed in the n. interstitialis striae terminalis extending from the preoptic region to the hypothalamic region. The bed nucleus at the level of n. medialis preopticus shows most dense staining. In the region of organum vasculosum laminae terminalis rostral to and surrounding the preoptic recess, weak staining of terminals can be seen. At this level the fasciculus medialis prosencephali shows heavy staining of fibers, which appears to be closely associated with the stained structures in the n. interstitialis striae terminalis as well as rostrally with the n. accumbens.

Immunoreactive enkephalin terminals are found in some pyramidal cells of the cerebral cortex distributed through the area cinguli, area occipitalis, and area retrosplenialis. The dendrites of some of these cells even appear to be positively stained for enkephalins. In some cells positive staining encircles the whole cell surface.

In the amygdala, medium to strong staining of the fibers and terminals is observed in the n. centralis, weak staining is seen in the n. medialis amygdalideus at its caudal end at the level of the central hypothalamus. At this level n. medialis amygdalideus is divided into two parts. The dorsal part is stained positively, but the ventral part does not stain.

In the hippocampus, throughout its extension, pyramidal cells of area CA-2 are surrounded by heavily stained enkephalin fibers and terminals. In contrast, the other areas of hippocampus, (CA-1, CA-3, CA-4), dentate gyrus, and subiculum do not show any evidence of positive staining for enkephalin.

In the telencephalon, [Met⁵]- or [Leu⁵]-enkephalin immunoreactive cell bodies are observed in the n. accumbens, the n. caudate-putamen, the n. interstitialis striae terminalis, and the central nucleus of the amygdala.

b. *Diencephalon.* A weak staining of fibers and terminals is observed in the dorsal part of the n. medialis preopticus in close proximity to the bed nucleus of the striae terminalis. At this level of the anterior hypothalamic area, enkephalin-positive terminals are seen in the perifornicular region as well as the fasciculus medialis prosencephali. Immunoreactive cell bodies are also observed in the n. paraventricularis and the n. supraopticus, in the perifornicular region and the lateral hypothalamus. In the lateral hypothalamus and perifornicular region, enkephalin cell bodies are smaller as compared with the enkephalin-positive cell bodies in supraoptic and paraventricular nuclei. Immunoreactive enkephalin fibers and terminals exist in the n. ventromedialis hypothalami, the n. dorsomedialis hypothalami, as well as the n. premammillaris ventralis. In the median eminence, the external layer contains enkephalin terminals with dense secretory granules. Also the areas adjacent to the nucleus subthalamicus and to Forel's H₁ and H₂ area contain enkephalin in fibers and terminals. In the mammillary region the n. mammillaris prelateralis shows enkephalin-positive fibers.

c. *Thalamus.* In several nuclear groups of the thalamus, weak to medium intensity staining of fibers and terminals is observed. The nuclear groups include the n. anterior medialis thalami, n. anterior ventralis thalami, n. ventralis medialis thalami, n. ventralis dorsalis thalami, n. reticularis thalami, n. parafascicularis, n. periventricularis rotundocellularis, n. medialis thalami, pars laterali, and n. thalami ventralis as well as the griseum centrale, n. habenulae lateralis, and the area adjacent to the lemniscus medialis.

d. *Mesencephalon.* Immunoreactive enkephalin fibers and terminals are observed in the griseum centrale surrounding the aqueduct, the formatio reticularis, the zona compacta of the substantia nigra, and the structures between the substantia nigra and the lemniscus medialis. In the n. interpeduncularis, heavy staining of fibers, terminals, and cell bodies is seen. At least 15–20 enkephalin cell bodies can be seen in one section. At the level of the colliculus caudalis, weak staining is observed in the periaqueductal substantia grisea and the n. raphe dorsalis. Enkephalin-positive terminals surround the aqueduct and also exist dorsally, lateral to the midline within the cortex colliculi caudalis. At this level the n. cuneiformis as well as some portion of the nuclei lemniscus dorsalis, lateralis, and medialis show positive staining.

At the level of the pons, enkephalin-positive fibers and terminals are found in the n. tegmentalis dorsalis, locus caeruleus, n. parabrachialis lateralis and medialis, n. lemniscus ventralis, ventrolateral part of the n. lemniscus dorsalis, n. centralis superior, n. raphes pontis, as well as the n. reticularis pontis oralis, n. reticularis, tegmenti pontis, and n. trochlearis.

Further caudally, enkephalin fibers and terminals are found in the nuclei cochlearis dorsalis and ventralis, substantia gliosa cochlearis, n. raphes, including the n. raphes pontis and n. raphes pallidus, and the n. tractus spinalis nervi trigemini. Cell bodies containing enkephalin are found in the n. cochlearis dorsalis, the n. vestibularis medialis, the n. vestibularis spinalis as well as the central gray. Enkephalin fibers and terminals are seen throughout the reticular formation in motor nuclei of cranial nerves IV, VII, X, and XII. Occasionally, enkephalin cell bodies can be seen within reticular formation.

The n. ambiguus contains enkephalin fibers and terminals. The lateral border of the n. reticularis magnocellularis contains enkephalin fibers. The n. tractus solitarii throughout its extension in the medulla oblongata contains immunoreactive fibers and terminals. This is continuous with the enkephalin-positive fibers in the n. dorsalis motoris nervi vagi. Furthermore, it is continuous laterally with the subnucleus zonalis, which caps the n. caudalis tractus spinalis nervi trigemini. The subnucleus zonalis contains enkephalin fibers and terminals. The enkephalin fibers and terminals in the n. subzonalis appear to be connected with the network of enkephalin fibers and terminals existing in the substantia gelatinosa of the spinal cord. Some enkephalin cell bodies are observed in the n. tractus spinalis nervi trigemini. At the lower end of the brain stem, n. commissuralis contains fibers and terminals that appear to be continuous with the enkephalin fibers and terminals in the n. tractus solitarii dorsally and the n. hypoglossi ventrally. The n. cuneatus medialis does not reveal any positive staining.

e. Spinal Cord. In the spinal cord, laminae I, II, VI, VII, and X show enkephalin fibers and terminals. The dense network of stained fibers can be seen in laminae I and II. Only the lateral portions of the laminae appears to contain enkephalin-positive fibers. These fibers are continuous with those of laminae VI, VII, and X. Some examples of immunohistochemical staining for enkephalin in the nervous system are illustrated in Figs. 4–6.

As mentioned above, several other groups have reported a distribution similar to that reported here. In some studies the distribution of enkephalins has been compared with that of other peptides, in particular β-endorphin, substance P, and neurotensin, and also with the distribution of opioid receptors as revealed by autoradiography.

Comparison of the distribution of [Met⁵]-enkephalin and substance P shows that the distribution of cell bodies and nerve endings containing

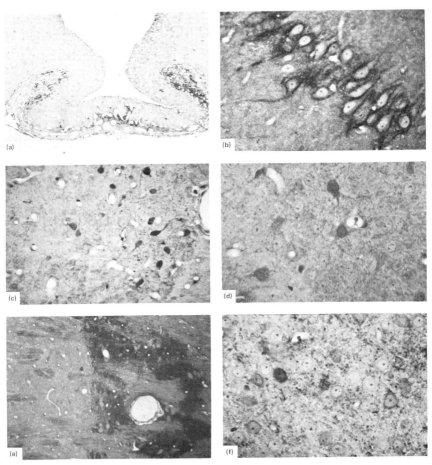

FIG. 4. Immunoperoxidase staining of rat brain using anti-[Leu⁵]-enkephalin antisera. (a) Median eminence; (b) hippocampus; (c) interpeduncular nucleus; (d) nucleus accumbens; (e) globus pallidus; (f) central amygdaloid nucleus. Unpublished observations of M. Sar, W. Stumpf, R. J. Miller, K.-J. Chang, and P. Cuatrecasas.

both these peptides have been observed to overlap in many areas of the central nervous system thought to be involved in the transmission of pain sensations (Hökfelt et al., 1977b). These areas include the periaqueductal central gray, the n. raphe magnus, the marginal layer of the substantia gelatinosa of the spinal trigeminal nucleus, and the dorsal horn of the spinal cord. The authors of this study suggest that the enkephalin-containing neurons are probably interneurons within the spinal cord, as enkephalin immunofluorescence is not depleted after transsection of the cord at the thoracic level or after unilateral dorsal rhizotomy. The authors hypothesize that stimulation-produced analgesia is related to the activation of spinal and spinal trigeminal enkephalinergic interneurons forming axo–axonic synapses with substance P containing pain afferents in the superficial laminae of the dorsal horn and spinal trigeminal nucleus. It is interesting to note that substance P has been reported to produce naloxone-reversible analgesia in the rat (Stewart et al., 1976); in addition, interactions between enkephalin and substance P at the biochemical level have been reported. Thus the electrically stimulated release of substance P from the spinal cord can be inhibited by enkephalins (Jessell and Iversen, 1977).

Uhl et al. (1977) have drawn attention to the fact that staining for enkephalin and neurotensin overlaps considerably in the nervous system. Areas containing high concentrations of both peptides include the substantia gelatinosa zones of the spinal cord and trigeminal nuclear complex. The n. tractus solitarius, the vagal nucleus, the periventricular thalamus, the central amygdala, the median eminence, the mediobasal hypothalamus, the stria terminalis, and the interstitial nucleus of the stria terminalis. However, it is not known at present what functional significance, if any, may be ascribed to this proximity of distribution. In addition, no interaction has as yet been demonstrated between the two systems.

The same group of workers have also compared the distribution of enkephalin immunofluorescence to that of the opioid receptor as revealed by their autoradiographic studies utilizing tritiated opioids, primarily [^{3}H]-diprenorphine (Simantov et al., 1977b). It is quite clear that in most cases the distribution of the two entities corresponds closely. However, there are cases where the two do not match up. For example, although the caudate-putamen displays a high density of opioid receptor grains, it shows only a low, patchy distribution of enkephalin immunofluorescence. The staining is localized mainly in the dorsal and ventral region whereas the distribution of opioid receptors is rather uniform. The authors therefore suggest that many of the opioid

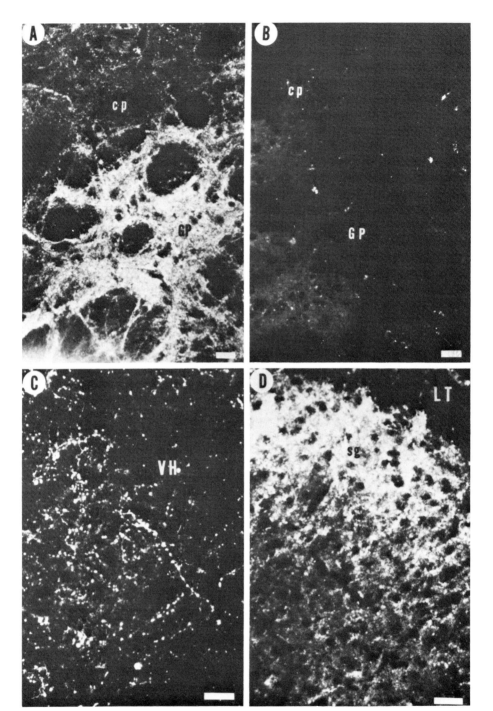

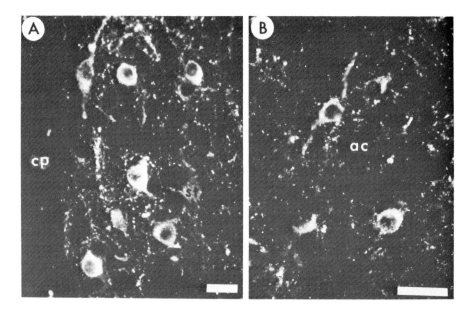

FIG. 6. Immunofluorescence micrographs of [Leu⁵]-enkephalin immunoreactivity from brain of colchicine-pretreated rats. (A) Nucleus interstitialis of the stria terminalis (st); cp, caudate-putamen. (B) Central amygdaloid nucleus (ac). Pictures by courtesy of Dr. George Uhl. Bar = 25 μm.

receptors in this region may be presynaptic in nature. The existence of such presynaptic opioid receptors has been previously demonstrated in another system (La Motte *et al.*, 1976). A similar situation occurs in the cerebral cortex, where considerable levels of opioid receptors are found but only scattered enkephalin immunoreactivity. In the spinal cord, the ventral gray matter and an area surrounding the central canal display fluorescent enkephalin fibers, but no detectable opioid receptor grains. In such a case, the authors suggest that they may be localizing enkephalinergic fibers "en passant" that may synapse elsewhere (Fig. 7).

Some work has begun on elucidating the pathways linking the vari-

FIG. 5. Immunofluorescence micrographs: (A and B) the globus pallidus (GP) and nucleus caudate-putamen (cp); (C) the cervical spinal cord showing the ventral ham (VH); and (D) Lissauer's tract (LT) and the substantia gelatinosa (sg). Staining was carried out with anti-[Leu⁵]-enkephalin antisera. (B) is a control in which antisera were absorbed overnight with 1 mM [Leu⁵]-enkephalin. Adapted from Simantov *et al.* (1977b). Pictures by courtesy of Dr. George Uhl. Bar = 25 μm.

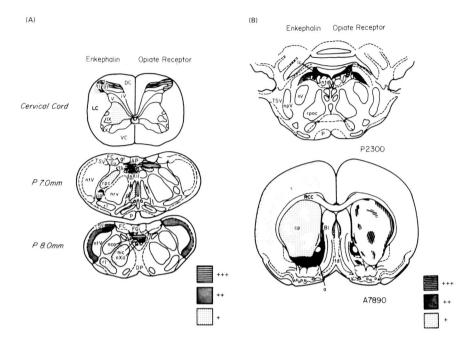

FIG. 7. Comparison of enkephalin immunoreactivity and opioid receptor distribution in rat brain. (A) Abbreviations: AP, area postrema; cu, nucleus cuneatus; DC, dorsal column; DP, decussatio pyramidis; FC, fasciculus cuneatus; FG, fasciculus gracilis; gr, nucleus gracilis; io, nucleus olivaris inferior; LC, lateral column; nco, nucleus commissuralis; nic, nucleus intercalatus; nrv, nucleus reticularis medullae oblongatae pars ventralis; ntV, nucleus tractus spinalis nervi trigemini; nXII nucleus origins nervi hypoglossi; P, tractus corticospinalis; rl, nucleus reticularis lateralis; rpc, nucleus reticularis parvocellularis; ts, tractus solitarius; TSV, tractus spinalis nervi trigemini; VC, ventral column. (B) Abbreviations: a, nucleus accumbens; cp, nucleus caudatus-putamen; lc, locus caeruleus; npV, nucleus principalis nervi trigemini; ntd, nucleus tegmenti dorsalis Gudden; nV, nucleus origins nervi trigemini; P, tractus corticospinalis, RCC, radiatio corporis callosi; rpoc, nucleus reticularis pontis caudalis; td, nucleus tractus diag. nolis (Broca); TSV, tractus spinalis nervi trigemini. Adapted from Simantov *et al.* (1977b).

ous sets of cell bodies and terminals so far described in the brain. Three groups of lesioning experiments have been reported: (a) Elde, Hokfelt and colleagues reported that lesions in the hypothalamic paraventricular nucleus decreased enkephalin immunoreactivity in the median eminence and have therefore suggested the existence of a paraventricular/perifornical–median eminence enkephalinergic pathway (Elde *et al.*, 1978). (b) C. Cuello (personal communication) has found that placing a knife cut between the caudate and globus pallidus reduces enkephalin immunoreactivity in the globus pallidus. Now the globus pallidus appears to contain enkephalinergic terminals exclusively, whereas the caudate contains terminals and a number of cell bodies as well. Thus it may be that an enkephalinergic pathways exists with cell bodies in the caudate and terminals in the globus pallidus. Support for this hypothesis comes from data showing that injection of kainic acid into the striatum reduces enkephalin content (Hong et al., 1977c). Kainic acid probably acts by destroying neuronal cell bodies close to the point of injection (Coyle and Schwartz, 1976; McGreer and McGreer, 1976). (c) Lesions of the central amygdala have been shown to cause a depletion of enkephalin immunoreactivity in the stria terminalis and in the interstitial nucleus of the stria terminalis. It therefore appears that an enkephalinergic pathway exists, running from cell bodies in the central amygdaloid nucleus and giving rise to terminals in the interestitial nucleus of the stria terminalis (Uhl et al., 1978).

It should be noted that enkephalin staining in the central nervous system is unaffected by hypophysectomy, again indicating that central enkephalin is not derived from the pituitary. This is in agreement with the data from radioimmunoassay discussed above.

Recently [Met[5]]-enkephalin immunoreactivity has been successfully localized at the electron microscopic level and compared to the localization of substance P and tyrosine hydroxylase in the locus caeruleus and A_2 regions (Pickel et al., 1978). In this study both [Met[5]]-enkephalin and substance P were seen to be localized in both large and small vesicles, exclusively found in axons and axon terminals (Fig. 8). Tyrosine hydroxylase, on the other hand, labeled only dendrites and dendritic spines. Staining of serial sections suggests that enkephalin and/or substance P nerve terminals form synapses on tyrosine hydroxylase containing dendrites. Thus, in both the locus caeruleus and A_2 regions, enkephalin- and substance P-labeled terminals form asymmetric contacts with catecholamine-containing neurons, an arrangement that is consistent with the fact that both enkephalin and substance P exert effects on the catecholaminergic system.

2. β-Endorphin/β-Lipotropin

As indicated previously, it has been demonstrated by radioimmunoassay that both β-lipotropin and β-endorphin probably exist in the central nervous system. Recently, some data have been reported on the distribution of these substances as revealed by immunohistochemistry. There are some areas of overlap between the reported

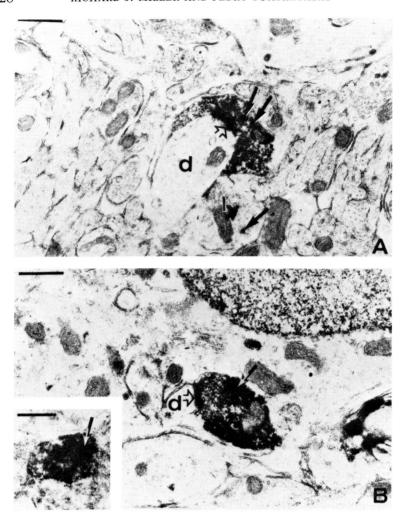

FIG. 8. Ultrastructural localization of [Met^5]-enkephalin in A$_2$ region of the medulla. (A) Axon terminal labeled specifically with enkephalin forms an asymmetric contact (open arrow) with dendrite (d). An intense accumulation of reaction product is associated with large granular vesicles (arrows). Small vesicles are also labeled. An unlabeled axon terminal forming a synapse with the same dendrite contains both dense granular vesicle (arrow) and smaller clear vesicles. Lead precipitate (l) is also seen. Bar = 0.5 μm. (B) Enkephalin-labeled axon terminal containing both large dense vesicles (black and white arrow) and smaller clear or dense vesicles forms an asymmetric contact (open arrow) with the small dendrite or dendritic spine (d). Inset in (B) shows a small axon labeled with enkephalin. Labeled granular particles (arrow) are not as evident as in the substance P-labeled axons. Bar = 0.5 μm. Picture by courtesy of Dr. Virginia Pickel.

distribution of β-lipotropin/β-endorphin and that of enkephalin, but there are also major differences. It is not completely clear whether antisera or β-endorphin and β-lipotropin stain exactly the same cells, although the patterns are very similar and this seems likely to be the case (Bloom *et al.*, 1978; Watson *et al.*, 1977a) (Fig. 9). In general, these two peptides are not nearly as widely distributed as the enkephalins. The difference in staining patterns of neuronal perikarya is particularly striking. Enkephalin-positive cell bodies are very widely distributed in the central nervous system. However, in the case of β-lipotropin and β-endorphin, positive cell bodies have been reported so far only in the basal hypothalamus. One group of β-endorphin-positive cells is found dorsolateral to the arcuate nucleus in its middle to posterior third while the second group is more lateral and anterior in the basal hypothalamus. Some cells form a continuous line across the floor of the third ventricle. It seems, therefore, that antisera to β-endorphin and to [Met⁵] and [Leu⁵]-enkephalin on the whole stain different cell populations (Bloom *et al.*, 1978). The processes of the β-endorphin cell bodies

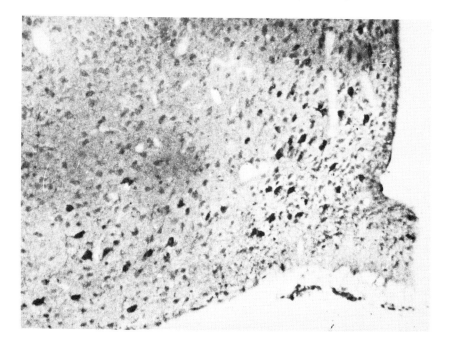

FIG. 9. Immunoperoxidase localization of β-endorphin-containing cell bodies in the rat hypothalamus. Picture by courtesy of Dr. Floyd Bloom.

in the basal hypothalamus are restricted to mainly midline terminal fields near the ventricular surfaces. Fibers are dense in the anterior hypothalamus, especially within the stria terminalis. Also within the hypothalamus, the paraventricular supraoptic and suprachiasmatic nuclei are clearly innervated, as is the median eminence. Other areas of innervation are the locus caeruleus, dorsal raphe, and midline structures within the thalamic and pontine periaqueductal gray, especially the anterior paraventricular nucleus. Under some conditions, staining can also be seen in other structures, particularly cortical areas of the limbic system, hippocampus, cerebellum, cingulate gyrus, and prepyriform and rhinencephalic cortex. However, in this case the staining can be blocked by preincubating the antiserum with myelin basic protein. This interesting crossreactivity of β-endorphin antisera to myelin basic protein has been discussed above.

The reported distribution of β-lipotropin staining in the brain is similar to that reported for β-endorphin, especially insofar as cell bodies are concerned (Watson et al., 1977a). Area of overlap between the staining of β-lipotropin or β-endorphin and that of enkephalin include the hypothalamus, periaqueductal gray, lateral septal nucleus, lateral reticular formation, zona compacta of the substantia nigra, and the periventricular nucleus of the thalamus. However, the above discussion clearly shows that there are also striking differences in distribution patterns, the globus pallidus being the most remarkable. Considering that this area has the highest enkephalin content in the brain, its paucity of β-lipotropin or β-endorphin is surprising. Other areas, however, such as the central amygdaloid nucleus, also show these staining differences.

One especially interesting recent observation is that the hypothalamic cell bodies that stain for β-endorphin/β-lipotropin also stain with antisera to ACTH (F. Bloom, personal communication). This observations fits in with staining and biochemical data from the pituitary showing that β-lipotropin and ACTH are synthesized as part of a large precursor molecule (MW $\simeq$ 31,000) known as "Big ACTH" (see above). ACTH itself has been detected in the brain by radioimmunoassay (Krieger et al., 1977a,b). Thus, it appears that the same biosynthetic mechanisms may be operative in the nervous system, although "Big ACTH" itself has not yet been unequivocally identified in nervous tissue.

It is useful, at this stage, to examine the evidence pertaining to the possible precursor relationships of β-lipotropin and β-endorphin to [Met^5]-enkephalin. It is clear that β-endorphin and [Met^5]-enkephalin antisera do not stain the same cells for the most part. It cannot be argued from this observation, however, that β-endorphin does not exist in the same cells as [Met^5]-enkephalin. The relevant factor here would be the rate of conversion of β-endorphin to [Met^5]-enkephalin. Thus, one does not observe dopamine by histofluorescence in noradrenergic neurons although dopamine is certainly the biosynthetic precursor to norepinephrine. However, if β-endorphin is ultimately derived from "Big ACTH," one might expect cells that stain for [Met^5]-enkephalin to stain for ACTH even if they do not stain for β-endorphin. This is certainly not the case in the central nervous system and in the gut (see below). Although one might argue that cells that rapidly convert β-endorphin to [Met^5]-enkephalin might also have some means of rapidly destroying ACTH, it is merely speculation at this point.

To conclude, therefore, there seem to be two separate neuronal systems—one staining for the enkephalins and the other staining for β-lipotropin or β-endorphin and also for ACTH. Whether a rapidly turning over pool of β-endorphin will ultimately be found to exist in enkephalinergic neurons awaits the relevant biochemical studies.

B. PITUITARY

High concentrations of β-endorphin are found in the pituitary glands of several species. Staining with anti-β-endorphin antibody is localized primarily in the intermediate lobe, where every cell stains heavily, and in scattered cells in the anterior lobe (Bloom et al., 1977a) (Fig. 10). These same cells also stain for ACTH and anti-α-endorphin, and anti-β-lipotropin antibodies also give the same staining patterns. All these data are consistent with the proposed mechanism of biosynthesis of ACTH and β-lipotropin already discussed at length above.

Staining with enkephalin antisera is slightly more complicated. We have observed staining of cells in the intermediate and anterior lobes with antisera to both [Met^5]- and [Leu^5]-enkephalins, although the former is more effective. These cells, again, also stain for ACTH; i.e., the pattern is the same as with β-endorphin. In addition, using the same antisera, Bloom and colleagues have also identified fiberlike elements in the neurohypophysis that are not stained with antisera to β-endorphin or ACTH (Bloom et al., 1978). This suggests that staining with antienkephalin antisera is not due merely to crossreactivity with the high concentrations of β-endorphin found in the gland. Some workers, however, have not obtained any staining with antienkephalin antibodies in the pituitary at all (Elde et al., 1976). Seeing that the pituitary by radioimmunoassay and also by fluorescent microanalytical analysis, does appear to contain enkephalin, it is not immediately ob-

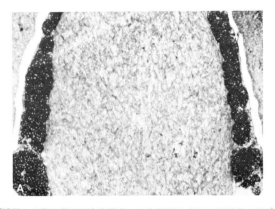

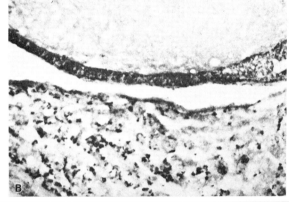

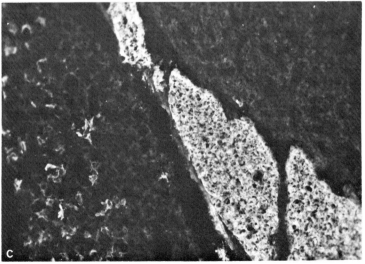

vious why no staining was seen. Possibly, it is because only [Met^5]-enkephalin appears to be made in the pituitary and antibodies to [Leu^5]-enkephalin were used. However the antibodies still had sufficient crossreactivity to [Met^5]-enkephalin that staining would have been expected. It is more likely that the antisera used were not sufficiently sensitive to pick up the levels of pituitary enkephalin.

C. GASTROINTESTINAL TRACT

It is most interesting that many neuroactive peptides are found to be localized in two main places: the central nervous system and the gastrointestinal tract. It is possible that some cells in these two tissues have a common embryological precursor (Pearse, 1976). Thus, not only enkephalin, but also several other peptides, such as substance P, are found in both localizations. The localization of enkephalin in the gut is perhaps not surprising in view of the known pharmacological effects of narcotics in this tissue. Opioid receptors have previously been demonstrated in homogenates of guinea pig myenteric plexus (Creese and Snyder, 1975). Moreover, radioimmunoassay data have illustrated the presence of enkephalins in this tissue (see above). In collaboration with Drs. I. Linnoilla and R. DiAugustine of the NIEHS, North Carolina, we have mapped out the localization of enkephalin immunoreactivity in the gut of guinea pig, hamster, and rat. This localization may be summarized as follows (Fig. 11).

Immunostaining was observed along the gastrointestinal tract as small spots and varicose fibers representing terminal nerve fibers. The immunopositive fibers were most numerous in the stomach, duodenum, and rectum of the guinea pig. In the wall of the stomach they appeared as long, beaded strings mainly dispersed along the external muscle fibers with occasional fragmentary fibers seen in the muscularis mucosae. The positive fibers throughout the stomach appeared to be more numerous and more heavily stained with [Met^5]-enkephalin than with [Leu^5]-enkephalin antiserum, which failed to react with fibers in the cardia region. In the duodenum or rectum, however, no such differences in the intensity or distribution could be observed between the two antisera. Positive fibers formed a dense plexus in the duodenum around unstained ganglion cell bodies of Meissner's plexus; individual

FIG. 10. Localization of endorphins and enkephalin in pituitary. (A) [Met^5]-enkephalin, rat pituitary; immunoperoxidase stain. Unpublished observations of M. Sar, W. Stumpf, R. J. Miller, K.-J. Chang, and P. Cuatrecasas. (B) β-Endorphin, kitten pituitary; immunoperoxidase stain. (C) α-Endorphin, rat pituitary; immunofluorescent stain. (B) and (C) Pictures by courtesy of Dr. Floyd Bloom.

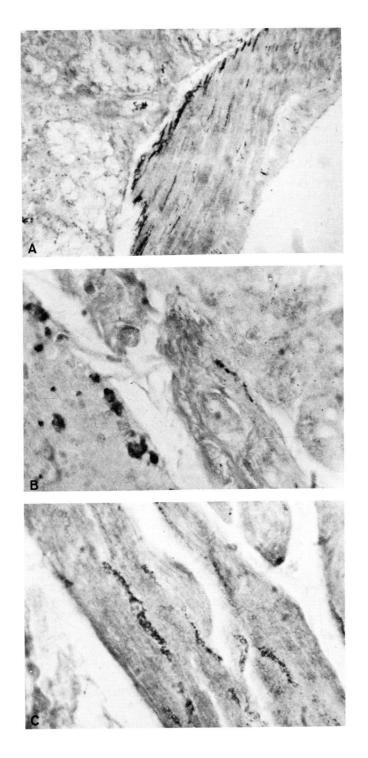

fibers were also seen in the circular muscle layer, running parallel with the muscle cells and occasionally surrounding a submucosal gland. In the lower part of the rectum, numerous stained beaded fibers were demonstrated in the circular muscle layer, often closely surrounding an unstained cell. Only a few immunopositive fibers were located in the longitudinal muscle layer. In the rectosigmoid region, a few scattered immunopositive fibers were seen in both external muscle layers.

In the jejunum and ileum of the guinea pig the immunostained fibers were numerous and were observed mainly in Meissner's plexus and in the circular muscle layer. Some structures staining as small spots were occasionally observed in Auerbach's plexus. No nerve fibers or other structures could be demonstrated in the cecum with these enkephalin antisera. In the colon of the guinea pig, nerve fibers were located among the circular muscle layers and appeared to be better stained with [Leu^5]- than with [Met^5]-enkephalin antiserum. In the esophagus of the guinea pig, few immunopositive nerve fibers could be found using [Met^5]-enkephalin antiserum. Immunopositive nerve fibers were observed in the walls of common bile duct and gallbladder, but not in the pancreas of the guinea pig. In spite of the application of several different fixation methods, no positive nerve cell bodies or epithelial cells could be identified in the gastrointestinal tract with enkephalin antisera. In the hamster, and particularly in the rat, the staining of the nerve fibers of gastrointestinal tract wall was considerably less intense than that observed with the guinea pig.

No immunostaining was observed for the gastrointestinal tract (or pituitary gland) following incubations with control serum (normal rabbit serum). The preincubation of [Leu^5]-enkephalin antiserum with [Leu^5]- or [Met^5]-enkephalin completely inhibited immunostaining in the gastrointestinal tract. [Met^5]-enkephalin antiserum was inactivated by [Met^5]- but not [Leu^5]-enkephalin. No immunopositive staining of nerve fibers or cells in the gastrointestinal tract was seen with antisera against (1–24) ACTH, (1–39) ACTH, or α-MSH. The presence of enkephalin in the gut fits in well with the known effects of morphine on gastrointestinal motility. The antidiarrheal effects of morphine and related opioids occur by enhancing the activity of intestinal circular muscle (Plant and Miller, 1926). Increased circular muscle activity produces a synchronous segmentation, and this in turn causes a reduc-

FIG. 11. Enkephalin localization in guinea pig gastrointestinal tract. (A) Duodenum; immunoperoxidase stain, anti-[Leu^5]-enkephalin. (B) Duodenum; immunoperoxidase stain, anti-[Met^5]-enkephalin. (C) Pylorus of the stomach; immunoperoxidase stain, anti-[Met^5]-enkephalin.

tion of intestinal propulsive movements (Ludwick *et al.*, 1968, 1970). In contrast, intestinal longitudinal muscle is usually not affected or is slightly relaxed after administration of opioids (Bass and Wiley, 1965).

One other report has appeared concerning staining of the gut for enkephalin immunoreactivity in the baboon and man (Polak *et al.*, 1977). This paper also reported staining nerve fibers with a similar distribution to those described above. However, in addition staining was seen in numerous endocrine cells in the midzone of the central mucosa. An extremely surprising observation, however, was that the endocrine cells also stained for gastrin and were tentatively identified as G cells. That such cells were not seen in the guinea pig may be due to interspecies differences, which occur extensively among the gastrointestinal endocrine cells of different species. As noted above, the enkephalin-containing cells in the guinea pig do not stain for ACTH (or α-MSH), as is probably the case for most enkephalin-containing cells in the nervous system. The labeling of the gut enkephalin-containing cells with antigastrin antibody raises the possibility that the biosynthesis of enkephalin may be linked to gastrin rather than ACTH. This possibility has not, however, been investigated as yet.

VI. Interaction with Other Neurotransmitter Systems

The various localizations of the opioid peptides described above may be compared with what is known about the distribution of other neurotransmitters in the central nervous system, particularly the biogenic amines. Such a comparison suggests that there may be an anatomical basis for interaction between the opioid peptides and these other systems. Some data already obtained point to this likelihood.

One may be struck, for example, by the number of instances in which the distribution of enkephalin and dopamine overlap. Such areas of overlap include the nucleus accumbens, basal hypothalamus, the central amygdaloid nucleus, and the striatum. However, it is true that in the striatum enkephalin is localized mainly in the globus pallidus, whereas dopamine is localized in the caudate and putamen. So far, reports on the interaction of opioid peptides with dopaminergic systems are rather confusing. The most basic observation is a report demonstrating the presence of opioid receptors as monitored by [^{3}H][Leu^5]-enkephalin or [^{3}H]-naloxone binding on dopaminergic neurons in the striatum (Pollard *et al.*, 1977). Unilateral lesions of the nigrostriatal dopaminergic pathway induced by injecting 6-OH-dopamine or by electrocoagulation of the substantia nigra produced a decrease in receptor binding in striatal membranes compared to the unlesioned side of the animal. One might now ask if such opioid receptors have any function in the control of dopamine metabolism or release. Here, reports are a little at variance with one another. It has been reported that the electrically stimulated release of dopamine from striatal slices can be inhibited by β-endorphin in a naloxone-reversible fashion (Loh et al., 1976b). One might therefore expect dopamine metabolism in the striatum as assessed by turnover experiments to be slowed by β-endorphin or enkephalins. However, the opposite has been reported in several studies (Van Loon and Kim, 1977; Fuxe et al., 1977; Izumi et al., 1977). In the hypothalamus, on the other hand, opioid peptides do decrease dopamine turnover (Ferland et al., 1977). This latter observation is certainly in line with the hypothesis that the effects of opioids and opioid peptides on prolactin release are mediated in the hypothalamus by an inhibitory effect on dopaminergic transmission. Not only can opioid peptides affect dopamine metabolism, but dopaminergic antagonists, i.e., neuroleptics, have been shown to affect concentrations of [Met^5]-enkephalin in the striatum although not in the hypothalamus. Acute haloperidol treatment failed to alter [Met^5]-enkephalin levels, but chronic treatment with chlorpromazine, haloperidol, or pimozide caused an increase in striatal concentrations (Hong et al., 1977b). Clozapine, which is supposed to produce a minimal amount of Parkinsonian side effects, did not raise striatal enkephalin levels. In studies with normal rats, L. L. Iversen et al. (personal communication) did not observe any effect of neuroleptics on the electrically stimulated release of enkephalin from slices of the globus pallidus. However, they did not examine release in animals that had been chronically treated with neuroleptics.

Several reports have been published on the ability of intracerebrally injected opioid peptides to produce hypermotility, an effect also produced by morphine. Pert and Sivet (1977) reported that both [D-Ala^2, MetNH$_2$^{5}]-enkephalin and apomorphine injected into the nucleus accumbens of rats produced hypermotility. The apomorphine effect, but not the peptide effect, could be inhibited by haloperidol, and the effect of the peptide was selectively blocked by naloxone. The authors therefore suggested that two independent systems may mediate these effects, one dopaminergic and one "enkephalinergic." In contrast, Baxter et al. (1977a) reported that intraventricular injection of [D-Ala^2, D-Leu^5]-enkephalin in mice produced hypermotility, but in this case these effects or similar ones produced by morphine were blocked by intraperitoneal injections of chlorpromazine, a result indicating that they were mediated by dopaminergic systems. The effect of [D-Ala^2,D-Leu^5]-enkephalin was extremely potent, being nearly 50 times more potent than morphine. Similar results were reported by Wei et al. (1977)

who found that [D-Ala,^{2},D-Leu^5]-enkephalin was far more effective than either morphine or [D-Ala^2,MetHN$_2$^{5}]-enkephalin in producing hypermotility. In addition, it was also shown that β-endorphin produced hardly any hypermotility at doses where it produced profound analgesia and that β-endorphin and [D-Ala^2,D-Leu^5]-enkephalin were equally effective in producing analgesia.

Dill and Costa (1977) reported results again implicating the nucleus accumbens in mediating some of the behavioral effects of morphine on opioid peptides. Thus, the analgesia and catalepsy elicited by subcutaneous morphine was blocked by the intracranial bilateral injection of naltrexone when the opioid antagonist was injected into the nucleus accumbens. Injection of naltrexone into the caudate had no such effects. In addition, morphine injected directly into the nucleus accumbens produced catalepsy and analgesia; however, injection of morphine into the caudate was ineffective. It is surprising that morphine injection into the nucleus accumbens in this study produced analgesia, and this may suggest some spreading of the drug from the site of injection.

Apart from interactions with dopaminergic systems, there are also indications of interactions of enkephalinergic systems with other neurotransmitters. In the case of norepinephrine there is the classic example of the mouse vas deferens, where opioid agonists and, in particular, opioid peptides are known to cause a decrease in the electrically stimulated outflow of norepinephrine from the tissue (Waterfield et al., 1977). In the CNS the stimulated release of norepinephrine from hypothalamic slices can be inhibited by [Met^5]-enkephalin in a naloxone-reversible fashion (Taube et al., 1976). Cholinergic mechanisms also appear to be altered by opioid peptides. Again, one has a classic example in the case of the electrically stimulated guinea pig myenteric plexus. This time opioids and opioid peptides serve to inhibit the release of acetylcholine from the stimulated tissue (Waterfield et al., 1977). Centrally, opioids and opioid peptides decrease the turnover of acetylcholine in various brain regions, including the cortex, hippocampus, nucleus accumbens, and globus pallidus (Moroni et al., 1977). At a biochemical level, the nicotinic antagonist d-tubocurarine has been shown to inhibit the binding of [^{3}H][Met^5]-enkephalin to opioid receptors in synaptic membranes at high concentrations (Somoza and Portal, 1977).

Opioid peptides may also interact with other "peptidergic" systems. The close parallel between the distribution of enkephalin and substance P in some instances has been discussed above. Some reports have suggested that substance P can produce analgesia in a naloxone-reversible fashion, suggesting that it may be acting by releasing endogenous opioid material (Stewart et al., 1976). In a particularly interesting series of studies, Jessell and Iversen (1977) showed that the potassium-stimulated release of substance P from the rat trigeminal nucleus could be blocked by β-endorphin, [D-Ala^2,MetNH$_2$^{5}]-enkephalin or various narcotic agonists in a stereospecific, naloxone-reversible fashion. The potassium-stimulated release of substance P from the substantia nigra, however, was not inhibited in this way, again indicating the specificity of the effect.

It also seems possible that enkephalins may regulate their own synthesis and release via some presynaptic mechanism. This possibility was raised by Simantov and Snyder (1976c), who reported an increase in brain opioid peptide activity in morphine-addicted rats. However, Fratta et al. (1977) were unable to confirm these results when measuring [Met^5]-enkephalin concentration selectivity by radioimmunoassay. These authors were also unable to show any change in [Met^5]-enkephalin content following repeated administration of foot shock to animals. This is, again, in contrast to prior studies which had suggested that such treatment does increase the content of some unidentified brain opioid fraction (Madden et al., 1977).

Finally, Baxter et al. (1977b) reported that after intraventricular injection of 5 μg of [D-Ala^2,D-Leu^5]-enkephalin in rats, immediate electroencephalogram (EEG) spiking was induced followed by facial and forelimb clonus. Moreover, other recent observations suggest that endogenous opioid peptides may play a role in epileptogenesis. Intracerebroventricular injection of [Met^5]-enkephalin or β-endorphin produced a rapid onset of epileptiform discharges in the EEG of rats (Bloom et al., 1978; Urca et al., 1977). This seizure activity appears to be restricted primarily to limbic structures and not to extend into motor systems. Such observations are preliminary but extremely tantalizing and illustrate one area on which the discovery of opioid peptides may lead to the introduction of novel therapies to treat various disorders.

VII. NEUROENDOCRINE EFFECTS

It has been known for some time that morphine and other opioid drugs may increase the release of prolactin, growth hormone, and vasopressin in animals following peripheral or intraventricular administration (George and Way, 1955, 1959; Ferland et al., 1976; Kokka et al., 1972; Tolis et al., 1975; Weitzman et al., 1977). It is not completely clear whether these are direct effects on the pituitary or mediated via the hypothalamus. The discovery of the opioid peptides and the localization

TABLE IV

RELEASING EFFECTS OF OPIOID PEPTIDES ON ANTERIOR PITUITARY HORMONES[a]

Agent	In vivo			In vitro	Reference
	Intra-ventricular	Intra-venous	Ip/sc		
[Leu⁵]	↑PL/GH↑				Cocchi et al. (1977)
β-End	↑PL/GH↑				
[Met⁵]	↑PL/GH↑				
[D-Ala²,MetNH₂⁵]	↑PL/GH↑				
[D-Ala²,Met⁵]	↑PL/GH↑				
[NAcTyr¹Met⁵]	N.E.				
[D-Tyr¹Met⁵]	N.E.				
α-End		PL↑			Dupont et al. (1977a)
[D-Ala²,α-End]		PL↑			
[D-Ala²,Met⁵]		PL↑			Cusan et al. (1977)
[D-Ala²,MetNH₂⁵]		PL↑			
[Leu⁵]			PL↑		May et al. (1977)
[Met⁵]			N.E.		
β-End	↑PL/GH↑				
[D-Ala²,MetNH₂⁵]	↑PL/GH↑				
α-End	↑PL/GH N.E.				Chihara et al. (1977)
γ-End	↑PL/GH N.E.				
[Met⁵]	↑PL/GH N.E.				
[D-Trp²,MetNH₂⁵]				N.E. PL/GH↑	Bowers et al. (1977)
[D-Phe²,MetNH₂⁵]				↑GH,↑LH,↑FSH	

Peptide					Reference
$[Met^5]$		PL↑	PL↑	PL↑	Lien et al. (1976)
$[Leu^5]$				PL↑	
β-End		GH↑			Dupont et al. (1977c)
$[Met^5]$		GH↑			
β-End	↑PL/GH↑	PL↑		N.E.	Rivier et al. (1977)
α-End		N.E.		N.E.	
$[Met^5]$		N.E.		N.E.	
β-End	↑PL/GH↑	↑PL/GH↑			Dupont et al. (1977b,c)
$[Met^5]$	↑PL/GH↑	↑PL/GH↑			
$[Met^5]$				PL↑	Hall et al. (1976)
$[Leu^5]$				PL↑	
$[Met^5]$	PL↑	PL↑			Ferland et al. (1977)
$[Met^5]$			↑PL,GH↑, ↓LH,TSH↓		Bruni et al. (1977)
$[MetNH_2^5]$		N.E. GH/PL N.E.		N.E. GH/PL N.E.	Shaar et al. (1977)
$[d\text{-}Ala^2,MetNH_2^5]$		↑GH/PL↑		N.E. GH/PL N.E.	
$[d\text{-}Ala^2,LeuNH_2^5]$		↑GH/PL↑		N.E. GH/PL N.E.	

[a] PL, prolactin; GH, growth hormone; FSH, follicle-stimulating hormone; N.E., no effect; ↑, increase; ↓, decrease; Ip/sc, intraperitoneal or subcutaneous; LH, lutenizing hormone; TSH, thyroid-stimulating hormone.

of enkephalinergic neurons in the median eminence has made these observations of great interest. There have now been several reports on the effects of opioid peptides on the release of prolactin and growth hormone and one on the release of vasopressin. These results have differed somewhat according to the route of administration used, but in general the results show that opioid peptides are effective in causing the release of prolactin, growth hormone, and vasopressin; in addition, it appears that the release of LH and TSH is depressed. These results are summarized in Table IV. It also seems that in general the prolactin response is rather more sensitive than the growth hormone response. In addition, β-endorphin is usually considerably more potent than [Met^5]- or [Leu^5]-enkephalin. However, pentapeptides being very rapidly metabolized in comparison to β-endorphin, this is not surprising. In fact, when stable enkephalin analogs are utilized, they show high potency. Although not all workers have checked to see whether the effects they observe are naloxone reversible, those workers who have done so have found naloxone to be effective, indicating that the effects are truly mediated by opioid receptors.

Recently, we studied the ability of a wide range of structural analogs of enkephalin to produce prolactin release in the rat. Table V summarizes the results of this study.

Eleven of 19 synthetic enkephalin analogs increased plasma prolactin levels following intraventricular injection (Table V). [Met^5]- and [Leu^5]-enkephalins increased plasma prolactin levels at 10 minutes but not at 30 minutes. They were of equivalent potency. Seven of the enkephalin analogs (Nos. 3–9 in Table V) increased prolactin levels in both the 10-minute and 30-minute samples. All were of equivalent potency with the exception of Tyr-D-Ala-Gly-pClPhe-D-LeuNHEt, which produced greater plasma prolactin levels than any other analog at both 10 and 30 minutes. Four compounds increased plasma prolactin levels in only the 10-minute sample (Nos. 10–13 in Table V). Eight compounds (Nos. 14–21 in Table V) were inactive.

As might be expected, analogs with a [D-Ala^2]-substitution, which conveys metabolic stability (see below), produced the most *prolonged* increases in plasma prolactin levels. However, the capacity to produce prolonged increases in prolactin secretion is not tightly coupled to opioid receptor affinity. Three of the 4 enkephalins that produced increased plasma prolactin only at 10 minutes had opioid receptor affinities of 2 to $9 \times 10^{-9} M$, whereas the fourth such compound had an affinity constant of only $5 \times 10^{-5} M$. On the other hand, most of the compounds that produced prolonged increases in plasma prolactin

TABLE V
Effect of Enkephalin and Enkephalin Analogs on Plasma Prolactin Levels in Male Rats[a]

	Plasma prolactin (ng/ml)			Opioid receptor affinity (M)
	Preinjection	10 Min	30 Min	
1. Tyr-Gly-Gly-Phe-Met	13.0 ± 4.5	32.0 ± 10.3	5.7 ± 1.8	2×10^{-8}
2. Tyr-Gly-Gly-Phe-Leu	11.9 ± 3.4	28.1 ± 5.0	8.0 ± 2.9	1.1×10^{-8}
3. Tyr-D-Ala-Gly-Phe-D-LeuNHEt	18.7 ± 10.6	36.1 ± 7.1	29.0 ± 9.4	1×10^{-8}
4. Tyr-D-Ala-Gly-Phe	10.1 ± 3.9	32.6 ± 4.4	32.4 ± 1.9	7×10^{-8}
5. Tyr-D-NMeAla-Gly-Phe-D-LeuOMe	6.2 ± 1.0	36.2 ± 3.5	20.5 ± 5.4	9×10^{-8}
6. Tyr-D-Ala-Gly-Phe-D-Leu	2.2 ± 0.8	41.5 ± 9.5	23.0 ± 4.3	2.6×10^{-9}
7. Tyr-D-Ala-Gly-pClPhe-D-LeuNHEt	13.4 ± 6.3	62.0 ± 20.6	47.4 ± 14.3	8×10^{-8}
8. NMeTyr-D-Ala-Gly-Phe-D-MetNH$_2$	10.4 ± 4.3	30.5 ± 7.2	32.5 ± 6.6	3×10^{-7}
9. NMeTyr-D-Ala-Gly-Phe-D-LeuNH$_2$	10.3 ± 5.6	30.7 ± 6.0	29.8 ± 2.8	2×10^{-8}
10. Tyr-D-Ala-Gly-Phe-Met-Thr	12.4 ± 2.8	34.0 ± 6.9	12.8 ± 5.3	5.6×10^{-9}
11. Tyr-D-Ala-Gly-pClPhe-DLeuOMe	10.3 ± 6.0	37.0 ± 7.6	16.0 ± 3.3	2×10^{-9}
12. Tyr-D-Trp-Gly-Phe-Leu	11.7 ± 2.1	23.4 ± 5.9	14.0 ± 3.2	9×10^{-9}
13. Tyr-Gly-Gly-TyrOMe-LeuOMe	12.8 ± 2.7	30.9 ± 6.4	12.6 ± 4.7	5×10^{-5}
14. Tyr-D-Trp-Gly-Phe-D-Leu	15.4 ± 3.5	16.1 ± 3.3	12.4 ± 3.4	8×10^{-6}
15. Tyr-D-Ala-Gly-Phe-D-Met	12.5 ± 5.2	18.9 ± 5.3	8.6 ± 3.3	1×10^{-8}
16. Tyr-Gly-Ala-Phe-Leu	21.0 ± 4.9	18.1 ± 2.4	11.3 ± 3.0	8×10^{-6}
17. Tyr-Gly-Gly-D-Phe-Leu	5.1 ± 2.4	7.4 ± 2.1	3.3 ± 0.9	$>10^{-4}$
18. Tyr-D-Ala-Gly-Leu-Leu	11.3 ± 4.5	19.5 ± 6.4	11.5 ± 6.2	$>10^{-4}$
19. D-Tyr-D-Ala-Gly-Phe-Leu	19.2 ± 6.0	24.1 ± 5.0	13.0 ± 2.8	3×10^{-4}
20. D-Ala-Gly-LeuOMe	23.9 ± 4.2	29.8 ± 4.9	26.9 ± 5.0	$>10^{-4}$
21. Phe-D-Ala-Gly-Phe-Leu	12.5 ± 5.9	19.4 ± 5.8	7.3 ± 4.2	1×10^{-7}

[a] Unpublished observations of H. Meltzer, R. J. Miller, R. Fessler, V. Fang, and M. Simonovic.

levels had opioid receptor affinity constants between $1 \times 10^{-7} M$ and $9 \times 10^{-8} M$.

In general, the ability of the various analogs to release prolactin correlates closely with their *effectiveness* in the opioid receptor binding assay and other assays of biological activity, such as the guinea pig ileum, mouse vas deferens, and mouse hot-plate test for analgesia (Beddell *et al.*, 1977a; Miller *et al.*, 1978b). Thus, previous studies have shown that D-amino acid substitution in the 5-position improves biological activity in many assays, whereas such substitution in the 1 or 4 position reduces biological activity. Inspection of Table V reveals that this is usually, but not always, true with regard to prolactin secretion. However, there are some interesting differences between the sets of data. For example, the analog [D-Ala^2,D-Met^5]-enkephalin is rather ineffective in stimulating prolactin release. In contrast, it is very potent as an analgesic on intraventricular injection (Miller *et al.*, 1978b). Moreover, the analog [D-Ala^2,D-Leu^{5}NHEt]-enkephalin is effective in producing prolactin release and as an analgesic but does not have particularly high opioid receptor affinity (Miller *et al.*, 1978b). Several such observations have been made during investigations of the pharmacology of the opioid peptides and have been used to support the suggestion that multiple classes of opioid receptors exist. However, it is also quite possible that in this case other factors such as the different hydrophobic character of each peptide may play an important role in their relative ability to stimulate prolactin secretion.

In addition, [D-Ala^2,D-Leu^5]-enkephalin, 0.5 mg/kg iv, significantly increased plasma prolactin (Table VI). Pretreatment with naloxone, the opioid antagonist, effectively blocked the stimulation of prolactin release induced by this enkephalin at 10 minutes.

TABLE VI

EFFECT OF INTRAVENOUS ENKEPHALIN AND NALOXONE ON RAT PLASMA
PROLACTIN LEVELS[a,b]

Treatment	Plasma prolactin (ng/ml)		
	0 Min	10 Min	30 Min
Saline + [D-Ala^2,D-Leu^5]	9.0 ± 8.0	25.6 ± 1.3	4.0 ± 3.0
Naloxone + [D-Ala^2,D-Leu^5]	4.0 ± 0.6	3.0 ± 1.0	3.6 ± 3.5

[a] H. Meltzer *et al.* (1978).

[b] Naloxone, 5 mg/kg, iv, or saline was injected iv 15 minutes before [D-Ala^2,D-Leu^5], 0.5 mg/kg, iv. Results are mean ± SEM.

These results certainly raise the possibility that one of the main functions of the opioid peptides *in vivo* may be as neuroendocrine modulating substances. As mentioned above, the localization of these substances in the median eminence and, in the case of enkephalin, in fiberlike processes in the neurohypophysis, provides a good anatomical basis for such a supposition (see above). One might, therefore, expect that under normal conditions an enkephalinergic system might be active in helping to maintain a tonic release of prolactin and growth hormone. It is, therefore, of particular interest to examine the effects of opioid antagonists, such as naloxone or naltrexone, in the normal animal, as such agents would be expected to cause a decrease in circulating prolactin and growth hormone. Where such an effect has been looked for, it has in general been found. Thus, both Shaar *et al.* (1977) and Bruni *et al.* (1977) reported that naloxone decreased circulating prolactin and growth hormone in the rat. In addition, the latter group of workers also reported that naloxone increased circulating LH and FSH concentrations. A most interesting series of experiments was carried out by Grandison and Guidotti (1977). These workers found that naltrexone inhibited prolactin secretion both in normal rats and in those with a deafferented hypothalamus, but not from isolated pituitaries *in vitro*. This indicated that the site of action of the opioid system was probably the hypothalamus. Moreover, prolactin secretion induced by foot-shock, stress, or injection of β-endorphin into the mediobasal hypothalamus is also blocked by naltrexone. However, the increase in prolactin secretion induced by haloperidol is not inhibited. These results indicate that an endogenous opioid peptide system acting in the hypothalamus may be involved in the control of prolactin release and that this system may in fact act by inhibiting the release of hypothalamic dopamine, which then has a direct action on the pituitary.

Several other workers have also attempted to identify the locus of action of the effects of opioids by examining their effects on hormone release from primary pituitary cultures or from pituitary fragments. The results obtained are somewhat contradictory. Ien *et al.* (1976) first found that both [Met⁵]- and [Leu⁵]-enkephalins were effective in releasing prolactin from pituitary cultures, whereas Rivier *et al.* (1977) found that neither morphine nor β-endorphin was effective in this system. Since that time two further groups have reported that enkephalin or synthetic analogs could release prolactin from pituitary fragments, whereas three others have found no effects (Table IV). Thus at this point the issue is still unresolved but seems to be tilting in favor of an action in the hypothalamus rather than a direct action on the pituitary.

VIII. Electrophysiological Effects

Several limited reports have appeared so far which provide electrophysiological data to support the notion that enkephalins act on opioid receptors in the central nervous system. Of particular interest are experiments where enkephalins have been microiontophoresed onto cells in areas that have previously been shown to possess opioid receptors. In the rat, for example, it has been shown that [Met^5]-enkephalin will depress spontaneous and glutamate-induced firing of single neurons in the frontal cortex, caudate nucleus, periaqueductal gray, and nucleus accumbens (Frederickson and Norris, 1976; McCarthy et al., 1977). Relatively few cells were excited, and all depressant effects could be reversed by naloxone. In addition, McCarthy et al. (1977) showed similar effects in the nucleus accumbens using [Leu^5]-enkephalin. In a particularly interesting study, Hill et al. (1976) found that the predominant effect of [Met^5]-enkephalin microiontophoresed onto neurons in the cerebral cortex, thalamus, and dorsal medulla was depression, and in addition they showed that neurons in the thalamus whose firing rate was specifically increased by noxious stimuli could be slowed by iontophoretically applied [Met^5]-enkephalin. This action could be completely reversed by naloxone. Similar studies have been carried out in the brain stem of the rat and cat. In both cases it was found that most neurons were depressed by [Met^5]- and [Leu^5]-enkephalin, although in a small number of instances the depression was followed by excitation and in the rat some neurons showed only excitation (Gent and Wolstencroft, 1976; Bradley et al., 1976). Only the effects obtained by the latter workers, however, were reversed by naloxone.

One study has involved iontophoresis of large endorphins as well as enkephalins (Nicoll et al., 1977). In this study both excitation and inhibition were obtained with opioid peptides, although the precise percentage of each type of response depended on the area examined. Both excitations and inhibitions were reversible with naloxone. Responses were observed using α- and β-endorphins and [Met^5]- and [Leu^5]-enkephalins, and compared with the effect of normorphine. Few responses were seen in the cerebellum. In the cerebral cortex, brain stem, caudate nucleus, and thalamus, naloxone-reversible inhibition was generally observed. In contrast, hippocampal pyramidal cells were strongly excited by all peptides, again in a naloxone-reversible manner. It is interesting to note that all these areas except for cerebellum contain appreciable quantities of enkephalin immunoreactivity as well as opioid receptors as revealed by autoradiography. Effects seen with

β-endorphin were considerably longer lasting than with enkephalin. As Nicoll *et al.* pointed out, this is probably due to the rapid inactivation of enkephalin relative to β-endorphin. Some quantitiative differences were also seen between β-endorphin and [Met[5]]-enkephalin as rather more excitations were seen with the former in the cortex and brain stem. In contrast to the excitation reported by Nicoll *et al.*, Segal (1977) reported that [Leu[5]]-enkephalin (and morphine) inhibited the excitation of hippocampal neurons by glutamate. However, as more of these actions were reversed by naloxone, it is hard to know what to make of them.

In studies in the spinal cord, Duggan *et al.* (1976) observed that [Met[5]]-enkephalin and also [MetNH$_2$[5]]-enkephalin were able to reduce the increase in firing of cells in the substantia gelatinosa of laminae IV and V of the cat produced by noxious stimuli. [MetNH$_2$[5]]-enkephalin was more effective than [Met[5]]-enkephalin. The peptide has less marked effects on neurons that were stimulated to fire by nonnoxious stimuli. All effects were reversed by naloxone. When [Met[5]]-enkephalin was iontophoresed onto Renshaw cells in the spinal cord of cats, the effects seen were all excitatory. Morphine was also able to excite these cells. However, in all other respects, the effects of [Met[5]]-enkephalin and morphine differed. Thus, morphine could reverse the action of glycine in depressing several neurons where [Met[5]]-enkephalin was ineffective in this respect. Moreover, [Met[5]]-enkephalin decreased the sensitivity of neurons to acetylcholine, whereas morphine enhanced the sensitivity of neurons to both acetylcholine and L-glutamate (Davies and Dray, 1976). One study examined cross-tolerance between the effects of [Met[5]]-enkephalin and morphine on rat cortical neurons (Zieglgansberger *et al.*, 1976). Both morphine and [Met[5]]-enkephalin were found to depress the rate of firing of cortical neurons whether fired by L-glutamate or firing spontaneously. However, neither morphine nor [Met[5]]-enkephalin were effective in rats that had been previously more tolerant to morphine. Hill *et al.* (1976) showed that repeated application of [Met[5]]-enkephalin to central neurons did not lead to desensitization, as has been reported to occur after repeated application of morphine (Bradley and Dray, 1974; Satoh *et al.*, 1974). However, in view of that fact that [Met[5]]-enkephalin is rapidly degraded, it is possible that sufficient concentrations were not achieved for sufficient periods of time to produce desensitization.

Apart from the above studies in the CNS, [Met[5]]- and [Leu[5]]-enkephalins have been shown to inhibit the firing of neurons in the myenteric plexus of the guinea pig ileum. [Met[5]]-enkephalin was found

to be approximately 5 times more potent than [Leu⁵]-enkephalin in
this respect (North and Williams, 1976).

IX. STRUCTURAL PHARMACOLOGY OF THE ENKEPHALINS

Considering the relatively short period of time that has elapsed since
the discovery of the opioid peptides, an enormous amount of data on
their pharmacology has been published. Two main reasons for all this
activity are apparent. The first is that the opioid peptides are of considerable fundamental interest to the scientific community. The second is
that several large pharmaceutical companies have become interested
in these molecules, as they represent an entirely new approach to the
synthesis of narcotics and related compounds. The argument has been
put forward that if enkephalins were addictive like morphine, then we
should all be addicted to our own enkephalin. Although this argument
may seem rather naive, it is still reasonable to say that these peptides
are now of fundamental pharmacological interest. The advances made
in this field in a short period of time are extremely significant for a
number of reasons. We shall attempt to summarize these and as much
of the available data as possible in what follows.

When one considers the possibility of making a centrally acting drug
based on the enkephalin molecule, two main problems must be faced.
To begin with, the pentapeptide is extremely unstable and its half-life
in the blood will be extremely short. Second, peptides are known not to
cross the blood–brain barrier at all easily. In order to solve these problems the structure of the enkephalin molecule has been altered considerably. Several hundred structural analogs have so far been reported.
One of the most interesting features to come out of the structure/
activity relationships of the enkephalins is that alterations to the
molecule change the different pharmacological effects of the molecule
to differing extents, yielding analogs that have fairly selective effects
in different systems. Moreover, analogs have now been produced that
are both stable and also produce analgesia after systemic administration. By analogy with the pharmacology of morphine, the following
effects of enkephalins will be considered with respect to their
structure/activity relationships: (a) opioid receptor interactions in
binding assay *in vitro;* (b) effects in bioassays such as the mouse vas
deferens and guinea pig ileum; (c) antinociceptive effects; (d) antidiarrheal effects (e) endocrine effects; (f) electrophysiological effects;
(g) conformation of the molecule; (h) other effects. Of these, (e) and (f)
have already been discussed above.

It should be noted that because of its limited potential for pharmaceutical development owing to its large size, structure/activity studies for β-endorphin have not been explored to nearly the same extent as for enkephalin. However, some structural analogs of β-endorphin have been synthesized, and they will be mentioned where appropriate.

A. OPIOID RECEPTOR INTERACTIONS

The most fundamental observations in examining the opioidlike properties of enkephalins and β-endorphins are those that consider the interaction of these peptides with opioid receptors *in vivo*. There are two biochemical systems available for monitoring this interaction. The first is the opioid receptor binding assay, and the second is the effect of narcoticlike substances on adenylate cyclase and cyclic-AMP concentrations in certain cell lines in culture, such as the NG108-15 neuroblastoma X glioma hybrid cell line.

The methodology for performing opioid receptor binding assays in rat brain homogenates or with synaptic membranes utilizing tritiated narcotic agonists and antagonists has been described by several groups in great detail. After the elucidation of the structure of [Met^5]- and [Leu^5]-enkephalin, several laboratories examined their effects in opioid receptor binding assays (Bradbury *et al.*, 1976b; Buscher *et al.*, 1976; Dewey *et al.*, 1976; Miller *et al.*, 1977; Pert *et al.*, 1976b,c). The values obtained for the affinities of these peptides varied a great deal between values that were comparable to morphine to values about three orders of magnitude less. One can now say with hindsight that this was due to the rapid degradation of the peptides by the brain membranes used in the assay. When precautions are taken, however, to protect the peptides by using either low temperatures or protease inhibitors such as bacitracin, then it is clear that the enkephalins do have high affinity for the opioid receptor, which is at least as high as [Met^5]-enkephalin (Miller *et al.*, 1977). In general, the affinity of [Leu^5]-enkephalin has been reported to be somewhat less than [Met^5]-enkephalin.

One of the earliest observations of significance in the structure/activity studies on the enkephalins concerned the effect of substituting a D-amino acid in position 2 instead of a glycine (Beddell *et al.*, 1977a,b; Coy *et al.*, 1976; Feldberg and Smyth, 1976, 1977; Pert *et al.*, 1976b,c; Walker *et al.*, 1977). It was found that substitution of a D-alanine in the 2-position, for example, produced a molecule that retained high affinity for the opioid receptor and in addition seemed to possess great stability. For example, peptides with the [D-Ala^2] substitution proved to be effective in the opioid binding assay even without the addition of bacitracin or when assays were run at room temperature, conditions under which the natural peptides were rapidly destroyed. The importance of D-amino acid substitution in this position is probably a further indication that metabolism takes place by removal of the N-terminal tyrosine. In fact, the stability of [D-Ala^2]-containing peptides has been confirmed by direct biochemical experiments using enkephalin-hydrolyzing enzymes found in plasma or brain homogenates. One indication of this increased stability can be seen in Fig. 12, which illustrates the relative effects of [Leu^5]-enkephalin and [D-Ala^2,D-Leu^5]-enkephalin in the guinea pig ileum bioassay. It can be seen that in the case of [Leu^5]-enkephalin inhibition of the guinea pig ileum twitch is obtained, but this is transitory and the contractions of the ileum return to their original magnitude after some time. In the case of [D-Ala^2, D-Leu^5]-enkephalin, however, inhibition is obtained, and this is found to be stable until the peptide is washed out of the gut bath. Figure 13 illustrates the effects of D-amino acid substitutions in each position of the enkephalin molecule in terms of overall activity. It can be seen that substitution of a D-amino acid in positions 2 or 5 or in both positions simultaneously leads to a molecule that contains substantial activity. In fact [D-Ala^2,D-Leu^5]-enkephalin is a potent and completely stable analog that shows high activity in a number of pharmacological tests. Table VII illustrates the effect of D-amino acid substitutions in each position of enkephalin on the affinity of the resulting molecule for the opioid receptor and also on its effect on the mouse vas deferens.

Apparently substitution of D-amino acids in the 2-position can have a variety of effects. One effect already mentioned is on the stability of the molecule. The second effect is on the affinity of the molecule for the opioid receptor. Thus, although all D-amino acid substitutions in this

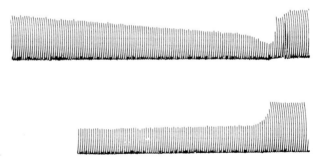

FIG. 12. Inhibition of contractions of the electrically stimulated guinea pig ileum by opioid peptides. Upper trace: [Leu^5]-enkephalin. Lower trace: [D-Ala^2, D-Leu^5]-enkephalin.

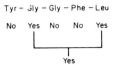

Tyr – ɔly – Gly – Phe – Leu

No   Yes   No   No   Yes

Yes

FIG. 13. D-Amino acid specificity for [Leu⁵]-enkephalin.

position seem to stabilize the molecule, not all such substitutions preserve the high receptor affinity. For example D-tryptophan or D-valine in this position lowers affinity considerably (Bedell et al., 1977a; Pert et al., 1976c). On the other hand, [D-Met²], [D-Thr²], or [D-Ser²] seem to preserve high affinity (Dutta et al., 1977; Bajusz et al., 1976, 1977; Székely et al., 1977; Yamashiro et al., 1977). The third important feature is that some of these substitutions may in part have some property on the molecule that enables it to cross the blood–brain barrier more easily. This certainly seems to be true for the case of [D-Met²] analogs, for example (Székely et al., 1977). The basis for this effect, however, is quite unknown.

Apart from D-amino acid substitutions, a considerable number of other chemical modifications of the enkephalin structure have been reported. Some general principles derived from the large number of peptide analogs reported may be summarized as follows.

1. As the length of the side chain of the amino acid in position 5 decreases, i.e., the amino acid becomes less lipophilic, there is a decrease in potency in the mouse vas deferens and in opioid receptor affinity. Of some consequence in relation to the preparation and storage of [Met⁵]-enkephalin solutions is the reduced activity of the methionine sulfoxide analogs. However, it should also be noticed that some analogs containing methionine sulfoxide show very high activity on peripheral administration (Römer et al., 1977).

One novel modification to be introduced into position 5 is alteration of the methionine carboxyl to the carbonyl analog [Met-ol]. This alteration considerably enhances receptor affinity. The introduction of a methionine sulfoxide in addition to the carbonyl modification also produces very marked increases in parenteral activity, As this substitution (i.e., modification of the sulfoxide moiety) somewhat reduces receptor affinity, this is an example of a structural alteration leading to decreased receptor affinity but producing enhanced analgesic potency in vivo. Such observations have been quite common with many enkephalin analogs and are discussed in greater detail below.

2. The low potency of [Tyr⁴]-enkephalin and also of the analog Tyr-D-Ala-Gly-Leu-Leu suggests that for high activity the 4-position must

TABLE VII

STEREOSPECIFICITY OF ENKEPHALIN[a]

Structural formula					Activity on vas deferens, $10^{-7}/IC_{50}\ M$	Receptor binding, $10^{-7}/IC_{50}\ M$
Tyr-	Gly-	Gly-	Phe-	Leu	8.17	9.09
D-Tyr-	Gly-	Gly-	Phe-	Leu	0.034	—
Tyr-D-Ala-		Gly-	Phe-	Leu	57.3	31.3
D-Tyr-D-Ala-		Gly-	Phe-	Leu	0.15	0.051
Tyr-D-Ala-		Gly-	Phe-D-Leu		263.0	38.5
D-Tyr-D-Ala-		Gly-	Phe-D-Leu		0.064	<0.010
Tyr-	Gly-	Gly-	Phe-	Leu	8.17	9.09
Tyr-	Ala-	Gly-	Phe-	Leu	0.006	0.020
Tyr-D-Ala-		Gly-	Phe-	Leu	57.3	31.3
Tyr-	Gly-D-Ala-		Phe-	Leu	0.021	0.002
Tyr-	Ala-D-Ala-		Phe-	Leu	0.009	<0.010
Tyr-D-Ala-D-Ala-			Phe-	Leu	0.075	0.026
Tyr-	Gly-	Gly-	Phe-	Leu	0.018	0.011
Tyr-	Gly-	Ala-	Phe-	Leu	0.009	<0.010
Tyr-	Gly-D-Ala-		Phe-	Leu	2.58	1.26
Tyr-	Gly-	Gly-	Phe-	Leu	8.17	9.09
Tyr-	Gly-	Ala-	Phe-	Leu	0.18	<0.011
Tyr-	Gly-D-Ala-		Phe-	Leu	0.021	0.002
Tyr-D-Ala-		Gly-	Phe-	Leu	57.3	31.3
Tyr-D-Ala-		Ala-	Phe-	Leu	2.50	1.26
Tyr-D-Ala-D-Ala-			Phe-	Leu	0.075	0.026
Tyr-	Ala-	Gly-	Phe-	Leu	0.006	0.02
Tyr-	Ala-	Ala-	Phe-	Leu	0.009	<0.010
Tyr-	Ala-D-Ala-		Phe-	Leu	0.009	<0.010
Tyr-	Gly-	Gly-	Phe-	Leu	8.17	9.09
Tyr-	Gly-	Gly-D-Phe-		Leu	0.002	<0.011
Tyr-D-Ala-		Gly-	Phe-	Leu	57.3	31.3
Tyr-D-Ala-		Gly-D-Phe-		Leu	0.043	0.011
Tyr-	Gly-	Gly-	Phe-	Leu	8.17	9.09
Tyr-	Gly-	Gly-	Phe-D-Leu		9.66	4.00
Tyr-D-Ala-		Gly-	Phe-	Leu	57.3	31.3
Tyr-D-Ala-		Gly-	Phe-D-Leu		263.0	38.5
Morphine					0.215	28.6

[a] From Beddell *et al.* (1977b).

be accommodated by a nonphenolic aromatic hydrophobic amino acid. In support of this notion it has been reported that analogs containing the [Trp⁴] substitution retain high activity (Schiller *et al.*, 1977). Apart from [Tyr⁴] analogs, the substitution of pNH₂Phe in position 4 also leads to low activity. However, analogs with pClPhe⁴ or pNO₂Phe⁴ substitutions are extremely potent. Analogs with pCH₃OPhe⁴ substitutions are of intermediate potency.

The substitution of [NMePhe⁴] also apparently enhances receptor affinity considerably (Römer *et al.*, 1977).

3. The glycine at position 3 appears to be essential for high biological activity. It is difficult to explain this in terms of peptide conformation alone, as no conformation is known for a small peptide that shows absolute stringency for glycine. It is also unlikely that a glycine-containing peptide would be more stable metabolically than a peptide containing alanine at position 3 unless special degradative mechanisms were involved. Thus it is suggested that [Gly³] is involved in close and specific interaction with the receptor, and provides a degree of flexibility to the peptide by virtue of the absence of a sterically hindered side chain. In keeping with this hypothesis is the decreases in biological activity and receptor affinity seen with [Ala³], [Sar³], and [Pro³] analogs. There do appear to be some exceptions, however, as one analog, Tyr-D-Ala-Asn-Phe-Leu, has proved to have relatively high activity in the guinea pig ileum and antidiarrhea tests selectively. The basis of this effect is not clear, but it could represent some fundamental differences in tissue specificity. Indeed, on the basis of differing effects of enkephalin analogs in differing assay systems, Lord *et al.* (1977) have proposed that some heterogeneity of opioid receptors may exist. The only substitution that has so far been reported to be acceptable in position 3 instead of a glycine is azaglycine.

4. The substitution of [Gly²] by a natural amino acid lowers biological activity and decreases opioid receptor affinity. It is of interest that substitution by Sar, Pro, or Ala in either the 2- or the 3-position are relatively and respectively the same. All lead to molecules that have reduced receptor affinity.

5. The modification of [Tyr¹] by the addition of a single carbon unit, either attached to the phenolic function as in *O*-methyltyrosine or inserted in the main peptide chain as with β-homotyrosine, reduces activity or binding. The importance of the free group in the aromatic ring is emphasized by the decrease of receptor affinity found with the [Phe¹] analog. On the other hand, activity is retained if the phenolic function is derivatized with a labile moiety such as an acetyl. It should be noted that the [Tyr¹] and [Phe⁴] are not interchangeable.

6. Increasing the length of the peptides has rather unpredictable results. Extending the chain at the N-terminus with an arginine decreases biological activity and receptor affinity. Lengthening the chain by placing a Thr in position 6 retains activity when an L-amino acid is in position 5 but reduces it when a D-amino acid is in position 5.

7. Esterification of the peptides tends to reduce receptor affinity and activity in the mouse vas deferens assay although its effect in the guinea pig ileum assay appear to increase potency in the case of several analogs.

8. There is a progressive decrease in opioid receptor affinity and activity in the mouse vas deferens assay in passing from analogs bearing a primary amino terminal residue through a secondary to a tertiary amine. Again in the guinea pig ileum the relative potency of such analogs is not so predictable (e.g., Lord et al., 1977).

9. The activity of tetrapeptides is interesting. It is clear that although they are less potent than the corresponding pentapeptides, tetrapeptides do retain full intrinsic activity in preparations such as the guinea pig ileum. If analogs are prepared that are protected from metabolism, such as Tyr-D-Ala-Gly-Phe, then such compounds have quite appreciable analgesic activity when injected intracerebrally. Certain tetrapeptides are also very potent in the antidiarrheal test.

10. As mentioned previously comparatively little is known about the structure activity relationships of the β-endorphin molecule. One analog containing the [D-Ala^2] substitution has been reported. It does not appear that this molecule has much more activity than the parent molecule (H. Loh, personal communication). However, as β-endorphin already possesses significant metabolic stability, the [D-Ala^2] substitution would not be expected to have very substantial effects in this respect. [D-Ala^2,D-Leu^5]-β-endorphin has also been synthesized. This molecule, unlike its enkephalin counterpart, is rather less effective than its parent molecule but still retains reasonable bioactivity (H. Loh, personal communication).

As well as examining the ability of opioid peptides to inhibit the binding of drugs such as [^{3}H]naloxone or [^{3}H]etorphine to the opioid receptor, some workers have examined the binding of the enkephalins themselves to the opioid receptor (Simantov and Snyder, 1976c; Audigier et al., 1977; Lord et al., 1976, 1977; Miller et al., 1978c; Morin et al., 1976). This has necessitated the use of labeled enkephalins or endorphins. So far no successful binding assays have been reported utilizing labeled β-endorphin or β-lipotropin. However, several binding assays utilizing tritiated or iodinated enkephalins have been reported, e.g., [^{3}H-][Met^5]-enkephalin (Simantov and Snyder, 1976c), [^{3}H][Leu^5]-

enkephalin (Lord *et al.*, 1976, 1977), [³H][D-Ala²,Leu⁵]-enkephalin (Miller *et al.*, 1978c), [¹²⁵I][D-Ala²,Leu⁵], [¹²⁵I][D-Ala²,D-Leu⁵]-enkephalin (Miller *et al.*, 1978c). The iodinated derivatives would seem to have certain advantages inasmuch as they are of higher specific activity and also have higher resistance to metabolism because they contain the [D-Ala²] substitution. Results in these binding assays seem to show that the binding site for the enkephalins is similar, but not identical, to that for [³H]naloxone, for example (Fig. 14). Thus in many ways enkephalin behaves in the same way as a typical opioid agonist. When saturation binding assays are performed, Scatchard analysis reveals the presence of two binding sites, one with K_D of about 8×10^{-10} M and the other of about 10^{-9} M (Simantov and Snyder, 1976c; Lord *et al.*, 1977; Miller *et al.*, 1978c). The binding of enkephalin is selectively reduced by physiological concentrations of sodium ions and enhanced by manganese ions. The biochemical properties of the binding site in brain membranes, as analyzed by the binding of [¹²⁵I][D-Ala²,Leu⁵]-enkephalin, resemble the properties already reported for [³H]naloxone binding. Thus binding is sensitive to temperature, sulfhydryl reagents, and proteolytic enzymes such as trypsin. Binding is also extremely sensitive to treatment with phospholipase A, but far less sensitive to treatment with other phospholipases or neuraminidase (R. J. Miller and K.-J. Chang, unpublished observations). From an examination of the kinetics of binding, Simantov and Snyder (1976c) found that [³H][Met⁵]-enkephalin behaved rather more like etorphine than naloxone,

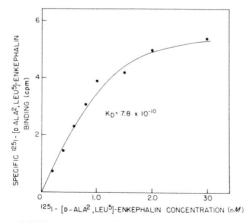

FIG. 14. Binding of ¹²⁵I-labeled [D-Ala², Leu⁵]-enkephalin in rat brain membranes. Unpublished observations of R. J. Miller, K.-J. Chang, and P. Cuatrecasas.

as its association and dissociation rates were relatively slow. Diprenorphine behaved similarly. However, the dissociation rates of [³H]dihydromorphine and [³H]naloxone are considerably faster.

Apart from binding in the brain, stereospecific binding has also been observed in the guinea pig ileum and in certain cell lines in culture, but not in the mouse vas deferens (R. J. Miller and K.-J. Chang, unpublished observations). One cell line that shows specific binding of ¹²⁵I-labeled [D-Ala²,D-Leu⁵]-enkephalin is NG108-15, a neuroblastoma × glioma hybrid line that has been previously reported to possess opioid receptors (Klee et al., 1976). In addition, N4TG1, a neuroblastoma cell line, also possesses a considerable number of opioid receptors. In a recent study we have utilized this cell line to examine the hypothesis that sulfatide is an integral part of the opioid receptor. Preliminary studies suggest, however, that N4TG1 cells do not make any sulfatide, and therefore in this system at any rate opiate receptors appear to exist in the absence of sulfatide (G. Dawson, personal communication).

Some studies also have concerned themselves with the ability of opioids and opioid peptides to inhibit the enzyme adenylate cyclase in homogenates of NG108-15 cells or the levels of cAMP in whole NG108-15 cells.

It has been shown that enkephalins and other opioid peptides will inhibit both basal and prostaglandin E-stimulated adenylate cyclase activity in these cells as well as cAMP concentrations in whole cells (Klee and Nirenberg, 1976; Brandt et al., 1976a, 1977; Goldstein et al., 1977; Traber et al., 1977). Again, as had been previously shown with morphine, prolonged exposure of the cells to the drug in the culture medium leads to an increase in adenylate cyclase activity, which has been suggested as a model of tolerance and related phenomena (Lampert et al., 1976; Brandt et al., 1976b). Some structure activity studies using NG108-15 cells show that the relative effects of the opioid peptides on inhibition of cAMP concentrations in whole cells or on adenylate cyclase in cell membranes is closely correlated to their opioid receptor affinities (Agarwal et al., 1977; Wahlström et al., 1977).

Some preliminary reports have also appeared suggesting that opioids and opioid peptides also increase concentrations of cGMP in NG108-15 cells and in slices of the striatum. However, this system has not yet been extensively investigated (Minneman and Iversen, 1976; Brandt et al., 1976b).

Some interesting differences have been found with respect to the potency of various drugs in displacing bound radioactive ligands from the opioid receptor. If the potency of a series of drugs in displacing

[^{3}H]naloxone binding is compared to their potency in displacing ^{3}H- or ^{125}I-labeled enkephalin binding in either cells or brain membranes, it is quite clear that the potencies of drugs in the two series vary a great deal and so does the order of potency, although certain features such as stereospecificity are still apparent. In general most narcotics are less able to displace bound enkephalin than to displace bound naloxone (Simantov and Snyder, 1976b; Lord et al., 1976, 1977; Miller et al., 1978b) (Table VIII). There are some exceptions to this, however; etorphine, for example, is equally effective in displacing both types of ligand (Simantov and Snyder, 1976b; Miller et al., 1978b). In contrast, it is

TABLE VIII

COMPARISON OF THE EFFECTS OF VARIOUS NARCOTIC DRUGS AND OPIOID PEPTIDES IN INHIBITION OF STEREOSPECIFIC BINDING OF [^{3}H]NALOXONE OR [^{125}I][D-ALA^2,LEU^5]-ENKEPHALIN BINDING TO OPIOID RECEPTORS IN RAT BRAIN OR OF [^{125}I][D-ALA^2,D-LEU^5]-ENKEPHALIN TO OPIOID RECEPTORS IN N4TG1 (NEUROBLASTOMA) CELLS[a]

Drug	[^{3}H]Naloxone binding rat brain	[^{125}I][D-Ala^2,Leu^5]-enkephalin binding rat brain	[^{125}I][D-Ala^2,D-Leu^5]-enkephalin binding N4TG1 cells
Naloxone	4×10^{-9}	2×10^{-9}	9×10^{-9}
Nalorphine	3×10^{-9}	7×10^{-9}	4×10^{-8}
Levorphanol	1.5×10^{-9}	3.6×10^{-9}	1.4×10^{-8}
Etorphine	8×10^{-10}	5×10^{-10}	8×10^{-10}
Morphine	3×10^{-9}	4×10^{-8}	7×10^{-8}
Levallorphan	2×10^{-9}	9×10^{-10}	6×10^{-9}
Pentazocine	9×10^{-8}	2×10^{-8}	1×10^{-7}
Phenazocine	4×10^{-9}	7×10^{-9}	8×10^{-9}
Phentanyl	1×10^{-9}	5×10^{-8}	4×10^{-7}
Pethidine	1×10^{-6}	2×10^{-5}	9×10^{-5}
Dextrorphan	3×10^{-5}	$>10^{-6}$	7×10^{-5}
Methadone	1×10^{-8}	8×10^{-8}	9×10^{-8}
Etonitazene	8×10^{-9}	5×10^{-7}	2×10^{-6}
Codeine	7×10^{-5}	8.5×10^{-6}	5×10^{-5}
[Met^5]-enkephalin	2.0×10^{-8}	6×10^{-9}	9.8×10^{-10}
[Leu^5]-enkephalin	1.1×10^{-8}	9.6×10^{-9}	2.2×10^{-9}
[D-Ala^2,D-Leu^5]-enkephalin	2.6×10^{-9}	1×10^{-9}	7×10^{-10}
[D-Ala^2,Leu^5]-enkephalin	3.2×10^{-9}	9×10^{-10}	1×10^{-9}
β-Endorphin	8×10^{-9}	2×10^{-9}	8×10^{-10}
β-Lipotropin	$>10^{-6}$	$>10^{-6}$	$>10^{-6}$

[a] Unpublished observations of K.-J. Chang, R. J. Miller, and P. Cuatrecasas.

found that enkephalins are in general more effective in displacing bound enkephalins than bound [^{3}H]naloxone. Again there are exceptions; β-endorphin is equally effective against both types of ligand (Simantov and Snyder, 1976b; Lord et al., 1977). Although a clear pattern is not yet apparent, it might be reasonable to suppose that naloxone and the enkephalins are binding to slightly different "overlapping" regions of the receptor. A theoretical model of the opiate receptor has been proposed containing at least three specific ligand binding sites (Feinberg et al., 1976). It may therefore be that etorphine and β-endorphin cover both regions accessible to naloxone and the enkephalins. However, other explanations have also been forthcoming. For example, Lord et al. (1977) prefer to account for the binding data by invoking a heterogeneity of opioid receptor sites.

Tables VII and IX show that a good correlation exists between the activity of analogs in the mouse vas deferens assay and in the opioid receptor binding assay. The correlation does not appear as good with the guinea pig ileum. It is interesting to note that all enkephalin analogs tested so far show considerably greater activity relative to morphine on the mouse vas deferens than on the guinea pig ileum. Such effects have also been reported by other workers (Hughes et al., 1975b; Lord et al., 1977; Waterfield et al., 1977). Previously it was proposed that subclasses of opioid receptors may exist (Martin, 1967). Indeed classes of narcotics have been found that are relatively more potent in the guinea pig ileum than in the mouse vas deferens (Hutchinson et al., 1976). These authors used these data in support of the hypothesis that multiple opioid receptors exist. Recently the same group reported the differential effects of certain enkephalin analogs in the guinea pig ileum and mouse vas deferens and have used such data to extend the multiple-receptor hypothesis (Lord et al., 1977). In addition to the bioassay data, further experiments utilizing opioid receptor binding assays based on the binding of radioactive enkephalins to the opiate receptor may also be interpreted in the light of the multiple-receptor hypothesis, as discussed above.

In relation to bioassay data, certain other observations are of interest. In contrast to opioid pentapeptides, Waterfield et al. (1977) found that β-endorphin was equipotent relative to morphine on the guinea pig ileum and mouse vas deferens. These authors also showed that [Met^5]-enkephalin could suppress the outflow of acetylcholine from the guinea pig ileum and of norepinephrine from the mouse vas deferens. Similarly it has been demonstrated that [Met^5]-enkephalin will reduce the release of [^{3}H]-norepinephrine from electrically stimulated slices of the rat occipital cortex (Taube et al., 1976).

TABLE IX[a]
OPIATE RECEPTOR AFFINITY RELATIVE TO MORPHINE (MORPHINE = 1)

Analog					Relative affinity
Tyr	D-Ala	Gly	pClPhe	D-Leu	3.5
Tyr	D-Ala	Gly	pClPhe	D-LeuOMe	1.75
Tyr	D-Ala	Gly	Phe	D-Leu	1.34
Tyr	D-Ala	Gly	Phe	Leu	1.09
Tyr	D-Ala	Gly	Phe	Met	0.97
Tyr	D-Ala	Gly	Phe	MetOMe	0.7
Tyr	D-Ala	Gly	Phe	Met Thr	0.62
Tyr	D-Ala	Gly	Phe	D-Met	0.44
Tyr	D-Ala	Gly	Phe	Leu Thr	0.44
Tyr	D-Ala	Gly	Phe	Nle	0.4
Tyr	D-Ala	Gly	Phe	LeuOMe	0.4
Tyr	D-Ala	Gly	Phe	D-LeuOMe	0.4

MOUSE VAS DEFERENS. POTENCY RELATIVE TO MORPHINE (MORPHINE = 1)

	Analog					Relative potency
	Tyr	D-Ala	Gly	pClPhe	D-Leu	1695
	Tyr	D-Ala	Gly	Phe	D-Leu	1227
	Tyr	D-Ala	Gly	Phe	Leu Thr	461
	Tyr	D-Ala	Gly	Phe	Leu	267
	Tyr	D-Ala	Gly	Phe	Met	229
	Tyr	D-Ala	Gly	Phe	Met Thr	229
NMe	Tyr	D-Ala	Gly	Phe	D-Leu	229
	Tyr	D-Ala	Gly	Phe	D-Met	228
	Tyr	D-Ala	Gly	pClPhe	D-LeuOMe	226
	Tyr	D-Ala	Gly	Phe	Nle	209
	Tyr	D-Ala	Gly	Phe	D-LeuOpClPh	177

GUINEA PIG ILEUM. POTENCY RELATIVE TO MORPHINE (MORPHINE = 1)

	Analog					Relative potency
	Tyr	D-Ala	Gly	Phe	D-LeuOMe	6.04
	Tyr	D-Ala	Gly	Phe	D-Leu	1.95
	Tyr	D-Ala	Gly	Phe	D-MetOMe	1.76
	Tyr	D-Ala	Gly	Phe	MetOMe	1.38
	Tyr	D-Ala	Asn	Phe	Leu	1.28
	Tyr	D-Ala	Gly	pClPhe	D-Leu	1.0
NMe	Tyr	Gly	Gly	Phe	Leu	0.93
	Tyr	D-Ala	Gly	Phe	D-Met	0.92
	Tyr	D-Ala	Gly	Phe	Leu Thr	0.87
NMe	Tyr	Gly	Gly	Phe	LeuOMe	0.75
	Tyr	D-Ala	Gly	Phe	D-Leu	0.66
	Tyr	D-Ala	Gly	Phe	Met Thr	0.63
NMe₂	Tyr	D-Ala	Gly	Phe	LeuOMe	0.65

(continued)

TABLE IX (*Continued*)
ANALGESIC ACTIVITY (HOT PLATE) ED_{50} FOR MICE μg/MOUSE
INTRAVENTRICULARLY INJECTED

Analog					ED_{50} μg/mouse
NMe Tyr	D-Ala	Gly	Phe	D-MetNH$_2$	0.005
Tyr	D-Ala	Gly	Phe	D-LeuNHEt	0.01
NMe Tyr	D-Ala	Gly	Phe	D-Met	0.007
NMe Tyr	D-Ala	Gly	Phe	D-MetOMe	0.02
NMe Tyr	D-Ala	Gly	Phe	D-LeuNH$_2$	0.05
Tyr	D-Ala	Gly	Phe	D-LeuOpClPh	0.05
NMe Tyr	D-Ala	Gly	Phe	D-LeuOMe	0.05
NMe Tyr	D-Ala	Gly	Phe	D-Leu	0.07
Tyr	D-Ala	Gly	pClPhe	D-Leu	0.07
NMe Tyr	D-Ala	Gly	Phe	D-MetNHEt	0.07
Tyr	D-Ala	Gly	Phe	D-LeuOMe	0.07
Tyr	D-Ala	Gly	Phe	D-LeuNHEt	0.1
Tyr	D-Ala	Gly	Phe	D-Leu D-Thr	0.1
Tyr	D-Ala	Gly	Phe	D-Leu Phe Gly	0.1
Tyr	D-Ala	Gly	Phe	D-Leu Thr	0.1
Tyr	D-Ala	Gly	Phe	Met Thr	0.24
Tyr	D-Ala	Gly	Phe	D-Leu	0.5
Tyr	D-Ala	Gly	Phe	D-Met	0.5
Tyr	D-Ala	Gly	Phe	D-Leu Thr	0.5
Tyr	D-Ala	Gly	Phe	Thr	0.5
Tyr	D-Ala	Gly	Phe	D-LeuOMe	0.5

ANTIDIARRHEAL ACTIVITY. ED_{50} mg/kg SUBCUTANEOUSLY

Analog					ED_{50} mg/kg
NMe Tyr	D-Ala	Gly	Phe	D-LeuNH$_2$	0.3
NMe Tyr	D-Ala	Gly	Phe	D-MetNHEt	0.7
NMe Tyr	D-Ala	Gly	Phe	D-MetNH$_2$	0.8
Tyr	D-Ala	Gly	pClPhe	D-LeuNHEt	1.0
NMe Tyr	D-Ala	Gly	Phe	D-Met	2.0
NMe Tyr	D-Ala	Gly	Phe	D-MetOMe	2.0
Tyr	D-Ala	Gly	Phe	D-Met	2.0
Tyr	D-Ala	Gly	Phe	D-Leu	3.0
Tyr	D-Ala	Asn	Phe	Leu	3.0
Tyr	D-Ala	Gly	Phe	Thr	3.0
Tyr	Ile	Asn	Met	Leu	8.0

^{a} Unpublished observations of R. J. Miller, K.-J. Chang, P. Cuatrecasas, C. Beddell, L. Lowe, S. Wilkinson, and R. Follenfant.

Analysis of all enkephalin analogs tested so far has not produced any strong evidence for an antagonist. One report suggested that the peptide H_2N-Arg-Tyr-Gly-Phe-Met-OH had antagonist properties (Ungar et al., 1976). However, this has not been confirmed in any system in which it has been examined (Law et al., 1977). The other indication of possible antagonist activity comes from examination of the so-called "sodium shift" associated with the receptor affinity of opioid drugs. It is well established that opioid agonists have a lower affinity for the opiate receptor in the presence of physiological concentrations of sodium ions than in their absence. The ratio of the IC_{50} of a drug in the [^{3}H]naloxone binding assay in the presence of 100 mM Na^+ ions to that in its absence is known as the "sodium shift" (Pert and Snyder, 1974). Extensive experiments with a large range of narcotics have shown that pure agonists have shifts of >10, pure antagonists have shifts of unity, and partial agonists have shifts in the range 1–10. [Leu^5]-enkephalin and its analogs generally have sodium shifts of >10 indicating that they are full agonists. The sodium shifts for several [Met^5]-enkephalin analogs are in the 1–10 range, and it might therefore be predicted that they would possess some antagonist activity (Beddell et al., 1977a; Bradbury et al., 1976a). However, this has not proved to be the case in any system so far examined. It must be said, however, that only a small number of the compounds currently available have been fully tested for antagonist activity.

It seems that sodium shift data do not predict agonist/antagonist activity in opioid peptides as accurately as they do for more conventional narcotics. However, it is quite clear that opioid peptides do produce sodium shifts of differing magnitudes, and one is left with the problem of what significance these may have. One intriguing possibility arises from the observation of Stein and colleagues (Belluzzi and Stein, 1977) that rats will self-administer [Leu^5]-enkephalin, but not [Met^5]-enkephalin. As it is well known that partial agonists (e.g., pentazocine) are not self-administered as readily as pure opioid agonists, these data suggest that sodium shift may be in some way predictive of "abuse potential." Two recent reports have concerned themselves with the activity of N-allyl derivatives of enkephalins (Hahn et al., 1977; C. B. Pert et al., 1977). It was proposed from various conformational speculations and by analogy with the activity of N-allyl derivatives of conventional narcotics that such compounds might be opioid antagonists. Both papers present various pieces of data suggesting that such N-allyl enkephalins do possess some antagonist activity. However the main effect seems to have been just to decrease the activity of the molecule in most respects, i.e., in both agonist and antagonist activities. The results were therefore not very convincing. Thus, although it may be the case that *N*-allyl enkephalins do possess some antagonist characteristics, it is still true to say that no opioid peptide antagonist has been produced that has the characteristics of a drug like naloxone or naltrexone.

Most investigations as to the effects of enkephalins in the periphery has been in relation to their antidiarrheal effects. Here it has been found that many of the enkephalin analogs so far produced have antidiarrheal effects (Miller *et al.*, 1978b). Some of the peptides are extremely potent and are as effective as morphine or loperamide. It should be noted that the peptides were administered intraperitoneally or subcutaneously. It is not known whether such effects are seen after oral administration of peptides. Some of the most effective peptides in the antidiarrheal test are reported in Table IX. The structure/activity relationships exhibited by compounds in this screen do not appear to be obviously related to their opioid receptor affinity. Clearly, other factors are also involved here or else the receptor mediating such effects is clearly different from that assayed by [^{3}H]naloxone binding in the brain. The effects of enkephalin analogs on gut motility are readily reversed by naloxone.

B. CONFORMATION OF THE ENKEPHALINS

Owing to the intrinsic opioidlike activity of the enkephalins and endorphins, several authors have speculated on the manner in which such peptides may fold up in order to attain a structure similar to that of the morphine or a similar drug. Three main types of approach have been utilized in these studies: (1) speculation as to the conformation of enkephalin at the opiate receptor resulting from model building and comparison with models of narcotic drugs or speculations resulting from the analysis of structure/activity relationships of a series of peptide analogs; (2) speculation as to the conformation of enkephalin in solution resulting from NMR data; (3) conformational analysis.

Horn and Rogers (1976) suggested that the N-terminal tyramine portion of enkephalin may be serving the same role as similar profiles found in several narcotics, such as levorphanol, metazocine, and profadol. All such drugs contain an important hydroxyl function and tertiary amino function within the molecule. It is suggested that the hydroxyl group of [Tyr^1] in enkephalin serves the same role as that in the narcotics described and that the primary amino group of [Tyr^1] serves the same role as the tertiary amino function. Some credence can be given to the role of the hydroxyl function because derivitization of this group in many enkephalin analogs leads to a considerable reduction in potency. One test of this model would be the synthesis of N-allyl derivatives of enkephalins. Such molecules ought to have partial agonist or antagonist properties by analogy with nalorphine and naloxone. However, as indicated previously, this does not necessarily seem to hold up (Hahn et al., 1977; C. B. Pert et al., 1977). By comparison with models of oripavine and morphine, Bradbury et al. (1976a) proposed that the two glycines in positions 2 and 3 of enkephalin occupy positions 2 and 3 of a β_1-bend with a hydrogen bond between the carbonyl group of the tyrosine residue and the amino group of the phenylalanine. Experimental support for this concept has recently come from the work of Schiller et al. (1977). These authors synthesized [Trp⁴,Met⁵]-enkephalin and found it to have high activity, being only 3.5 times less potent than the parent molecule. From measurements of the efficiency of energy transfer from [Tyr¹] to [Trp⁴] from both tyrosine fluorescence quenching and relative enhancement of tryptophan fluorescence, it was found that the average intramolecular [Tyr¹]-[Trp⁴] distance was 10.0 ± 1.1 Å. This is very close to the distance of [Tyr¹]-[Trp⁴] found in either 4–1 or 5–2 hydrogen-bonded β_1-models of this enkephalin analog and also close to the phenol–phenyl separation in oripavine type molecules.

From conformational energy calculations, Isogai et al. (1977) deduced a preferred conformation for [Met⁵]-enkephalin in free solution. This conformation contains a βII'-bend centered on [Gly³]-[Phe⁴] and is stabilized by a hydrogen bond between the hydroxyl group of the tyrosyl side chain and the backbone carbonyl group of either [Gly³] or [Phe⁴]. However, as these authors themselves pointed out and as is also pointed out by Momany (1977), this lowest energy conformation of [Met⁵]-enkephalin is not consistent with the biological activity of several enkephalin analogs. This restructure would predict increased conformational stability by introduction of D-alanine at position 3 rather than position 2. However, quite the opposite is found in practice. It therefore seems that the lowest energy conformation of [Met⁵]-enkephalin is probably not the conformer that interacts with the opioid receptor.

Beddell et al. (1977b) considered the biological activity of a large number of enkephalin analogs, particularly those involving substitution of D-amino acids in each position sequentially. These authors argued as follows.

The various conformations of a peptide can be described in terms of torsion angles of each bond in the peptide chain. Assuming that the peptide group is trans and planar, and considering the allowed contact distance between atoms, then a two-dimensional plot of ϕ and ψ the torsion angles about the other bonds in the peptide chain may be constructed (Fig. 15). The regions of accessible conformational space for a glycine and an L-alanine residue are shown in Fig. 15. Consider the conformations shown in Table X. The configurations allowed at each residue position in these conformations may be estimated by plotting the ϕ and ψ values. Each residue is plotted according to its being glycine, an L-amino acid or a D-amino acid. A D-residue is plotted on the map for an L-residue by inverting the ϕ and ψ angles before plotting. It can be seen that a D-residue at position 1 and an L-residue at position 2 are disallowed. Table XI summarizes the results of this study for the conformations in Table X, mirror-related conformations being denoted by a prime. The top line of Table XII summarizes the activity and binding data from Table VII. The configurations at each position in the peptide that favor activity and binding are shown. For example, at position 1, L-tyrosine favors activity and binding and D-tyrosine does

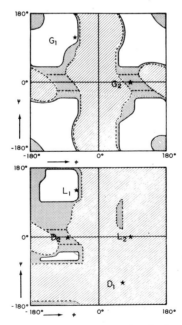

FIG. 15. Conformational maps for glycine (tgs) and L-alanine. Disallowed combinations of ϕ and Ψ are hatched. For these, atoms would be too close. Allowed areas are clear. Stippled areas (allowed) correspond to these approaches (e.g., hydrogen bonds). The two residues (1,2) in a β11-bend conformation are plotted according to each being glycine (G) and L-amino acid (L) or a D-amino acid (D).

TABLE X

TORSION ANGLES FOR SOME HYDROGEN-BONDED PEPTIDE CONFORMATIONS[a]

Conformation	Position						Reference
	1	1	2	2	3	3	
γ-turn	172	128	68	−61	−131	162	Némethy and Printz (1972)
Inverse γ-turn	70	−170	−86	57	−155	−60	Matthews (1972)
V-turn	−80	80	80	−80			Lewis et al. (1973)
β1-bend	−60	−30	−90	0			Lewis et al. (1973)
β11-bend	−60	120	80	0			Lewis et al. (1973)
β111-bend	−60	−30	−60	−30			Lewis et al. (1973)
2_7-helix	−75	70					Ramakrishnan and Ramachandran (1965)
2.2_7^R-helix	−78	59					Ramakrishnan and Ramachandran (1965)
3_{10}^R-helix	−49	−26					Ramakrishnan and Ramachandran (1965)
α^R-helix	−48	−57					Ramakrishnan and Ramachandran (1965)
$\gamma\alpha^R$-helix	84	78					Ramakrishnan and Ramachandran (1965)

[a] The ϕ and ψ angles for the minimum number of residues needed to describe each conformation are shown, successive residues being indicated by subscript.

TABLE XI

STEREOSELECTIVITY OF VARIOUS HYDROGEN-BONDED PEPTIDE CONFORMATIONS
ESTIMATED FROM RAMACHANDRAN PLOTS[a]

Conformation	Position 1[b]	Position 2[b]	Position 3[b]
γ-turn	G(L)	D	L
γ-turn	G(D)	L	D
Inverse γ-turn	D(L)	L	L
Inverse γ'-turn	L(D)	D	D
V-turn	L	D	
V'-turn	D	L	
β1-bend	A	L	
β1'-bend	A	D	
β11-bend	L	D	
β11'-bend	D	L	
β111-bend	A	A	
β111'-bend	A	A	
$2_7, 2.2_7{}^{R}$-helices	L		
$2_7', 2.2_7{}^{L}$-helices	D		
$3_{10}{}^{R}, \alpha^{R}$-helices	A		
$3_{10}{}^{L}, \alpha^{L}$-helices	A		
γ^{R} helix, γ^{L}-helix	G		

[a] Conformations at the boundary between allowed and disallowed regions are presumed to be allowed.

[b] G, glycine only; L, L-residue or glycine only; D, D-residue or glycine only; A, any residue configuration (that is, L, D, G); ( ), within 15° of allowed region, may be possible.

not. At position 2, on the other hand, the reverse is the case. Activity and binding are low when L-alanine is present, but high when D-alanine or glycine are present, provided that substitutions elsewhere in the molecule do not inhibit activity and binding. Apart from the optical configuration allowed at each position in the peptide, glycine is regarded as permitted in all cases, since there is no area on the conformational map accessible to an L- or D-residue that excludes glycine. It is assumed that if loss of activity results from a replacement of an L- or D-residue by glycine, this is due to a loss of interaction with the receptor rather than destabilization of the peptide conformation. Clearly one is neglecting possible stabilizing interactions between the residue side chains within the peptide. In the remainder of Table XII we consider each conformation in turn in each successive possible alignment in the peptide chain and show the configurational specificity appropriate to the conformation. The right-hand column of Table XII indicates agreement or contradiction between configurational specificity of a conformation in a given alignment with the peptide residues and that

TABLE XII

COMPARISON BETWEEN THE OBSERVED CONFIGURATIONAL SELECTIVITY OF ENKEPHALIN
(TOP LINE) AND THAT PREDICTED IF ENKEPHALIN WERE TO ADOPT ANY OF THE
HYDROGEN-BONDED CONFORMATIONS DESCRIBED IN TABLE XI

| Structure | Position[a] | | | | | Validity[b] |
	1	2	3	4	5	
Enkephalin	L+	D+	G	L	A+	
γ-turn	G(L)	D	L	L	L	x(?)
		G(L)	D	L		x
			G(L)	D	L	x
γ-turn	G(D)	L	D			x
		G(D)	L	D		x
			G(D)	L	D	x
Inverse γ-turn		D(L)	L	L		√
Inverse γ-turn		L(D)	D	D		x
V-turn		L	D			x
			L	D		x
V'-turn		D	L			√
			D	L		√
β1-bend		A	L			√
			A	D		√
β1'-bend		A	D			√
			A	D		x
β11-bend		L	D			√
			L	D		√
β11'-bend		D	L			√
			D	L		√
β111 or 111'-bend		D	L			√
			A	A		√
$2_7,2.2_7{}^R$-helices	L	L	L	L	L	x
$2_7,2.2_7{}^l$-helices	D	D	D	D	D	x
γ^R helix, γ^l-helix	G	G	G	G	G	x
$3_{10}{}^{R\ L}$ or						
$^R\alpha'{}^{l}$-helices	A	A	A	A	A	√

[a] +L or D includes G. A is L, D, or G.
[b] √, allowed; x, disallowed.
Letters in parentheses indicate disagreement with enkephalin.

deduced for enkephalin from activity and binding data. Violation occurs when the activity and binding data allow an L- or D-configuration for a residue and this is disallowed in the conformation. Table XIII summarizes the resultant possible conformations for enkephalin; the last two, however, explain very little. The inverse γ-turn, the V-turn, and the β11'-bend can explain the preference for a D-residue in position

TABLE XIII

Summary of the Conformations for Enkephalin Indicated as Valid in Table XII[a]

Structure	Position				
	1	2	3	4	5
Enkephalin	L+	D+	G	L	A[a]
Inverse γ-turn		D(L)	L	L	
V'-turn		D	L		
			D	L	
β1-bend		A	L		
			A	L	
β1'-bend		D	L		
			D	L	
β11'-bend		D	L		
			D	L	
β111 or 111'-bend		A	A		
			A	A	
$3_{10}{}^{R,L}$ or $\alpha^{R,L}$-helices	A	A	A	A	A

[a] A is L, D, or G.

2. These and the β1-bend could also account for the preference for an L-residue in position 4. However, the inverse γ-turn can simultaneously explain both. Finally, no conformation can explain the preference for glycine in position 3.

Although the inverse γ-turn explains the data most completely, it would be premature to conclude that this is the conformation of enkephalin at the receptor, but it represents a useful starting hypothesis for future studies. For example, certain assumptions have been made here that may not be valid, such as the planar nature of the peptide group. Bradbury *et al.* (1976d) have advocated a β-bend at positions 2 and 3. Jones *et al.* (1976) and Roques *et al.* (1976) have advocated a β1-turn in positions 3 and 4 from proton magnetic resonance data from enkephalin solutions. Our studies would not necessarily exclude either of these conformations.

X. ANALGESIC EFFECTS

One of the most striking effects of narcotic drugs is their ability to produce analgesia. It is therefore of particular interest to know whether in fact the enkephalins are truly analgesic compounds that might be implicated in the perception of pain. Soon after the structure of enkephalin was elucidated, synthetic pentapeptides were injected intraventricularly into mouse and rat brain and some analgesic effects were observed. These effects, however, were modest and extremely transient in comparison to morphine, for example (Belluzzi *et al.*, 1976; Buscher *et al.*, 1976). In retrospect this was not all surprising, owing to the rapid metabolism of the peptides. When stable compounds are used such as β-endorphin or nonmetabolized analogues of the enkephalins, the results are much more impressive (Feldberg and Smyth, 1976, 1977; Baxter *et al.*, 1977a,b; Coy *et al.*, 1976; Miller *et al.*, 1978b; Pert *et al.*, 1976b; Walker *et al.*, 1977; Wei *et al.*, 1977). When the analgesic activity of β-endorphin is compared to that [Met^5]-enkephalin, the former is several thousand times more active in spite of the fact that the two compounds have similar affinities for the opiate receptor. This, as mentioned above, is presumably due to the rapid metabolism of the pentapeptide. When stabilized pentapeptides are used, however, they appear to be at least as potent as β-endorphin (Miller *et al.*, 1978b; Wei *et al.*, 1977). This was shown clearly by Pert (1976), who found that [D-Ala^2, MetNH$_2$^{5}]-enkephalin and β-endorphin were both very potent relative to morphine and also much more potent than [D-Leu^5]-enkephalin as analgesics. The fact that many enkephalin analogs and endorphins are considerably more potent than morphine in producing analgesia subsequent to intracerebral injection is rather reminiscent of the relative potencies of these substances on the mouse vas deferens rather than the guinea pig ileum (see above). This may indicate that the receptor mediating these analgesic effects resembles that in the mouse vas deferens rather than the guinea pig ileum. However, other explanations are possible. Table IX shows a series of some of the more potent peptide analogs in producing analgesia after intracerebral injection. It can be seen that some of these are extremely potent—up to 100 times more potent than [D-Ala^2,D-Leu^5]-enkephalin, which has been shown to be equipotent with β-endorphin (Wei *et al.*, 1977). However as β-endorphin was not run under the same conditions as the compounds in Table IX it is not possible to say whether some of these analogs are in fact more potent than β-endorphin, although this seems likely. Indeed Römer *et al.* (1977) reported that several synthetic analogs were considerably more potent than β-endorphin. It can be seen that the order of potency found for compounds in this series differs somewhat from that found in the opioid receptor binding assay. Several of the most effective enkephalins have modified N- or C-termini and in general appear to be more hydrophobic in character. It is also interesting that several tetrapeptides that contain the [D-Ala^2] substitution are also effective in this test.

From the point of view of drug development, workers have been at pains to try to develop enkephalin analogs that produce analgesia on peripheral administration. Hopes that this might be achieved are high, seeing that β-endorphin, which has 31 amino acids, has been shown to produce analgesia when administered peripherally (Tseng et al., 1976a). Apart from this observation, De Wied (1974) and colleagues (Gispen et al., 1975) have shown consistently over the last several years that peptides related in structure to ACTH can produce central effects when injected peripherally in extremely small doses. Initially, few analgesic effects were reported when stable enkephalins were administered subcutaneously or intraperitoneally. However, recent reports show that such molecules are in fact effective when administered intravenously or by other routes. Thus, apart from β-endorphin (Tseng et al., 1976a), [D-Ala^2,D-Leu^5]- and [D-Met^2,ProNH$_2$^{5}]-enkephalin have been shown to have considerable analgesic activity when given intravenously (Bajusz et al., 1976, 1977; Wei et al., 1977). Moreover, the former group of workers have synthesized a series of compounds based on the substitution [D-Met^2,ProNH$_2$^{5}] and have shown such derivatives to be very effective when administered subcutaneously as well as intravenously (Bajusz et al., 1976, 1977; Székely et al., 1977). Thus [D-Met^2,ProNH$_2$^{5}]-enkephalin was as potent as morphine in producing analgesia when administered subcutaneously in rats and was somewhat more potent when given intravenously.

Another recent report of enkephalin analogs exhibiting activity following parenteral administration comes from Dutta et al. (1977). These analogs possessed either the [D-Ala^2] or [D-Ser^2] substitution. In addition, the most potent analogs also possessed either [ProNHEt^5] or substitutions. The authors also make two other interesting points. First, that the ability of analogs to produce analgesia did not correlate at all well with their activity on the guinea pig ileum. This observation is in line with those made by others. It is clear that an in vitro assay, such as the guinea pig ileum assay, can be expected to correlate with central effects only when the compounds being compared have equal ability to enter the brain. The other possible explanation, as mentioned above, is that the receptors mediating effects in the guinea pig ileum and those mediating analgesia are different. This likelihood is further supported by the observations of Dutta et al., who claim that many of their peripherally active analgesic enkephalins do not appear to depress respiration at all. This important observation must be followed up, as respiratory depression is one of the most untoward side effects of narcotics such as morphine.

The most promising report, however, has come from Römer et al.

(1977). These workers have produced analogs that are effective orally in the rat, as well as intravenously and subcutaneously. The structure of the most potent compound produced was [D-Ala^2,NMePhe^{4}Met(0)-ol^5]. This analog was more potent than morphine when administered intravenously or subcutaneously and somewhat less potent when administered orally. Continued administration of this compound over several days produced tolerance, however. In spite of the fact that this particular analog looks as though it may not offer any great improvement over currently available narcotics, its efficacy is of great theoretical importance because usually peptides are thought to cross the blood–brain barrier only with difficulty.

One of the main hopes aroused by the discovery of the opioid peptides was that some form of nonaddictive analgesic might be produced based upon such a compound. Some argued that this seemed possible because if such compounds were addictive then we would all be addicted to our own endogenous opioid peptides. It is, therefore, of particular interest to find out what the addictive potential of the enkephalins and endorphins may be.

The overall impression obtained from reports so far indicates that opioid peptides are in fact "additive." This is best documented for β-endorphin, owing to its stability. Thus tolerance to the antinociceptive, catatonic, and hypothermic effects of β-endorphin have been observed after repeated intraventricular injections (Tseng et al., 1977). β-Endorphin will also suppress morphine withdrawal effects and shows cross-tolerance with morphine (Tseng et al., 1976b, 1977).

Limited experiments have been performed with stable enkephalin analogs. For example, Pert (1976) has shown that repeated intraventricular injections of [D-Ala^2,MetNH$_2$^{5}]-enkephalin produce tolerance in rats, and naloxone will precipitate a withdrawal syndrome in animals made tolerant to this peptide. Baxter and colleagues (1977b) have shown that [D-Ala^2,D-Leu^5]-enkephalin will suppress withdrawal symptoms in animals addicted to morphine. Tolerance to [Met^5]-enkephalin itself is harder to demonstrate owing to the speed at which it is metabolized. Blasig and Herz (1976) and Bhargava (1977), however, have shown that animals that were made tolerant to morphine after pellet implantation were cross-tolerant to [Met^5]-enkephalin and would inhibit the naloxone-precipitated withdrawal syndrome (Bhargava, 1977). In an elegant series of experiments, Wei and Loh were able to precipitate a withdrawal syndrome in animals in which [Met^5]-enkephalin had been perfused for 70 hours through the periaqueductal gray/4th ventricle area by means of an osmotic minipump inserted subcutaneously (Wei and Loh, 1976). Finally, as mentioned above, the orally effective enkephalin analog [D-Ala^2,NMePhe^4,Met(0)-01^5]-en-kephalin produces tolerance in animals following repeated adminis-tration (Römer et al., 1977). Repeated administration of β-endorphin within a 24-hour period intraventricularly in cats was found to pro-duce tolerance (Hosobuchi et al., 1977). However, this tolerance was reduced immediately by systemic administration of the serotonin pre-cursor 5-hydroxytryptophan. It was further shown that 5-hydroxy-tryptophan potentiates the analgesic effect of a low dose of β-endorphin. These observations again illustrate the close connection between the analgesic effects produced by narcotics, their side effects, and central serotonergic action.

Two other models have also been used to look at tolerance and de-pendence phenomena with opioid peptides. In the guinea pig ileum or mouse vas deferens preparation taken from animals made tolerant to morphine by pellet implantation the pharmacological responses in these tissues show tolerance to morphine and cross-tolerance to en-kephalin (Waterfield et al., 1976; Schulz and Herz, 1976). In addition, the cell culture system utilizing NG108-15 cells has been mentioned above.

Thus in all systems so far examined that are indicative of addiction potential, it appears that opioid peptides do indeed cause the normal spectrum of tolerance and withdrawal behaviors, indicating that drugs produced from such molecules may not be free of these problems. It is important to stress, however, that only relatively few synthetic analogs have so far been examined for these properties. As has been shown above, different enkephalin analogs certainly exhibit differences in the spectrum of their activities. Moreover, the recent observations that several enkephalins and β-endorphin can produce analgesia when administered peripherally shows that much more work is needed in this area, using peripheral routes of administration in order to see whether any derivatives may have no, or at least acceptably low, addictive potential. Indeed, it would be surprising if among the large number of opioid peptides differences in their ability to produce these effects were not found. To conclude, enkephalin analogs have now been produced that show all the usual effects of narcotic drugs both "good" and "bad." In addition, analogs have been produced that are both pro-tected from degradation and are effective by several peripheral routes of administration.

XI. Some Conclusions

When one considers the above discussion, one cannot help but be impressed not only by the enormous amount of data that have accumulated in this area in the last 2 years, but also by the way in which the research has developed in many unexpected ways. After all, this was a problem that started out as being something of a neuropharmacological speculation. One was looking for a molecule in the nervous system that looked like morphine. Not only did the morphinelike molecule prove to exist, but its structure was a complete surprise. In addition, the structure of enkephalin proved to be related to that of a peptide hormone already sequenced, that is β-lipotropin. β-Lipotropin in its turn proved to be related biosynthetically to corticotropin. One is therefore now at a stage where some of the most interesting problems in the field relate to the biosynthesis of peptide hormones examined by experiments in *in vitro* cell-free protein-synthesizing systems. Opiate neuropharmacologists could never have imagined two years ago as they observed the effects of a drug in an isolated guinea pig ileum preparation that they would ultimately be concerned with problems of the microanalysis of peptide hormone sequences.

One may care to speculate at this point as to what might be expected to develop in the near future and also as to what areas are currently of the greatest interest. First, as already mentioned, the biosynthetic relationships of the opioid peptides and corticotropin seem to reveal more and more surprises. In a related area it will be most interesting to see whether the opioid peptide systems described in the hypothalamus ultimately prove to be of fundamental importance in the regulation of pituitary hormone release. Moreover, although release of β-endorphin itself from the pituitary has been shown to be regulated in concert with that of corticotropin, one still has no idea what the β-endorphin does once it has been released. Thus β-endorphin in the blood stream currently has the status of a hormone looking for a function. The elucidation of such a function is certainly a problem of great current interest. One can therefore see that there are many areas in what may be called neuroendocrinology where opioid peptides most probably play crucial roles.

A second area of general interest focus on the central effects of the opioid peptides. In order to probe the role of enkephalinergic systems in analgesia, for example, workers have looked for central effects of haloxone. In general, most groups of investigators have found naloxone to produce hyperalgesia in animals and man, indicating some tonic central analgesic effects, presumably mediated by opioid peptide systems (Lasagna, 1965; Jacob *et al.,* 1974; Walker *et al.,* 1977). In addition, acupuncture analgesia has also been reported to be blocked by naloxone (Mayer *et al.,* 1977). However, not all results agree about these points, and recent results suggest that this may be because different segments of the population respond to naloxone in different ways

(Buschbaum *et al.*, 1977; Goldstein *et al.*, 1976; El-Sobky *et al.*, 1976). Such results in turn suggest that opioid peptide systems may be involved in the control of mood. This suggestion fits in well with the speculation that such systems may also mediate some of the aberrant mental states found in psychoses (Jacquet and Marks, 1977; Bloom *et al.*, 1977b; Gunne *et al.*, 1977; Terenius *et al.*, 1977). The profound behavioral effects elicited by the opioid peptides also supports this contention (Fig. 16). However, it must be stressed that at this time this remains merely speculation. Results attempting to show effects of naloxone or β-endorphin in schizophrenia or depression have left many observers as confused as the individuals on whom these drugs are being tested (Davis *et al.*, 1977; Gunne *et al.*, 1977; Volavka *et al.*, 1977). To be fair, however, good clinical work is extraordinarily difficult and time-consuming to carry out, and because it deals with human subjects it necessarily lags behind basic research. The results of this work will certainly be awaited with great anticipation. One other problem relating to the central nervous system springs to mind. It will be remembered that the globus pallidus contains remarkably high concentrations of enkephalins. It is not at all clear what function is subserved by these vast reserves of opioid peptide in the basal ganglia. Some initial data point to a function in the control of locomotion. Here again is problem of particular interest.

Finally, one should perhaps try to put the whole opioid peptide field

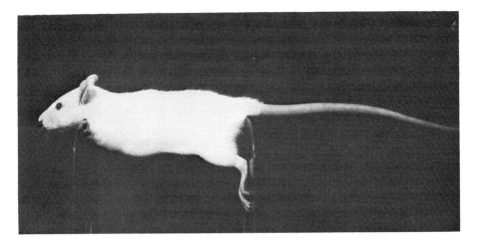

Fig. 16. Behavioral effect of intraventricular injection of β-endorphin ($14.9 \times 10^{-9} M$) in the rat. Thirty minutes after injection, the rat appeared as in the photograph. Rat pinup by courtesy of Dr. Floyd Bloom. Adapted from Bloom *et al.* (1977a).

into context. The enkephalins, it turns out, are just the tip of a very large peptide iceberg. A very large family of peptide hormones has been found to be localized in both the gut and the nervous system. Peptides such as somatostatin, substance P, vasoactive intestinal polypeptide, gastrin, neurotensin, and cholecystokinin are all found in the nervous system as well as the gut. A rationale for this dual localization has been provided by Pearse (1976), who has pointed out the common embryological ancestry of peptide-containing cells in these two tissues. Most of the hormones alluded to have been shown to have pharmacological effects on the gastrointestinal tract, and many of them have also been shown to produce central effects. The current vogue for enkephalin research has served to focus our interest on this whole idea. As time goes on neuropeptides will certainly be shown to be more and more important in the control of various modes of behavior. Neuropharmacologists have now demonstrated, using enkephalin as a model, that systemically active centrally effective compounds can be produced, based on the structure of peptides. The realization that the nervous system contains an abundance of peptidergic neuronal systems may therefore usher in a new era of neuropharmacology.

ACKNOWLEDGMENTS

The authors wish to thank the following workers, who contributed data prior to publication or in other ways aided us in preparing this article: Floyd Bloom, Kwen-Jen Chang, Solomon Snyder, George Uhl, Virginia Pickel, Madhab Sar, Walter Stumpf, Illona Linnoilla, Herb Meltzer, Leslie Iversen, Claudio Cuello, Dick DiAugustine, and Pat Grabovac, who typed the manuscript.

REFERENCES

Agarwal, N. S., Hruby, V. J., Katz, R., Klee, W., and Nirenberg, M. (1977). *Biochem. Biophys. Res. Commun.* **76,** 129.

Akil, H., Mayer, D. J., and Liebeskind, J. C. (1976). *Science* **14,** 961.

Audigier, Y., Malfroy-Camine, B. R., and Schwarz, J. C. (1977). *Eur. J. Pharmacol.* **41,** 247.

Austen, B. M., Smyth, D. G., and Snell, C. R. (1977). *Nature (London)* **269,** 619.

Bajusz, S., Ronai, A. Z., Székely, J., Dunai-Kovacs, Z., Berzetei, I., and Graf, L. (1976). *Acta Biochim. Biophys. Acad. Sci. Hung.* **11,** 305.

Bajusz, S., Ronai, A. Z., Székely, J., Graf, L., Dunai-Kovacs, Z., and Berzetei, L. (1977). *FEBS Lett.* **76,** 91.

Bass, P., and Wiley, J. B. (1965). *Am. J. Physiol.* **208,** 908.

Baxter, M. G., Goff, E., Miller, A. A., and Saunders, I. A. (1977a). *Br. J. Pharmacol.* **59,** 455.

Baxter, M. G., Follenfant, R. L., Miller, A. A., and Sethna, D. M. (1977b). *Br. J. Pharmacol.* **60,** 523.

Beddell, C., Clark, B., Hardy, G. W., Lowe, L. G., Ubatuba, F., Vane, J. R., Wilkinson, S., Chang, K.-J., Cuatrecasas, P., and Miller, R. J. (1977a). *Proc. R. Soc. London, Ser. B* **198,** 249.

Beddell, C., Chang, K.-J., Cuatrecasas, P., Clark, R. B., Lowe, L. A., Miller, R. J., and Wilkinson, S. (1977b). *Br. J. Pharmacol.* **61**, 351.

Belluzzi, J. D., and Stein, L. (1977). *Nature (London)* **265**, 556.

Belluzzi, J. D., Grant, N., Garsky, V., Sarantakis, J., Wise, C. D., and Stein, L. (1976). *Nature (London)* **260**, 625.

Bhargava, H. N. (1977). *Eur. J. Pharmacol.* **41**, 81.

Blasig, J., and Herz, A. (1976). *Naunyn-Schmiedeberg's Arch. Pharmacol.* **294**, 297.

Bloom, F. E., Battenberg, E., Rossier, J., Ling, N., Lappaluoto, J., Vargo, T. N., and Guillemin, R. (1977a). *Life Sci.* **20**, 43.

Bloom, F. E., Segal, D., Ling, N., and Guillemin, R. (1977b). *Science* **194**, 629.

Bloom, F. E., Rossier, J., Battenberg, E., Bayon, A., French, E., Henrickson, S. J., Siggins, G. R., Segal, D., Browne, R., Ling, N., and Guillemin, R. (1978). *Adv. Psychopharmacol.* **18** (in press).

Bowers, C. Y., Chang, J.-K., and Fong, B. W. (1977). *Proc. Endocr. Soc.* **232** (abstr.).

Bradybury, A. F., Smyth, D. G., and Snell, C. R. (1976a). *Ciba Found. Symp.* **41**, 61.

Bradybury, A. F., Smyth, D. G., Snell, C. R., Birdsall, N. J. M., and Hulme, E. C. (1976b). *Nature (London)* **260**, 793.

Bradbury, A. F., Feldberg, W. F., Smyth, D. G., and Snell, C. R. (1976c). *In* "Opiates and Endogenous Opioid Peptides" (H. Kosterlitz, ed.), p. 9. North-Holland Publ., Amsterdam.

Bradbury, A. F., Smyth, D. G., and Snell, C. R. (1976d). *Nature (London)* **260**, 793.

Bradley, P. B., and Dray, A. (1974). *Br. J. Pharmacol.* **50**, 47.

Bradley, P. B., Briggs, J., Gayton, R. J., and Lambert, L. A. (1976). *Nature (London)* **261**, 425.

Brandt, M., Gullis, R. J., Fischer, K., Buchen, C., Hamprecht, B., Moroder, L., and Wunsch, E. (1976a). *Nature (London)* **262**, 311.

Brandt, M., Fischer, K., Moroder, L., Wunsch, E., and Hamprecht, B. (1976b). *FEBS Lett.* **68**, 38.

Brandt, M., Buchen, C., and Hamprecht, B. (1977). *FEBS Lett.* **80**, 251.

Bruni, J. F., Van Vugt, D., Marshall, S., and Meites, J. (1977). *Life Sci.* **21**, 461.

Buschbaum, M., Davis, G. C., and Bunney, W. E. (1977). *Nature (London)* **270**, 621.

Buscher, H. H., Hill, R. C., Römer, D., Cardinaux, A., Closse, A., Hauser, D., and Pless, J. (1976). *Nature (London)* **261**, 423.

Chang, J.-K., Fong, B. W., Pert, A., and Pert, C. B. (1976). *Life Sci.* **18**, 1473.

Cheung, A., and Goldstein, A. (1976). *Life Sci.* **19**, 1005.

Cheung, A., Stavinoha, W. B., and Goldstein, A. (1977). *Life Sci.* **20**, 1285.

Chihara, K., Arimura, A., and Coy, D. H. (1977). *Proc. Endocr. Soc.* **94** (abst.).

Cocchi, D., Santagostino, A., Gil-Ad, I., Ferris, S., and Muller, E. E. (1977). *Life Sci.* **20**, 2041.

Cox, B. M., Opheim, K. E., Teschemacher, H., and Goldstein, A. (1975). *Life Sci.* **16**, 1777.

Cox, B. M., Gentleman, S., Su, T.-P., and Goldstein, A. (1976a). *Brain Res.* **115**, 285.

Cox, B. M., Goldstein, A., and Li, C. H. (1976b). *Proc. Natl. Acad. Sci. U.S.A.* **73**, 1821.

Coy, D. H., Kastin, A. J., Schally, A. V., Martin, O., Garon, M. G., Labrie, F., Walker, J. M., Fertel, R. J., Bernstein, G. G., and Sandman, C. P. (1976). *Biochem. Biophys. Res. Commun.* **73**, 632.

Coyle, J. T., and Schwartz, R. (1976). *Nature (London)* **263**, 244.

Creese, I., and Snyder, S. H. (1975). *J. Pharmacol. Exp. Ther.* **194**, 205.

Crine, P., Benjannet, S., Seidah, N. G., Lis, M., and Chrétien, M. (1977a). *Proc. Natl. Acad. Sci. U.S.A.* **74**, 1403.

Crine, P., Benjannet, S., Seidah, N. G., Lis, M., and Chrétien, M. (1977b). *Proc. Natl. Acad. Sci. U.S.A.* **74**, 4276.

Cuatrecasas, P. (1971). *Proc. Natl. Acad. Sci. U.S.A.* **68**, 1264.

Cuello, A. C., and Paxinos, G. (1978). *Nature (London)* **271**, 180.

Cusan, L., Dupont, A., Kledzik, G. S., Labrie, F., Coy, D. H., and Schally, A. V. (1977). *Nature (London)* **268**, 564.

Davies, J., and Dray, A. (1976). *Nature (London)* **262**, 603.

Davis, G. C., Bunney, W. E., De Fraites, E. G., Kleinman, J. E., van Kammen, D. P., Post, R. M., and Wyatt, R. J. (1977). *Science* **197**, 74.

Day, A. R., Lujan, M., Dewey, W. L., Harris, L. S., Redding, J. A., and Freer, R. J. (1976). *Res. Commun. Chem. Pathol. Pharmacol.* **14**, 597.

Desbuquois, B., Krug, E., and Cuatrecasas, P. (1974). *Biochim. Biophys. Acta* **343**, 101.

Dewey, W. L., Thy, T., Day, A., Lujan, A., Harris, L. S., and Freer, R. J. (1976). *In* "Opiates and Endogenous Opioid Peptides" (H. Kosterlitz, ed.), p. 103. North-Holland Publ., Amsterdam.

De Wied, D. (1974). *In* "The Neurosciences: Third Study Program" (F. O. Schmitt and E. G. Worden, eds.), p. 653. M.I.T. Press, Cambridge, Massachusetts.

Dill, R. E., and Costa, E. (1977). *Neuropharmacology* **16**, 323.

Duggan, A. W., Hall, J. G., and Headley, P. R. (1976). *Nature (London)* **269**, 456.

Dupont, A. *et al.* (1977a).

Dupont, A., Cusan, L., Garon, M., Labrie, F., and Li, C. H. (1977b). *Proc. Natl. Acad. Sci. U.S.A.* **74**, 358.

Dupont, A., Cusan, L., Labrie, F., Coy, D. H., and Li, C. H. (1977c). *Biochem. Biophys. Res. Commun.* **75**, 76.

Dupont, A., Cusan, L., Garon, M., Alvarado-Urbina, G., and Labrie, F. (1977d). *Life Sci.* **21**, 907.

Dutta, A. S., Gormley, J. J., Haywood, C. F., Morley, J. S., Shaw, J. S., Stacey, G. J., and Turnbull, M. T. (1977). *Life Sci.* **21**, 559.

Eipper, B. A., and Mains, R. E. (1976). *Biochemistry* **14**, 3836.

Eipper, B. A., Mains, R. E., and Guenzi, D. (1976). *J. Biol. Chem.* **251**, 4121.

Elde, R., Hökfelt, T., Johansson, O., and Terenius, L. (1976). *Neuroscience* **1**, 349.

Elde, R., Hökfelt, T., Johansson, O., Ljungdahl, A., Nilsson, G., and Jeffcoate, S. L. (1978). *In* "Centrally Acting Peptides" (J. Hughes, ed.). Macmillan, New York, (in press).

El-Sobky, A., Dostrovsky, J. O., and Wall, P. D. (1976). *Nature (London)* **263**, 783.

Feinberg, A. P., Creese, I., and Snyder, S. H. (1976). *Proc. Natl. Acad. Sci. U.S.A.* **73**, 4215.

Feldberg, W., and Smyth, D. G. (1976). *J. Physiol. (London)* **260**, 31.

Feldberg, W., and Smyth, D. G. (1977). *Br. J. Pharmacol.* **60**, 445.

Ferland, L., Labrie, F., Coy, D. H., Arimura, A., and Schally, A. V. (1976). *Mol. Cell. Endocrinol.* **41**, 797.

Ferland, L., Fuxe, K., Feroch, P., Gustafsson, J. B., and Skelt, P. (1977). *Eur. J. Pharmacol.* **63**, 89.

Fratta, W., Yang, H.-Y., Hong, J., and Costa, E. (1977). *Nature (London)* **268**, 452.

Frederickson, R. C. A., and Norris, F. H. (1976). *Science* **194**, 440.

Fuxe, K., Ferland, L., Agnati, L. F., Eneroth, P., Gustafsson, J. A., Labrie, F., and Skelt, P. (1977). *Acta Pharmacol. Toxicol.* **41**, Suppl. IV, 48.

Gent, J. P., and Wolstencroft, J. H. (1976). *Nature (London)* **261**, 426.

George, R., and Way, E. L. (1955). *Br. J. Pharmacol. Chemother.* **10**, 260.

George, R., and Way, E. L. (1959). *J. Pharmacol. Exp. Ther.* **125**, 111.

Giagnoni, G., Sabol, S. L., and Nirenberg, M. (1977). *Proc. Natl. Acad. Sci. U.S.A.* **74**, 2259.

Gintzler, A. R., Levy, A., and Spector, S. (1976). *Proc. Natl. Acad. Sci. U.S.A.* **73**, 2132.

Gispen, W. H., van Wimermsa Greidanus, T. B., Waters-Ezrin, C., Zimmerman, E., Krivoy, W. A., and De Wied, D. (1975). *Eur. J. Pharmacol.* **33**, 99.

Goldstein, A., Pryor, G. T., Otis, L. S., and Larsen, F. (1976). *Life Sci.* **18**, 599.

Goldstein, A., Cox, B. M., Klee, W. A., and Nirenberg, M. (1977). *Nature (London)* **265**, 362.

Grandison, L., and Guidotti, A. (1977). *Nature (London)* **270**, 357.

Guillemin, R., Ling, N., and Burgus, R. (1976). *C.R. Hebd. Seances Acad. Sci.* **282**, 783.

Guillemin, R., Ling, N., and Vargo, T. (1977a). *Biochem. Biophys. Res. Commun.* **77**, 361.

Guillemin, R., Vargo, T., Rossier, J., Minick, S., Ling, N., Rivier, C., Vale, W., and Bloom, F. E. (1977b). *Science* **197**, 1367.

Gunne, M., Lindström, L., and Terenius, L. (1977). *J. Neurol. Trans.* **40**, 13.

Hahn, E. F., Fishman, J., Shiwaka, Y., Foldes, E. F., Nagashima, H., and Duncalf, D. (1977). *Res. Commun. Chem. Pathol. Pharmacol.* **18**, 1.

Hakanson, R., Owman, C. H., Sjöberg, W.-O., and Sporrong, B. (1970). *Histochemie* **21**, 189.

Hall, T. R., Adois, J. P., Smith, A. F., and Meites, J. (1976). *IRCS Libr. Compend.* **4**, 559.

Hambrook, J. M., Morgan, B. A., Rance, M. J., and Smith, C. F. L. (1976). *Nature (London)* **262**, 782.

Hill, R. G., Pepper, C. M., and Mitchell, J. F. (1976). *Nature (London)* **262**, 604.

Hökfelt, T., Elde, R., Johansson, O., Terenius, L., and Stein, L. (1977a). *Neurosci. Lett.* **5**, 25.

Hökfelt, T., Ljungdahl, D., Terenius, L., Elde, R., and Nilsson, G. (1977b). *Proc. Natl. Acad. Sci. U.S.A.* **74**, 3081.

Hong, J. S., Yang, H-Y., Fratta, W., and Costa, E. (1977a). *Brain Res.* **135**, 383.

Hong, J. S., Yang, H.-Y., Fratta, W., and Costa, E. (1977b). *Soc. Neurosci. Symp.* 293 (abstr.).

Hong, J. S., Yang, H.-Y., and Costa, E. (1977c). *Neuropharmacology* **16**, 451.

Horn, A. S., and Rogers, J. K. (1976). *Nature (London)* **260**, 795.

Hosobuchi, Y., Meglio, M., Adams, J. E., and Li, C. H. (1977). *Proc. Natl. Acad. Sci. U.S.A.* **74**, 4017.

Hughes, J. (1975). *Brain Res.* **88**, 295.

Hughes, J., Smith, T. W., Morgan, B. A., and Fothergill, L. H. (1975a). *Life Sci.* **16**, 1753.

Hughes, J., Smith, T. W., Kosterlitz, H. W., Fothergill, L. H., Morgan, B. A., and Morris, H. (1975b). *Nature (London)* **255**, 577.

Hutchinson, M., Kosterlitz, H. W., Lesli, F. M., Waterfield, A. A., and Terenius, L. (1976). *Br. J. Pharmacol.* **55**, 541.

Isogai, Y., Némethy, G., and Scheraga, H. A. (1977). *Proc. Natl. Acad. Sci. U.S.A.* **74**, 414.

Izumi, K., Motomatsu, T., Chrétien, M., Butterworth, R. F., Lis, M., Seidah, N., and Barbeau, A. (1977). *Life Sci.* **20**, 1149.

Jacob, J. J., Tremblay, F. C., and Colombel, M. C. (1974). *Psychopharmacologia* **37**, 217.

Jacquet, Y. F., and Marks, N. (1977). *Science* **194**, 631.

Jessell, T., and Iversen, L. L. (1977). *Nature (London)* **268**, 549.

Jones, C. R., Gibbons, W. A., and Garsky, V. (1976). *Nature (London)* **262**, 779.

Klee, W. A., and Nirenberg, M. (1976). *Nature (London)* **263**, 609.

Klee, W. A., Lampert, M., and Nirenberg, M. (1976). *In* "Opiates and Endogenous Opioid Peptides" (H. Kosterlitz, ed.), p. 153. North-Holland Publ., Amsterdam.

Kobayashi, R., Palkovits, M., Miller, R. J., Chang, K.-J., and Cuatrecasas, P. (1978). *Life Sci.* (in press).

Kokka, N., Garcia, J. F., George, R., and Elliot, H. W. (1972). *Endocrinology* **90**, 735.

Kosterlitz, H. W., and Waterfield, A. A. (1975). *Annu. Rev. Pharmacol.* **15**, 29.

Kosterlitz, H. W., and Watt, A. J. (1968). *Br. J. Pharmacol. Chemother.* **33**, 266.

Krieger, D. T., Liotta, D., and Brownstein, M. J. (1977a). *Proc. Natl. Acad. Sci. U.S.A.* **74,** 648.

Krieger, D. T., Liotta, D., Suda, T., Palkovits, M., and Brownstein, M. J. (1977b). *Biochem. Biophys. Res. Commun.* **76,** 930.

Kuhar, M. J., Pert, C. B., and Snyder, S. H. (1973). *Nature (London)* **245,** 447.

Kurahashi, K. (1974). *Annu. Rev. Biochem.* **43,** 445.

LaBella, F., Queen, G., Senyshyn, J., Lis, M., and Chrétien, M. (1977). *Biochem. Biophys. Res. Commun.* **75,** 350.

La Motte, C., Pert, C. B., and Snyder, S. H. (1976). *Brain Res.* **117,** 407.

Lampert, A., Nirenberg, M., and Klee, W. (1976). *Proc. Natl. Acad. Sci. U.S.A.* **73,** 3165.

Lane, A. C., Rance, M. J., and Walter, D. S. (1977). *Nature (London)* **269,** 75.

Lasagna, L. (1965). *Proc. R. Soc. Med.* **58,** 978.

Law, P. Y., Wei, E. T., Tseng, L. F., Loh, H. H., and Way, E. L. (1977). *Life Sci.* **20,** 251.

Lazarus, L. H., Ling, N., and Guillemin, R. (1976). *Proc. Natl. Acad. Sci. U.S.A.* **73,** 2156.

Lewis, P. N., Momany, F. A., and Scheraga, H. A. (1973). *Biochim. Biophys. Acta* **303,** 211.

Li, C. H. (1964). *Nature (London)* **201,** 924.

Li, C. H. (1977). *Arch. Biochem. Biophys.* **183,** 592.

Li, C. H., Barnafi, L., Chrétien, M., and Chung, D. (1965). *Nature (London)* **208,** 1093.

Li, C. H., Rao, A. J., Doneen, B. A., and Yamashiro, D. (1977). *Biochem. Biophys. Res. Commun.* **75,** 576.

Lien, E. L., Fenichel, R. L., Garsky, V., Sarantakis, D., and Grant, D. H. (1976). *Life Sci.* **19,** 837.

Ling, N., and Guillemin, R. (1976). *Proc. Natl. Acad. Sci. U.S.A.* **73,** 3308.

Linnoilla, I., SiAugustine, R., Miller, R. J., Chang, J-K., and Cuatrecasas, P. (1978). *Neuroscience* (in press).

Loh, H. H., Tseng, L. F., Wei, E., and Li, C. H. (1976a). *Proc. Natl. Acad. Sci. U.S.A.* **73,** 2895.

Loh, H. H., Brase, D. A., Sumpath-Khana, S., Mar, J. B., Way, E. L., and Li, C. H. (1976b). *Nature (London)* **264,** 567.

Lohmar, P., and Li, C. H. (1967). *Endocrinology* **82,** 898.

Lord, J. A. H., Waterfield, A. A., Hughes, J., and Kosterlitz, H. W. (1976). *In* "Opiates and Endogenous Opioid Peptides" (H. Kosterlitz, ed.), pp. 275–280. North-Holland Publ., Amsterdam.

Lord, J. A. H., Waterfield, A. A., Hughes, J., and Kosterlitz, H. W. (1977). *Nature (London)* **267,** 495.

Ludwick, J. R., Wiley, J. B., and Bass, P. (1968). *Gastroenterology* **54,** 41.

Ludwick, J. R., Wiley, J. B., and Bass, P. (1970). *Am. J. Dig. Dis.* **15,** 347.

McCarthy, P. S., Walker, R. J., and Woodruff, G. N. (1977). *J. Physiol (London)* 40 (abstr.).

McGeer, E. G., and McGeer, P. L. (1976). *Nature (London)* **263,** 517.

Madden, I. V., Akil, H., Patrick, R. L., and Barchas, J. D. (1977). *Nature (London)* **265,** 358.

Mains, R. E., and Eipper, B. A. (1976). *J. Biol. Chem.* **251,** 4115.

Mains, R. E., Eipper, B. A., and Ling, N. (1977). *Proc. Natl. Acad. Sci. U.S.A.* **74,** 3014.

Martin, W. R. (1967). *Pharmacol. Rev.* **19,** 421.

Matthews, B. W. (1972). *Macromolecules* **5,** 818.

May, P., Rittler, J., Proper, S., Theodoropoulas, M., and Kochu, S. (1977). *Proc. Endocr. Soc.* **62** (abstr.).

Mayer, D. J., and Price, D. D. (1976). *Pain* **2,** 379.

Mayer, D. J., Price, D. D., and Rafii, A. (1977). *Brain Res.* **121**, 368.

Meek, J., Yang, H.-Y., and Costa, E. (1977). *Neuropharmacology* **16**, 151.

Meltzer, H. V., Miller, R. J., Fessler, R. G., Simonovic, M., and Fang, U.S. (1978). *Life Sci.* **22**, 1931.

Miller, R. J., Chang, K.-J., Cuatrecasas, P., and Wilkinson, S. (1977). *Biochem. Biophys. Res. Commun.* **74**, 1311.

Miller, R. J., Chang, K.-J., Cooper, B., and Cuatrecasas, P., (1978a). *J. Biol. Chem.* **253**, 1778.

Miller, R. J., Chang, K.-J., Cuatrecasas, P., Wilkinson, S., Lowe, L., Beddell, C., and Follenfant, R. (1978b). *In* "Centrally Acting Peptides" (J. Hughes, ed.), Macmillan, New York (in press).

Miller, R. J., Chang, K.-J., Cuatrecasas, P., and Leighton, J. (1978c). *Life Sci.* **22**, 379.

Minneman, K., and Iversen, L. L. (1976). *Nature (London)* **262**, 313.

Momany, F. A. (1977). *Biochem. Biophys. Res. Commun.* **75**, 1098.

Morgan, R. A., Smith, C. F. C., Waterfield, A. A., Hughes, J., and Kosterlitz, H. W. (1976). *J. Pharm. Pharmacol.* **28**, 660.

Morin, O., Garon, M. R., Delean, A., and Labrie, F. (1976). *Biochem. Biophys. Res. Commun.* **73**, 940.

Moroni, F., Cheney, D. L., and Costa, E. (1977). *Nature (London)* **267**, 267.

Nakanishi, S., Tau, S., Hirata, Y., Matsukura, S., Imura, H., and Numa, S. (1976). *Proc. Natl. Acad. Sci. U.S.A.* **73**, 4319.

Némethy, G., and Printz, M. P. (1972). *Macromolecules* **5**, 755.

Nicoll, R. A., Siggins, G., Ling, N., Bloom, F. E., and Guillemin, R. (1977). *Proc. Natl. Acad. Sci. U.S.A.* **74**, 2584.

North, A. R., and Williams, J. T. (1976). *Nature (London)* **264**, 460.

Orth, D. N., Nicholson, W. E., Mitchell, W. M., Island, D. P., Shapiro, M., and Byyny, M. L. (1973). *Endocrinology* **92**, 385.

Pasternak, G., Goodman, R., and Snyder, S. H. (1975). *Life Sci.* **16**, 1765.

Pasternak, G., Simantov, R., and Snyder, S. H. (1976). *Mol. Pharmacol.* **12**, 504.

Paton, W. D. M. (1957). *Br. J. Pharmacol.* **12**, 119.

Pearse, A. G. E. (1976). *Nature (London)* **262**, 92.

Pert, A. (1976). *In* "Opiates and Endogenous Opioid Peptides" (H. Kosterlitz, ed.), pp. 87–94. North-Holland Publ., Amsterdam.

Pert, A., and Sivet, C. (1977). *Nature (London)* **265**, 645.

Pert, A., Simantov, R., and Snyder, S. H. (1977). *Brain Res.* **136**, 523.

Pert, C. B., and Snyder, S. H. (1973a). *Science* **179**, 1011.

Pert, C. B., and Snyder, S. H. (1973b). *Proc. Natl. Acad. Sci. U.S.A.* **70**, 2243.

Pert, C. B., and Snyder, S. H. (1974). *Mol. Pharmacol.* **10**, 868.

Pert, C. B., Pert, A., and Tallman, J. (1976a). *Proc. Natl. Acad. Sci. U.S.A.* **73**, 2226.

Pert, C. B., Pert, A., Chang, J.-K., and Fong, B. T. W. (1976b). *Science* **194**, 330.

Pert, C. B., Bowie, D. L., Fong, B. T. W., and Chang, J.-K. (1976c). *In* "Opiates and Endogenous Opioid Peptides" (H. Kosterlitz, ed.), p. 79. North-Holland Publ., Amsterdam.

Pert, C. B., Bowie, D. L., Pert, A., Morrell, J., and Gross, E. (1977). *Nature (London)* **269**, 73.

Pickel, B., Joh, T., Reis, D. J., Leeman, S. E., and Miller, R. J. (1978). *Brain Res.* (in press).

Plant, O. H., and Miller, G. H. (1926). *J. Pharmacol. Exp. Ther.* **27**, 361.

Polak, J. M., Sullivan, S. N., Bloom, S. R., Facer, R., and Pearse, A. G. E. (1977). *Lancet* **1**, 972.

Puig, N., Gascon, P., Craviso, G. L., and Musacchio, J. M. (1977). *Science* **195**, 419.

Queen, G., Pinsky, C., and LaBella, F. C. (1976). *Biochem. Biophys. Res. Commun.* **72**, 1021.

Ramakrishnan, C., and Ramachandran, G. N. (1965). *Biophys. J.* **5**, 909.

Rees, L. H. (1975). *J. Endocrinol.* **67**, 143.

Reynolds, D. V. (1969). *Science* **164**, 444.

Rivier, C., Vale, W., Ling, N., Brown, M., and Guillemin, R. (1977). *Endocrinology* **100**, 238.

Roberts, J. L., and Herbert, E. (1977). *Proc. Natl. Acad. Sci. U.S.A.* **74**, 4826.

Römer, D., Buscher, H., Hill, R., Pless, J., Bauer, W., Cardinaux, F., Classe, A., Hauser, D., and Huguenin, R. (1977). *Nature (London)* **268**, 547.

Roques, B. P., Garbay-Jaureguiberry, C., Oberlin, R., Anteunis, M., and Lala, A. K. (1976). *Nature (London)* **262**, 778.

Ross, M., Dingledine, R., Cox, B. M., and Goldstein, A. (1977). *Brain Res.* **124**, 523.

Rossier, J., Bayon, A., Vargo, T. M., Ling, N., Guillemin, R., and Bloom, F. (1977a). *Life Sci.* **21**, 1847.

Rossier, J., Bayon, A., Vargo, T., Ling, N., Bloom, F. E., and Guillemin, R. (1977b). *Proc. Natl. Acad. Sci. U.S.A.* **74**, 5162.

Rubinstein, M., Stein, M., Garber, L. D., and Udenfriend, S. (1977a). *Proc. Natl. Acad. Sci. U.S.A.* **74**, 3052.

Rubinstein, M., Stein, M., and Udenfriend, S. (1977b). *Proc. Natl. Acad. Sci. U.S.A.* **74**, 4969.

Satoh, M., Zieglgansberger, W., Freis, W., and Herz, A. (1974). *Brain Res.* **82**, 378–382.

Schaumann, W. (1955). *Br. J. Pharmacol. Chemother.* **10**, 456.

Schiller, P. W., Yam, C. F., and Lis, M. (1977). *Biochemistry* **16**, 1831.

Schulz, R., and Herz, A. (1976). *Eur. J. Pharmacol.* **39**, 429.

Schulz, R., Wuster, M., and Herz, A. (1977a). *Life Sci.* **21**, 105.

Schulz, R., Wuster, M., Simantov, R., Snyder, S. H., and Herz, A. (1977b). *Eur. J. Pharmacol.* **41**, 347.

Scott, A. P., and Lowry, P. J. (1974). *Biochem. J.* **134**, 593.

Segal, M. (1977). *Neuropharmacology* **16**, 587.

Shaar, C. J., Frederickson, R. C. D., Dininger, N. D., and Jackson, L. (1977). *Life Sci.* **21**, 853.

Simantov, R., and Snyder, S. H. (1976a). *Proc. Natl. Acad. Sci. U.S.A.* **73**, 2515.

Simantov, R., and Snyder, S. H. (1976b). *In* "Opiates and Endogenous Opioid Peptides" (H. Kosterlitz, ed.), pp. 41–48. North-Holland Publ., Amsterdam.

Simantov, R., and Snyder, S. H. (1976c). *Nature (London)* **262**, 505.

Simantov, R., and Snyder, S. H. (1978). *Eur. J. Pharmacol.* (in press).

Simantov, R., Kuhar, M. J., Pasternak, G. W., and Snyder, S. H. (1976a). *Brain Res.* **106**, 189.

Simantov, R., Snowman, A. H., and Snyder, S. H. (1976b). *Brain Res.* **107**, 650.

Simantov, R., Goodman, R., Aposhian, D., and Snyder, S. H. (1976c). *Brain Res.* **111**, 204.

Simantov, R., Childers, S. R., and Snyder, S. H. (1977a). *Brain Res.* **135**, 358.

Simantov, R., Kuhar, M. J., Uhl, G., and Snyder, S. II. (1977b). *Proc. Natl. Acad. Sci. U.S.A.* **74**, 2167.

Simon, E. J., Hiller, J. M., and Edelman, I. C. (1973). *Proc. Natl. Acad. Sci. U.S.A.* **69**, 1835.

Smith, T. W., Hughes, J., Kosterlitz, H. W., and Sasa, R. P. (1976). *In* "Opiates and Endogenous Opioid Peptides" (H. Kosterlitz, ed.), pp. 57–62. North-Holland Publ., Amsterdam.

Snell, C. R., Jeffcoate, W., Lowry, P. J., Rees, L. H., and Smyth, D. G. (1977). *FEBS Lett.* **81**, 427.

Snyder, S. H. (1975). *Nature (London)* **257**, 185.

Snyder, S. H. (1977). *Chem. & Eng. News* **55**, 26.

Snyder, S. H., and Matthysse, S. (1975). *Neurosci. Res. Bull.* **13**.

Somoza, E., and Portal, C. M. G. (1977). *Life Sci.* **20**, 1815.

Stewart, J. M., Grillo, C. J., Neldner, K., Reeve, E. R., Krivoy, W. A., and Zimmerman, E. (1976). *Nature (London)* **262**, 784.

Székely, J., Ranai, A. Z., Dunai-Kovacs, Z., Miglecz, E., Berzetei, I., Bajusz, S., and Graf, L. (1977). *Eur. J. Pharmacol.* **43**, 293.

Taube, H. P., Borowski, E., Endo, T., and Starke, K. (1976). *Eur. J. Pharmacol.* **38**, 377.

Terenius, L. (1973). *Acta Pharmacol. Toxicol.* **33**, 377.

Terenius, L., and Wahlström, A. (1975a). *Acta Physiol. Scand.* **96**, 76.

Terenius, L., and Wahlström, A. (1975b). *Life Sci.* **16**, 1759.

Terenius, L., Wahlström, A., Lindberg, G., Karlsson, S., and Ragnasson, V., (1976). *Biochem. Biophys. Res. Commun.* **71**, 175.

Terenius, L., Wahlström, A., and Agren, H. (1977). *Psychopharmacologia* **54**, 31.

Teschemacher, H., Opheim, K. E., Cox, B. M., and Goldstein, A. (1975). *Life Sci.* **16**, 1771.

Tolis, G., Hickey, J., and Gujda, H. (1975). *J. Clin. Endocrinol. Metab.* **41**, 797.

Traber, J., Glaser, T., Brande, M., Klebensberger, W., and Hamprecht, B. (1977). *FEBS Lett.* **81**, 351.

Tseng, L. F., Loh, H. H., and Li, C. H. (1976a). *Nature (London)* **263**, 239.

Tseng, L. F., Loh, H. H., and Li, C. H. (1976b). *Proc. Natl. Acad. Sci. U.S.A.* **73**, 4187.

Tseng, L. F., Loh, H. H., and Li, C. H. (1977). *Biochem. Biophys. Res. Commun.* **74**, 390.

Tsou, K., and Jang, C.-S. (1964). *Sci. Sin.* **8**, 1099.

Uhl, G., Kuhar, M. J., and Snyder, S. H. (1977). *Soc. Neurosci. Symp.* 417 (abstr.).

Uhl, G., Kuhar, M. J., and Snyder, S. H. (1978). *Brain Res.* (in press).

Unger, G., Unger, A. L., and Malin, D. H. (1976). *In* "Opiates and Endogenous Opioid Peptides" (H. Kosterlitz, ed.), p. 121. North-Holland Publ., Amsterdam.

Urca, G., Frenk, H., Liebeskind, J. C., and Taylor, A. (1977). *Science* **197**, 83.

Van Loon, G. R., and Kim, C. (1977). *Res. Commun. Chem. Pathol. Pharmacol.* **18**, 171.

Volavka, J., Mallya, A., Baig, S., and Perez-Cruet, J. (1977). *Science* **196**, 1227.

Wahlström, A., Brandt, M., Moroder, L., Wunsch, E., Lindberg, G., Ragnasson, U., Terenius, L., and Hamprecht, B. (1977). *FEBS Lett.* **77**, 28.

Walker, J. M., Berntson, G., Sandman, C. D., Coy, D. H., Schally, A. V., and Kastin, A. J. (1977). *Science* **196**, 85.

Waterfield, A. A., Hughes, J., and Kosterlitz, H. W. (1976). *Nature (London)* **260**, 624.

Waterfield, A. A., Smokcum, R. W. J., Hughes, J., Kosterlitz, H. W., and Henderson, G. (1977). *Eur. J. Pharmacol.* **43**, 107.

Watson, S. J., Barchas, J. D., and Li, C. H. (1977a). *Proc. Natl. Acad. Sci. U.S.A.* **74**, 5155.

Watson, S. J., Akil, H., Sullivan, S., and Barchas, J. D. (1977b). *Life Sci.* **21**, 733.

Wei, E., and Loh, H. H. (1976). *Science* **193**, 1262.

Wei, E., Tseng, L. F., Loh, H. H., and Li, C. H. (1977). *Life Sci.* **21**, 321.

Weissman, B. A., Gershon, H., and Pert, C. B. (1976). *FEBS Lett.* **70**, 245.

Weitzmann, R. E., Risher, D. A., Minick, S., Ling, N., and Guillemin, R. (1977). *Endocrinology* **101**, 1643.

Yalow, R. S., and Berson, S. A. (1971). *Biochem. Biophys. Res. Commun.* **44**, 439.

Yalow, R. S., and Berson, S. A. (1973). *J. Clin. Endocrinol. Metab.* **36**, 415.

Yamashiro, D., Tseng, L. F., and Li, C. H. (1977). *Biochem. Biophys. Res. Commun.* **78**, 1124.

Yang, H.-Y., Hong, J.-S., and Costa, E. (1977). *Neuropharmacology* **16**, 303.

Yang, H.-Y., Hong, J.-S., Fratta, W., and Costa, E. (1978). *Adv. Psychopharmacol.* **18**, (in press.)

Zieglgansberger, W., Fry, J. P., Herz, A., Moroder, L., and Wunsch, E. (1976). *Brain Res.* **115**, 160.

VITAMINS AND HORMONES, VOL. 36

Hormonal Control of Hepatic Gluconeogenesis

S. J. PILKIS, C. R. PARK, and T. H. CLAUS

Department of Physiology, Vanderbilt University School of Medicine, Nashville, Tennessee

I. INTRODUCTION

Gluconeogenesis is the process whereby lactate, pyruvate, glycerol, and certain amino acids are converted to glucose and glycogen. The liver is the major site of gluconeogenesis, although the kidney becomes important during prolonged starvation. The most important function of gluconeogenesis is the maintenance of blood glucose levels during times when food intake is restricted and/or glycogen stores are depleted. It is the means whereby the lactate that is produced by glycolysis in erythrocytes and in exercising muscle is reconverted to glucose. Similarly, it conserves the glycerol that is released during lipolysis in adipose tissue and the alanine produced by amino acid metabolism and glycolysis in muscle. Gluconeogenesis also contributes significantly to the utilization of amino acids, which are either absorbed from the alimintary tract or released during protein breakdown in muscle and other tissues. When conditions of metabolic acidosis exist, such as during times of prolonged starvation, the contribution of renal gluconeogenesis to the total glucose produced increases from less than 20% to about 50% (Owen *et al.*, 1969). At the low pH, the conversion of glutamate and α-ketoglutarate to glucose is enhanced. This in turn leads to an increase in NH_3 production, which is used to counteract the acidosis (Goodman *et al.*, 1966; Steiner *et al.*, 1968).

Figure 1 shows the sequence of reactions by which lactate, pyruvate, and various gluconeogenic amino acids are converted to glucose in the hepatocyte. Amino acids and probably lactate enter the cell by various carrier-mediated plasma membrane transport systems. Lactate and most amino acids are converted to pyruvate in the cytoplasm of the cell.

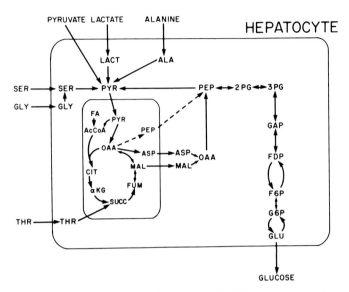

FIG. 1. Gluconeogenic pathway in the hepatocyte. The plasma membrane of the hepatocyte is represented by the large rectangle. The mitochondrion is depicted by the small rectangle. The dashed line represents the pathway for conversion of oxaloacetate to phosphoenolpyruvate in species that possess mitochondrial phosphoenolpyruvate carboxykinase. Abbrevations: LACT, lactate; PYR, pyruvate; ALA, alanine; SER, serine; GLY, glycine; FA, fatty acid; AcCoA, acetyl-CoA; CIT, citrate; αKG, α-ketoglutarate; SUCC, succinate; FUM, fumarate; MAL, malate; OAA, oxaloacetate; ASP, aspartate; THR, threonine; PEP, phosphoenolpyruvate; 2PG, 2-phosphoglycerate; 3PG, 3-phosphoglycerate; GAP, glyceraldehyde 3-phosphate; FDP, fructose 1,6-diphosphate; F6P, fructose 6-phosphate; G6P, glucose 6-phosphate; GLU, glucose.

Pyruvate enters the mitochondria by a transport system and is converted to oxaloacetate by pyruvate carboxylase or to acetyl-CoA by pyruvate dehydrogenase. The fate of the mitochondrial oxaloacetate varies in different species, depending in large part on the distribution of the enzyme phosphoenolpyruvate carboxykinase between cytoplasm and mitochondria (Tilghman *et al.*, 1976). In the rat and mouse liver, it is converted to malate and/or aspartate, and these metabolites are transported to the cytoplasm, where they are reconverted to oxaloacetate. The oxaloacetate is then converted to phosphoenolpyruvate by phosphoenolpyruvate carboxykinase, which is a cytosolic enzyme in rat and mouse liver. This complicated series of interconversions is apparently necessary because the mitochondrial membrane is presumably impermeable to oxaloacetate (however, see Gimpel *et al.*, 1973). In pigeon, chicken, and rabbit liver, phosphoenolpyruvate carboxykinase is in the mitochondria and oxaloacetate is directly converted to phosphoenolpyruvate and then transported to the cytoplasm. In the human, guinea pig, sheep, and cow liver, the enzyme is present both in the mitochondria and the cytoplasm, but the fraction of total phosphoenolpyruvate synthesis at each site is as yet uncertain. Cytosolic phosphoenolpyruvate can be disposed of by two routes. First, a portion is converted to pyruvate because of the presence of pyruvate kinase. This creates a complicated substrate cycle between pyruvate and phosphoenolpyruvate. Second, the remaining phosphoenolpyruvate is converted to fructose diphosphate by the enzymes of the Embden–Meyerhof pathway. Fructose diphosphate is then converted to fructose 6-phosphate by fructose diphosphatase. However, the presence of phosphofructokinase also creates a second substrate cycle between fructose diphosphate and fructose 6-phosphate. The fraction of fructose 6-phosphate not recycled is converted to glucose 6-phosphate by glucose-6-phosphate isomerase. The final step in the pathway is the conversion of glucose 6-phosphate to glucose by glucose-6-phosphatase. However, the presence of hexokinase and glucokinase in liver creates the potential for a third substrate cycle between glucose and glucose 6-phosphate.

Hormonal control of gluconeogenesis can be divided for convenience into three categories. The first involves regulation of substrate supply. All gluconeogenic substrates reach the liver in subsaturating concentration. Thus, regulation of substrate release into the blood from the extrahepatic tissues will directly affect hepatic glucose formation. This aspect of gluconeogenic control has been reviewed by Scrutton and Utter (1968), Exton *et al.* (1970), and Exton (1972) and will not be discussed here. The second category deals with the very important but relatively slow adaptive changes in enzyme activity due to regulation of protein synthesis and/or degradation. This topic will not be considered here in any detail. The third category is concerned with the minute-to-minute regulation of gluconeogenesis by glucagon, catecholamines, and insulin. This will be the central topic of this review. The hypothesis will be put forth that these hormones act in the pathway by affecting the phosphorylation state of several enzymes involved in the substrate cycles between pyruvate and phosphoenolpyruvate and fructose diphosphate and fructose 6-phosphate. The regulation of pyruvate kinase, fructose diphosphatase, and phosphofructokinase will be emphasized. While the emphasis will be on the minute-to-minute regulation of gluconeogenesis, it is clear that regulation *in vivo* occurs in all three categories simultaneously and in an integrated fashion.

II. Role of Cyclic AMP in Hormonal Control of Gluconeogenesis

The hormonal control of hepatic gluconeogenesis has been studied intensively since the early 1960s, during which time the isolated perfused liver system was fully developed. Schimassek and Mitzkat (1963), Garcia et al. (1964), Struck et al. (1965), and Exton and Park (1966) reported that glucagon stimulated gluconeogenesis in perfused rat liver, and Exton and Park (1966) demonstrated a similar effect of epinephrine. Using the isolated perfused liver system, Exton and Park (1966, 1969) postulated that the effect of these hormones was mediated by an elevation of cyclic AMP (cAMP) levels. The evidence for this was based on the following observations: (1) both glucagon and epinephrine caused rapid elevations of hepatic cAMP; (2) the concentration of hormone necessary to elicit elevation of cAMP levels was similar to that needed to stimulate gluconeogenesis; and (3) addition of exogenous cAMP mimicked the effect of the hormones. These observations are consistent with the concept of cAMP as the second messenger (see Robison et al., 1971). According to this concept, the hormone, or first messenger, carries the required information to the cell, where it binds to specific hormone receptors. This event in turn stimulates adenylate cyclase to convert ATP to cAMP. This intracellular or second messenger then transfers the information to the cell's enzymic machinery. In the case of gluconeogenesis, this information transfer is thought to be similar to that for glycogen metabolism. That is, cAMP activates a protein kinase, which by catalyzing the phosphorylation of one or more enzymes alters their activity.

Regulation of the level of cAMP could also explain the inhibitory effect of insulin on gluconeogenesis. Butcher et al. (1968) first showed that insulin lowered the level of cAMP in adipocytes exposed to epinephrine, and Exton et al. (1971) observed a similar lowering of cAMP by insulin in the isolated perfused liver exposed to glucagon and epinephrine. Similar data have been obtained in isolated hepatocyte preparations by Pilkis et al. (1975) and Claus and Pilkis (1976) as shown in Fig. 2. It can be seen that insulin 10 nM suppressed the response of gluconeogenesis to low concentrations of glucagon or cAMP, and that the suppression disappeared as the concentration of agonist increased. Insulin also suppressed the small stimulation by a maximally effective concentration (1 μM) of epinephrine. Since insulin lowered cAMP levels concomitantly, it suggested that insulin affected gluconeogenesis by lowering cAMP levels. The failure of insulin to suppress the effects of high concentrations of glucagon or cAMP was probably due to the fact that the intracellular level of the nucleotide

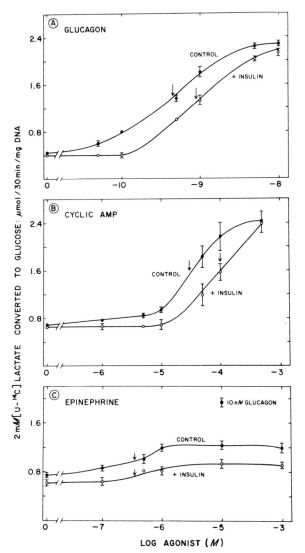

F<small>IG</small>. 2. Insulin antagonism of the concentration-dependent stimulation of gluco-
neogenesis by various agonists. Hepatocytes from fed rats were preincubated for 30
minutes without any additions and then incubated for 30 minutes with 2 mM
[U-^{14}C]lactate and the appropriate conditions. The insulin concentration was 10 nM.
The arrows indicate the concentration of agonist that gave a half-maximum response.
The data are from Claus and Pilkis (1976).

had become so great that reduction in its level by insulin was insufficient to make it rate-limiting for gluconeogenesis.

While it appears that glucagon effects in liver are mediated by cAMP, recent evidence indicates that catecholamine effects may or may not be. Sherline *et al.* (1972) showed that the effects of catecholamines on glycogenolysis in the perfused rat liver were mediated by both a β- and an α-mechanism. The α-mechanism was not associated with changes in cAMP levels. Tolbert *et al.* (1973) and Tolbert and Fain (1974) first showed that epinephrine could stimulate gluconeogenesis by an α-mechanism. That is, the catecholamine stimulation of gluconeogenesis was blocked by α-blocking agents, such as phentolamine and dihydroergotamine, but not by the β-blocker propranolol, which suppressed the increase in cAMP. Furthermore, the catecholamine stimulation of glucose synthesis was suppressed by α-blockers even though cAMP levels remained elevated. In addition, isoproterenol, a pure β-agonist, elevated cAMP levels but had no effect on gluconeogenesis. Phenylephrine, a synthetic catecholamine and α-agonist, also increased gluconeogenesis but did not elevate cAMP. Exton and Harper (1975) and Cherrington *et al.* (1976) have confirmed many of these observations and have shown that the α-effect of catecholamine in rat hepatocytes is not associated with an activation of cAMP-dependent protein kinase.

The physiological significance of stimulation of gluconeogenesis by an α-receptor mediated, cAMP-independent mechanism is unclear and an important role for the cAMP-mediated pathway of catecholamine action has not been excluded. It has been noted, for example, that a maximal stimulation of gluconeogenesis by the α-pathway in isolated rat hepatocytes from fed rats increases the rate by only about 60%, whereas glucagon in the same preparation stimulates 3- to 4-fold (Pilkis *et al.*, 1975). Furthermore, earlier studies by Exton and Park (1969b), using a perfused liver preparation from fed rats, showed that epinephrine caused almost as large a stimulation (2- to 3-fold) as glucagon. The reason for the difference in behavior of these preparations is not clear, but the difference may be due to damage to isolated hepatocytes and their receptors by collagenase treatment and Ca^{2+} deprivation. Furthermore, it is known from studies of lipolysis in fat tissue that the balance between α- and β-receptor effects shows striking species variability. It is therefore quite possible that catecholamines activate gluconeogenesis in some species by a predominantly β-receptor mechanism and in others by an α-mechanism.

There is also evidence that insulin can suppress gluconeogenesis by a mechanism that is independent of changes in cAMP (Claus and Pilkis,

1976). This is supported by three lines of evidence: (1) Glucagon (0.5 nM) stimulated glucose synthesis from 2 mM [U-^{14}C]lactate 40–50% in either the absence or the presence of extracellular Ca^{2+}. Insulin (10 nM) almost completely abolished the stimulation in both instances, even though it did not lower cAMP levels in the absence of Ca^{2+}. (2) Insulin was able to suppress gluconeogenesis stimulated by 10 μM epinephrine plus a β-blocking agent. Under these conditions, insulin did not lower the tissue level of cAMP, the rise of which had been largely or completely abolished by propranolol (10–100 μM). Neither insulin nor propranolol had any effect on cAMP levels in the absence of epinephrine. Insulin also suppressed the stimulation of gluco-neogenesis by phenylephrine, which had no measurable effect on cAMP levels. (3) Insulin suppressed the epinephrine-induced stimula-tion of gluconeogenesis even when added 20 minutes after the catecholamine. At this time, cAMP levels had already returned to near basal values and were not further reduced by insulin addition. When the two hormones were added together, insulin suppressed the rise of both cAMP and gluconeogenesis. Thus insulin suppresses the stimula-tion of gluconeogenesis by either the α- or the β-component of catecholamine actions. It seems, therefore, that there are at least two mechanisms by which insulin can suppress gluconeogenesis, one de-pendent and the other independent of changes in tissue level of cAMP. Which mechanism is most important physiologically is unclear, but may depend on which gluconeogenic agonist is involved and in which species. Similar cAMP-dependent and -independent effects of insulin on catecholamine activation of lipolysis in adipose tissue (Siddle and Hales, 1974) and muscle (Larner, 1968) have been observed.

It has been suggested recently by several laboratories that the α-component of catecholamine action on glycogenolysis in liver is mediated by alterations in Ca^{2+} flux (Van de Werve et al., 1977; Kep-pens et al., 1977; Assimacopoulos-Jeannet et al., 1977; Chan and Exton, 1977). This proposal is supported by the observations that: (1) phenyleph-rine did not activate cAMP-dependent protein kinase or elevate cAMP levels (Keppens et al., 1977; Cherrington et al., 1976; Birnbaum and Fain, 1977); (2) in the absence of calcium, phenylephrine did not activate phosphorylase (Van de Werve et al., 1977; Keppens et al., 1977; Assimacopoulos-Jeannet et al., 1977); (3) the calcium ionophore, A-23127, mimicked the effect of phenylephrine (Keppens et al., 1977; Assimacopoulos-Jeannet et al., 1977); (4) phenylephrine altered $^{45}Ca^{2+}$ flux (Keppens et al., 1977; Assimacopoulos-Jeannet et al., 1977); and (5) the effect of phenylephrine on Ca^{2+} flux was blocked by an α-blocker (Keppens et al., 1977; Assimacopoulos-Jeannet et al., 1977). Whether the α-component of catecholamine action on gluconeogenesis is mediated by calcium is unknown. It is also not known how insulin suppresses gluconeogenesis in a cAMP-independent manner.

III. SITES OF ACTION OF HORMONES ON HEPATIC GLUCONEOGENESIS

It was thought that the major rate-limiting step(s) were in the initial part of the gluconeogenic pathway, since maximal concentrations of lactate, pyruvate, or alanine produced rates of gluconeogenesis that are usually much less than those of substrates that entered at or above the triose phosphate level (Exton and Park, 1967; Ross et al., 1967a). Analysis of intermediary metabolites from rat livers perfused with high concentrations of lactate, pyruvate, or alanine led to the hypothesis that glucagon, cAMP, epinephrine, and insulin acted somewhere between pyruvate and phosphoenolpyruvate (Exton and Park, 1969; Williamson et al., 1969c; Mallette et al., 1969a). However, glucagon also appeared to affect reactions between fructose diphosphate and fructose 6-phosphate (Williamson et al., 1969c; Blair et al., 1973; Harris, 1975; Pilkis et al., 1976a). In addition, the transport of alanine across the plasma membrane was found to be stimulated by glucagon (Mallette et al., 1969a). The region of the pathway between pyruvate and phosphoenolpyruvate involves many steps, both cytosolic and mitochondrial (Fig. 1). Attempts to localize the step affected by measurement of the total concentration of intermediary metabolites have been unsuccessful, since many of the metabolites exist in both the cytosol and mitochondria. However, a number of mitochondrial steps have been proposed as sites of glucagon action. They include the reactions catalyzed by pyruvate carboxylase and pyruvate dehydrogenase, as well as pyruvate transport into mitochondria and dicarboxylate transport from the mitochondria. Cytosolic sites which have been proposed for hormone action include the enzymes of the pyruvate–phosphoenolpyruvate substrate cycle (phosphoenolpyruvate carboxykinase and pyruvate kinase) and those of the fructose diphosphate–fructose 6-phosphate cycle (fructose diphosphatase and phosphofructokinase). These sites will be discussed in detail in the following sections.

A. TRANSPORT ACROSS THE PLASMA MEMBRANE AS A POSSIBLE SITE OF HORMONE ACTION

There is no evidence that plasma membrane transport of lactate, pyruvate, or glycerol is under hormonal control in liver. These substances presumably enter the liver by rapid carrier-mediated transport. Hepatic amino acid transport, on the other hand, has been shown to be regulated by glucagon, insulin, catecholamines, cortisol, and growth hormone (see Exton, 1972). Glucagon has been shown to stimulate the net hepatic uptake of a number of amino acids (Mallette et al., 1969b; Marliss et al., 1970), but only in the case of alanine and lysine is there evidence for an effect on membrane transport per se (Mallette et al., 1969b). LeCam and Freychet (1976) have recently demonstrated a stimulatory effect of glucagon on the uptake of the amino acid analogs γ-aminoisobutyric (AIB) and cycloleucine in freshly prepared isolated hepatocytes. Glucagon stimulated AIB uptake against a concentration gradient. The hormone effect was rapid in onset, abolished by cycloheximide, mimicked by dibutyryl cAMP, and limited to the A-type transport system. Similar effects of glucagon have been reported in liver slices (Tews et al., 1970, 1975) and perfused rat liver (Chambers et al., 1968; Mallette et al., 1969b). Kletzien et al., (1976a) have also reported glucagon-stimulated AIB transport in primary cultures of hepatocytes, but the hormone effect was seen only after a 1- to 2-hour lag period. Prior or simultaneous addition of dexamethasone to glucagon-treated cells resulted in a strong potentiation of the glucagon enhancement of AIB transport. These investigators found that glucagon altered the $K_{0.5}$ for AIB transport. The mechanism of the glucagon effect is unknown, but it is presumably mediated by elevation of cAMP.

Epinephrine has been shown to increase hepatic accumulation of AIB in primary cultures of rat hepatocytes (Pariza et al., 1977). Interestingly, when hepatocytes were maintained in culture for several days, they responded to epinephrine with substantially larger increases in cAMP than those observed in freshly prepared hepatocytes. Propranolol blocked this rise in cAMP but had no effect on the epinephrine-induced stimulation of AIB transport. α-Blockers diminished the effect of epinephrine on AIB transport. These results suggest that epinephrine can enhance AIB transport by a cAMP-independent action.

The stimulation of amino acid transport may contribute to the effect of glucagon or epinephrine on gluconeogenesis. However, insulin suppressed alanine gluconeogenesis that had been stimulated by glucagon (Claus and Pilkis, 1976), but increased the rate of AIB uptake in primary cultures of adult rat hepatocytes (Kletzien et al., 1976b). Although insulin and glucagon apparently promote hepatocyte amino acid transport, the different actions of these hormones on gluconeogenesis are probably due to effects at other sites. Further experimentation is necessary to relate the effect of hormones on hepatic amino acid transport to regulation of glucose synthesis.

B. Possible Mitochondrial Sites of Hormone Action

1. *Pyruvate Carboxylase*

Pyruvate carboxylase plays a key role in gluconeogenesis since pyruvate must be converted to oxaloacetate for net glucose synthesis to occur. This mitochondrial enzyme requires acetyl-CoA for activity (Keech and Utter, 1963). The requirement for acetyl-CoA was the basis for a hypothesis (Utter *et al.,* 1964) that glucagon stimulates gluconeogenesis by increasing the levels of this effector (Struck *et al.,* 1966; Williamson *et al.,* 1966a,b; Ross *et al.,* 1967b; Soling *et al.,* 1968). The elevation of acetyl-CoA levels resulted from an increase in fatty acid oxidation triggered by the activation of lipolysis by a cAMP-sensitive lipase. Support for the hypothesis came from several observations. First, the addition of fatty acid (oleate) to perfused rat livers stimulated gluconeogenesis from three-carbon precursors and its effect was not additive with that of glucagon (Williamson *et al.,* 1969a,c). Second, both glucagon and oleate increased the redox state of the mitochondrial and cytoplasmic compartments in rat liver and increased the phosphate potential of the mitochondria (Siess and Wieland, 1976). Third, glucagon increased ketogenesis, albeit to a smaller extent than oleate (Williamson *et al.,* 1969c). However, these similarities in the effects of glucagon and oleate have not been universally observed. Exton *et al.* (1969) noted that glucagon frequently had little or no effect on ketogenesis even though it always stimulated gluconeogenesis. Ross *et al.* (1967a) and Exton *et al.* (1969) have observed that the effects of maximally effective concentrations of fatty acid and glucagon are additive. Additive effects were also observed with acetate, which elevates acetyl-CoA levels, and glucagon (Claus *et al.,* 1975). Thus glucagon appears to stimulate gluconeogenesis by some mechanism in addition to raising acetyl-CoA levels. This conclusion was further supported by the observation that glucagon still promoted gluconeogenesis when liver lipolysis was inhibited by glucodiazine (Frolich and Wieland, 1971).

The stimulatory effect of fatty acid on gluconeogenesis has also been attributed to the increased redox state of the mitochondria and cytoplasm. The increased $NADH:NAD^+$ ratio in the mitochondria would increase the export of malate from the mitochondria, which, upon reconversion to oxaloacetate in the cytoplasm, would provide NADH for the conversion of 3-phosphoglycerate to glyceraldehyde 3-phosphate (Williamson, 1966; Williamson *et al.*, 1969a). In support of this view, β-hydroxybutyrate, the sole fate of which in the liver is mitochondrial conversion to acetoacetate with the generation of NADH, was found to mimic the effect of fatty acid on lactate gluconeogenesis in the perfused rat liver (Arinze *et al.*, 1973). We have observed a similar effect of β-hydroxybutyrate in isolated rat hepatocytes. However, its effect was additive with that of glucagon (Claus and Pilkis, 1977). Thus it does not appear that glucagon enhances gluconeogenesis solely by changes in redox state.

That glucagon stimulates gluconeogenesis by a mechanism independent of changes in fatty acid oxidation is also supported by the different changes in levels of gluconeogenic intermediates that are brought about by glucagon and oleate. Ui *et al.* (1973a,b) and Siess *et al.* (1977) showed that glucagon markedly decreased the levels of glutamate and α-ketoglutarate and increased the levels of phosphoenolpyruvate. Oleate, on the other hand, elevated the level of glutamate, only slightly depressed that of α-ketoglutarate, and had no effect on phosphoenolpyruvate (Siess *et al.*, 1977). Oleate also elevated malate, acetyl-CoA, and citrate levels (Williamson *et al.*, 1969a,b; Siess *et al.*, 1977), whereas glucagon had little or no effect (Williamson *et al.*, 1969a; Exton and Park, 1969; Siess *et al.*, 1977). Thus changes in acetyl-CoA levels do not appear to mediate the acute effects of glucagon on gluconeogenesis. This is also supported by the observation that the addition of physiological levels of fatty acids did not stimulate gluconeogenesis (Exton *et al.*, 1969). However, they may contribute to the increase in gluconeogenesis that is brought about by starvation, diabetes, and corticosteroid treatment.

Pyruvate carboxylase activity can also be regulated by a number of other factors that include substrate availability, adenine nucleotides, other acyl-CoA derivatives, metal ions, and certain amino acids. The influence of substrate (pyruvate) availability is discussed later. Different conclusions as to the importance of regulation by adenine nucleotides have come from studies with the purified enzyme and intact rat liver mitochondria. Purified pyruvate carboxylase shows product inhibition by Mg-ADP$^-$ (McClure and Lardy, 1971). Maximum inhibition was observed when saturating pyruvate concentrations were present, whereas no inhibition was observed when lower concentrations of pyruvate were used. This suggested that inhibition by Mg-ADP$^-$ may be of little physiological importance. However, experiments with intact rat liver mitochondria have revealed that the rate of pyruvate carboxylation decreased as the intramitochondrial ADP concentration increased, and that the rate correlated with the ATP : ADP ratio whether high or low pyruvate concentrations were used as substrate (Stucki *et al.,* 1972; von Glutz and Walter, 1976). This suggests that changes in the ATP : ADP ratio may be physiologically important for the regulation of pyruvate carboxylation. Glucagon addition to intact hepatocytes resulted in an elevated intramitochondrial ATP : ADP ratio (Siess *et al.,* 1977; Bryla *et al.,* 1977), thus providing a mechanism by which the hormone could stimulate pyruvate carboxylase. The intramitochondrial ratio of ATP to ADP may be regulated, at least in part, by the adenine nucleotide transporter (Pfaff *et al.,* 1969). Fatty acids, via their CoA derivative, have been shown to inhibit ADP influx and ATP efflux and thus increase the ATP : ADP ratio and promote pyruvate carboxylation (Lopes-Cardozo *et al.,* 1972; Wojtczak *et al.,* 1972). Whether glucagon may act through a similar mechanism is unknown.

Several naturally occurring CoA esters can act as inhibitors of purified liver pyruvate carboxylase: they include malonyl-CoA, succinyl-CoA, and acetoacetyl-CoA (Utter and Scrutton, 1969; Barritt *et al.,* 1976). The first two inhibitors are competitive with respect to acetyl-CoA whereas the latter compound is noncompetitive. Cook *et al.* (1977) have reported that glucagon caused a rapid fall in the level of malonyl-CoA in isolated rat hepatocytes, presumably by inhibiting flux through acetyl-CoA carboxylase. However, it seems unlikely that malonyl-CoA would act as an inhibitor of pyruvate carboxylase *in vivo* since it has a negligible effect when the purified enzyme is assayed under physiological conditions (McClure and Lardy, 1971). Propionyl-CoA, β-hydroxybutyryl-CoA, and butyryl-CoA can act as activators of the avian liver enzyme (Utter and Scutton, 1969; Barritt *et al.,* 1976), but they apparently do not affect the rat liver enzyme (McClure and Lardy, 1971).

Pyruvate carboxylase requires both monovalent and divalent cations for activity (McClure *et al.,* 1971; McClure and Lardy, 1971). The intracellular concentration of K^+ should be sufficient to meet the need for a monovalent cation. The enzyme requires Mg^{2+} in excess of the amount needed to complex ATP, but it is uncertain whether changes in the free Mg^{2+} concentration in the mitochondria can affect enzyme activity under physiological conditions. Recent results suggest that there may be little change in the concentration of free magnesium *in vivo* (Veloso *et al.,* 1973). Calcium ion can be a potent inhibitor of the enzyme by competing with Mg^{2+} (McClure and Lardy, 1971; Wimhurst and Manchester, 1970). Calcium ion also inhibited pyruvate carboxylation in isolated rat liver mitochondria (Kimmich and Rasmussen, 1969), and this led to the proposal that Ca^{2+} may regulate gluconeogenesis (Friedmann and Rasmussen, 1970; Rasmussen, 1970). However, recent evidence suggested that Ca^{2+} inhibits pyruvate carboxylation only in media that contain a high concentration of sucrose. Replacement of the sucrose with mannitol relieved the inhibition (Morikofer-Zwez et al., 1973). Thus it appears unlikely that Ca^{2+} plays a role in regulating pyruvate carboxylation.

Pyruvate carboxylase activity can also be inhibited by glutamate (Scrutton and White, 1974). The high concentration required to inhibit activity $(K_i > 5$ m$M)$ was thought to preclude its physiological significance. However, Siess et al. (1977) recently reported that the intramitochondrial concentration of this amino acid was approximately 15 mM and that glucagon addition to hepatocytes dramatically reduced it to about 3 mM. It is possible that this amino acid may normally exert a restraining influence on pyruvate carboxylation. If it does, it may also provide an explanation for why the rate of pyruvate carboxylase measured in intact mitochondria is so much less than that of the isolated enzyme (Haynes, 1972).

While it is possible that hormones indirectly affect the activity of pyruvate carboxylase by altering the level of various effectors, there is no evidence that the enzyme undergoes phosphorylation or other covalent modification (Leiter et al., 1978). Measurement of pyruvate carboxylase activity in homogenates of livers treated with glucagon has not revealed any change.

2. Pyruvate Dehydrogenase

Pyruvate that enters mitochondria can be converted either to oxaloacetate by pyruvate carboxylase or to acetyl-CoA by pyruvate dehydrogenase (Fig. 1). Since the two enzymes compete for pyruvate, pyruvate dehydrogenase has been suggested as a site for regulation. Inactivation of the enzyme would facilitate carboxylation, and thus gluconeogenesis, whereas activation would enhance lipogenesis and depress gluconeogenesis. The enzyme is a high-molecular-weight complex containing three catalytic components. Pyruvate dehydrogenase itself and dihydrolipoyl dehydrogenase are bound to the dihydrolipoyl transacetylase, and together the three enzymes convert pyruvate to CO_2, acetyl-CoA, and NADH (Koike et al., 1963; Hayakawa et al., 1969; Glemzha et al., 1966; Reed and Oliver, 1968). The mammalian pyruvate dehydrogenase complex also contains two regulatory enzymes, pyruvate dehydrogenase kinase and pyruvate dehydrogenase phosphatase (Linn et al., 1969a,b). The kinase is tightly bound to the transacetylase whereas the phosphatase appears to be loosely associated with the complex (Linn et al., 1972; Barrera et al., 1972). The kinase utilizes Mg-ATP^{2-} as the substrate and inactivates pyruvate dehydrogenase by phosphorylation of a seryl residue in the α-subunit of pyruvate dehydrogenase (Linn et al., 1972; Reed et al., 1972b; Barrera et al., 1972). Adenosine diphosphate competes with Mg-ATP^{2-} for the kinase (Linn et al., 1969b, 1972; Martin et al., 1972). Pyruvate also appears to inhibit the kinase and thus prevents phosphorylation (Hucho et al., 1972). The kinase will not phosphorylate histones, and it does not require cAMP for activity (Hucho et al., 1972). Wieland and Siess (1970) reported that cAMP stimulated pyruvate dehydrogenase phosphatase activity, but others have found no effect (Reed et al., 1972a,b; Jungas, 1971). Pyruvate dehydrogenase phosphatase, which reactivates the enzyme by removing the covalently bound phosphate (Reed et al., 1972a,b; Wieland et al., 1972a,b) requires both magnesium (Reed et al., 1972a,b; Wieland and Siess, 1970; Coore et al., 1971; Wieland and Van Jagow-Westermann, 1969; Wieland et al., 1971) and calcium (Pettit et al., 1972; Denton et al., 1972). Calcium appears to act by promoting the binding of the phosphatase to the transacetylase and by increasing the affinity of the phosphatase for the phosphorylated pyruvate dehydrogenase (Pettit et al., 1972). Furthermore, it has been shown that acetyl-CoA and NADH stimulate the activity of pyruvate dehydrogenase kinase and that NADH also inhibits the phosphatase (Pettit et al., 1975). This suggests that the major effect of these reaction products may be on the phosphorylation state of the complex, rather than as feedback inhibitors as originally proposed (Garland and Randle, 1964; Bremer, 1969; Wieland, 1969).

The phosphorylation state of pyruvate dehydrogenase in the intact cell may be regulated by changes in the ratio of ATP:ADP, NADH:NAD$^+$, and/or acetyl-CoA:CoA. The energy state of the mitochondrial adenine nucleotides has been shown to affect the phosphorylation of pyruvate dehydrogenase in mitochondria from several tissues (Martin et al., 1972; Berger and Hommes, 1973; Wieland et al., 1973; Walajtys et al., 1974; Taylor et al., 1975; Chiang and Sacktor, 1975; Jope and Blass, 1975; Portenhauser et al., 1977). More recently, changes in the NADH:NAD$^+$ and/or acetyl-CoA:CoA ratio have also been shown to affect the phosphorylation state of the enzyme (Kerbey et al., 1976; Batenburg and Olson, 1976; Hansford, 1976; Portenhauser et al., 1977). The fraction of pyruvate dehydrogenase in the active form was increased by the addition of inhibitors of oxidative phosphorylation to isolated hepatocytes (Siess and Wieland, 1975) or by loading the hepatocytes with fructose, glycerol, or sorbitol (Siess and Wieland, 1976). Fructose loading in vivo also significantly increased the amount of active rat liver pyruvate dehydrogenase while it decreased the ATP concentration (Soling and Bernhard, 1971). Starvation lowered the ratio of active to inactive enzyme in rat heart and kidney (Wieland *et al.*, 1971) as well as in liver (Wieland *et al.*, 1972a). These changes were also probably due to alterations in the metabolite ratios, since starvation results in elevated ratios of acetyl-CoA/CoA and NADH/NAD$^+$ (Greenbaum *et al.*, 1971). The addition of high concentrations of pyruvate to perfused liver or isolated hepatocytes converted nearly all the enzyme to the active form (Patzelt *et al.*, 1973; Siess and Wieland, 1976; Claus and Pilkis, 1977). Its effect is probably related not to changes in the intramitochondrial metabolite ratios, but to its ability to inhibit pyruvate dehydrogenase kinase directly.

Various hormones have been shown to affect pyruvate dehydrogenase or pyruvate oxidation. Insulin increased and epinephrine decreased the ratio of active to inactive pyruvate dehydrogenase in adipose tissue (Jungas, 1971; Coore *et al.*, 1971; Severson *et al.*, 1976). Adrenocorticotropic hormone and dibutyryl cAMP inhibited the effect of insulin (Coore *et al.*, 1971). Insulin appeared to affect pyruvate dehydrogenase phosphatase (Mukherjee and Jungas, 1975), but its effect was not mediated by changes in cAMP (Coore *et al.*, 1971) or by an increase in the mitochondrial concentration of Ca^{2+} (Severson *et al.*, 1976). However, epinephrine may decrease pyruvate dehydrogenase activity by decreasing mitochondrial Ca^{2+} (Severson *et al.*, 1976). Pyruvate oxidation has been reported to be stimulated by dibutyryl cAMP in adipose tissue (Schimmel and Goodman, 1972), by glucagon or epinephrine in heart (Buse *et al.*, 1973), and by epinephrine in skeletal muscle (Buse *et al.*, 1973). An inhibition of pyruvate oxidation by glucagon has been inferred from the hormone-induced decrease in $^{14}CO_2$ production from 10 mM [1-^{14}C]pyruvate in isolated hepatocytes from starved rats (Zahlten *et al.*, 1973). However, glucagon also inhibited pyruvate gluconeogenesis as well as pyruvate oxidation under these special circumstances, and it now appears that the decreased rate of $^{14}CO_2$ production was due to the decreased rate of gluconeogenesis.

We have used dichloroacetate, an activator of pyruvate dehydrogenase (Whitehouse and Randle, 1973; Whitehouse *et al.*, 1974), to investigate the role of pyruvate dehydrogenase in the control of hepatic glucose synthesis by glucagon (Claus and Pilkis, 1977). Dichloroacetate did not prevent glucagon from inhibiting glucose synthesis from 10 mM pyruvate even though pyruvate dehydrogenase was completely activated. Instead, its effect was additive with that of glucagon. Thus, the inhibition of pyruvate gluconeogenesis is not due to inhibition of pyruvate dehydrogenase. Mapes and Harris (1976), using a different approach, reached the same conclusion. We also found that glucagon stimulated glucose synthesis from a variety of substrates regardless of whether the ratio of the active to inactive form of pyruvate dehydrogenase was low, intermediate, or high. Furthermore, glucagon had no effect on the activity of pyruvate dehydrogenase or on the estimated flux through the enzyme regardless of its state of activation. It is to be noted, however, that mitochondria isolated from glucagon- or epinephrine-treated rats and isolated hepatocytes show an enhanced rate of decarboxylation of pyruvate (Adams and Haynes, 1969; Yamazaki and Haynes, 1975; Garrison and Haynes, 1975; Titheradge and Coore, 1976b). Thus it appears that pyruvate dehydrogenase is not involved in the hormonal regulation of gluconeogenesis. A similar conclusion was reached by Yamazaki and Haynes (1975) and by Crabb *et al.* (1976).

3. *Pyruvate Transport*

There is some indirect evidence to suggest that carboxylation of pyruvate may be limited by the rate of entry into mitochondria. Haynes (1972) found an apparent K_m value of 0.04–0.08 mM when the rate of carboxylation in isolated rat liver mitochondria was measured as a function of the extramitochondrial pyruvate concentration. This was less than the value of 0.22 mM that he obtained for the pyruvate carboxylase reaction measured in sonicated extracts of mitochondria and less than the value of 0.14 mM for the purified rat liver enzyme (McClure and Lardy, 1971). Since entry of pyruvate into mitochondria is a carrier-mediated process (Papa *et al.*, 1969, 1971; Halestrap and Denton, 1975; Mowbray, 1974, 1975; Halestrap, 1975; Titheradge and Coore, 1975), the value of 0.04–0.08 mM pyruvate may represent the apparent K_m value for the carrier.

There is also some evidence that pyruvate entry is under hormonal regulation. Adam and Haynes (1969) found that liver mitochondria isolated from rats that had been treated with glucagon, epinephrine, or cortisol exhibited higher rates of pyruvate carboxylation and oxidation than mitochondria from control rats. However, the activity of pyruvate carboxylase assayed in sonicated extracts of mitochondria, were unaffected by hormone treatment. This suggested that the hormones increased a reaction that is common to both enzymes, i.e., pyruvate entry into the mitochondria. Similar results were obtained with mitochondria from isolated hepatocytes that had been exposed to glucagon, epinephrine, or cAMP (Garrison and Haynes, 1975). These results rule out extrahepatic factors as being responsible for the observed differences. Further support for the hypothesis was provided by the observation that mitochondria from hepatocytes treated with glucagon, epinephrine, or cAMP or liver mitochondria from rats injected with glucagon or epinephrine take up more pyruvate than do those from control rats (Adams and Haynes, 1969; Garrison and Haynes, 1975; Titheradge and Coore, 1976a,b). The catecholamine effect appears to be mediated by an α-receptor mechanism (Garrison and Borland, 1977). The glucocorticoid effect was additive with that of glucagon or triiodothyronine, which suggests that these hormones affect mitochondrial metabolism by separate mechanisms (Wakat and Haynes, 1977).

We also have obtained data suggesting that glucagon may affect mitochondrial pyruvate transport. We have looked at the effect of increasing concentrations of α-cyanocinnamate, a specific inhibitor of pyruvate transport (Halestrap, 1975; Halestrap and Denton, 1975; Titheradge and Coore, 1975), on the stimulation by glucagon of glucose synthesis from 1 mM [1-^{14}C]pyruvate in hepatocytes from fed rats (T. H. Claus, unpublished results). Figure 3 shows that almost twice as much inhibitor was needed to produce a 50% inhibition of glucose

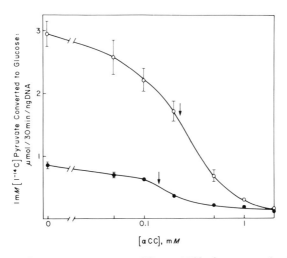

FIG. 3. Effect of α-cyanocinnamate (αCC) on [^{14}C] glucose synthesis from 1 mM [1-^{14}C]pyruvate in isolated hepatocytes from fed rats. Hepatocytes were incubated for 30 minutes without any additions and then incubated for an additional 30 minutes with 1 mM [1-^{14}C]lactate and various concentrations of αCC in the absence (●) or in the presence (○) for 10 nM glucagon. The arrows represent the concentration of αCC that gave half-maximal inhibition of gluconeogenesis. The values were 0.14 mM αCC in the absence of glucagon and 0.23 mM αCC in its presence (T. H. Claus, unpublished results).

synthesis in the presence of glucagon than in its absence. Similar results were obtained with 2 mM [1-^{14}C]lactate.

Titheradge and Coore (1976a,b) presented data to suggest that glucagon treatment of rats directly affects pyruvate transport, but Halestrap (1978) was unable to repeat their observations. Most of the data suggest that glucagon does not specifically affect pyruvate transport. Yamazaki (1975) showed that mitochondria from livers of glucagon-treated rats showed increased rates of respiration from malate, α-ketoglutarate, glutamate, succinate, as well as from pyruvate. This has been confirmed by Titheradge and Coore (1976b), Bryla et al. (1977) and Halestrap (1978). Mitochondria from rats treated with glucagon or cAMP also showed an increased rate of respiration with β-hydroxybutyrate as substrate and an increased uptake of ADP (Bryla et al., 1977). Since all of these substrates require specific transport systems in order to enter the mitochondrial matrix, it appears that glucagon may activate anion transport in general. This may be true for other hormones as well, since glucocorticoids (Wakat and Haynes, 1977) and epinephrine (Titheradge and Coore, 1976b) have similar effects on mitochondrial metabolism.

Other mitochondrial processes appear to be affected by glucagon treatment as well. Yamazaki et al. (1977a) have reported that glucagon treatment of rats yields mitochondria that have increased rates of citrulline synthesis. This finding has been confirmed in mitochondria isolated from hepatocytes that were exposed to glucagon (Bryla et al., 1977; Triebwasser and Freedland, 1977), and the increased rate correlated with an increase in ATP content (Bryla et al., 1977). Glucagon treatment also results in an enhanced mitochondrial ATPase activity in the presence of an uncoupler of oxidative phosphorylation and in an increased rate of K$^+$ uptake (Yamazaki et al., 1977b). The effect of glucagon on ATPase activity persists in sonicated mitochondria (Titheradge et al., 1978a,b). Norepinephrine stimulated mitochondrial ATPase activity more than did glucagon, its effect was α-mediated (Titheradge et al., 1978a,b).

Yamazaki (1975) suggested that the effects of glucagon on anion transport are consistent with either a general stimulation of mitochondrial transport systems or stimulation of the mitochondrial electron transport chain. Titheradge and Coore (1976b) found that glucagon treatment led to an increase in pH of the mitochondrial matrix, a finding confirmed by Halestrap (1978). This increase in hydroxyl ions, should stimulate anion transport, since hydroxyl ions exchange either directly or indirectly with the various anions. Titheradge and

Coore (1976b) proposed that this might be the mechanism by which glucagon increases anion transport, a point of view also favored by Halestrap (1978). Glucagon appears to stimulate transport by enhancing electron flow between cytochromes b and c, thus increasing proton efflux and matrix pH (Halestrap, 1978; Titheradge et al., 1978a,b).

Glucagon treatment of intact rats or of intact hepatocytes leads to changes in mitochondrial metabolism that persist throughout the time needed to isolate the organelle. This suggests that the hormone produces a stable, perhaps covalent, modification, but the site of its effect(s) is uncertain. Many of the changes in mitochondrial metabolism have been correlated with changes in cAMP (Garrison and Haynes, 1975). If all the effects of cAMP are mediated through the phosphorylation of specific proteins by the cAMP-dependent protein kinase, it would be predicted that glucagon would enhance the phosphorylation of mitochondrial protein(s) and that the mitochondria would contain such a kinase. Zahlten et al. (1972) reported that rat liver mitochondrial membranes were phosphorylated in vivo and that glucagon increased the phosphorylation. Halestrap (1978) reported that mitochondrial proteins were phosphorylated when isolated hepatocytes were incubated with labeled inorganic phosphate. One such protein had the same molecular weight as cytochrome c_1, which is found on the external surface of the inner mitochondrial membrane. Whether glucagon enhances the phosphorylation of any of the proteins was not reported. No reports of a cAMP-dependent protein kinase in mitochondria have appeared. A cAMP-independent protein kinase has recently been found on the inner membrane of mouse liver mitochondria (Varadanis, 1977), but it is possible that it represents the catalytic subunit of the cAMP-dependent protein kinase. Suggestive support for the presence of a cAMP-dependent protein kinase in mitochondria comes from the recent claim that the addition of cAMP and ATP to isolated mitochondria can mimic the effects of glucagon (Halestrap, 1978).

Epinephrine apparently does not affect mitochondrial metabolism by the same mechanism as glucagon, since it does not alter the matrix pH (Titheradge and Coore, 1976b). Instead, it apparently reduces the matrix volume (Titheradge and Coore, 1976b). That there are different mechanisms for the two hormones is also supported by the observation that the catecholamine effects are not cAMP mediated (Garrison and Borland, 1977). There is no information available on how catecholamines affect the matrix volume, nor are there any reports that these effects of catecholamines or glucagon can be counteracted by insulin.

4. *Mitochondrial Anion Transport*

Mitochondrial anion transport is an integral part of the gluconeogenic pathway from physiological substrates in the rat, since oxaloacetate cannot readily escape from the mitochondria. This gluconeogenic intermediate is converted to aspartate and/or malate, which are exported from the mitochondria and reconverted to oxaloacetate in the cytoplasm. With lactate as substrate, oxaloacetate is predominantly converted to aspartate, whereas when pyruvate is the substrate, malate serves as the carrier of both carbon and reducing equivalents (Haynes, 1965; Lardy, 1965; Krebs *et al.*, 1967; Struck *et al.*, 1965). A role for these mitochondrial transport systems in gluconeogenesis is supported by inhibitor studies with intact liver preparations. Thus, *n*-butylmalonate, a potent inhibitor of dicarboxylate transport in intact mitochondria (Robinson and Chappell, 1967) inhibited gluconeogenesis from pyruvate or lactate (Williamson *et al.*, 1970; Soling *et al.*, 1973). Similar results were obtained with fluoromalate (Berry and Kun, 1972). The inhibition of lactate gluconeogenesis was somewhat unexpected, but it has been postulated that malate is needed in the cytoplasm in order to exchange with intramitochondrial α-ketoglutarate, which in turn is necessary for the transamination of aspartate to oxaloacetate (Williamson *et al.*, 1970; Soling *et al.*, 1973). Aminooxyacetate, a transaminase inhibitor, strongly inhibits lactate gluconeogenesis, but produces only a small inhibition of pyruvate gluconeogenesis (Rognstad and Katz, 1970; Anderson *et al.*, 1971). Similar results were obtained by Berry and Kun (1972) using difluoroxaloacetate as the transaminase inhibitor.

Except for the studies on pyruvate transport cited above, the regulation of anion transport by hormones has received little attention. Mullhofer *et al.* (1974) found that both gluconeogenesis and the transport of hydrogen equivalents from the cytoplasm into the mitochondria via the α-glycerophosphate cycle were greatly increased in livers from rats treated with triiodothyronine, where mitochondrial α-glycerophosphate dehydrogenase is greatly increased (Lee *et al.*, 1959; Lee and Lardy, 1965). Dibutyryl cAMP had no effect on gluconeogenesis in this case, whereas the nucleotide stimulated gluconeogenesis and hydrogen equivalent transport in normal rats. They postulated that dibutyryl cAMP stimulates gluconeogenesis by enhancing malate efflux from the mitochondrion and by enhancing hydrogen equivalent flux through the α-glycerophosphate cycle. An effect of glucagon on malate efflux is also consistent with the observation that *n*-butyl malate reduced the magnitude of the glucagon stimulation of gluconeogenesis from 10 mM [U-^{14}C]lactate while having only a small effect on the basal rate (T. H. Claus, unpublished results). Parrilla *et al.* (1975, 1976) suggested that glucagon facilitated the transport of many anionic intermediates since the hormone increased the calculated mitochondria-to-cytoplasm concentration gradient for each of them. However, a direct measurement of the effect of glucagon on the distribution of the intermediates between the two compartments did not reveal any changes (Siess *et al.*, 1977).

C. POSSIBLE EXTRAMITOCHONDRIAL SITES OF HORMONE ACTION

Three enzymes specific for gluconeogenesis have been identified in cytosol of rat liver. They are phosphoenolpyruvate carboxykinase, which catalyzes the conversion of mitochondria-generated oxaloacetate to phosphoenolpyruvate; fructose-1,6-diphosphatase, which converts fructose 1,6-diphosphate to fructose 6-phosphate; and glucose-6-phosphatase, which hydrolyzes glucose 6-phosphate to free glucose and inorganic phosphate. These three gluconeogenic enzymes are opposed in the cell by three glycolytic enzymes, pyruvate kinase, phosphofructokinase, and hexokinase, respectively. The existence in the same cell of enzymes that catalyze opposing reactions raised the possibility of cycling between the substrates and products of the enzymes (Fig. 1). Since each of the reactions is nonequilibrium, energy must be expended during such cycling. These cycles were designated "futile" cycles because ATP was hydrolyzed without any change in reactants. This apparent futility led to the proposal that the activities of the opposing enzymes would be regulated such that when one was active, the other was inactive. However, Newsholme and Gevers (1967) have speculated that the simultaneous operation of the opposing enzymes would offer a very sensitive control system in which both the rate and direction of glucose metabolism could be regulated by very small changes in the concentration of effectors of one or all of the enzymes involved in the cycle. The small amount of energy that is expended by the cycles would not be wasted, but used to create a more efficient regulatory system than the "on-off" system originally proposed. Since they may not be "futile" cycles, the term substrate cycles has come into use.

1. *The Phosphoenolpyruvate–Pyruvate Substrate Cycle and Its Enzymes*

Recent studies have provided much evidence that the phosphoenolpyruvate–pyruvate cycle is very important in the regulation of gluconeogenesis. Earlier work employing crossover plots of metabolic intermediates had suggested that rate-limiting step(s) occur in this region of the pathway. The cycle is quite complex. The pyruvate produced by the action of pyruvate kinase must be carboxylated to oxaloacetate (Fig. 4) and then decarboxylated to phosphoenolpyruvate. The route of these conversions is dependent upon the location of phosphoenolpyruvate carboxykinase, which is distributed in various preparations between cytosol and mitochondria, depending on species, as described earlier. This cycle may therefore include mitochondrial membrane transport systems and a number of enzymes. One mole of ATP and one of GTP are consumed, and 1 mol of ATP is generated. Thus 1 mol of energy-rich phosphate is expended per cycle.

The first evidence that some phosphoenolpyruvate is recycled to pyruvate during gluconeogenesis was presented by Friedman *et al.* (1971a,b), using perfused rat liver, and by Rognstad and Katz (1972), using kidney cortex segments. Both groups used [2-^{14}C]pyruvate as substrate and determined the flux through pyruvate kinase by measuring the distribution of radioactivity among carbon atoms of lactate and pyruvate. Both groups found that in the fasting state about one-half as much phosphoenolpyruvate was recycled to pyruvate as was converted

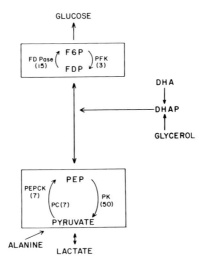

Fig. 4. Diagram of the hepatic gluconeogenic pathway. The substrate cycles that have been implicated in the hormonal control of gluconeogenesis are enclosed in boxes (PC., pyruvate carboxylase; PEPCK, phosphoenolpyruvate carboxykinase; PK, pyruvate kinase; FDPase, fructose diphosphatase, PFK, phosphofructokinase.) The numbers in parentheses are the enzyme activities in units per gram of liver measured under V_{max} conditions (Scrutton and Utter, 1968). Glycerol and dihydroxyacetone (DHA) are phosphorylated by glycerol kinase, ultimately yielding dihydroxyacetone phosphate (DHAP) that enters the pathway at the triose phosphate level.

to glucose. In the fed state, the situation was reversed, the rate of pyruvate kinase flux being four times that of glucose synthesis (Friedman et al., 1971a,b). With [2-^{14}C]lactate as substrate in kidney cortex segments, only 30% as much phosphoenolpyruvate was recycled to pyruvate as was converted to glucose (Rognstad and Katz, 1972).

A simpler approach to measuring flux through pyruvate kinase was devised by Rognstad (1975). Labeled NaHCO$_3$ was used instead of [2-^{14}C]pyruvate or lactate, since it will incorporate radioactivity into phosphoenolpyruvate prior to pyruvate. The amount of label found in lactate and pyruvate, along with the estimated specific activity of phosphoenolpyruvate, was used to calculate pyruvate kinase flux. In hepatocytes from starved rats, incubated with 20 mM pyruvate, the flux was estimated to be about 50% of the rate of gluconeogenesis (Rognstad, 1975). With 20 mM lactate as substrate, the flux through pyruvate kinase was estimated to be from 7 to 23% of the rate of gluconeogenesis in the starved case and about 50% in the fed case (Katz and Rognstad, 1976; Rognstad and Katz, 1977).

We have also estimated the flux through pyruvate kinase in isolated hepatocytes by measuring the rate of lactate and pyruvate production from dihydroxyacetone (Pilkis et al., 1976a,b). This compound is first converted to dihydroxyacetone phosphate by glycerol kinase and then to either glucose or to lactate and pyruvate (Fig. 4). Flux was about equal to the rate of gluconeogenesis in hepatocytes from fed or 24-hour starved rats, but was depressed with further starvation (Pilkis et al., 1976a). In hepatocytes from fed rats, glucagon caused a dose-dependent decrease in lactate production from dihydroxyacetone and a concomitant, quantitatively equivalent increase in glucose synthesis (Fig. 5). Glucagon also decreased the flux through pyruvate kinase in hepatocytes from starved rats (Pilkis et al., 1976a). Insulin relieved this inhibition when submaximal concentrations of glucagon were added to hepatocytes from fed rats (Pilkis et al., 1976b). Epinephrine produced only a small decrease in pyruvate kinase flux in hepatocytes from fed or starved rats (Pilkis et al., 1976a, Rognstad, 1976), and the effect was α-mediated (Pilkis et al., 1976a).

Some differences in the effect of these hormones on flux through pyruvate kinase were observed when lactate or pyruvate was the substrate, rather than dihydroxyacetone, and flux was measured by the NaH^{14}CO$_3$ method. Neither glucagon nor epinephrine affected flux when 20 mM lactate was the substrate in hepatocytes from starved rats, even though both hormones increased glucose synthesis (Rognstad and Katz, 1977). When 20 mM pyruvate was the substrate in hepatocytes from starved rats, glucagon and cAMP inhibited pyruvate

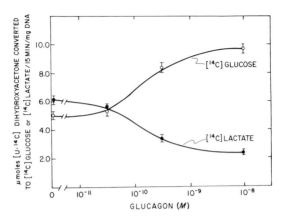

FIG. 5. Effect of glucagon on conversion of [^{14}C]dihydroxyacetone to [^{14}C]lactate and [^{14}C]glucose in hepatocytes from fed rats. Cells were incubated for 30 minutes with 1.5 mM [^{14}C]dihydroxyacetone, and labeled glucose and lactate were determined. The data are from Pilkis *et al.* (1976a).

kinase flux by about 45% (Rognstad, 1975, 1976), whereas epinephrine was only marginally effective (Rognstad, 1976). Both glucagon and cAMP also inhibited pyruvate gluconeogenesis, whereas epinephrine had a variable effect. The glucagon effect on glucose synthesis from pyruvate was unaffected by the absence of calcium ions (Rognstad, 1976). In hepatocytes from fed rats, both glucagon and epinephrine increased lactate gluconeogenesis (Rognstad and Katz, 1977). In this case, glucagon caused a dose-dependent decrease in flux, while epinephrine appeared to increase it. Other studies showed that pyruvate kinase flux was increased almost 10-fold during gluconeogenesis from 20 mM lactate in hepatocytes from fasted, triiodothyronine-treated rats (Rognstad, 1977).

The reason why the hormone effects on flux through pyruvate kinase are not always the same with dihydroxyacetone as substrate as with lactate is not clear. One possibility is that flux through pyruvate kinase is regulated to a greater extent by the level of fructose diphosphate when dihydroxyacetone is the substrate (see next section) whereas other effectors may predominate when lactate is the substrate. Another possibility may be that different populations of parenchymal cells are involved with each substrate. Katz and Jungermann (1976) have proposed that there are two types of hepatocytes, one being predominantly glycolytic (the pericentral zone), and one predominantly gluconeogenic (the periportal zone). Guder *et al.* (1976) found in livers from fed rats that the activity of pyruvate kinase was higher in the pericentral zone than in the periportal zone whereas the opposite distribution was found for phosphoenolpyruvate carboxykinase. When rats were starved for 48 hours, the difference between the two zones was reduced, largely because the activity of pyruvate kinase decreased, and that of phosphoenolpyruvate carboxykinase increased, in the pericentral zone. Similar distributions and effects of fasting has been observed for glucose-6-phosphatase, glucokinase, and fructose diphosphatase (Sasse *et al.*, 1975; Katz *et al.*, 1977).

It is as yet uncertain just how important are changes in pyruvate kinase flux as a means of regulating gluconegenesis. All the studies on pyruvate kinase flux have been done with concentrations of physiological substrates that produce maximum rates of gluconeogenesis or with nonphysiological substrates. Regulation of pyruvate kinase flux may be more (or less) important under conditions which produce submaximal rates of gluconeogenesis, i.e., conditions that mimic those found *in vivo*. This question can be finally resolved only by direct measurement of the extent of recycling between pyruvate and phosphoenolpyruvate with substrate concentrations in the physiological range. However, studies on the phosphorylation of the enzyme, both *in vitro* and *in vivo*, provide strong evidence that pyruvate kinase plays a central role in the hormonal regulation of gluconeogenesis.

a. Hepatic Pyruvate Kinase. There is approximately ten times more pyruvate kinase activity in rat liver than phosphoenolpyruvate carboxykinase (Fig. 4). This suggests that pyruvate kinase must be substantially inhibited in order for gluconeogenesis to occur. This consideration, and the observation that hormones can affect flux through pyruvate kinase, has fostered a great deal of research on the properties of this enzyme. Many studies conducted in various species and tissues suggest that there are three isozymes of pyruvate kinase in mammalian tissues (Seubert and Schoner, 1971; Imamura *et al.*, 1972; Ibsen, 1977). The liver type (L-type) is found as the major species in hepatocytes and as a minor isozyme of kidney cortex and intestine and perhaps of the erythrocytes. The muscle type (M-type) is thought to occur only in striated muscle, heart, and brain. The kidney type (K-type) is found in all other adult and fetal tissues and in tumors. With some exceptions, such as in frog and chicken liver, where it is predominant, the K-isozyme is present only in small amounts in liver. Chicken liver was thought to contain only the K-form, but recent work has revealed the presence of the L-form as well (Eigenbrodt and Schoner, 1977a). Hybrids of the K- and L-forms have in general not been detected, except in extracts of *Rana pipiens* liver (Schloen *et al.*, 1974). Table I illustrates some of the differences and similarities between the three different classes of isozyme. The L-isozyme exhibits sigmoidal kinetics with regard to its

TABLE I

COMPARISON OF THE PROPERTIES OF THE L-, K-, M-, AND PHOSPHORYLATED L-ISOZYME OF PYRUVATE KINASE IN RAT TISSUES

Characteristic	L-type[a]	Phospho-L-isozyme[b]	K-type[c]	M-type[d]
Tissue distribution	Liver, kidney, and erythrocytes	Liver	Kidney and many adult cells. Predominant in fetal tissues and tumors	Muscle and brain
Subunit structure	Tetramer	Tetramer	Tetramer	Tetramer
Molecular weight	228,000	228,000	216,000	250,000
Chronic adaptation				
Starvation	Decreased	?	Unchanged	Unchanged
High-carbohydrate diet	Increased	?	Unchanged	Unchanged
Diabetes	Decreased	?	Unchanged	Unchanged
Kinetics with regard to PEP ($K_{0.5}$)	Sigmoidal (0.6 mM)	Sigmoidal (1.2 mM)	Sigmoidal (0.4 mM)	Hyperbolic (0.07 mM)
Hill coefficient for PEP	2.0	2.7–2.9	1.4–1.5	1.0
Activation by FDP	Yes	Yes, but less sensitive than L-isozyme	Yes	No
Inhibition by alanine ($K_{i,app}$)	1 mM	0.3 mM	0.45 mM	—
Inhibition by ATP ($K_{i,app}$)	1 mM	0.4 mM	3 mM	3 mM
Allosteric activation by hydrogen ions	Yes	Yes	?	No
Phosphorylation by protein kinases	Yes	—	Yes (chicken liver; no (pig kidney)	No
Acute hormonal regulation	Yes	Yes	?	No

[a] From Seubert and Schoner (1971); Imamura et al. (1972); Ibsen (1977).

[b] Ljungström et al. (1974, 1976); Berglund et al. (1977); Pilkis et al. (1978a,b); Feliu et al. (1976, 1977); Riou et al. (1976).

[c] Imamura et al. (1972).

[d] Kayne and Price (1972); Imamura et al. (1972).

substrate, phosphoenolpyruvate. When the allosteric activator fructose diphosphate is added or the pH is lowered, the enzyme exhibits normal Michaelis–Menten kinetics (Bailey *et al.*, 1968; Jimenez de Asua *et al.*, 1970; Carminatti *et al.*, 1968; Llorente *et al.*, 1970; Rozengurt *et al.*, 1969; Schoner *et al.*, 1970; Seubert *et al.*, 1968; Susor and Rutter, 1968; Tanaka *et al.*, 1965; Taylor and Bailey, 1967; Gancedo *et al.*, 1967; Haeckel *et al.*, 1968; Hess *et al.*, 1966; Hunsley and Suelter, 1969; Koler and Vanbellinghen, 1968). The M-isozyme has hyperbolic kinetics with phosphoenolpyruvate as substrate and is not activated by fructose diphosphate (Imamura *et al.*, 1972). The K-isozyme has properties intermediate between those of the M- and L-types. There is some degree of sigmoidicity in the phosphoenolpyruvate concentration curve, and fructose diphosphate does stimulate the activity of the K-isozyme, but not nearly as effectively as that of the L-isozyme (Imamura, *et al.*, 1972). Differences between the different isozymes also exist with regard to inhibition by ATP and alanine (see Table I). The M-, K-, and the L-isozymes are homotetramers, with a subunit molecular weight of about 50,000 (Seubert and Schoner, 1971; Imamura *et al.*, 1972).

Since the three forms have distinct kinetic and physical properties and apparently are not interconvertible, it has been assumed that they are products of three distinct genes. This is supported by differences in amino acid composition (Cardenas *et al.*, 1975; Kutzbach *et al.*, 1973) and by the independence of changes in activity of the L- and K-isozymes when one or the other is induced (Table I). However, Marie *et al.* (1976b) have suggested that the M-isozyme is a modified form of the K-isozyme since the two forms crossreact immunologically. Eigenbrodt and Schoner (1977a) have reported that antibodies against the

TABLE II

EFFECT OF PROTEIN KINASE INHIBITOR (PKI) ON INACTIVATION OF
PYRUVATE KINASE BY CYCLIC AMP[a]

Condition	V/V_{max} (0.4/4.0)
Control	0.319
cAMP for 6 min	0.218
cAMP for 20 min	0.120
cAMP for 20 min, PKI at 0 min	0.322
cAMP for 20 min, PKI at 6 min	0.217

[a] Hepatocyte extracts were prepared and incubated with 5 mM Mg-ATP as described in Fig. 8. cAMP was present at 0.2 μM. Pyruvate kinase activity was measured at 0.4 and 4.0 mM phosphoenolpyruvate. PKI was present at a concentration of 500 U/ml (Claus and Pilkis, 1978b).

L-isozyme from chicken liver inactivate the L-isozyme from rat and partially inactivate the K-isozymes from chicken and rat. Resolution of these differences will require determination of the amino acid sequence of each form.

While the L-, K-, and M-isozymes are not interconvertible, various interconvertible forms of the L- and of the K-isozyme have been identified by isoelectric focusing (Hess and Kutzbach, 1971; Ibsen and Trippet, 1974; Ibsen et al., 1975; Marie et al., 1976b). These forms are thought to be due to difference in the amount of fructose diphosphate bound to the enzyme. One form of the L-isozyme, with an isoelectric point (pI) of 5.3 (pig) and 5.4–5.5 (rat), is a tetramer that shows hyperbolic kinetics with respect to phosphoenolpyruvate and is not activated by fructose diphosphate (Hess and Kutzbach, 1971; Ibsen and Trippet, 1974; Ibsen et al., 1975; Muroya et al., 1976). This form can be converted to a form with a pI of 5.6–5.7 after either purification (Hess and Kutzbach, 1971), electrofocusing (Ibsen and Trippet, 1974; Muroya et al., 1976), incubation with fructose diphosphatase (Ibsen et al., 1975), or starvation (Ibsen and Trippet, 1974). The resulting enzyme has sigmoidal kinetics with respect to phosphoenolpyruvate and is activated by fructose diphosphate. The addition of fructose diphosphate converts this form back to the low pI form. Further purification produces a form with an even higher pI, which can then be converted to the low-pI form by electrofocusing in the presence of fructose diphosphate (Ibsen and Trippet, 1974; Ibsen et al., 1975). Using the terminology of Jacob and Monod, Ibsen and co-workers (1975) concluded that the low pI was the R-conformer and the high pI form was the T-conformer of an R–T tetramer set. Hess and Kutzbach (1971) have postulated that the different forms of the pig L-isozyme are a function of differing amounts of fructose diphosphate bound to the enzyme. They suggest that the low pI had 2 mol of fructose diphosphate bound per mole of enzyme, the intermediate form had 1 mol bound, and the high-pI form had none. This concept is supported by the report that pyruvate kinase possesses high- and low-affinity binding sites for fructose diphosphate (Muroya et al., 1976; Irving and Williams, 1973). Although Ibsen has pointed out that incubation with fructose diphosphatase does not generate the high-pI form, it is conceivable that fructose diphosphate that is tightly bound to pyruvate kinase is not hydrolyzed by fructose diphosphatase. It does not appear likely that the different pI forms of the L-isozyme are a reflection of different degrees of phosphorylation of the enzyme (see below) since they are interconvertible in the absence of ATP.

Interconvertible forms of the K-isozyme have also been reported in various tissues (Ibsen and Trippet, 1972; Ibsen et al., 1975; Muroya et *al.*, 1976). The high-p*I* form of the K-isozyme appears to be a dimer with a high $K_{0.5}$ for phosphoenolpyruvate, and the other two forms are tetramers. There is some argument about the physiological significance of the different p*I* forms of this enzyme. It is possible that the variant of adipose tissue pyruvate kinase generated by treatment with EDTA, as described by Pogson (1968a,b; Pogson *et al.*, 1975), is a dimeric form of the K-isozyme. Ibsen *et al.* (1976) have demonstrated that incubation of extracts containing K-isozyme with EDTA generates dimers. The presence of small quantities of dimers (Ibsen and Trippet, 1972) or of very high $K_{0.5}$ forms in fresh tissue extracts (Van Berkel *et al.*, 1974) provides evidence that alterations in the tetramer–dimer equilibrium may have physiological significance. Changes in erythrocyte pyruvate kinase during aging or storage may also be due to dimerization (Ibsen *et al.*, 1971; Paglia and Valentine, 1970). Feliu and Sols (1976) have argued that dimerization of the K-isozyme may be significant for regulation in ascites tumor cells. Van Berkel *et al.* (1973) and Badwey and Westhead (1975) have demonstrated that sulfhydryl oxidation converted the L-isozyme to a very high-$K_{0.5}$ form. In the case of the erythrocyte enzyme, a number of forms are generated by this treatment including tetramers, dimers, and monomers. It has been proposed that alanine, in a concentration-dependent manner, causes dimer formation and inactivation (Hofmann *et al.*, 1975) whereas fructose diphosphate, and to a lesser degree, phosphoenolpyruvate, favor tetramer formation and inactivation (Hofmann *et al.*, 1975; Ibsen *et al.*, 1975). However, in spite of the various ways by which tetramer–dimer interconversions may occur, the tetrameric forms of both the L- and K-isozymes predominate in tissue extracts of the rat, and it is probable that these are the forms that exist *in vivo*.

The pyruvate kinase of the erythrocyte is interesting because of its apparently close relationship to the L-isozyme. It crossreacts immunologically with the latter, but not with the K- or M-isozyme (Marie *et al.*, 1976a; Lincoln *et al.*, 1975; Nakashima, 1974). Its kinetics with regard to substrate are similar to that of the L-isozyme (Marie *et al.*, 1976a). A number of observations suggest that the two enzymes are the products of a single gene. Incubation of the erythrocyte form with liver extract converts it to the L-form of the enzyme (Nakashima, 1974); the erythrocyte form in patients with hepatitis is identical to the L-isozyme (Nakashima *et al.*, 1974); and hepatic L-isozyme is deficient in patients with pyruvate kinase deficiency hemolytic anemia (Nakashima *et al.*, 1974; Bigley and Koler, 1968; Imamura *et al.*, 1973; Miwa *et al.*, 1975). Recently, the erythrocyte enzyme itself has been purified and resolved into two types (Marie *et al.*, 1977), one, a tetramer composed of four identical subunits, and the other, a hybrid of 2 L-type subunits and 2 subunits of slightly higher molecular weight. The specific activity of the latter was half that of the homotetramer. The hybrid could be converted to a homotetramer similar to the L-isozyme by treatment with trypsin. It was postulated that the erythrocyte enzyme is a proenzyme that can be transformed to the L-isozyme by postsynthetic proteolysis. This proenzyme is presumably not seen in liver because of the high rate of proteolysis in that organ. Fructose diphosphate binding to both forms was studied, and it was shown that the homotetramer had four binding sites for fructose diphosphate whereas the heterotetramer had only two (Garreau et al., 1977). These results may help to resolve many of the questions vis-à-vis the relationship between the erythrocyte and liver enzymes. It is not known whether such proenzymes exist in other tissues or what may be their physiological relevance. Dahlgvist-Edberghas (1978) reported that erythrocyte pyruvate kinase cannot be phosphorylated, presumably because the site of phosphorylation has been removed by proteolytic cleavage.

L-Type pyruvate kinase is allosterically inhibited by ATP and alanine and activated by fructose diphosphate (Seubert and Schoner, 1971; Imamura et al., 1972). The presence of physiological concentrations of these effectors can have profound effects on the degree of cooperativity that the enzyme shows as well as on the $K_{0.5}$ for phosphoenolpyruvate. With physiological concentrations of alanine, ATP, and phosphoenolpyruvate, it might be predicted that the enzyme would be completely inhibited unless it were activated by fructose diphosphate. In fact, the active form of pyruvate kinase in vivo is probably an enzyme–fructose diphosphate complex. The amount of this complex depends on the concentration of free fructose diphosphate in the cytosol. This in turn depends on the amount of fructose diphosphate bound to other enzymes in liver, such as aldolase, fructose diphosphatase, and perhaps phosphofructokinase. Marco and Sols (1970) have calculated that the concentration of free fructose diphosphate is very small compared to that which is bound; at best 10% of the total fructose diphosphate, at a concentration of 20–50 μM, is available to pyruvate kinase. Any change in the affinity of pyruvate kinase for fructose diphosphate, or in the binding of the compound to other enzymes, would have a great influence on the activity of pyruvate kinase. As will be detailed below, hormonal control of fructose diphosphate levels may be an important aspect of the regulation of flux through pyruvate kinase and of gluconeogenesis.

The K-isozyme is subject to regulation by the same effectors as the L-isozyme, although the role of ATP inhibition is somewhat uncertain

(Ibsen et al., 1975). In general, the M-isozyme is thought not to be regulated by allosteric effectors. However, the enzyme from the rat is inhibited by phenylalanine in what may be an allosteric manner, and this inhibition is reversed by alanine and fructose diphosphate (Carminatti et al., 1971; Ibsen and Marles, 1976; Ibsen and Trippet, 1973, 1974; Kayne and Price, 1972; Weber, 1969). The rat M-isozyme may also exist in several conformational forms (Ibsen and Trippet, 1972; Kayne and Price, 1972).

Recently it was demonstrated that the activity of pyruvate kinase can be regulated by a phosphorylation–dephosphorylation mechanism. Ljungström et al. (1974) first demonstrated that the purified rat L-isozyme can be phosphorylated by $[\gamma\text{-}^{32}P]ATP$ in a reaction catalyzed by cAMP-dependent protein kinase. The activity of the enzyme is decreased by phosphorylation, especially at low phosphoenolpyruvate concentrations. About 4 M of phosphate are incorporated per mole of enzyme. The relationship of moles of phosphate incorporated to inhibition of activity has not been completely worked out, but it has been observed that incorporation of 1.5–2.0 M of phosphate per mole of rat liver pyruvate kinase is sufficient to inhibit over 90% of the activity in the presence of 0.15 mM phosphoenolpyruvate (Titanji et al., 1976). In similar studies with the purified pig liver enzyme, incorporation of 1.5 M causes only 25% inhibition, and incorporation of 3 M results in 75% inhibition of enzyme activity (Ljungström et al., 1976). The initial phosphate content of the enzymes used in these studies was not reported. Riou et al. (1976) and Pilkis et al. (1978b) have confirmed the observation that phosphorylation of purified rat liver pyruvate kinase by cAMP-dependent protein kinase results in inhibition of activity measured at low phosphoenolpyruvate concentrations. As shown in Fig. 6, phosphorylation results in an increase in the $K_{0.5}$ for phosphoenolpyruvate from 0.6 mM to 1.2 mM. No change in activity was obtained when the enzyme was assayed at high phosphoenolpyruvate concentrations or in the presence of optimal concentrations of fructose diphosphate. Similar results have been obtained by Ljungström et al. (1974, 1976) with the pig liver enzyme. However, Titanji et al. (1976) have obtained phosphorylation-induced inactivation of rat liver pyruvate kinase in the presence of high phosphoenolpyruvate concentrations, which is overcome by fructose diphosphate. In general, phosphorylation of the enzyme causes a shift of the phosphoenolpyruvate concentration curve to the right and results in an increase in the Hill coefficient (Table I, Fig. 6). The effect of phosphorylation is overcome by saturating concentrations of phosphoenolpyruvate or by fructose diphosphate (Ljungström et al., 1974, 1976; Titanji et al., 1976; Riou et al., 1976).

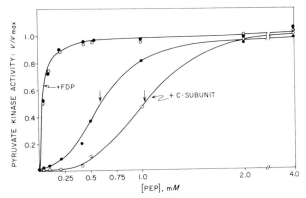

FIG. 6. Inactivation of hepatic pyruvate kinase by phosphorylation. Homogeneous rat hepatic pyruvate kinase (Riou *et al.*, 1978) was incubated with 1 m*M* Mg-ATP and a homogeneous preparation of the catalytic subunit of cAMP-dependent protein kinase from beef heart for 30 minutes at 30°C. The reaction was terminated by the addition of saturated $(NH_4)_2SO_4$, and the enzyme pellet was washed with more $(NH_4)_2SO_4$ as described by Pilkis *et al.* (1978a). Pyruvate kinase activity was then assayed as a function of phosphoenolpyruvate concentration in the presence and in the absence of fructose diphosphate (20 µ*M*). V/V_{max} represents the activity at any particular phosphoenolpyruvate concentration divided by the maximal rate.

Hydrogen ions will also overcome the inhibition due to phosphorylation (Ljungström *et al.*, 1976). This is consistent with the observation that fructose diphosphate promotes binding of phosphoenolpyruvate only at high pH, indicating that dissociation of a proton is required for allosteric control (Rozengurt *et al.*, 1969). Thus, no deviation from Michaelis–Menten kinetics can be demonstrated at pH 6.9, using either the phosphorylated or nonphosphorylated enzyme in the presence or the absence of fructose diphosphate (Ljungström *et al.*, 1976). In contrast to the above, ATP and alanine have greater effects on the phosphorylated than on the nonphosphorylated protein (Ljungström *et al.*, 1976; Riou *et al.*, 1976) (Table I). In fact, the inhibitory effect of phosphorylation is most clearly seen when the enzyme is assayed with low concentrations of phosphoenolpyruvate in the presence of millimolar concentrations of ATP and alanine (Riou *et al.*, 1976).

Phosphorylation of the pig or rat liver enzyme reduces activation by fructose diphosphate (Ljungström *et al.*, 1976; Riou *et al.*, 1976; Van Berkel *et al.*, 1977a). This is best seen when the enzyme is assayed in the presence of physiological concentrations of alanine and ATP (Riou *et al.*, 1976). The phosphorylation of the enzyme reduces affinity for fructose diphosphate, which, in turn, may be responsible for the increase in the $K_{0.5}$ for phosphoenolpyruvate. These considerations should be kept in mind in evaluating the effects of phosphorylation of the purified enzyme that have been observed using enzyme preparations containing high concentrations of fructose diphosphate (Titanji *et al.*, 1976; Ljungström *et al.*, 1976). The inactivation of pyruvate kinase in crude extracts by phosphorylation may also be modified by fructose diphosphate, since the extracts have been shown to contain different forms of the L-isozyme with varying amounts of the bound effector (Hess and Kutzbach, 1971). If the only effect of phosphorylation were to reduce binding of fructose diphosphate, no effect of phosphorylation would be observed in the absence of fructose diphosphate. However, the apparent decrease in fructose diphosphate binding may be secondary to the decreased affinity for phosphoenolpyruvate. To date there have been no direct studies of ligand binding to the phosphorylated and nonphosphorylated forms of the enzyme.

Table I compares some properties of the phosphorylated and non-phosphorylated forms of the L-isozyme. Phosphorylation appears to modify the ease with which the enzyme undergoes conformational changes in response to its effectors. The end result is to shift the equilibrium between the active and inactive forms. This hypothesis is illustrated in Fig. 7, where it is postulated that increasing concentrations of phosphoenolpyruvate and fructose diphosphate cause a conformational change in the enzyme leading to a more closely associated quaternary structure and to increased activity. Phosphorylation of the enzyme subunits tends to impede this conformational change, result-

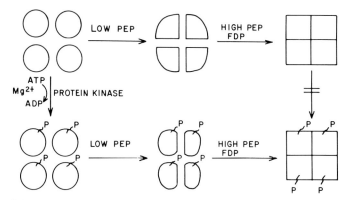

FIG. 7. Schematic representation of the effect of phosphorylation on the equilibrium between the active and inactive forms of pyruvate kinase. The circles represent the inactive form of the pyruvate kinase subunit. The squares depict the active form. Other symbols represent transitional forms of the subunit. P represents phosphate groups on the enzyme subunit. The active tetrameric form is depicted as not undergoing phosphorylation as suggested by the data of Eigenbrodt and Schoner (1977b,c).

ing in a "looser" quaternary structure at low concentrations of phosphoenolpyruvate, and to decreased enzyme activity. High concentrations of phosphoenolpyruvate and fructose diphosphate can overcome this effect of phosphorylation. No evidence for an effect of phosphorylation on the dissociation of the L-isozyme has been reported, although such an effect has been reported for the K-isozyme from chicken liver (Eigenbrodt and Schoner, 1977b).

The site of phosphorylation on the enzyme has been determined. Humble *et al.* (1975) showed that alkali-inactivated pig liver pyruvate kinase and a cyanogen bromide peptide from the same enzyme could be phosphorylated by [γ-^{32}P]ATP in the presence of cAMP-dependent protein kinase. They also isolated a peptide from rat liver pyruvate kinase and showed that the minimum structural requirements for phosphorylation were met by the pentapeptide Arg-Arg-Ala-Ser-Val (Hjelmquist *et al.*, 1974). Evidence from other laboratories suggest that this or very closely related sequences are on the sites of phosphorylation in other proteins that serve as substrates for cyclic AMP-dependent protein kinases (Daile and Carnegie, 1974; Kemp *et al.*, 1975; Daile *et al.*, 1975). The concentration of pentapeptide which gave half-maximal rates of phosphorylation was 0.08 mM while that of a heptapeptide (Leu-Arg-Arg-Ser-Val-Ala) was 0.01 mM (Zetterqvist *et al.*, 1976). The concentration of native enzyme that gives half-maximal rates of phosphorylation by the cAMP-dependent protein kinase *in vitro* appears to be higher than the above. An exact value could not be obtained, since the rate continued to increase even when micromolar concentrations of pyruvate kinase were added (Berglund *et al.*, 1977a). Riou *et al.* (1978) have demonstrated that the rat liver enzyme is phosphorylated *in vivo*, but it is not known whether the site(s) phosphorylated *in vivo* corresponds to the above pentapeptide.

In studies to date, the rat and pig liver pyruvate kinases appear to be phosphorylated by a cyclic AMP-dependent protein kinase (Titanji *et al.*, 1976; Berglund *et al.*, 1977a; Ljungström *et al.*, 1976; Riou *et al.*, 1976). Phosphorylation has been studied using a homogeneous preparation of bovine liver or heart catalytic subunit of the cAMP-dependent protein kinase and homogeneous rat liver pyruvate kinase (Pilkis *et al.*, 1978b). In many cases, however, very crude preparations of protein kinase were used, and it is possible that they contained cyclic AMP-independent as well as cAMP-dependent protein kinases. Pilkis *et al.* (1978a) have investigated the possibility that an independent kinase could be involved by studying phosphorylation in rat hepatocyte homogenates that had been gel filtered on Sephadex G-25 in order to remove all low-molecular-weight compounds. The addition of cAMP and Mg-ATP to these extracts produced a time-dependent inactivation

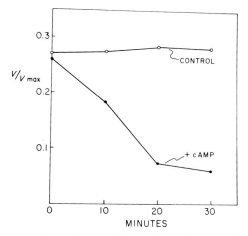

Fig. 8. Times course of the effect of cAMP on inactivation of pyruvate kinase in hepatocyte homogenates. Sephadex-treated hepatocyte extracts were incubated with 5 mM Mg-ATP $\pm$ 50 μM cAMP. The reaction was terminated by addition of saturated $(NH_4)_2SO_4$, and the resulting pellet was washed, suspended, and assayed for pyruvate kinase activity (Pilkis et $al.$, 1978a). V/V_{max} represents the ratio of activity measured at 0.4 mM to 4.0 mM phosphoenolpyruvate.

of pyruvate kinase, whereas the addition of Mg-ATP alone had no effect (Fig. 8). The cAMP-induced inactivation was characterized by an increase in the $K_{0.5}$ for phosphoenolpyruvate (Fig. 9) and could be completely blocked by the addition of protein kinase inhibitor, a compound

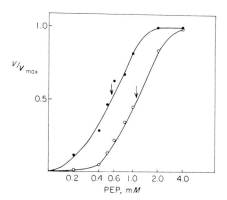

Fig. 9. Phosphoenolpyruvate concentration curves for control and inactivated pyruvate kinase from hepatocyte homogenates. Sephadex-treated extracts were incubated for 30 minutes with and without cAMP, and washed $(NH_4)_2SO_4$ fractions were prepared. Pyruvate kinase activity was assayed as a function of phosphoenolpyruvate concentration. V/V_{max} represents the ratio of activity measured at any given substrate concentration to that measured at 4 mM phosphoenolpyruvate. O—O, Extracts incubated with cAMP.

specific for the catalytic subunit of cAMP-dependent protein kinase (Walsh *et al.*, 1971). These results demonstrate cAMP-dependent phosphorylation but do not rule out the existence of an intermediate kinase that requires the cAMP-dependent protein kinase for activation. This would be analogous to the cascade system that activates phosphorylase. If such an intermediate kinase existed, addition of protein kinase inhibitor to a Sephadex-treated extract after inactivation has been initiated by cAMP should not stop further inactivation of pyruvate kinase. However, the inhibitor, added 6 minutes after the cAMP, does completely suppress any further inactivation of pyruvate kinase (Table II).

The inactivation of rat liver pyruvate kinase in hepatocyte homogenates by submaximal concentrations of cAMP can be suppressed by the addition of physiological concentrations of fructose diphosphate or phosphoenolpyruvate (Table III) (Feliu *et al.*, 1977; Pilkis *et al.*, 1978a). However, neither alanine nor pyruvate had any effect. The mechanism whereby these substances affect inactivation of pyruvate kinase is unknown. Eigenbrodt and Schoner (1977c) have reported that fructose diphosphate inhibited and alanine stimulated the cAMP-independent

TABLE III

EFFECT OF VARIOUS AGENTS ON THE CYCLIC AMP-INDUCED INACTIVATION OF PYRUVATE KINASE IN HEPATOCYTE HOMOGENATES[a]

Additions	$-cAMP$	V/V_{max} $+ 0.2 \mu M$ cAMP	$+ 2 \mu M$ cAMP
Mg-ATP (5 mM)	0.30 ± 0.02	0.17 ± 0.01	0.11 ± 0.02
+ FDP (10 μM)		0.15 ± 0.02	
(20 μM)		0.25 ± 0.01	
(50 μM)	0.30 ± 0.01	0.24 ± 0.01	0.15 ± 0.02
(100 μM)	0.30 ± 0.02	0.27 ± 0.02	
+ PEP (0.1 mM)		0.18 ± 0.01	
(0.2 mM)		0.22 ± 0.01	
(0.5 mM)	0.31 ± 0.02	0.24 ± 0.01	0.13 ± 0.02
+ Alanine (0.1 mM)		0.19 ± 0.02	
(1 mM)		0.20 ± 0.02	
(10 mM)	0.30 ± 0.02	0.18 ± 0.01	0.11 ± 0.02
+ Pyruvate (0.1 mM)		0.17 ± 0.02	
(1 mM)	0.29 ± 0.02	0.20 ± 0.02	
(10 mM)	0.28 ± 0.03	0.20 ± 0.02	0.14 ± 0.02

[a] Sephadex-treated extracts were prepared and incubated with 5 mM Mg-ATP as described by Pilkis *et al.* (1978a). The incubation time was 25 minutes. The activity is expressed as the ratio of activity measured at 0.4 mM/4.0 mM (V/V_{max}). The results are the average $\pm$ standard deviation of four experiments.

phosphorylation of chicken liver pyruvate kinase by affecting the dimer-to-tetramer equilibrium of the enzyme. Alanine favored formation of the dimer (MW 98,000) whereas fructose diphosphate favored tetramer (MW 165,000) formation. Thus, in the case of the chick liver K-isozyme, the dimer is apparently more readily phosphorylated than the tetramer. It is not known whether the L-isozyme from pig or rat liver undergoes any tetramer-to-dimer transitions under the influence of allosteric effectors. However, Berglund et al. (1977a) reported that alanine increased the rate of phosphorylation of purified pig liver pyruvate kinase by a partially purified preparation of cAMP-dependent protein kinase. This stimulatory effect was seen at alkaline pH, but it is not clear whether the phosphate was incorporated into the same site as normally seen or whether there was any associated alteration in enzyme activity. Fructose diphosphate had no effect on the phosphorylation. Although these effectors may directly affect the activities of the kinases and/or phosphatases for pyruvate kinase, it seems more likely that they produce in the enzyme structure conformational changes that result in a substrate that is more (or less) susceptible to phosphorylation and/or dephosphorylation. Evaluation is clouded by the fact that experiments have not been performed with purified protein kinases in most cases and it is not possible to distinguish between effects on phosphorylation or dephosphorylation of pyruvate kinase. However, the ability of allosteric effectors to modify the phosphorylation state of pyruvate kinase extends considerably the flexibility and sensitivity of its regulation.

The enzyme(s) responsible for the dephosphorylation of pyruvate kinase have received little attention. A histone phosphatase, which is capable of dephosphorylating [^{32}P]pyruvate kinase, has been purified from rat liver (Titanji et al., 1976, 1977). The dephosphorylation produced an activation of the enzyme. Van Berkel et al. (1977a) reported that inactive pyruvate kinase in crude homogenates could be reactivated by incubation with divalent cations. A phosphoprotein phosphatase with a rather broad substrate specificity has also been isolated from chicken liver (Eigenbrodt and Schoner, 1977b,c). It was able to dephosphorylate and reactivate the K-isozyme and the rate of dephosphorylation was increased by fructose diphosphate. Thus, it appears that pyruvate kinase resembles glycogen synthase D in that the inactive phosphoenzyme can be activated by dephosphorylation or by the presence of hexose phosphates: fructose diphosphate for pyruvate kinase and glucose 6-phosphate for glycogen synthase.

Neither the M-isozyme from rabbit muscle (Pilkis et al., 1978a) nor the K-isozyme from pig kidney appear to be phosphorylated (Berglund *et al.*, 1977b; Humble *et al.*, 1975). However, Eigenbrodt and Schoner (1977a,b,c) have shown that the K-isozyme from chicken liver can be phosphorylated by a cAMP-independent protein kinase. This phosphorylation produced an inhibition of enzyme activity even when measured with saturating concentrations of phosphoenolpyruvate. Thus the nature of the change in activity is different from that observed for the L-isozyme from rat and pig liver, where activity is affected only in the presence of low substrate concentration. It is likely that the site of phosphorylation of the K-isozyme is different from that on the L-isozyme. It is not known whether chicken liver pyruvate kinase can be phosphorylated by a cAMP-dependent kinase, but such would be consistent with the observation that glucagon stimulates gluconeogenesis in chicken liver (Dikson *et al.*, 1975). However, it has also been claimed that glucagon does not affect pyruvate kinase activity in isolated hepatocytes from the chicken (Ochs and Harris, 1977). Additional studies on the hormonal control of gluconeogenesis and pyruvate kinase in this species are needed.

Taunton *et al.* (1972) first reported that hormones could acutely affect the activity of pyruvate kinase. They showed that injection of glucagon or epinephrine into the portal vein of rats caused a rapid decrease in the activities of both pyruvate kinase and phosphofructokinase while stimulating the activity of fructose diphosphatase. Insulin injection caused the opposite effects on the three enzymes (Taunton *et al.*, 1974; Stifel *et al.*, 1974). These observations suggested that regulation of the substrate cycles between pyruvate and phosphoenolpyruvate and between fructose diphosphate and fructose 6-phosphate were important for regulation of gluconeogenesis. These results stimulated much research on the effect of hormones on these enzymes. Most of the attention has focused on pyruvate kinase.

A number of laboratories have demonstrated that addition of glucagon to the isolated perfused rat liver (Blair *et al.*, 1976) or to isolated hepatocytes (Friedrichs, 1976; Van Berkel *et al.*, 1976, 1977a,b; Riou *et al.*, 1976; Pilkis *et al.*, 1976a,b; Feliu *et al.*, 1976; Foster and Blair, 1976) leads to an inhibition of pyruvate kinase activity. Riou *et al.* (1976) compared the kinetics of the enzyme in extracts of glucagon-treated cells with those of the purified enzyme that had been phosphorylated *in vitro*. They found several similarities. First, there was an apparent decrease in the affinity of the enzyme for phosphoenolpyruvate. Second, both preparations were more sensitive to inhibition by ATP and alanine. Third, both enzymes were less sensitive to activation by fructose diphosphate. Riou *et al.* (1978) have also obtained direct evidence to support the hypothesis that glucagon stimulates the phosphorylation of this enzyme by demonstrating that the hormone stimulates ^{32}P incorporation into the enzyme *in vivo*. Glucagon administration increased the moles of phosphate incorporated per mole of enzyme from 0.5 to 1.5. This increase in enzyme-bound phosphate was associated with an inhibition of pyruvate kinase activity and an increase in cAMP (Riou *et al.*, 1978). Ljungström and Ekman (1977) have obtained similar data using rat liver slices. The stoichiometry of the *in vivo* phosphorylation is uncertain and must await determination of the total phosphate content of the enzyme.

The effect of glucagon on pyruvate kinase reduces flux through the enzyme, diminishes recycling, and increases conversion of phosphoenolpyruvate to glucose. This effect is consistent with the results of Exton and Park (1969), who found a fall in pyruvate and a rise in phosphoenolpyruvate steady-state concentrations in livers perfused with the hormone or cAMP. Claus *et al.* (1975) have studied the effect of glucagon on the rate of [^{14}C]glucose synthesis from various concentrations of labeled lactate, pyruvate, and alanine in isolated hepatocytes. Figure 10 shows that the greatest stimulation by glucagon (2- to 4-fold) was observed at low substrate concentrations whereas only a 1.6- to 2.4-fold stimulation was observed at very high substrate concentrations. Similar results were obtained with dihydroxyacetone as substrate, although the maximum stimulation was less than that observed with lactate, pyruvate, or alanine (Pilkis *et al.*, 1976a). The greater stimulation of glucose synthesis from lactate, pyruvate, and alanine can be explained as follows. All carbon from these substrates will be subject to whatever rate of cycling is taking place at the phosphoenolpyruvate level, whereas at least half of the carbon from dihydroxyacetone goes directly to glucose without exposure to cycling through phosphoenolpyruvate. Thus, the hormone effects would be expected to be larger with physiological substrates, but the rates, particularly in the absence of glucagon, would be slower than with dihydroxyacetone.

Glucagon does not stimulate the uptake of dihydroxyacetone (Pilkis *et al.*, 1976a,b), suggesting that the hormone increases the efficiency of substrate conversion to glucose. The data in Fig. 10 suggest that glucagon may have a similar effect with physiological substrates since the major effect of the hormone was to lower by 75% the concentration of substrate necessary for a half-maximal rate of incorporation into glucose. Similar results were seen with dihydroxyacetone as substrate (Pilkis *et al.*, 1976a). All of these results are consistent with an inhibition of flux through pyruvate kinase.

Catecholamines have also been reported to inhibit hepatocyte pyruvate kinase. The inhibition is quite small compared to that seen with

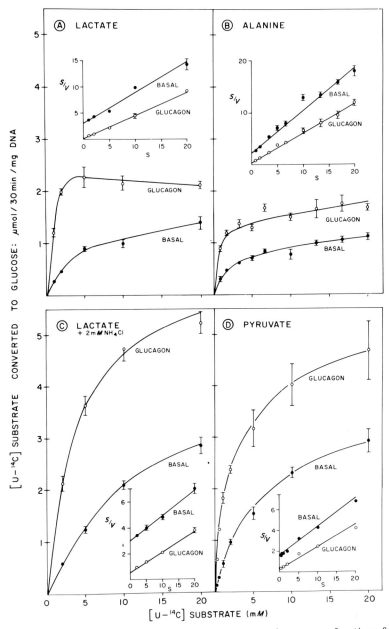

FIG. 10. Incorporation of U-^{14}C-labeled substrates into glucose as a function of their concentrations. Cells prepared from fed rats were first incubated for 30 minutes without any additions and then incubated for 30 minutes with substrate in the absence (●) or the presence (○) of 10 nM glucagon. *Insert:* Hanes plot of the data where S is the substrate concentration (mM) and V is the rate of conversion to glucose (μM/30 min per milligram of DNA). Data are from Claus *et al.* (1975).

glucagon (Feliu *et al.*, 1976) and correlates well with the relatively small increases in hepatic cAMP and hepatic glucose synthesis (Exton and Park, 1972; Pilkis *et al.*, 1975). It is not clear whether the catecholamine effect is mediated by an α- or β-receptor mechanism. The inhibition is associated with an increase in the $K_{0.5}$ for phosphoenolpyruvate (Feliu *et al.*, 1976) which suggests phosphorylation of pyruvate kinase. However, this has not yet been established.

Insulin has been shown to prevent both the catecholamine-induced inhibition of the enzyme and inhibition induced by submaximal glucagon concentrations (Blair *et al.*, 1976; Feliu *et al.*, 1976; Claus and Pilkis, 1978b). This effect of insulin is associated with a decrease in the $K_{0.5}$ for phosphoenolpyruvate, which suggests that insulin either suppresses phosphorylation of the enzyme, increases dephosphorylation, or both. The effect of insulin could be explained under some conditions by a fall in the level of cAMP. However, insulin has also been shown to suppress catecholamine- and glucagon-stimulated gluconeogenesis by mechanisms that are independent of nucleotide concentration (Claus and Pilkis, 1976), though it is not known whether the latter involve pyruvate kinase activity. No direct demonstration that insulin modulates the phosphorylation state of the enzyme in intact cells has been reported. However, it is attractive to postulate that insulin also acts at this site in the gluconeogenic pathway.

Pyruvate kinase activity can also be modulated by hormone-induced changes in the intracellular level of various allosteric effectors, particularly fructose diphosphate. In the experiments of Fig. 11, hepatocytes were incubated in the absence or the presence of 5 mM dihydroxyacetone. The substrate raised the intracellular concentration of fructose diphosphate 4-fold, but had no effect on the levels of ATP and phosphoenolpyruvate (Claus and Pilkis, 1978a,b). When pyruvate kinase was assayed, the $K_{0.5}$ for phosphoenolpyruvate was found to be 0.06 mM in homogenates of the cells incubated with dihydroxyacetone and 0.4 mM in the absence of substrate (Claus and Pilkis, 1978a,b). When these homogenates were treated with $(NH_4)_2SO_4$, which removes all low-molecular-weight effectors including the tightly bound fructose diphosphate, the $K_{0.5}$ for phosphoenolpyruvate was 0.4 mM in both cases (Fig. 12). This value is about the same as that obtained with the purified enzyme (Claus and Pilkis, 1978a,b; Riou *et al.*, 1978).

Fructose diphosphate may play an important role in the regulation of pyruvate kinase in hepatocytes from rats starved for 24 hours. We have shown that flux through pyruvate kinase can be controlled by the level of fructose diphosphate when dihydroxyacetone is the substrate (Claus and Pilkis, 1978a,b). With lactate as substrate, the flux through

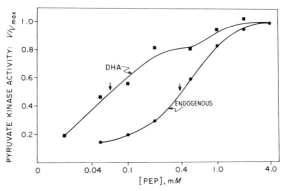

FIG. 11. The effect of phosphoenolpyruvate (PEP) concentration on the activity of pyruvate kinase in homogenates of hepatocytes from 18-hour-starved rats. Hepatocytes were incubated for 20 minutes without any additions and then for 10 minutes with and without 5 mM dihydroxyacetone. The cells were rapidly centrifuged, the medium was aspirated, and the cells were homogenized in 10 mM potassium phosphate–1 mM mercaptoethanol–40% (v/v) glycerol, pH 7.7. The homogenate was centrifuged for 30 minutes at 20,000 g, and the supernatant fluid was assayed for pyruvate kinase activity. Activity is expressed relative to the rate obtained with 4 mM PEP. At this saturating concentration of substrate, the same rate was obtained in all cases. The arrows represent the $K_{0.5}$ for PEP in each case.

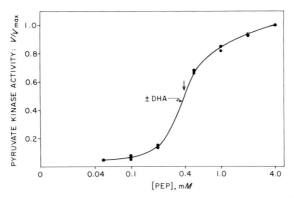

FIG. 12. The effect of phosphoenolpyruvate (PEP) concentration on the activity of pyruvate kinase in (NH$_4$)$_2$SO$_4$-treated homogenates of hepatocytes from 18-hour-starved rats. The incubation of the hepatocytes and the preparation of the homogenate are described in Fig. 11. The homogenate was treated with 60% (NH$_4$)$_2$SO$_4$ (final concentration) and centrifuged; the pellet was redissolved in the same homogenization buffer described in Fig. 11. Activity is expressed as in Fig. 11. The arrows represent the $K_{0.5}$ for PEP in each case.

pyruvate kinase is only 25–30% of that in hepatocytes from fed rats (Rognstad and Katz, 1977). Figure 13 shows that the amount of enzyme is not appreciably decreased by starvation nor is control by glucagon altered. It is conceivable, however, that the decrease in pyruvate kinase flux is due to a fall in the level of fructose diphosphate. Lawson *et al.* (1975) have calculated that the free fructose diphosphate concentration in liver decreases with starvation. Since cAMP levels are elevated in livers from starved rats (Exton *et al.*, 1970), owing presumably to higher glucagon and lower insulin levels, it is possible that pyruvate kinase may also be more phosphorylated in the starved than in the fed rat. The decrease in pyruvate kinase flux, together with the induction of more phosphoenolpyruvate carboxykinase, may be responsible for the high rate of gluconeogenesis in starvation. This combination of changes could explain why addition of glucagon has little further effect on gluconeogenesis from lactate in isolated hepatocytes from 24-hour-starved rats (Claus and Pilkis, 1976; Rognstad and Katz, 1977).

It is interesting that glucagon is still quite effective in stimulating glucose synthesis from dihydroxyacetone in cells from starved rats (Pilkis *et al.*, 1976a). In this case, it seems likely that the elevated level of fructose diphosphate both activates pyruvate kinase (Fig. 11) and/or inhibits phosphorylation, thus promoting recycling. Under these conditions, glucagon lowers fructose diphosphate levels (see later) and pro-

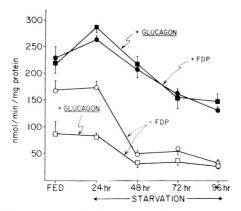

FIG. 13. Effect of starvation and glucagon on the activity of hepatocyte pyruvate kinase. Hepatocytes were prepared from rats starved for various periods (0–96 hours). The cells were incubated with and without 10 nM glucagon for 10 minutes, and pyruvate kinase activity was assayed in homogenates of these cells. The enzyme was assayed at 0.1 mM phosphoenolpyruvate (○, □) and with 4 mM phosphoenolpyruvate plus 20 μM fructose diphosphate (●, ■).

motes enzyme phosphorylation with a resulting increase in glucose synthesis (Pilkis *et al.*, 1976a).

The various factors that can influence pyruvate kinase activity are summarized in Fig. 14. The addition of glucagon to hepatocytes leads to inactivation when the enzyme is assayed with low substrate concentrations, but not at high substrate concentrations or in the presence of micromolar concentrations of fructose diphosphate. The effect of glucagon is mediated by a cAMP-induced increase in protein kinase activity and by a decrease in fructose diphosphate levels (Fig. 15) (Blair *et al.*, 1973; Pilkis *et al.*, 1976a,b). The fall in the concentration of the latter reduces pyruvate kinase activity by inducing a conformational change. This change presumably converts the protein to a more favorable substrate for inactivation by the protein kinase and/or to a less favorable substrate for activation by a protein phosphatase. The inactivation of pyruvate kinase by these concerted changes brings about a rise in phosphoenolpyruvate, which may then act as a negative feedback inhibitor of further phosphorylation of pyruvate kinase. The effect of phosphoenolpyruvate may also be brought about by a conformational change in the pyruvate kinase, which makes it a less favorable substrate for the protein kinase and/or a better substrate for the phosphatase (Feliu *et al.*, 1977; Pilkis *et al.*, 1978a). Thus, enzyme activity can be regulated by phosphorylation, changes in the level of allosteric effectors, and by the ability of allosteric effectors to influence phosphorylation state (Fig. 14).

At this writing a number of questions remain: (1) Is there a specific

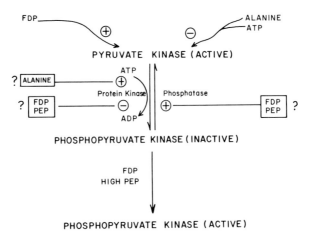

FIG. 14. Factors affecting the activity and phosphorylation of hepatic pyruvate kinase.

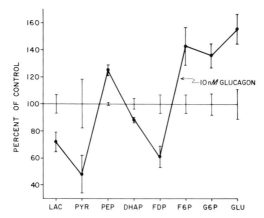

FIG. 15. Effect of glucagon on the levels of glycolytic intermediates in hepatocytes. Hepatocytes from fed rats were incubated for 15 minutes with 2 mM dihydroxyacetone in the absence and in the presence of 10 nM glucagon. The data were adapted from those of Pilkis *et al.* (1976a,b).

phosphatase for dephosphorylation of pyruvate kinase? (2) Is this phosphatase activity controlled by hormones? (3) Does phosphorylation of the L-isozyme result in changes in its quaternary structure as reported for the K-isozyme (Eigenbrodt and Schoner, 1977b,c)? (4) Do the effects of fructose diphosphate and phosphoenolpyruvate on the phosphorylation state of the enzyme result from a decreased rate of phosphorylation or an increased rate of dephosphorylation of the enzyme, and are these effects important in physiological regulation? (5) Does phosphorylation of the enzyme change its affinity for phosphoenolpyruvate, for fructose diphosphate, or for both?

Another form of regulation of pyruvate kinase activity is by adaptive changes in the concentration of the enzyme protein. Few studies on this subject have appeared. Krebs and Eggleston (1965) demonstrated that starvation led to low levels of hepatic pyruvate kinase activity, as did experimental diabetes. The feeding of diets high in carbohydrate produced markedly elevated levels of enzyme activity. Tanaka *et al.* (1965) showed that these changes, as well as the increased activity observed after prolonged administration of insulin, were due to changes in the amount of the L-isozyme. The K-isozyme in liver was unaffected. It has been postulated that the synthesis of the L-isozyme in liver is under the control of insulin, although activity of the enzyme in livers of alloxan diabetic rats can be elevated by glycerol feeding (Taketa *et al.*, 1967). Kohl and Cottam (1977) also studied adaptation of the enzyme during starvation and refeeding. They found ten times more pyruvate kinase measured as immunoprecipitable protein than by activity measurements in livers from fasted-refed rats. This suggested to them that a covalent modification of the enzyme may be an initial step in its degradation since the antibody used in these studies may have reacted differently with a modified enzyme. It may also be that the immunochemical method used may not specifically measure pyruvate kinase. Nevertheless, these studies raise the possibility that phosphorylation of pyruvate kinase may alter its degradation *in vivo.* In this regard, Bergström *et al.* (1975) have shown that phosphorylated pyruvate kinase is subject to proteolytic attack *in vitro,* but that enzyme activity is unaffected. The phosphorylated enzyme was more susceptible to digestion by subtilisin than the nonphosphorylated enzyme, and it was suggested that phosphorylation may increase the rate of enzyme degradation *in vivo.* Certainly, additional work on the question of how the turnover of pyruvate kinase protein is regulated would be worthwhile.

b. *Phosphoenolpyruvate Carboxykinase.* Phosphoenolpyruvate carboxykinase (PEPCK) was first discovered in chicken liver mitochondria by Utter and Kurahashi (1953). The enzyme has since been found to be present in high concentrations in liver and kidney cortex in all species (Utter and Kolenbrander, 1972), in white adipose tissue in some species (Tilghman *et al.,* 1976) and in lung tissue and brain (Tilghman *et al.,* 1976). Its concentration in gluconeogenic tissues is high, and it plays an essential role in gluconeogenesis from three or four carbon precursors. Although livers of all species studied to date contain both a mitochondrial and a cytosolic form of the enzyme, the intracellular distribution of PEPCK varies from species to species. The avian liver enzyme is located almost exclusively in the mitochondria (Chiao, 1976), whereas in rodent liver it is 95% or more cytosolic (Nordlie and Lardy, 1963). Most other species possess both mitochondrial and cytosolic forms, which are often roughly equal in amount (Soling and Kleineke, 1976). This is the case for human liver (Wieland *et al.,* 1968). Both forms of the enzyme appear to be a single polypeptide chain of molecular weights ranging from 71,000 for the avian liver enzyme (Chiao, 1976) to possibly 85,000 for the rat liver enzyme (Tilghman *et al.,* 1976). However, the two forms of PEPCK have been shown to be distinct proteins on the basis of immunological and chemical studies (Ballard and Hanson, 1969; Ballard, 1971; Diesterhaft *et al.,* 1971).

Only the cytosolic enzyme in rat liver is responsive to dietary and hormonal changes. The level of the enzyme is raised by fasting and diabetes and by the administration of glucagon, epinephrine, norepinephrine, glucocorticoids, and tryptophan when these agents are administered for periods of hours or days to the intact animals. The level is reduced by prolonged administration of insulin (see Tilghman *et al.*, 1976, for review). These effects are due to changes in enzyme synthesis except for tryptophan, which also decreases the rate of degradation (Tilghman *et al.*, 1976). Fasting has been reported to increase the cytosolic form of the guinea pig enzyme as well (Soling *et al.*, 1970). However, Elliott and Pogson (1977) have recently reported that the activity of the mitochondrial enzyme is doubled after 48 hours of starvation.

While there is ample evidence for the hormonal regulation of PEPCK levels, the evidence that PEPCK is acutely affected by hormones is only indirect. When rat livers were perfused with glucagon, cAMP, or epinephrine and the amount of glycolytic intermediates were measured, a "crossover" was observed between pyruvate and phosphoenolpyruvate (Exton and Park, 1969; Ui *et al.*, 1973a). However, these changes appear to be adequately explained by changes in pyruvate kinase activity. Attempts to measure a change in the kinetic properties of PEPCK in homogenates of livers treated with glucagon have been unsuccessful. We have also been unable to phosphorylate the purified enzyme with the catalytic subunit of cAMP-dependent protein kinase. Wicks *et al.* (1972) also reported that the enzyme was not phosphorylated. However, the addition of ATP and Mg^{2+} to kidney cortex homogenates activated PEPCK (Graf *et al.*, 1976). Attempts to find metabolic effectors for PEPCK also appear to have been unsuccessful, although it can be postulated that variations in the concentration of oxaloacetate can regulate the activity of the enzyme. The $K_{0.5}$ for oxaloacetate was originally thought to be too high for the enzyme to participate in gluconeogenesis. But more recent studies have placed the value in the 1- to 10 μM range (Ballard, 1970; Walsh and Chen, 1971; Jomain-Baum *et al.*, 1976), which is about the same as the concentration of oxaloacetate (5–10 μM) in perfused rat liver cytosol (Williamson *et al.*, 1969b). On the other hand, the $K_{0.5}$ for Mn-GTP^{2-} has been estimated to be 16 μM (Jomain-Baum *et al.*, 1976), whereas the GTP concentration in the whole liver is 100–600 μM (Chance *et al.*, 1965; Clifford *et al.*, 1972). If the nucleotide were evenly distributed in the liver, PEPCK would be nearly saturated with GTP. This would suggest that GTP does not have a regulatory role in phosphoenolpyruvate formation, as was suggested from studies with isolated guinea pig liver mitochondria (Garber and Ballard, 1970; Ishihara and Kikuchi, 1968).

Another type of control of PEPCK appears to involve metal ions. The enzyme requires two metal ions in order to form phosphoenolpyruvate at maximum rates (Foster et al., 1967; Holten and Nordlie, 1965; Utter and Kolenbrander, 1972). Magnesium is required in approximately stoichiometric amounts to the nucleotide (GTP or ITP), and micromolar concentrations of a divalent transition metal ion such as Fe^{2+}, Mn^{2+}, Co^{2+}, or Cd^{2+} activate the enzyme (Snoke et al., 1971). When PEPCK was assayed in rat liver cytosol, the addition of the transition metal ions activated the enzyme 2- to 3-fold (Snoke et al., 1971; Bentle et al., 1976). If the cytosol was first incubated with the transition metal ion, even greater effects were observed, and Fe^{2+} was the most effective activator. Evidence has been presented that Fe^{2+} is the natural activator in rat liver cytosol. When rat liver PEPCK was purified to homogeneity, the enzyme lost sensitivity to Fe^{2+} but not to Mn^{2+} stimulation (Bentle et al., 1976). Addition of rat liver cytosol to the purified enzyme restored the response to Fe^{2+}. This observation prompted the search for and the discovery of a protein that permits Fe^{2+} to activate the purified enzyme 3- to 4-fold (Bentle and Lardy, 1977). This protein, called PEPCK ferroactivator, has a molecular weight of approximately 100,000. A subunit molecular weight of 23,600 was obtained by sodium dodecyl sulfate electrophoresis. The activity of PEPCK with Fe^{3+}, Mn^{2+}, Co^{2+}, Cd^{2+}, Mg^{2+}, or Ca^{2+} was not affected by the ferroactivator. These data suggest that the rate of phosphoenolpyruvate synthesis by gluconeogenic tissues may be regulated by the availability of intracellular Fe^{2+} to the ferroactivator and PEPCK. Support for this view comes from studies of the tissue distribution of the ferroactivator and the effects of diabetes and starvation on it (MacDonald et al., 1978). The highest concentrations of ferroactivator were found in liver, kidney, and erythrocytes, and intermediate levels were found in the heart and pancreas. Except for erythrocytes and heart, the tissue distribution parallels that reported for PEPCK. Starvation and diabetes increased the amount of ferroactivator found in liver and kidney, and insulin treatment of diabetic rats returned the amount of ferroactivator to normal. Thus the ferroactivator showed adaptive behavior which paralleled that of PEPCK. Whether or not this protein participates in an acute activation of PEPCK in response to a hormone such as glucagon is unknown. The hormone could make more Fe^{2+} available or the activator may be interconverted between a phospho and a dephospho form. The presence of significant amounts of this protein in nongluconeogenic tissues suggests that it may have other functions.

2. The Fructose 6-Phosphate–Fructose Diphosphate Substrate Cycle and Its Enzymes

The importance of the fructose diphosphate cycle in the regulation of gluconeogenesis from physiological substrates is less certain than it is for the phosphoenolpyruvate–pyruvate cycle. The rate of gluconeogenesis from 3-carbon precursors is not limited directly by the reactions in this region of the pathway. There is five times greater fructose diphosphatase than phosphofructokinase activity in liver, so that changes in the flux through phosphofructokinase may not have as large effects on gluconeogensis as changes in flux through pyruvate kinase (Fig. 4). However, phosphofructokinase and fructose diphosphatase activities may regulate gluconeogenesis indirectly by controlling the hepatic level of fructose diphosphate, a potent activator of pyruvate kinase. The addition of glucagon or cAMP to rat hepatocytes or perfused rat liver causes a decrease in the level of fructose diphosphate (Fig. 15) (Williamson et $al.$, 1969c; Blair et $al.$, 1973; Harris, 1975; Pilkis et $al.$, 1976a) and thus promotes inactivation of the enzyme, as discussed earlier. The mechanism whereby glucagon lowers fructose diphosphate levels must involve a stimulation of fructose diphosphatase and/or an inhibition of phosphofructokinase activity.

Evidence that both enzymes of this cycle are operative in liver in $vivo$, and in perfused liver or isolated hepatocytes has been reviewed by Katz and Rognstad (1976). Hormone effects have been studied by following the metabolism of glucose labeled in various positions with tritium and/or ^{14}C. M.G. Clark et $al.$ (1973) estimated the rate of substrate cycling in rat liver in $vivo$ by following the metabolism of intraperitoneally injected [5-^{3}H, U-^{14}C]glucose. When the net flux of substrate was in the direction of glucose synthesis, phosphorylation of fructose 6-phosphate by phosphofructokinase was equal to the rate of substrate cycling. Fructose 6-phosphate phosphorylation was estimated by the amount of tritium found in the intrahepatic water. When the net flux was in the direction of glycolysis, the rate of dephosphorylation of fructose diphosphate was equal to the difference in the rate of fructose 6-phosphate phosphorylation and the rate of glycolysis, and it could be estimated from the decrease in the ^{3}H : ^{14}C ratio in hexose 6-phosphate. The authors found that the rate of phosphorylation of fructose 6-phosphate was inversely proportional to the rate of dephosphorylation of fructose diphosphate. The rate of phosphorylation of fructose 6-phosphate was about 60% greater than the rate of lactate gluconeogenesis in fed rats, but only about 40% greater in starved rats. Clark et $al.$ (1974b) also found that glucagon and cAMP affect the substrate cycle in isolated hepatocytes by inhibiting flux through phosphofructokinase whereas flux through fructose diphosphatase was stimulated. Similar effects were reported by Katz et $al.$ (1975). Kneer et $al.$ (1974) found that epinephrine and cGMP had the same effect on this substrate cycle as did glucagon. Since the effect of epinephrine was blocked by phenoxybenzamine but not by propranolol, it was concluded that epinephrine expressed its activity through the α-receptor. However, Dunn *et al.* (1976), suggested that glucagon activated fructose diphosphatase with little change in phosphofructokinase.

Katz and Rognstad have pointed out the possibilities for serious quantitative errors in the [^{3}H,^{14}C]glucose method of measuring this substrate cycle (Katz *et al.*, 1975; Rognstad *et al.*, 1975; Katz and Rognstad, 1976). Hué and Hers (1974a) have questioned even the existence of this cycle, suggesting that the production of tritiated water from [5-^{3}H]glucose is attributable to a transaldolase exchange reaction and to the operation of the pentose cycle. Rognstad and Katz (1976) devised a method that uses [1-^{14}C]galactose instead of tritiated glucose and found that glucagon did inhibit flux through phosphofructokinase while increasing flux through fructose-1,6-diphosphatase. Epinephrine was only half as effective as glucagon, and its effects were at least in part due to the cAMP-mediated β-adrenergic mechanism. Thus the weight of evidence supports the existence in rat liver of a fructose 6-phosphate–fructose diphosphate cycle that can be regulated by hormones.

a. Hepatic Fructose Diphosphatase. The highest activities of fructose diphosphatase occur in tissues having high rates of gluconeogenesis, such as liver and kidney. This is not surprising since fructose diphosphatase activity must be present for glucose formation to occur. This is strikingly evident in patients who lack this enzyme and as a result suffer from ketotic hypoglycemia, metabolic acidosis, and hepatomegaly (Pagliara *et al.*, 1970; Melançon *et al.*, 1973; Baker and Winegrad, 1970). These abnormalities are promptly corrected by administration of glucose and perhaps of folate (Hopgood *et al.*, 1977; Greene *et al.*, 1972). The enzyme is also found in muscle tissue (Black *et al.*, 1972; Krebs and Woodford, 1967; Salas *et al.*, 1964), although in general its activity is low and its physiological role unclear. It has been proposed that the high activity of fructose diphosphatase in bumblebee flight muscle is important for thermogenesis via the fructose 6-phosphate–fructose diphosphate substrate cycle (Newsholme *et al.*, 1972). The presence of fructose diphosphatase in mammalian and avian skeletal muscle may also serve a general function to sustain thermogenesis though this is uncertain (M. D. Clark *et al.*, 1973; Newsholme and Crabtree, 1976). Fructose diphosphatase has also been detected in brain, but its function is unknown (Scrutton and Utter, 1968).

The number of genes responsible for the synthesis of fructose diphosphatase is unclear. Immunological studies of fructose diphosphatase from muscle, liver, and kidney indicate that the liver and kidney enzymes are identical but the muscle enzyme is distinctly different

(Horecker *et al.*, 1975). The muscle enzyme also differs from the liver and kidney enzyme with regard to isoelectric point and inhibition by AMP (Esner *et al.*, 1969). It is more sensitive to inhibition by AMP than the liver enzyme and is activated by both creatine phosphate and citrate.

Most studies on the regulatory and kinetic properties of hepatic fructose diphosphatase have been restricted to the enzyme from rabbit and rat liver (see Horecker *et al.*, 1975, for review). Hepatic fructose diphosphatase is a cytosolic enzyme that is subject to a multiplicity of hormonal and metabolic controls including allosteric inhibition by AMP (Taketa and Pogell, 1963, 1965; Mendicino and Vasarkely, 1963; Underwood and Newsholme, 1965a; Rosenberg *et al.*, 1973; Datta *et al.*, 1974; Nimmo and Tipton, 1975; Tejwani *et al.*, 1976a; Riou *et al.*, 1977), substrate inhibition by fructose diphosphate (Taketa and Pogell, 1965; Nakashima *et al.*, 1970), and activation by a number of substances, such as histidine (Pogell *et al.*, 1968), chelators, and fatty acids (Carlson *et al.*, 1973). Many of the initial studies on the hepatic and kidney fructose diphosphatase were performed with purified enzyme that possessed a pH optimum of about 9. This represented the so-called "alkaline" enzyme. Traniello *et al.*, (1971) showed that this was not the native enzyme but arose from proteolytic cleavage of a small peptide (MW 6000) from the enzyme subunit during purification. The native enzyme had a pH optimum of less than 8. It was more sensitive to AMP inhibition than the alkaline enzyme and was a tetramer, each subunit having a molecular weight of about 35,000 instead of 29,000. The key to purification of the enzyme was a heat step at neutral pH, which tended to avoid release and activation of lysosomal proteases responsible for cleavage of the enzyme (Pogell and McGilvery, 1952; Hers and Kusaka, 1953; Byrne, 1961; Nakashima and Horecker, 1971). Homogeneous preparations of the intact enzyme from rat and rabbit liver (Tashima *et al.*, 1972; Carlson *et al.*, 1973; Byrne *et al.*, 1971; Ulm *et al.*, 1975; Traniello, 1974; Tejwani *et al.*, 1976a; Riou *et al.*, 1977) and swine kidney (Mendicino *et al.*, 1975; Marcus, 1967) have since been obtained.

There are reports that proteolytic modification of the enzyme may occur *in vivo*. Pontremoli *et al.* (1973b) have reported that seasonal differences in the total activity of rabbit liver fructose diphosphatase can be correlated with lysosomal activity as measured by the amount of free protease activity in the liver. In the summer, there was low protease activity and the enzyme had a subunit molecular weight of 35,000, whereas in the winter, protease activity was high and small quantities of the 29,000 molecular weight form were observed. Pontremoli *et al.* (1973a) studied effects of cold and fasting on rabbit liver and kidney fructose diphosphatases. They found that 18 hours of exposure to cold or starvation for 36 hours resulted in changes in fructose diphosphatase similar to those seen in winter rabbits. Differences in the amino acid analysis of the liver enzyme that had been purified from either fed or starved rabbits also suggest that the enzyme undergoes some proteolytic modification. When fructose diphosphatase was prepared from fed rabbits, it contained 4 M of tryptophan per mole of enzyme, and this tryptophan was presumably located somewhere near the N-terminal end of the enzyme subunit. However, the enzyme from starved rabbits contained no tryptophan, and the N-terminal amino acid was acetylated (Abrams et al., 1975; Benkovic et al., 1974; El-Dorry et al., 1977). Benkovic et al. (1974) have suggested that the latter enzyme may be the first species produced by lysosomal proteases and that further proteolysis produces the "alkaline" enzyme.

The nature of the proteolytic cleavage in vitro has also been studied (Traniello, et al., 1971; Pontremoli et al., 1973a,b, 1974). Limited digestion of the native enzyme from rabbit (Dzugaj et al., 1976) or sheep liver (Zalitis, 1976) with low concentrations of subtilisin appears to mimic the proteolytic events that occur during the preparation of the alkaline enzyme since the altered enzyme had a pH optimum around 9 and was less sensitive to inhibition by AMP than was the native enzyme. Similar results have been found for the purified rat liver enzyme (S. J. Pilkis, unpublished results). Subtilisin digestion results in the cleavage of a 6000 MW peptide from the N-terminal end of the enzyme subunit, which can only be dissociated from the 29,000 MW fragment under denaturing conditions (Dzugaj et al., 1976; Zalitis, 1976). Further evidence was provided by Pontremoli et al. (1973b), who showed that incubation of the purified neutral enzyme with lysosomes from liver results in changes in catalytic properties identical to those obtained with subtilisin.

It is possible that there are several steps in the conversion of neutral to alkaline fructose diphosphatase. The first may be splitting of a small peptide containing tryptophan. This process may occur in vivo during starvation or cold exposure but does not alter catalytic activity. This may be followed by a modification leading to loss of AMP sensitivity as has been well documented. This process, presumably at the lysosome level is associated with a change in subunit molecular weight from 36,000 to 29,000 and may occur in vivo to some degree in winter rabbits. The observation that the purified neutral enzyme from rats and rabbits is acetylated is not completely consistent with the hypothesis that a small tryptophan containing peptide is split off from the enzyme. Alternatively the findings of tryptophan in enzyme preparations from fasted rabbits may be due to as yet undetected contaminating proteins.

It has been proposed that fructose diphosphatase must exist in the cell as an activated form since the enzyme purified from rat or rabbit liver is inactive at neutral pH unless an activator is added. Many substances and mechanisms of activation have been advanced including sulfhydryl modification, chelation of metal ions, and activation by 3-phosphoglycerate, fatty acids, phospholipid, and protein factors. Pontremoli *et al.* (1965) have shown that reaction of two sulfhydryl groups per mole of enzyme with *p*-hydroxymercuribenzoate increases the activity of the enzyme at pH 7.5. A similar effect can be obtained by forming mixed disulfides of the enzyme with acyl carrier protein, coenzyme A (Nakashima *et al.*, 1969, 1970), homocystine, and cystamine (Pontremoli *et al.*, 1967). It is unlikely that sulfhydryl modification is a relevant control mechanism *in vivo*. Fructose diphosphatase is strongly activated by EDTA, which probably removes the zinc ions that are tightly bound to the enzyme (Tejwani *et al.*, 1976b). Tejwani *et al.* (1976b) have demonstrated that Zn^{2+} binds to the enzyme and inhibits its activity. In general, EDTA lowers the pH optimum from about 8 to 7.2 (Pontremoli and Horecker, 1971). This effect is most striking with the enzyme from *Candida utilis,* which is inactive at PH 7.5 to 8 in the absence of EDTA (Rosen *et al.*, 1965). In the case of rat liver fructose diphosphatase, EDTA stimulates enzyme activity 10- to 15-fold at pH 7.2 (Tejwani *et al.*, 1976a; J. P. Riou and S. J. Pilkis, unpublished results). Other chelators, such as histidine (Hers and Eggermont, 1961; McGilvery, 1961; Pogell *et al.*, 1968), 3-phosphoglycerate, and fatty acids (Carlson *et al.*, 1973), also activate the enzyme and shift the pH optimum downward, probably by chelation of Zn^{2+} or other metals. It has been proposed that alterations in the intracellular levels of effectors such as those noted above control the activity of fructose diphosphatase *in vivo* (Tejwani *et al.*, 1976b; Horecker *et al.*, 1975). The activation by a protein factor from rat liver homogenates (Pogell *et al.*, 1968) may be due to chelation, since it was subsequently found to be due to its free fatty acid content (Carlson *et al.*, 1973). Fatty acid may be the active factor in the γ-globulin fraction of rabbit serum (Baxter *et al.*, 1972). The effects of most of these naturally occurring chelators, particularly free fatty acids, are probably not important physiologically, their intracellular concentrations not being great enough. One possible exception is histidine (Horecker *et al.*, 1975). The effect of phospholipids on rabbit liver fructose diphosphatase (Allen and Blair, 1972) may also be related to metal ion chelation.

Pogell *et al.* (1968) have reported that rabbit liver fructose diphosphatase can be specifically activated by phosphofructokinase. However, Söling and Kleineke (1976) have shown that serum albumin was more effective than a homogeneous preparation of rat liver phosphofructokinase, and they concluded that the activation by proteins was a nonspecific effect. Thus, it does not appear likely that enzyme–enzyme interaction between fructose diphosphatase and phosphofructokinase plays a significant role in the physiological regulation of fructose diphosphatase activity.

Inhibition of fructose diphosphatase by adenine nucleotides has been reported. AMP is a potent allosteric inhibitor of the enzyme except in the case of slime mold (Rosen, 1966) and bumble bee flight muscle (Newsholme et al., 1972). Given the hepatic concentration of AMP (500 μM) and the K_i for inhibition ($K_i \sim 20 \mu M$), one would expect AMP to exert a strong inhibitory effect in the intact cell and that flux through fructose diphosphatase might be regulated by changes in the intracellular concentration of AMP. However, those factors that alter flux through the enzyme in intact cells did not affect the AMP concentration (Start and Newsholme, 1968; Clark et al., 1974b). If metabolic control is exerted by this substance, other factors must be involved. The inhibitory effect of AMP on the enzyme is potentiated by fructose diphosphate (Pontremoli et al., 1968), but potentiation is observed only with concentrations of fructose diphosphate in excess of in vivo levels of this metabolite. Inhibition by ATP and ADP can be observed with purified as well as crude preparations of fructose diphosphatase if the enzyme is diluted after incubation with the nucleotides (Taketa and Pogell, 1963; Jones, 1972). The K_m for fructose diphosphate was not changed by ATP (Taketa et al., 1971). The inhibition by ATP of the rabbit and guinea pig enzyme can be prevented by 3-phosphoglycerate (Pogell et al., 1971; Jones, 1972). In addition, a large number of unrelated compounds all prevented to some degree the inhibition of the rabbit liver enzyme by ATP and ADP (Taketa et al., 1971). This lack of specificity casts some doubts on the physiological significance of the ATP and ADP inhibition. The purified rat liver enzyme did not appear to be affected by ATP (J. P. Riou and S. J. Pilkis, unpublished results).

Fructose diphosphatase from guinea pig liver is not stimulated by EDTA but is inhibited by ATP, fructose diphosphate, and AMP (Jones, 1972) in a manner similar to that reported for the rabbit and rat liver enzyme. Citrate potentiates the inhibition by high concentrations of AMP and it has been suggested that changes in citrate concentration could lead to large changes in the activity of this enzyme. In view of the reported differences in its kinetic properties compared to the rat and rabbit liver enzymes, additional studies on the purified guinea pig enzyme merit further attention.

Fructose diphosphatase may also be subject to long-term adaptive changes in the amount of enzyme protein (Weber et al., 1965). Fructose diphosphatase activity has been reported to be increased during starvation and diabetes (Weber et al., 1965). However, others have failed to observe any changes (Soling et al., 1970; Willms et al., 1970) or have found a decrease in activity after starvation (Horecker et al., 1975). In general, adaptive changes in total enzyme activity do not appear to be striking.

As regards the acute effect of hormones on the activity of hepatic fructose diphosphatase, Taunton et al. (1974) have reported that portal vein injection of glucagon or epinephrine in rats increases activity of the enzyme in liver homogenates prepared 4 minutes after hormone administration. Insulin counteracts the effects of glucagon and epinephrine. These provocative results have not been confirmed but other studies with intact cells do suggest that flux through the fructose diphosphate step is increased by glucagon. The mechanism of these effects is unknown, but the hormone effects are not accounted for by changes in putative allosteric effectors (Clark et al., 1974b). Thus, it is attractive to postulate that glucagon and catecholamines affect enzyme activity by a phosphorylation mechanism.

Modification of fructose diphosphatase activity by phosphorylation–dephosphorylation was first suggested by Mendicino et al. (1966). They reported that a crude preparation of kidney fructose diphosphatase was inactivated when incubated with ATP and cAMP. Riou et al. (1977) have shown that ^{32}P is incorporated into the rat liver enzyme in vivo. They have also shown that a homogeneous preparation of the catalytic subunit of cAMP-dependent protein kinase from bovine liver or heart catalyzes the phosphorylation of a purified preparation of the enzyme. The phosphate is incorporated in seryl residues, and 4 M of phosphate are incorporated per mole of enzyme (Fig. 16). Rabbit skeletal muscle enzyme is not phosphorylated under the same conditions. A 40% increase in activity is associated with the phosphorylation, but only when the enzyme was assayed in the absence of EDTA (Fig. 17). Phosphorylation had no effect on the K_i for AMP inhibition. Similar increases in enzyme activity have been observed in homogenates of hepatocytes incubated with glucagon (J. P. Riou and S. J. Pilkis, unpublished results). The small changes in enzyme activity with phosphorylation may reflect ignorance of the factors that control enzyme activity in the cell. It is also possible that the enzyme is proteolytically modified during isolation so that the effect of phosphorylation is masked.

In summary, the evidence suggests that glucagon modifies fructose diphosphatase activity, and an attractive hypothesis is that the hormone acts by a phosphorylation mechanism. However, glucagon has

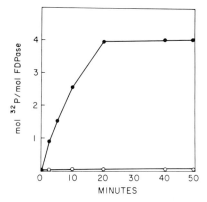

FIG. 16. Time course of phosphorylation of fructose diphosphatase (FDPase) by the catalytic subunit of cAMP-dependent protein kinase from bovine heart. Rat liver FDPase (●) or rabbit muscle FDPase (○) was added at a concentration of 1.6 μM and incubated with 8500 units of catalytic subunit (0.9 μM). At the indicated times, 5-μ1 aliquots were withdrawn and the ^{32}P incorporation into FDPase was determined.

not yet been shown to affect phosphorylation of the enzyme *in vivo*. Since fructose diphosphatase activity in liver is present in excess of phosphofructokinase activity, the most logical site of regulation of flux at this level would be control of fructose diphosphatase. Studies on the hormonal control of the enzyme and on the possibility that activation of the enzyme in intact cells is related to its phosphorylation state deserve additional attention.

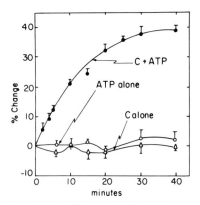

FIG. 17. Effect of phosphorylation of fructose diphosphatase on catalytic activity. Fructose diphosphatase was incubated with catalytic subunit of cAMP-dependent protein kinase as described in Fig. 16. At the indicated times the enzyme was assayed in the absence of EDTA (Riou *et al.*, 1977).

b. Phosphofructokinase. Phosphofructokinase is similar to pyruvate kinase in that there appear to be several isozymic forms (Tsai and Kemp, 1973). It has been postulated that rabbit heart and muscle contain predominantly a single isozyme (phosphofructokinase A) and the liver and red blood cell predominantly another (phosphofructokinase B). Brain contains a third type, designated phosphofructokinase C. Tissues other than liver, heart, and skeletal muscle contain isozymes A and B. These results were based on immunological and electrophoretic studies, and few comparisons of the kinetic and structural properties of these forms have been reported. Liver phosphofructokinase has been purified from pig (Massey and Deal, 1973, 1975), rat (Dunaway and Weber, 1974; Brand and Söling, 1974), sheep (Brock, 1969), chicken (Kono and Uyeda, 1971, 1973), and rabbit (Ramaiah and Tejwani, 1970; Kemp, 1971, 1975; Massey and Deal, 1975). The rat liver enzyme consists of four apparently identical subunits with a molecular weight of 82,000 (Brand and Söling, 1974). The liver enzyme, like that of the heart (Mansour, 1965; Mansour *et al.*, 1966) and muscle (Paetkau *et al.*, 1968; Paetkau and Lardy, 1967), tends to form aggregates with molecular weights of the order of several million (Brand and Söling, 1974; Trujillo and Deal, 1977). This aggregation is an equilibrium process influenced by enzyme concentration, the presence of allosteric effectors, the oxidation–reduction state of the sulfhydryl groups, and temperature (Bloxham and Lardy, 1973; Mansour, 1972; Ramaiah, 1974). The aggregation state of phosphofructokinase may also influence its kinetic behavior. Reinhart (1977) observed that the rat liver enzyme gave nonlinear rates of activity when it was diluted whereas linear rates were obtained when high concentrations of enzyme were used. The sigmoidal kinetics with fructose 6-phosphate seen with the muscle enzyme have been postulated to be due to reassociation of the enzyme by the substrate (see Bloxham and Lardy, 1973). It has also been shown that the purified rabbit muscle enzyme exhibits slow changes in specific activity that reflect the association of inactive dimers into active tetramers (Bock and Frieden, 1976a,b; Frieden *et al.*, 1976).

Phosphofructokinase from liver (Brand and Söling, 1974; Massey and Deal, 1973, 1975) exhibits homotropic cooperativity with regard to its substrate fructose 6-phosphate. 5'-Adenosine monophosphate, ADP, and cyclic 5-AMP are allosteric activators of the liver enzyme, and ATP and citrate are allosteric activators of the liver enzyme, and ATP and citrate are allosteric inhibitors (Brand and Soling, 1974). The muscle enzyme can be affected by these and many other effectors (for review, see Mansour, 1972; Bloxham and Lardy, 1973). Kemp (1971) has reported that rabbit liver phosphofructokinase is less sensitive to inhibition by ATP and citrate but more sensitive to inhibition by 2,3-diphosphoglycerate than the skeletal muscle enzyme. The ATP inhibition of phosphofructokinase decreases markedly as the pH increases from 6.5 to 8.0. Citrate potentiates the inhibitory effect of ATP on hepatic phosphofructokinase from sheep (Passoneau and Lowry, 1964) and rats (Underwood and Newsholme, 1965b). Both 5'-AMP and fructose 6-phosphate can overcome the increased sensitivity to ATP inhibition induced by the presence of citrate (Passoneau and Lowry, 1964; Underwood and Newsholme, 1965b). Brand and Söling (1974) have presented evidence that the reaction for the rat liver enzymes is an ordered BiBi mechanism where fructose 6-phosphate binds first, followed by Mg-ATP. Both a Ping-Pong and a random sequential mechanism have been suggested for the muscle enzyme (Uyeda, 1970, 1972; Lee and Griffin, 1972; Hanson et al., 1973).

Control of phosphofructokinase by enzyme–enzyme interactions has been suggested by Uyeda and Luby (1974), who reported that chicken liver fructose diphosphatase potentiated ATP inhibition of phosphofructokinase from both rabbit muscle and chicken liver. Other proteins were without effect, but it was not possible to demonstrate that fructose diphosphatase actually interacted with phosphofructokinase. Söling and Bernhard (1976) have since shown that fructose diphosphatase removed tightly bound fructose diphosphate from phosphofructokinase. Thus the inhibition of phosphofructokinase by fructose diphosphatase did not represent enzyme–enzyme interaction, but resulted from removal of fructose diphosphate.

The activity of liver phosphofructokinase can also be affected by phosphorylation (Brand and Söling, 1975; Brand et al., 1976). The rat liver enzyme can be phosphorylated by a cAMP-independent kinase, with a resulting increase in activity of the enzyme. The phosphate was incorporated into seryl residues, and 4 M of phosphate were incorporated per mole of enzyme. It was postulated that phosphorylation affects the association–dissociation equilibrium between the enzyme subunits. The dephosphorylated phosphofructokinase dissociated into subunits, and phosphorylation of the enzyme caused association of the previously inactive subunits to form an active tetramer. In the presence of high concentrations of fructose diphosphate, the inactive nonphosphorylated subunits also reassociated to form an active tetramer. If fructose diphosphate was removed, the enzyme dissociated into inactive monomers again. Phosphorylation of the enzyme was more rapid in the presence of fructose diphosphate than in its absence. It has also been demonstrated that purified muscle phosphofructokinase can be isolated in a phosphorylated form, but no effect of phosphorylation on its activity could be detected (Hofer and Furst, 1976; Hussey *et al.*, 1977). There are no reports of whether or not the liver enzyme is phosphorylated *in vivo*.

Glucagon and catecholamines have been reported to depress the activity of hepatic phosphofructokinase within minutes after their administration to intact rats (Taunton *et al.*, 1974; Stifel *et al.*, 1974). The same hormones inhibit flux through the enzyme in intact hepatocytes (Clark *et al.*, 1974b; Kneer *et al.*, 1974; Rognstad and Katz, 1976). The observation that liver phosphofructokinase activity can be altered by cAMP-independent phosphorylation supports the hypothesis that these hormones affect flux by changes in the phosphorylation state of the enzyme. However, the effect of phosphorylation to activate phosphofructokinase is opposite to the effects of the hormones on flux. Also, glucagon is thought to act by stimulating a cAMP-dependent protein kinase, which presumably would lead to phosphorylation of the enzyme and stimulation of its activity. It is of course possible that in intact cells phosphofructokinase is not phosphorylated by a cAMP-dependent kinase, and thus glucagon action would not result in its phosphorylation. It may be that glucagon and epinephrine promote the dephosphorylation of phosphofructokinase, either by activating a phosphatase or inhibiting the cAMP-independent kinase. Experiments to ascertain whether the cAMP-dependent kinase can affect any component of this system would be of great interest.

Liver phosphofructokinase activity can also be regulated through effects on the amount of enzyme protein (Weber *et al.*, 1965). Dunaway and Weber (1974) found that the levels of this enzyme in the rat decreased 60–70% during starvation or when the rats were made diabetic with alloxan or streptozotocin. Refeeding the starved rats restored the level within 72 hours, and insulin treatment for 72 hours increased the levels 6- to 8-fold over that in the diabetic. The decreased amount of the enzyme in the starved rats was the consequence of an increased rate of degradation. Dunaway and Segal (1974, 1976) have isolated a peptide that appears to play a role in regulating the turnover of phosphofructokinase *in vivo*. The peptide was decreased in fasting and diabetes and was subsequently induced by glucose or insulin, respectively. They have postulated that this peptide is a stabilizing factor that affects the conformation of the enzyme such that it is less susceptible to lysosomal and thermal inactivation.

3. The Glucose–Glucose 6-Phosphate Substrate Cycle

More than 20 years ago it was noted that [^{14}C]glucose was utilized, even in the absence of net glucose uptake by rat liver slices (Ashmore *et al.*, 1957). The same group also suggested that the enzymes of this substrate cycle, glucokinase, and glucose-6-phosphatase, could operate simultaneously in liver to control blood glucose levels as well as the direction and magnitude of liver carbohydrate metabolism (Cahill *et al.*, 1959). More direct evidence for the existence of this substrate cycle in liver has come from studies on the metabolism of [2-^{3}H]glucose. The labeled glucose is incorporated into glucose 6-phosphate by hexokinase/glucokinase and the rate of this reaction can be estimated from the rate of tritiated water formation and the specific radioactivity of the [^{3}H]glucose. Tritium is lost from the C-2 position of glucose 6-phosphate when it is converted to fructose 6-phosphate in the reaction catalyzed by hexose phosphate isomerase. This methodology has been used to estimate the rate of glucose phosphorylation by rat liver *in vivo* (Clark *et al.*, 1974a), by perfused liver (Clark *et al.*, 1975), and by isolated rat hepatocytes (D. G. Clark *et al.*, 1973; Rognstad *et al.*, 1973; Clark *et al.*, 1974b; Katz and Rognstad, 1976; Katz *et al.*, 1975). Results of these studies indicate that the rate of glucose phosphorylation *in vivo* is about a third the rate of glucose 6-phosphate hydrolysis, but is similar to that of fructose 6-phosphate phosphorylation in the 2-day-old suckling rat (Clark *et al.*, 1974a). The rate is high in hepatocytes from high carbohydrate or meal-fed rats, but is depressed during starvation or diabetes (Katz *et al.*, 1975). The rate of glucose phosphorylation is independent of the rate of gluconeogenesis, but is proportional to the extracellular glucose concentration (D. G. Clark *et al.*, 1973).

Although the activities of glucokinase and glucose 6-phosphatase do not appear to be acutely sensitive to hormones, their simultaneous operation may be important for the regulation of carbohydrate metabolism by the liver. Hué and Hers (1974b) have proposed that the major advantage of this substrate cycle may be to allow large changes in the net flux of carbon either toward glucose or glucose 6-phosphate, which are controlled solely by substrate concentration. For example, a small elevation in blood glucose levels leads to a large increase in glucose uptake by the liver and to a decrease in glucose 6-phosphate levels. The decrease in the level of this intermediate is attributed to an activation by glucose of glycogen synthetase and increased incorporation into glycogen. Thus when glucose levels rise, the phosphorylation of glucose increases, the dephosphorylation of glucose 6-phosphate decreases due to a lower concentration of glucose 6-phosphate, and the net uptake of glucose is enhanced. Katz and Rognstad (1976) have pointed out that glucose 6-phosphate is a focal point for the synthesis of glucose or glycogen, for glycogenolysis and glycolysis, and for the pentose cycle. Since the concentration of this intermediate is normally at equilibrium with fructose 6-phosphate and glucose 1-phosphate, these authors have proposed that carbohydrate metabolism in the liver may be regulated at the level of hexose phosphate by the coordinated control of the glucose–glucose 6-phosphate and the fructose 6-phosphate–fructose diphosphate cycles.

The addition of glucagon to hepatocytes from starved rats did not affect the rate of glucose phosphorylation (Clark *et al.*, 1974b). Effects of catecholamines and insulin have not been reported, but it appears that this substrate cycle may not be of great importance for the hormonal regulation of gluconeogenesis. The fact that there is at least four times more glucose-6-phosphatase activity may also support that notion. Since there is no evidence that hormones acutely affect the glucose cycle or that the enzymes of the cycle are phosphorylated, the properties of glucokinase/hexokinase and glucose-6-phosphatase will not be discussed. The reader is referred to the excellent reviews by Weinhouse (1976) and Nordlie (1976) for details of these enzymes.

IV. Summary and Overview

The actions of glucagon, insulin, and catecholamines on gluconeogenesis were originally thought to be mediated by changes in the intracellular level of cAMP. It was assumed that changes in this nucleotide affected the ability of the cAMP-dependent protein kinase to catalyze the phosphorylation of one or more than one rate-limiting enzyme in the pathway. In recent years, a number of discoveries have made it necessary to modify that hypothesis. Several laboratories have clearly shown that in addition to a cAMP-dependent mechanism, catecholamines can also promote hepatic gluconeogenesis in the rat by a mechanism independent of changes in the nucleotide. It has also been demonstrated that insulin can under certain conditions suppress gluconeogenesis that had been stimulated by either glucagon or catecholamines by a mechanism that does not involve changes in cAMP. Thus it is clear that the second messenger hypothesis must be modified to include other intracellular messengers as well as cAMP. The nature of the cAMP-independent messengers of hormone action is uncertain, but changes in Ca^{2+} distribution have been suggested. It is also uncertain whether the action of these other messengers is mediated by a phosphorylation–dephosphorylation mechanism.

Since 1969, when it was postulated that the action of these hormones affected a site(s) in the gluconeogenic pathway somewhere between pyruvate and phosphoenolpyruvate, the precise site has been sought by many investigators. This portion of the pathway involves both cytosolic and mitochondrial steps. Several discoveries have greatly aided the search for the affected reaction(s). First, it was discovered that glucagon and catecholamines could stimulate glucose synthesis from substrates that entered the pathway beyond the mitochondrial steps. This stimulated the search for cytosolic enzymes that might be affected, and it subsequently led to the observation that the hormones act at the fructose 6-phosphate–fructose diphosphate substrate cycle to stimulate flux through fructose diphosphatase and to inhibit flux through phosphofructokinase. Second, it was discovered that hepatic pyruvate kinase could be phosphorylated *in vitro* by a cAMP-dependent protein kinase with a concomitant inhibition of enzyme activity. These observations provided for the first time a mechanism for glucagon stimulation of gluconeogenesis consistent with the role of cAMP in affecting a reaction between pyruvate and phosphoenolpyruvate. Third, both phosphofructokinase and fructose diphosphatase can be phosphorylated *in vitro* by protein kinase with associated alterations in the kinetic properties of the enzymes. These important observations provide a possible mechanism for the regulation of substrate cycling at the fructose 6-phosphate–fructose diphosphate level.

It is the thesis of this review that the major effect of glucagon, catecholamines, and insulin on gluconeogenesis is to alter the flux of carbon through the phosphoenolpyruvate–pyruvate substrate cycle by affecting the activity of pyruvate kinase. These hormones also affect the fructose 6-phosphate–fructose diphosphate substrate cycle by altering the activity of fructose diphosphatase and perhaps phosphofructokinase. It is postulated that hormones modulate the activity of these enzymes by altering their phosphorylation state. Alterations in flux through pyruvate kinase can lead directly to a crossover between phosphoenolpyruvate and pyruvate. Alterations in the fructose 6-phosphate–fructose diphosphate cycle, which is not located in the rate-limiting portion of the pathway, can affect the activity of pyruvate kinase by altering the levels of fructose diphosphate, a potent activator of the enzyme. It appears that this metabolite not only affects pyruvate kinase activity directly, but also influences the phosphorylation state of the enzyme. Thus fructose diphosphate may serve as a link between the two substrate cycles.

Glucagon and catecholamines may also affect gluceoneogenesis by alterations in the rate of phosphoenolpyruvate production. These hormones have been shown to produce changes in mitochondrial metabolism that would favor gluconeogenesis, and these effects persist after isolation of the organelle. The hormones do not appear to affect the activity of pyruvate carboxylase or pyruvate dehydrogenase, but they do produce a general increase in anion transport by the mitochondria. Glucagon, via cAMP, appears to stimulate proton efflux from the mitochondria by activating cytochrome c_1. This activation may involve an increase in the phosphorylation state of the cytochrome, which is located on the outer surface of the inner mitochondrial membrane. This suggestion would be consistent with the reported stimulation by glucagon of the phosphorylation of mitochondrial membrane protein. Epinephrine does not increase proton efflux, but instead reduces the mitochondrial matrix volume by an unknown mechanism. The actions of both hormones promote the efflux of dicarboxylate anions from the mitochondria, which would lead to an increase in cytosolic phosphoenolpyruvate formation. Activation of phosphoenolpyruvate carboxykinase would also increase phosphoenolpyruvate production, but no acute effects of hormones on this enzyme have been found. A ferroprotein activator of this enzyme has recently been identified, and future studies may reveal that hormones acutely affects its activity, perhaps by changes in its phosphorylation state. While hormones may affect phosphoenolpyruvate production by these mechanisms, it appears that a major effect of these hormones on gluconeogenesis is to regulate the disposal of phosphoenolpyruvate by pyruvate kinase.

The strongest evidence supporting the hypothesis that pyruvate kinase is a major site of hormone action comes from studies with glucagon. All available evidence suggests that this hormone acts solely by a cAMP-dependent mechanism. Glucagon inhibits both flux through pyruvate kinase in intact cells and its activity in homogenates of hepatocytes treated with the hormone. The hormone-induced changes in enzyme activity are identical to those induced by phosphorylation of the enzyme with the cAMP-dependent protein kinase. Also, glucagon stimulates the *in vivo* phosphorylation of the enzyme. The addition of glucagon to hepatocytes also lowers the level of fructose diphosphate by increasing flux through fructose diphosphatase and/or inhibiting flux through phosphofructokinase. Although there is no direct evidence that the lower levels of fructose diphosphate contribute to the hormone-induced inhibition of pyruvate kinase, it is known that this metabolite can control the activity of the enzyme in the cell in certain circumstances, and that it can affect the ability of glucagon to phosphorylate pyruvate kinase in the intact hepatocyte.

Catecholamines appear to affect the same reactions in the gluconeogenic pathway as does glucagon, but by a cAMP-independent mechanism. In hepatocytes from fed rats, catecholamines have smaller effects on pyruvate kinase activity than does glucagon, and these results correlate well with the smaller effects on gluconeogenesis. In perfused livers from fed rats, the effects of glucagon and catecholamines on gluconeogenesis are more nearly equivalent. The reason for this difference is not clear, but it may be due to some alteration of the catecholamine receptor during preparation of the hepatocytes. However, catecholamine effects on gluconeogenesis are elicited only with very high concentrations of the hormone in either isolated hepatocytes or the isolated perfused liver. Thus the physiological significance of their effects is uncertain, although it has been suggested that stimulation of the sympathetic nerves within the liver may produce such high concentrations at the nerve endings.

Insulin opposes the action of both maximal concentrations of catecholamines and submaximal concentrations of glucagon on pyruvate kinase activity. Since insulin has identical effects on glucose synthesis, it is reasonable to assume that an important site of insulin action in the gluconeogenic pathway is at the pyruvate kinase step. How insulin acts at this site is unclear. Since insulin can suppress hormone-stimulated glucose synthesis by both cAMP-dependent and independent mechanisms, insulin may act either by activating a specific phosphatase for pyruvate kinase and/or by suppressing protein kinase activity.

There is currently no direct evidence that glucagon, catecholamines, or insulin affect the phosphorylation state of either fructose diphosphatase or phosphofructokinase. However, there is some evidence that is consistent with this possibility. The intravenous administration of glucagon or catecholamines can increase the activity of fructose diphosphatase and decrease that of phosphofructokinase. Insulin administration has opposite effects on these two enzymes. Glucagon and catecholamines can affect flux through these enzymes in intact cells in accordance with these activity changes. Since *in vitro* phosphorylation of fructose diphosphatase leads to activation of the enzyme, it is reasonable to postulate that glucagon and catecholamine administration leads to phosphorylation of the enzyme in intact cells. Such an effect would explain the hormone induced increase in flux through fructose diphosphatase and the glucagon induced fall in fructose diphosphate levels. Phosphofructokinase can also be phosphorylated *in vitro* by a cAMP-independent protein kinase, but phosphorylation increases enzyme activity. Since glucagon and catecholamines inhibit flux through phosphofructokinase and reduce its activity, it seems unlikely that these hormones promote phosphorylation of this enzyme.

Some properties of these three enzymes are summarized in Table IV. They are tetrameric enzymes that behave allosterically with regard to

TABLE IV

COMPARISON OF SOME PROPERTIES OF HEPATIC PYRUVATE KINASE,
FRUCTOSE DIPHOSPHATASE, AND PHOSPHOFRUCTOKINASE

	Pyruvate kinase[a] (L-isozyme)	Fructose diphosphatase[b]	Phospho-fructokinase[c]
Subunits	Tetramer	Tetramer	Tetramer
Phosphorylated by:			
cAMP-dependent protein kinase	Yes	Yes	?
cAMP-independent protein kinase	No	?	Yes
Moles phosphate/mole subunit	1.0	1.0	1.0
Activity of the phosphoenzyme	Inhibited	Enhanced	Enhanced
ATP	Inhibitor	Inhibitor	Inhibitor
FDP	Activator	Substrate (inhibitor)	Activator
Effect of phosphorylation + FDP	None	—	None
Acute effect of hormones on activity in liver			
Glucagon	Inhibition	Stimulation	Inhibition
Catecholamine	Inhibition	Stimulation	Inhibition
Insulin[d]	Stimulation	Inhibition	Stimulation

[a] From Ljungström et al. (1974); Riou et al. (1976); Pilkis et al. (1978a,b); Taunton et al. (1972, 1974); Feliu et al. (1976); Blair et al. (1976).

[b] From Horecker et al. (1975); Riou et al. (1977); Taunton et al. (1972, 1974).

[c] From Brand and Söling (1974, 1975); Brand et al. (1976); Taunton et al. (1972, 1974).

[d] Insulin acts to suppress the effects of submaximal concentrations of glucagon and maximal concentrations of catecholamine on these enzyme activities. It has no effect when added alone.

substrates and/or effectors. They are inhibited by ATP and are affected by fructose diphosphate. They can be phosphorylated in vitro, 4 M of phosphate being incorporated per mole of enzyme. Pyruvate kinase activity is inhibited by phosphorylation, and fructose diphosphatase and phosphofructokinase activities are enhanced. In the case of pyruvate kinase and phosphofructokinase, the effect of phosphorylation on enzyme activity is overcome by fructose diphosphate. It has been suggested that phosphorylation leads to the dissociation of pyruvate kinase to a dimer but to the association of phosphofructokinase to a tetramer. In rat liver, the phosphorylation of pyruvate kinase and fructose diphosphatase is catalyzed by cAMP-dependent protein kinase whereas that of phosphofructokinase is catalyzed by a cAMP-independent protein kinase. It is unknown whether the phosphorylation of fructose diphosphatase can be catalyzed by a cAMP-independent kinase or whether cAMP-dependent kinases can catalyze the phosphorylation of phosphofructokinase.

Although our knowledge of how, and at what sites, hormones affect gluconeogenesis has greatly increased in the last few years, there are still many areas that merit further study. These include the identification of the intracellular messengers for catecholamines and insulin; the elucidation of the mechanism and significance of hormonal regulation at the level of the mitochondria; the quantitation of substrate cycling at both the phosphoenolpyruvate–pyruvate and the fructose 6-phosphate–fructose diphosphate cycles; further characterization of the phosphorylation and hormonal control of phosphofructokinase and fructose diphosphatase; and the identification, isolation, and characterization of the protein kinases and phosphatases involved in the phosphorylation and dephosphorylation of pyruvate kinase, phosphofructokinase, and fructose diphosphatase. Knowledge from these and other studies should provide new insights into the mechanism of action of hormones on hepatic gluconeogenesis.

REFERENCES

Abrams, B., Sasaki, T., Datta, A., Melloni, E., Pontremoli, S., and Horecker, B. L. (1975). Arch. Biochem. Biophys. 169, 116–125.

Adam, P. A. J., and Haynes, R. C., Jr. (1969). J. Biol. Chem. 244, 6444–6450.

Allen, M. B., and Blair, J. McD. (1972). Biochem. J. 130, 1167.

Anderson, J. H., Nicklas, W. J., Blank, B., Refino, C., and Williamson, J. R. (1971). In "Regulation of Gluconeogenesis" (H. D. Söling and B. Willms, eds.), pp. 293–315. Academic Press, New York.

Arinze, I. J., Garber, A. J., and Hanson, R. W. (1973). J. Biol. Chem. 248, 2266–2274.

Ashmore, J., Cahill, G. F., Jr., Baird-Hastings, A., and Zottu, S. (1957). J. Biol. Chem. 224, 225–235.

Assimacopoulos-Jeannet, F. D., Blackmore, P. F., and Exton, J. H. (1977). J. Biol. Chem. 252, 2662–2669.

Badwey, J. A., and Westhead, E. W. (1975). In "Isozymes" (C. L. Markert, ed.), Vol. 1, pp. 509–521. Academic Press, New York.

Bailey, E., Stirpe, F., and Taylor, C. B. (1968). Biochem. J. 108, 427.

Baker, L., and Winegrad, A. I. (1970). Lancet 2, 13–16.

Ballard, F. J. (1970). Biochem. J. 120, 809–814.

Ballard, F. J. (1971). Biochim. Biophys. Acta 242, 470–472.

Ballard, F. J., and Hopgood, M. F. (1973). Biochem. J. 136, 259–264.

Barrera, C. R., Namihira, G., Hamilton, L., Munk, P., Eley, M. H., Linn, T. C., and Reed, L. J. (1972). Arch. Biochem. Biophys. 148, 342–358.

Barritt, G. J., Zander, G. L., and Utter, M. (1976). In "Gluconeogenesis: Its Regulation in Mammalian Species" (R. W. Hanson and M. A. Mehlman, eds.), pp. 3–46. Wiley, New York.

Batenburg, J. J., and Olson, M. S. (1976). J. Biol. Chem. 251, 1364–1370.

Baxter, R. C., Carlson, C. W., and Pogell, B. M. (1972). Fed. Proc., Fed. Am. Soc. Exp. Biol. 31, 837.

Benković, S. J., Frey, W. A., Libley, C. B., and Vilafranca, T. J. (1974). Biochem. Biophys. Res. Commun. 57, 196.

Bentle, L. A., and Lardy, H. A. (1977). J. Biol. Chem. 252, 1431–1440.

Bentle, L. A., Snoke, R. E., and Lardy, H. A. (1976). J. Biol. Chem. 251, 2922–2928.

Berger, R., and Hommes, F. A. (1973). Biochim. Biophys. Acta 314, 1–7.

Berglund, L., Ljungström, O., and Engström, L. (1977a). J. Biol. Chem. 252, 613–619.

Berglund, L., Ljungström, O., and Engström, L. (1977b). J. Biol. Chem. 252, 6108–6111.

Bergström, G., Ekman, P., Dahlqvist, U., Humble, E., and Engström, L. (1975). FEBS Lett. 56, 288–291.

Berry, M. N., and Kun, E. (1972). Eur. J. Biochem. 27, 395–400.

Bigley, R. H., and Koler, R. D. (1968). Am. Hum. Genet. 31, 383–388.

Birnbaum, M. J., and Fain, J. N. (1977). J. Biol. Chem. 252, 528–535.

Black, W. J., VanTol, A., Farnando, T., and Horecker, B. L. (1972). Arch. Biochem. Biophys. 151, 576.

Blair, J. B., Cook, D. E., and Lardy, H. A. (1973). J. Biol. Chem. 248, 3601.

Blair, J. B., Cimbala, M. H., and Foster, J. L. (1976). J. Biol. Chem. 251, 3756–3762.

Bloxham, D., and Lardy, H. A. (1973). In "The Enzymes" (P. D. Boyer, ed.), 3rd ed., Vol. 8, pp. 229–278. Academic Press, New York.

Bock, P. E., and Frieden, C. (1976a). J. Biol. Chem. 251, 5630–5636.

Bock, P. E., and Frieden, C. (1976b). J. Biol. Chem. 251, 5637–5643.

Brand, I., and Söling, H. D. (1974). J. Biol. Chem. 249, 7824–7831.

Brand, I., and Söling, H. D. (1975). FEBS Lett. 57, 163–168.

Brand, I. A., Muller, M. K., Unger, C., and Söling, H. D. (1976). FEBS Lett. 68, 271–274.

Bremer, J. (1969). Eur. J. Biochem. 8, 535–540.

Brock, D. J. H. (1969). Biochem. J. 113, 234.

Bryla, J., Harris, E. J., and Plumb, J. A. (1977). FEBS Lett. 80, 443–448.

Buse, M. G., Biggers, J. F., Drier, C., and Buse, J. F. (1973). J. Biol. Chem. 248, 697–706.

Butcher, R. W., Baird, C. E., and Sutherland, E. A. (1968). J. Biol. Chem. 243, 1705–1712.

Byrne, W. L. (1961). In "Fructose-1,6-Diphosphatase and Its Role in Gluconeogenesis" (R. W. McGilvery and B. M. Pogell, eds.), pp. 89–100. Am. Inst. Biol. Sci., Washington, D.C.

Byrne, W. L., Rajagopolan, G. T., Griffin, L. D., Ellis, E. H., Harris, T. M., Hochachka, P., Reid, L., and Giller, A. M. (1971). Arch. Biochem. Biophys. 146, 118–133.

Cahill, G. F., Jr., Asmore, J., Renold, A. E., and Hastings, A. B. (1959). Am. J. Med. 26, 264–282.

Cardenas, J. M., Dyson, R. D., and Strandholm, T. T. (1975). In "Isozymes" (C. L. Markert, ed.), Vol. 1, pp. 523–541. Academic Press, New York.

Carlson, C. W., Baxter, R. C., Ulm, E. F., and Pogell, B. M. (1973). J. Biol. Chem. 248, 5555–5561.

Carminatti, H., Jiménez de Asua, L., Recondo, E., Posserson, S., and Rozengurt, E. (1968). J. Biol. Chem. 243, 3051.

Carminatti, H., Jiménez de Asua, L., Leiderman, B., and Rojengurt, E., (1971). J. Biol. Chem. 246, 7284–7288.

Chambers, J. W., George, R. H., and Bass, A. D. (1968). Endocrinology 83, 1185–1192.

Chan, T. M., and Exton, J. H. (1977). *J. Biol. Chem.* **252**, 8645–8651.

Chance, B., Schoener, B., Krejci, K., Russmann, W., Wesemann, W., Schnitger, H., and Bucher, T. (1965). *Biochem. J.* **341**, 325–333.

Cherrington, A. D., Assimacopoulos, F. D., Harper, S. C., Corbin, J. D., Park, C. R., and Exton, J. H. (1976). *J. Biol. Chem.* **251**, 5209.

Chiang, P. K., and Sacktor, B. (1975). *J. Biol. Chem.* **250**, 3399–3408.

Chiao, Y.-B. (1976). *Fed. Proc., Fed. Am. Soc. Exp. Biol.* **35**, Abstr. No. 1522.

Clark, D. G., Rognstad, R., and Katz, J. (1973). *Biochem. Biophys. Res. Commun.* **54**, 1141–1148.

Clark, D. G., Lee, D., Rognstad, R., and Katz, J. (1975). *Biochem. Biophys. Res. Commun.* **67**, 212–219.

Clark, M. G., Williams, C. H., Pfeifer, W. F., Bloxham, D. P., Holland, P. C., Taylor, C. A., and Lardy, H. A. (1973). *Nature (London)* **245**, 99–101.

Clark, M. G., Bloxham, D. P., Holland, P. C., and Lardy, H. A. (1974a). *J. Biol. Chem.* **249**, 279–290.

Clark, M. G., Kneer, N. M., Bosch, A. L., and Lardy, H. A. (1974b). *J. Biol. Chem.* **249**, 5695–5703.

Claus, T. H., and Pilkis, S. J. (1976). *Biochim. Biophys. Acta* **421**, 246–262.

Claus, T. H., and Pilkis, S. J. (1977). *Arch. Biochem. Biophys.* **182**, 52–63.

Claus, T. H., and Pilkis, S. J. (1978a). *Fed. Proc., Fed. Am. Soc. Exp. Biol.* **37**, 1303.

Claus, T. H., and Pilkis, S. J. (1978b). Submitted for publication.

Claus, T. H., Pilkis, S. J., and Park, C. R. (1975). *Biochim. Biophys. Acta* **404**, 110–123.

Clifford, A. J., Riumallo, J. A., Baliga, B. S., Munro, H. N., and Brown, P. R. (1972). *Biochim. Biophys. Acta* **277**, 443–458.

Cook, G. A., Nielsen, R. C., Hawkins, R. A., Mehlman, M. A., Lakshmanan, M. R., and Veech, R. L. (1977). *J. Biol. Chem.* **252**, 4421–4424.

Coore, H. G., Denton, R. M., Martin, B. R., and Randle, P. J. (1971). *Biochem. J.* **125**, 115–127.

Crabb, D. W., Mapes, J. P., Boersma, R. W., and Harris, R. A. (1976). *Arch. Biochem. Biophys.* **173**, 658–665.

Dahlguist-Edberg, U. (1978). *FEBS Lett.* **88**, 139–143.

Daile, P., and Carnegie, P. R. (1974). *Biochem. Biophys. Res. Commun.* **61**, 852–858.

Daile, P., Carnegie, P. R., and Young, J. D. (1975). *Nature (London)* **257**, 416–418.

Datta, A. G., Abrams, B., Sasaki, T., and Van den Berg, T. W. (1974). *Arch. Biochem. Biophys.* **165**, 641–645.

Denton, R. M., Randle, P. J., and Martin, B. R. (1972). *Biochem. J.* **128**, 161–163.

Diesterhaft, M., Shrago, E., and Sallach, H. J. (1971). *Biochem. Med.* **5**, 297–303.

Dikson, A. J., Anderson, C. E., and Langslow, D. R. (1975). *Fed. Eur. Biochem. Soc. Meet. [Proc.].* Vol. 38, Abstr. 1462.

Dunaway, G. A., and Segal, H. L. (1974). *Biochem. Biophys. Res. Commun.* **56**, 689–696.

Dunaway, G. A., and Segal, H. L. (1976). *J. Biol. Chem.* **251**, 2323–2329.

Dunaway, G. A., and Weber, G. (1974). *Arch. Biochem. Biophys.* **162**, 620–628.

Dunn, A., Chenoweth, M., and Beuer, K. (1976). *Fed. Proc., Fed. Am. Soc. Exp. Biol.* **35**, 1427.

Dzugaj, A., Chu, D. K., El-Dorry, H. A., Horecker, B. L., and Pontremoli, S. (1976). *Biochem. Biophys. Res. Commun.* **70**, 638–646.

Eigenbrodt, E., and Schoner, W. (1977a). *Hoppe-Seyler's Z. Physiol. Chem.* **358**, 1033–1046.

Eigenbrodt, E., and Schoner, W. (1977b). *Hoppe-Seyler's Z. Physiol. Chem.* **358**, 1047–1054.

Eigenbrodt, E., and Schoner, W. (1977c). *Hoppe-Seyler's Z. Physiol. Chem.* **358**, 1055–1066.

El-Dorry, H., Chu, D. K., Dzugaji, A., Botelho, L. H., Pontremoli, S., and Horecker, B. L. (1977). *Arch. Biochem. Biophys.* **182**, 763–773.

Elliott, K. R. F., and Pogson, C. I. (1977). *Biochem. J.* **164**, 352–361.

Esner, M., Shapiro, S., and Horecker, B. L. (1969). *Arch. Biochem. Biophys.* **129**, 377.

Exton, J. H. (1972). *Metab., Clin. Exp.* **21**, 945–990.

Exton, J. H., and Harper, S. C. (1975). *Adv. Cyclic Nucleotide Res.* **5**, 519–532.

Exton, J. H., and Park, C. R. (1966). *Pharmacol. Rev.* **18**, 181–188.

Exton, J. H., and Park, C. R. (1967). *J. Biol. Chem.* **242**, 2622–2636.

Exton, J. H., and Park, C. R. (1968). *J. Biol. Chem.* **243**, 4189–4196.

Exton, J. H., and Park, C. R. (1969). *J. Biol. Chem.* **244**, 1424–1433.

Exton, J. H., and Park, C. R. (1972). *Handb. Physiol., Sect. 7: Endocrinol.* **1**, 437–455.

Exton, J. H., Corbin, J. D., and Park, C. R. (1969). *J. Biol. Chem.* **244**, 4095–5102.

Exton, J. H., Mallette, L. E., Jefferson, L. S., Wong, E. H. A., Friedmann, N., Miller, T. B., Jr., and Park, C. R. (1970). *Recent Prog. Horm. Res.* **26**, 411–461.

Exton, J. H., Lewis, S. B., Ho, R. J., Robison, G. A., and Park, C. R. (1971). *Ann. N.Y. Acad. Sci.* **185**, 85–100.

Feliu, J. E., and Sols, A. (1976). *Mol. Cell. Biochem.* **13**, 31–44.

Feliu, J. E., Hué, L., and Hers, H. G. (1976). *Proc. Natl. Acad. Sci. U.S.A.* **73**, 2762–2766.

Feliu, J. E., Hué, L., Hers, H. G. (1977). *Eur. J. Biochem.* **81**, 609–617.

Foster, D. O., Lardy, H. A., Ray, P. D., and Johnston, J. B. (1967). *Biochemistry* **6**, 2120–2128.

Foster, J. L., and Blair, J. (1976). *Fed. Proc., Fed. Am. Soc. Exp. Biol.* **35**, 1428.

Freiden, C., Gilber, H. R., and Bock, P. (1976). *J. Biol. Chem.* **251**, 5644–5647.

Friedman, B., Goodman, E. H., Jr., Saunders, H. L., Kostos, V., and Weinhouse, S. (1971a). *Metab., Clin. Exp.* **20**, 2–12.

Friedman, B., Goodman, E. H., Jr., Saunders, H. L., Kostos, V., and Weinhouse, S. (1971b). *Arch. Biochem. Biophys.* **143**, 566–578.

Friedmann, N., and Rasmussen, H. (1970). *Biochim. Biophys. Acta* **222**, 241.

Friedrichs, D. (1976). *In* "Use of Isolated Liver Cells and Kidney Tubules in Metabolic Studies" (J. M. Tager, H. D. Soling, and J. R. Williamson, eds.), pp. 444–447. North-Holland Publ., Amsterdam.

Fröhlich, J., and Wieland, O. H. (1971). *Eur. J. Biochem.* **19**, 557–562.

Gancedo, T. M., Gancedo, C., and Sols, A. (1967). *Biochem. J.* **102**, 23c.

Garber, A. J., and Ballard, F. J. (1970). *J. Biol. Chem.* **245**, 2229–2240.

Garcia, A., Williamson, J. R., and Cahill, G. F., Jr. (1964). *Fed. Proc., Fed. Am. Soc. Exp. Biol.* **23**, 520.

Garland, P. B., and Randle, P. J. (1964). *Biochem. J.* **91**, 6C.

Garreau, H., Columelli, S., Marie, J., and Kahn, A. (1977). *FEBS Lett.* **78**, 95–97.

Garrison, J. C., and Borland, K. (1977). *Fed. Proc., Fed. Am. Soc. Exp. Biol.* **36**, 318.

Garrison, J. C., and Haynes, R. C., Jr. (1975). *J. Biol. Chem.* **250**, 2769–2777.

Gimpel, J. A., de Haan, E. J., and Tager, J. M. (1973). *Biochim. Biophys. Acta* **292**, 582–591.

Glemzha, A. A., Lilber, L. S., and Severin, S. E. (1966). *Biokhimiya* **31**, 1033–1040.

Goodman, A. D., Fuisz, F. E., and Cahill, G. F., Jr. (1966). *J. Clin. Invest.* **45**, 612–619.

Graf, B., Peters, H. H., Bore-Nath, A., Steiller, G., and Weiss, G. (1976). *Abstr., Int. Congr. Biochem. 10th, 1976*, p. 373.

Greenbaum, A. L., Gumaa, K. A., and McLean, P. (1971). *Arch. Biochem. Biophys.* **143**, 617–663.

Greene, H., Stifel, F. B., and Herman, R. (1972). *Am. J. Dis. Child.* **124**, 415–418.
Guder, W. G., Schmidt, U., Funk, B., Wevs, J., and Purschel, S. (1976). *Hoppe-Seyler's Z. Physiol. Chem.* **357**, 1793–1800.
Haeckel, R., Hess, B., Lauterborn, W., and Wuster, K. H. (1968). *Hoppe-Seyler's Z. Physiol. Chem.* **349**, 699.
Halestrap, A. P. (1975). *Biochem. J.* **148**, 85–96.
Halestrap, A. P. (1978). *FEBS-Symp.* **42**, 61–70.
Halestrap, A. P., and Denton, R. M. (1975). *Biochem. J.* **148**, 313–316.
Hansford, R. G. (1976). *J. Biol. Chem.* **251**, 5483–5489.
Hanson, R. G., Rudolph, F. B., and Lardy, H. A. (1973). *J. Biol. Chem.* **248**, 7852–7859.
Harris, R. A. (1975). *Arch. Biochem. Biophys.* **169**, 168–180.
Hayakawa, T., Kanzaki, T., Kitamura, T., Fukuyoshi, Y., Sakurai, Y., Koike, K., Suematsu, T., and Koike, M. (1969). *J. Biol. Chem.* **244**, 3660–3670.
Haynes, R. C., Jr. (1965). *J. Biol. Chem.* **240**, 4103–4106.
Haynes, R. C., Jr. (1972). *In* "Energy Metabolism and the Regulation of Metabolic Processes in Mitochondria" (M. A. Mehlman and R. W. Hanson, eds.), pp. 239–252. Academic Press, New York.
Hers, H. G., and Eggermont, E. (1961). *In* "Fructose-1,6-Diphosphatase and Its Role in Gluconeogenesis" (R. W. McGilvery and B. M. Pogell, eds.), pp. 14–19. Am. Inst. Biol. Sci., Washington, D.C.
Hers, H. G., and Kusaka, T. (1953). *Biochim. Biophys. Acta* **11**, 427–437.
Hess, B., and Kutzbach, C. (1971). *Hoppe-Seyler's Z. Physiol. Chem.* **352**, 453–458.
Hess, B., Hoeckel, R., and Brand, K. (1966). *Biochem. Biophys. Res. Commun.* **24**, 824.
Hjelmqvist, G., Andersson, J., Edlund, B., and Engström, L. (1974). *Biochem. Biophys. Res. Commun.* **6**, 559–563.
Hofer, H. W., and Furst, M. (1976). *FEBS Lett.* **62**, 118–122.
Hofmann, E., Kurgano, B. I., Schellenberger, W., Schultz, J., Sparmann, G., Wenzel, K.-W., and Zimmerman, G. (1975). *Adv. Enzyme Regul.* **13**, 247–277.
Holten, D. D., and Nordlie, R. C. (1965). *Biochemistry* **4**, 723–731.
Hopgood, N. J., Holzman, I., and Drash, A. L. (1977). *Am. J. Dis. Child.* **131**, 418–421.
Horecker, B. L., Melloni, E., and Pontremoli, S. (1975). *Adv. Enzymol.* **42**, 193–226.
Hucho, F., Randall, D. D., Roche, T. E., Burgett, M. W., Pelley, J. W., and Reed, L. J. (1972). *Arch. Biochem. Biophys.* **151**, 328–340.
Hué, L., and Hers, H. G. (1974a). *Biochem. Biophys. Res. Commun.* **58**, 532–539.
Hué, L., and Hers, H. G. (1974b). *Biochem. Biophys. Res. Commun.* **58**, 540–548.
Humble, E., Berglund, L., Titanji, V. P. K., Ljungström, O., Edlund, B., Zetterqvist, O., and Engström, L. (1975). *Biochem. Biophys. Res. Commun.* **66**, 614–621.
Hunsley, T. R., and Suelter, C. H. (1969). *J. Biol. Chem.* **244**, 4819.
Hussey, C. R., Liddle, P. F., Ardron, D., and Kellett, G. L. (1977). *Eur. J. Biochem.* **80**, 497–506.
Ibsen, K. (1977). *Cancer Res.* **37**, 341–353.
Ibsen, K. H., and Marles, S. W. (1976). *Biochemistry* **15**, 1073–1079.
Ibsen, K. H., and Trippet, P. (1972). *Biochemistry* **11**, 4442–4450.
Ibsen, K. H., and Trippet, P. A. (1973). *Arch. Biochem. Biophys.* **156**, 730–744.
Ibsen, K. H., and Trippet, P. A. (1974). *Arch. Biochem. Biophys.* **163**, 570–580.
Ibsen, K. H., Schillor, K. W., and Haas, T. A. (1971). *J. Biol. Chem.* **246**, 1233–1240.
Ibsen, K. H., Trippet, P., and Basne, J. (1975). *In* "Isozymes" (C. L. Markert, ed.), Vol. 1, pp. 543–559. Academic Press, New York.
Ibsen, K. H., Murray, L., and Marles, S. W. (1976). *Biochemistry* **15**, 1064–1073.
Imamura, K., Taniuchi, K., and Tanaka, T. (1972). *J. Biochem. (Tokyo)* **72**, 1001–1015.

Imamura, K., Tanakia, T., Nishima, T., Nakashima, K., and Miwa, S. (1973). *J. Biochem.* (*Tokyo*) **74**, 1165–1175.

Irving, M. G., and Williams, J. P. (1973). *Biochem. J.* **131**, 303–313.

Ishihara, N., and Kikuchi, G. (1968). *Biochim. Biophys. Acta* **153**, 733–748.

Jimenez de Asua, L., Rogengurt, E., and Carminatti, H. (1970). *J. Biol. Chem.* **245**, 3901.

Jomain-Baum, M., Schramm, V. L., and Hanson, R. W. (1976). *J. Biol. Chem.* **257**, 37–44.

Jones, C. T. (1972). *Biochem. J.* **130**, 23P.

Jope, R., and Blass, J. P. (1975). *Biochem. J.* **150**, 397–403.

Jungas, R. L. (1971). *Metab., Clin. Exp.* **20**, 43–53.

Katz, J., and Rognstad, R. (1976). *Curr. Top. Cell. Regul.* **10**, 237–289.

Katz, J., Wals, P. A., Golden, S., and Rognstad, R. (1975). *Eur. J. Biochem.* **60**, 91–101.

Katz, N., and Jungermann, K. (1976). *Hoppe-Seyler's Z. Physiol. Chem.* **357**, 359–375.

Katz, N., Teutsch, H. F., Jungermann, K., and Sasse, D. (1977). *FEBS Lett.* **83**, 272–276.

Kayne, F. J., and Price, N. C. (1972). *Biochemistry* **11**, 4415–4420.

Keech, D. B., and Utter, M. F. (1963). *J. Biol. Chem.* **238**, 2609–2614.

Kemp, B. E., Bylund, D. B., Huang, T.-S., and Krebs, E. G. (1975). *Proc. Natl. Acad. Sci. U.S.A.* **72**, 3448–3452.

Kemp, R. G. (1971). *J. Biol. Chem.* **246**, 245–252.

Kemp. R. G. (1975). *In* "Methods in Enzymology" (W. A. Wood, ed.), Vol. 42, p. 67. Academic Press, New York.

Keppens, S. S., Vandenheede, J. R., and DeWulf, H. (1977). *Biochim. Biophys. Acta* **496**, 448–457.

Kerbey, A. L., Randle, P. J., Cooper, R. H., Whitehouse, S., Pask, H. T., and Denton, R. M. (1976). *Biochem. J.* **154**, 327–388.

Kimmich, G. A., and Rasmussen, H. (1969). *J. Biol. Chem.* **244**, 190–199.

Kletzien, R. F., Pariza, M. W., Becker, J. E., and Potter, V. R. (1976a). *J. Cell. Physiol.* **89**, 641–646.

Kletzien, R. F., Pariza, M. W., Becker, J. E., Potter, V. R., and Butcher, V. R. (1976b). *J. Biol. Chem.* **251**, 3014–3020.

Kneer, N. M., Bosch, A. L., Clark, M. G., and Lardy, H. A. (1974). *Proc. Natl. Acad. Sci. U.S.A.* **71**, 4523–4527.

Kohl, A., and Cottam, L. (1977). *Arch. Biochem. Biophys.* **176**, 671–682.

Koike, M., Reed, L. J., and Carroll, W. R. (1963). *J. Biol. Chem.* **238**, 30–39.

Koler, R. D., and Vanbellinghen, P. (1968). *Adv. Enzyme Regul.* **6**, 127.

Kono, N., and Uyeda, K. (1971). *Biochem. Biophys. Res. Commun.* **42**, 1095.

Kono, N., and Uyeda, K. (1973). *J. Biol. Chem.* **248**, 8592–8603.

Krebs, H. A., and Eggleston, L. V. (1965). *Biochem. J.* **94**, 3c.

Krebs, H. A., and Woodford, M. (1967). *Biochem. J.* **94**, 436–445.

Krebs, H. A., Gascoyne, T., and Netton, B. M. (1967). *Biochem. J.* **102**, 275–282.

Kutzbach, C., Beschofberger, J., Hess, B., and Zimmerman-Telschow, H. (1973). *Hoppe-Seyler's Z. Physiol. Chem.* **354**, 1473–1489.

Lardy, H. A. (1965). *Harvey Lect.* **60**, 261–278.

Larner, J. (1968). *Adv. Enzyme Regul.* **6**, 409–423.

Lawson, J. W. R., Guynn, R. W., Cornell, N., and Veech, R. L. (1976). *In* "Glucogenesis: Its Regulation in Mammalian Species" (R. W. Hanson and M. A. Mehlman, eds.), pp. 481–512. Wiley, New York.

Lea, A., and Griffin, C. C. (1972). *Arch. Biochem. Biophys.* **149**, 361–368.

LeCam, A., and Freychet, P. (1976). *Biochim. Biophys. Res. Commun.* **72**, 843–901.

Lee, Y. P., and Lardy, H. H. (1965). *J. Biol. Chem.* **240**, 1427–1436.

Lee, Y. P., Takemori, H. E., and Lardy, H. A. (1959). *J. Biol. Chem.* **234,** 3051–3054.
Leiter, A. B., Weinberg, M., Isohaslir, F., Utter, M. F., and Linn, T. (1978). *J. Biol. Chem.* **253,** 2716–2723.
Lincoln, D. R., Black, J. A., and Rittenberg, M. B. (1975). *Biochim. Biophys. Acta* **410,** 279–284.
Linn, T. C., Pettit, F. H., Hucho, F., and Reed, L. J. (1969a). *Proc. Natl. Acad. Sci. U.S.A.* **64,** 221–234.
Linn, T. C., Pettit, F. H., and Reed, L. J. (1969b). *Proc. Natl. Acad. Sci. U.S.A.* **62,** 234–241.
Linn, T. C., Pettey, J. W., Pettit, F. H., Hucho, F., Randall, D. D., and Reed, L. J. (1972). *Arch. Biochem. Biophys.* **148,** 327–342.
Ljungström, O., and Ekman, P. (1977). *Biochem. Biophys. Res. Commun.* **78,** 1147–1155.
Ljungström, O., Hjelmquist, G., and Engström, L. (1974). *Biochim. Biophys. Acta* **358,** 289–298.
Ljungström, O., Berlund, L., and Engström, L. (1976). *Eur. J. Biochem.* **68,** 497–506.
Llorente, P., Marco, R., and Sols, A. (1970). *Eur. J. Biochem.* **13,** 45–52.
Lopes-Cardozo, M., Vaartjes, W. J., and Van den Berg, S. G. (1972). *FEBS Lett.* **28,** 265–270.
McClure, W. R., and Lardy, H. A. (1971). *J. Biol. Chem.* **246,** 3591–3596.
McClure, W. R., Lardy, H. A., and Kneifel, H. P. (1971). *J. Biol. Chem.* **246,** 3569.
MacDonald, M. J., Bentle, L. A., and Lardy, H. A. (1978). *J. Biol. Chem.* **253,** 116–124.
McGilvery, R. W. (1961). *In* "Fructose-1,6-Diphosphatase and Its Role in Gluconeogenesis" (R. W. McGilvery and B. M. Pogell, eds.), pp. 3–13. Am. Inst. Biol. Sci., Washington, D. C.
Mallette, L. E., Exton, J. H., and Park, C. R. (1969a). *J. Biol. Chem.* **244,** 5713–5723.
Mallette, L. E., Exton, J. H., and Park, C. R. (1969b). *J. Biol. Chem.* **244,** 5724–5728.
Mansour, T. E. (1965). *J. Biol. Chem.* **240,** 2165–2172.
Mansour, T. E. (1972). *Curr. Top. Cell. Regul.* **5,** 1–46.
Mansour, T. E., Wakid, N., and Sprouse, H. M. (1966). *J. Biol. Chem.* **241,** 1512.
Mapes, J. P., and Harris, R. A. (1976). *J. Biol. Chem.* **251,** 6189–6196.
Marco, R., and Sols, A. (1970). *In* "Metabolic Regulation and Enzyme Action" (A. Sols and S. Grisolia, eds.), p. 63. Academic Press, New York.
Marcus, F. (1967). *Arch. Biochem. Biophys.* **122,** 393–399.
Marie, J., Kahn, A., and Bowin, P. (1976a). *Biochim. Biophys. Acta* **438,** 393–406.
Marie, J., Kahn, A., and Bowin, P. (1976b). *Hum. Genet.* **31,** 35–45.
Marie, J., Garreau, H., and Kahn, A. (1977). *FEBS Lett.* **78,** 91–94.
Marliss, E. G., Aoki, T. T., Unger, R. H., Soeldner, J. S., and Cahill, G. F., Jr. (1970). *J. Clin. Invest.* **49,** 2256–2270.
Martin, B. R., Denton, R. M., Pask, H. T., and Randle, P. J. (1972). *Biochem. J.* **129,** 763–773.
Massey, T. H., and Deal, W. C. (1973). *J. Biol. Chem.* **248,** 56.
Massey, T. H., and Deal, W. C. (1975). *In* "Methods in Enzymology" (W. A. Wood, ed.), Vol. 42, p. 99. Academic Press, New York.
Melancon, S. B., Khachadurian, A. K., Nadler, H. L., and Brown, B. I. (1973). *J. Pediatr.* **82,** 650.
Mendicino, T., and Vasarkely, F. (1963). *J. Biol. Chem.* **11,** 3528–3534.
Mendicino, T., Beaudreau, C., and Bhattacharyya, R. N. (1966). *Arch. Biochem. Biophys.* **116,** 436.
Mendicino, T., Abow Issa, H., Medicus, R., and Kratowich, N. (1975). *In* "Methods in Enzymology" (W. A. Wood, ed.), Vol. 42, pp. 375–397. Academic Press, New York.

Miwa, S., Nakashima, K., and Skinohara, L. (1975). *In* "Isozymes" (C. L. Markert, ed.), Vol. 2, pp. 487–500. Academic Press, New York.

Morikofer-Zwez, S., Kunin, A. S., and Walter, R. (1973). *J. Biol. Chem.* **248**, 7588–7594.

Mowbray, J. (1974). *FEBS Lett.* **44**, 344–347.

Mowbray, J. (1975). *Biochem. J.* **148**, 41–47.

Mukherjee, C., and Jungas, R. L. (1975). *Biochem. J.* **148**, 229–235.

Mullhofer, G., Low, E., Wollenberg, P., and Kramer, R. (1974). *Hoppe-Seyler's Z. Physiol. Chem.* **355**, 239–254.

Muroya, N., Nagao, Y., Mayasaki, K., Nishikawa, K., and Horio, T. (1976). *J. Biochem. (Tokyo)* **79**, 203–215.

Nakashima, K. (1974). *Clin. Chim. Acta* **55**, 245–254.

Nakashima, K., and Horecker, B. L. (1971). *Arch. Biochem. Biophys.* **146**, 153–160.

Nakashima, K., Pontremoli, S., and Horecker, B. L. (1969). *Proc. Natl. Acad. Sci. U.S.A.* **64**, 947.

Nakashima, K., Horecker, B. L., Traniello, S., and Pontremoli, S. (1970). *Arch. Biochem. Biophys.* **139**, 190.

Nakashima, K., Miwa, S., Oda, S., Tanaka, T., Imanwa, K., and Nishina, T. (1974). *Blood* **43**, 437–448.

Newsholme, E. A., and Crabtree, B. (1976). *Biochem. Soc. Symp.* **41**, 61–109.

Newsholme, E. A., and Gevers, W. (1967). *Vitam. Horm. (N.Y.)* **25**, 1–87.

Newsholme, E. A., Crabtree, B., Higgins, S. J., Thornton, S. D., and Start, C. (1972). *Biochem. J.* **128**, 89.

Nimmo, H. G., and Tipton, K. F. (1975). *Biochem. J.* **145**, 323–334.

Nordlie, R. C. (1976). *In* Gluconeogenesis: Its Regulation in Mammalian Species" (R. W. Hanson and M. A. Mehlman, eds.), pp. 93–152. Wiley, New York.

Nordlie, R. C., and Lardy, H. A. (1963). *J. Biol. Chem.* **238**, 2259–2263.

Ochs, R., and Harris, R. A. (1977). *Fed. Proc., Fed. Am. Soc. Exp. Biol.* **36**, 690.

Owen, O. E., Felig, P., Morgan, A. P., Wahren, J., and Cahill, G. F., Jr. (1969). *J. Clin. Invest* **48**, 574–583.

Paetkau, V., and Lardy, H. A. (1967). *J. Biol. Chem.* **252**, 2035.

Paetkau, V., Younathan, E. S., and Lardy, H. A. (1968). *J. Mol. Biol.* **33**, 721–736.

Paglia, D. E., and Valentine, W. N. (1970). *J. Lab. Clin. Med.* **76**, 202–212.

Pagliara, A. S., Karl, I. E., Keating, J., Brown, B., and Kipnes, D. M. (1970). *J. Lab. Clin. Med.* **76**, 1020.

Papa, S., Lofrumento, N. E., Loglisci, M., and Quagliarello, E. (1969). *Biochim. Biophys. Acta* **189**, 311–314.

Papa, S., Francavilla, A., Paradies, G., and Henduri, B. (1971). *FEBS Lett.* **12**, 285–288.

Pariza, M. W., Butcher, F. R., Becker, J. E., and Potter, V. R. (1977). *Proc. Natl. Acad. Sci. U.S.A.* **74**, 234–237.

Parrilla, R., Jimenez, I., and Ayuso-Parrilla, M. S. (1975). *Eur. J. Biochem.* **56**, 375–383.

Parrilla, R., Jimenez, I., and Ayuso-Parrilla, M. S. (1976). *Arch. Biochem. Biophys.* **174**, 1–12.

Passoneau, J. V., and Lowry, O. H. (1964). *Adv. Enzyme Regul.* **2**, 265.

Patzett, C., Loffler, G., and Wieland, O. H. (1973). *Eur. J. Biochem.* **33**, 117–127.

Pettit, F. H., Roche, T. E., and Reed, L. J. (1972). *Biochem. Biophys. Res. Commun.* **49**, 563–571.

Pettit, F. H., Pelley, J. W., and Reed, L. J. (1975). *Biochem. Biophys. Res. Commun.* **65**, 575–582.

Pfaff, E., Heldt, H. H., and Klingenberg, M. (1969). *Eur. J. Biochem.* **10**, 484–493.

Pilkis, S. J., Claus, T. H., Johnson, R. A., and Park, C. R. (1975). *J. Biol. Chem.* **250,** 6238–6363.

Pilkis, S. J., Riou, J. P., and Claus, T. H. (1976a). *J. Biol. Chem.* **251,** 7841–7852.

Pilkis, S. J., Claus, T. H., Riou, J. P., and Park, C. R. (1976b). *Metab., Clin. Exp.* **25,** Suppl. 1, 1355–1341.

Pilkis, S. J., Pilkis, J., and Claus, T. H. (1978a). *Biochem. Biophys. Res. Commun.* **81,** 139–146.

Pilkis, S. J., Claus, T. H., Riou, J. P., Cherrington, A. D., Chaisson, J. E., Liljenquist, J. E., Lacy, W. W., and Park, C. R. (1978b). *FEBS Symp.* **42,** 13–29.

Pogell, B. M., and McGilvery, R. W. (1952). *J. Biol. Chem.* **197,** 293–302.

Pogell, B. M., Tanaka, A., and Siddons, R. C. (1968). *J. Biol. Chem.* **243,** 1356–1367.

Pogell, B. M., Taketa, K., and Saingadharan, M. G. (1971). *J. Biol. Chem.* **246,** 1947–1948.

Pogson, C. I. (1968a). *Biochem. J.* **110,** 67–77.

Pogson, C. I. (1968b). *Biochem. Biophys. Res. Commun.* **30,** 297–302.

Pogson, C. I., Longshaw, I. D., and Crisp, D. (1975). *In* "Isozymes" (C. L. Markert, ed.), Vol. 2, pp. 651–665. Academic Press, New York.

Pontremoli, S., and Horecker, B. L. (1971). *In* "The Enzymes" (P. D. Boyer, ed.), 3rd ed., Vol. 4, p. 611. Academic Press, New York.

Pontremoli, S., Luppis, B., Traniello, S., Rippa, M., and Horecker, B. L. (1965). *Arch. Biochem. Biophys.* **112,** 7.

Pontremoli, S., Traniello, S., Ensei, M., Shapiro, S., and Horecker, B. L. (1967). *Proc. Natl. Acad. Sci. U.S.A.* **58,** 286.

Pontremoli, S., Granzi, E., and Accorri, A. (1968). *Biochemistry* **7,** 3628.

Pontremoli, S., Melloni, E., Balestrereo, F., Franzi, A. T., DeFlora, A., and Horecker, B. L. (1973a). *Proc. Natl. Acad. Sci. U.S.A.* **70,** 303–305.

Pontremoli, S., Melloni, E., Solomino, F., Franzi, A. T., DeFlora, A., and Horecker, B. L. (1973b). *Proc. Natl. Acad. Sci. U.S.A.* **70,** 3674.

Pontremoli, S., Melloni, E., DeFlora, A., and Horecker, B. L. (1974). *Arch. Biochem. Biophys.* **163,** 435–441.

Portenhauser, R., Wieland, O. H., and Wenzel, H. (1977). *Hoppe-Seyler's Z. Physiol. Chem.* **358,** 657–658.

Ramaiah, A. (1974). *Curr. Top. Cell. Regul.* **8,** 298–345.

Ramaiah, A., and Tejwani, G. A. (1970). *Biochem. Biophys. Res. Commun.* **39,** 1149.

Rasmussen, H. (1970). *Science* **170,** 404–412.

Reed, L. J., and Oliver, R. M. (1968). *Brookhaven Symp. Biol.* **21,** 397–411.

Reed, L. J., Linn, T. C., Pettit, F. H., Oliver, R. M., Hucho, F., Pelley, J. W., Randall, D. D., and Roche, T. E. (1972a). *In* "Energy Metabolism and the Regulation of Metabolic Processes in Mitochondria" (M. P. Mehlman and R. W. Hanson, eds.), pp. 253–270. Academic Press, New York.

Reed, L. J., Linn, T. C., Hucho, F., Namihira, G., Barrera, C. R., Roche, T. E., Pelley, J. W., and Randall, D. D. (1972b). *In* "Metabolic Interconversion of Enzyme" (O. Wieland, E. Helmreich, and H. Holzen, eds.), pp. 281–293. Springer-Verlag, Berlin and New York.

Reinhart, G. D. (1977). *Fed. Proc., Fed. Am. Soc. Exp. Biol.* **36,** 3095.

Riou, J. P., Claus, T. H., and Pilkis, S. J. (1976). *Biochem. Biophys. Res. Commun.* **73,** 591–599.

Riou, J. P., Claus, T. H., Flockhart, D., Corbin, J., and Pilkis, S. J. (1977). *Proc. Natl. Acad. Sci. U.S.A.* **74,** 4615–4619.

Riou, J. P., Claus, T. H., and Pilkis, S. J. (1978). *J. Biol. Chem.* **253,** 656–659.

Robinson, B. H., and Chappell, J. B. (1967). *Biochem. Biophys. Res. Commun.* **28,** 249–255.

Robison, G. A., Butcher, R. W., and Sutherland, E. W. (1971). "Cyclic AMP." Academic Press, New York.

Rognstad, R. (1975). *Biochem. Biophys. Res. Commun.* **63,** 900–905.

Rognstad, R. (1976). *Int. J. Biochem.* **7,** 403–408.

Rognstad, R. (1977). *Biochem. Biophys. Res. Commun.* **78,** 881–888.

Rognstad, R., and Katz, J. (1970). *Biochem. J.* **116,** 483–491.

Rognstad, R., and Katz, J. (1972). *J. Biol. Chem.* **247,** 6047–6054.

Rognstad, R., and Katz, J. (1976). *Arch. Biochem. Biophys.* **177,** 337–345.

Rognstad, R., and Katz, J. (1977). *J. Biol. Chem.* **252,** 1831–1833.

Rognstad, R., Clark, D. G., and Katz, J. (1973). *Biochem. Biophys. Res. Commun.* **54,** 1149–1156.

Rognstad, R., Wals, P. A., and Katz, J. (1975). *J. Biol. Chem.* **250,** 8642–8647.

Rosen, O. (1966). *Arch. Biochem. Biophys.* **114,** 31.

Rosen, O. M., Rosen, S. M., and Horecker, B. L. (1965). *Arch. Biochem. Biophys.* **112,** 411.

Rosenberg, J. S., Tashima, Y., and Horecker, B. L. (1973). *Arch. Biochem. Biophys.* **154,** 283–293.

Ross, B. D., Hems, R., and Krebs, H. A. (1967a). *Biochem. J.* **102,** 942–951.

Ross, B. D., Hems, R., Freedland, R. A., and Krebs, H. A. (1967b). *Biochem. J.* **105,** 869–875.

Rozengurt, E., Jimenez de Asua, L., and Carminatti, H. (1969). *J. Biol. Chem.* **244,** 3142.

Salas, M., Vinuela, E., Salas, J., and Sols, A. (1964). *Biochem. Biophys. Res. Commun.* **2,** 150–155.

Sasse, D., Katz, N., and Jungermann, K. (1975). *FEBS Lett.* **57,** 83–88.

Schimassek, H., and Mitzkat, H. J. (1963). *Biochem. Z.* **337,** 510–518.

Schimmel, R. J., and Goodman, H. M. (1972). *Biochim. Biophys. Acta* **260,** 153–158.

Schloen, L. H., Kmiotek, E. H., and Sallach, H. J. (1974). *Arch. Biochem. Biophys.* **164,** 254–265.

Schoner, W., Haag, U., and Seubert, W. (1970). *Hoppe-Seyler's Z. Physiol. Chem.* **351,** 1071–1088.

Scrutton, M. C., and Utter, M. F. (1968). *Annu. Rev. Biochem.* **37,** 249–302.

Scrutton, M. C., and White, M. D. (1974). *J. Biol. Chem.* **249,** 5405–5415.

Seubert, W., and Schoner, W. (1971). *Curr. Top. Cell. Regul.* **3,** 237–267.

Seubert, W., Henning, H. V., Schoner, W., and L'Age, M. (1968). *Adv. Enzyme Regul.* **6,** 153–187.

Severson, D. L., Denton, R. M., Bridges, B. J., and Randle, P. J. (1976). *Biochem. J.* **154,** 209–233.

Sherline, P., Lynch, A., and Glinsmann, W. H. (1972). *Endocrinology* **91,** 680–690.

Siddle, K., and Hales, C. N. (1974). *Biochem. J.* **142,** 97–103.

Siess, E. A., and Wieland, O. H. (1975). *FEBS Lett.* **52,** 226–230.

Siess, E. A., and Wieland, O. H. (1976). *Biochem. J.* **156,** 91–102.

Siess, E. A., Brocks, D. G., Lattke, H. K., and Wieland, O. H. (1977). *Biochem. J.* **166,** 225–235.

Snoke, R. E., Johnston, J. B., and Lardy, H. A. (1971). *Eur. J. Biochem.* **24,** 342–346.

Söling, H. D., and Bernhard, G. (1971). *FEBS Lett.* **3,** 271–275.

Söling, H. D., and Bernhard, G. (1976). *Arch. Biochem. Biophys.* **182,** 563–571.

Söling, H. D., and Kleineke, J. (1976). *In* "Gluconeogenesis: Its Regulation in Mammalian Species" (R. W. Hanson and M. A. Mehlman, eds.), pp. 369–462. Wiley, New York.

Söling, H. D., Willms, B., Friedrichs, D., and Kleineke, J. (1968). *Eur. J. Biochem.* **4,** 364–372.

Söling, H. D., Willms, B., Kleineke, J., and Gehlhoff, M. (1970). *Eur. J. Biochem.* **16,** 289–302.

Söling, H. D., Kleineke, J., Willms, B., Janson, G., and Kuhn, A. (1973). *Eur. J. Biochem.* **37,** 233–243.

Start, C., and Newsholme, E. A. (1968). *Biochem. J.* **107,** 411.

Steiner, A. L., Goodman, A. D., and Treble, D. H. (1968). *Am. J. Physiol.* **215,** 211–217.

Stifel, F. B., Taunton, O. D., Greene, H. L., and Herman, R. H. (1974). *J. Biol. Chem.* **249,** 7239–7244.

Struck, E., Ashmore, J., and Wieland, O. (1965). *Biochem. Z.* **343,** 107–110.

Struck, E., Ashmore, J., and Wieland, O. H. (1966). *Adv. Enzyme Regul.* **4,** 219–224.

Stucki, J. W., Brawand, F., and Walter, P. (1972). *Eur. J. Biochem.* **27,** 181–191.

Susor, W. A., and Rutter, W. J. (1968). *Biochem. Biophys. Res. Commun.* **30,** 14.

Taketa, K., and Pogell, B. M. (1963). *Biochem. Biophys. Res. Commun.* **12,** 229–235.

Taketa, K., and Pogell, B. M. (1965). *J. Biol. Chem.* **240,** 651–662.

Taketa, K., Inoue, H., Honjo, K., Taneka, H., and Daikuhara, Y. (1967). *Biochim. Biophys. Acta* **136,** 214–222.

Taketa, K., Sarngadharon, M. G., Watanabe, A., Aoe, H., and Pogell, B. M. (1971). *J. Biol. Chem.* **236,** 5676–5683.

Tanaka, T., Sue, F., and Marimura, H. J. (1965). *Biochem. Biophys. Res. Commun.* **29,** 444.

Tashima, Y., Tholey, G., Drummond, G., Bertrand, H., Rosenberg, J. S., and Horecker, B. L. (1972). *Arch. Biochem. Biophys.* **149,** 118–126.

Taunton, O. D., Stifel, F. B., Greene, H. L., and Herman, R. H. (1972). *Biochem. Biophys. Res. Commun.* **48,** 1663–1670.

Taunton, O. D., Stifel, F. B., Greene, H. L., and Herman, R. H. (1974). *J. Biol. Chem.* **249,** 7228–7239.

Taylor, C. B., and Bailey, E. (1967). *Biochem. J.* **102,** 32c.

Taylor, S. I., Mukherjee, C., and Jungas, R. L. (1975). *J. Biol. Chem.* **250,** 2028–2035.

Tejwani, G. A., Pedrosa, F. O., Pontremoli, S., and Horecker, B. L. (1976a). *Arch. Biochem. Biophys.* **177,** 253–264.

Tejwani, G. A., Pedrosa, F. O., Pontremoli, S., and Horecker, B. L. (1976b). *Proc. Natl. Acad. Sci. U.S.A.* **73,** 2692–2695.

Tews, J. K., Woodcock, N. A., and Harper, A. E. (1970). *J. Biol. Chem.* **245,** 3026–3032.

Tews, J. K., Woodcock, N. A., Colosi, N. W., and Harper, A. E. (1975). *Life Sci.* **16,** 739–750.

Tilghman, S. M., Hanson, R. W., and Ballard, F. J. (1976). *In* "Gluconeogenesis: Its Regulation in Mammalian Species" (R. W. Hanson and M. A. Mehlman, eds.), pp. 47–91. Wiley, New York.

Titanji, V. P. K., Zetterqvist, O., and Engström, L. (1976). *Biochim. Biophys. Acta* **422,** 98–108.

Titheradge, M. A., and Coore, H. G. (1975). *Biochem. J.* **150,** 553–556.

Titheradge, M. A., and Coore, H. G. (1976a). *FEBS Lett.* **63,** 45–50.

Titheradge, M. A., and Coore, H. G. (1976b). *FEBS Lett.* **71,** 73–78.

Titheradge, M. A., Binder, S. B., Wakat, D. K., and Haynes, R. C., Jr. (1978a). *Fed. Proc., Fed. Am. Soc. Exp. Biol.* **37,** 433.

Titheradge, M. A., Binder, S. B., Yamazaki, R. K., and Haynes, R. C., Jr. (1978b). *J. Biol. Chem.* **253,** 3357–3360.

Tolbert, M. E. M., and Fain, J. N. (1974). *J. Biol. Chem.* **249,** 1162–1166.

Tolbert, M. E. M., Butcher, F. R., and Fain, J. N. (1973). *J. Biol. Chem.* **248**, 5686–5692.
Traniello, S. (1974). *Biochim. Biophys. Acta* **341**, 129–137.
Traniello, S., Pontremoli, S., Tashima, Y., and Horecker, B. L. (1971). *Arch. Biochem. Biophys.* **146**, 161–166.
Triebwasser, K. C., and Freedland, R. A. (1977). *Biochem. Biophys. Res. Commun.* **76**, 1159–1165.
Trujillo, J. L., and Deal, W. C. (1977). *Biochemistry* **16**, 3098–3104.
Tsai, M. Y., and Kemp. R. (1973). *J. Biol. Chem.* **248**, 785.
Ui, M., Claus, T. H., Exton, J. H., and Park, C. R. (1973a). *J. Biol. Chem.* **248**, 5344–5349.
Ui, M., Exton, J. H., and Park, C. R. (1973b). *J. Biol. Chem.* **248**, 5350–5359.
Ulm, E. H., Pogell, B. M., DeMaine, M. M., Libley, C. B., and Benkovic, S. J. (1975). *In* "Methods in Enzymology" (W. A. Wood, ed.), Vol. 42, pp. 369–375. Academic Press, New York.
Underwood, A. H., and Newsholme, E. A. (1965a). *Biochem. J.* **95**, 767–774.
Underwood, A. H., and Newsholme, E. A. (1965b). *Biochem. J.* **95**, 868–875.
Utter, M. F., and Kolenbrander, H. M. (1972). *In* "The Enzymes" (P. D. Boyer, ed.), 3rd ed., Vol. 6, pp. 117–168. Academic Press, New York.
Utter, M. F., and Kurahashi, K. (1953). *J. Am. Chem. Soc.* **75**, 758.
Utter, M. F., and Scrutton, M. C. (1969). *Curr. Top. Cell. Regul.* **1**, 253–296.
Utter, M. F., Keech, D. B., and Scrutton, M. C. (1964). *Adv. Enzyme Regul.* **2**, 44–68.
Uyeda, K. (1970). *J. Biol. Chem.* **245**, 2268–2275.
Uyeda, K. (1972). *J. Biol. Chem.* **247**, 1692–1698.
Uyeda, K., and Luby, L. J. (1974). *J. Biol. Chem.* **14**, 4562–4570.
Van Berkel, T. J. C., Koster, J. K., and Hulsmann, W. C. (1973). *Biochim. Biophys. Acta* **293**, 118–124.
Van Berkel, T. J. C., De Jonge, R., Koster, J. F., and Hulsmann, W. C. (1974). *Biochem. Biophys. Res. Commun.* **60**, 398–405.
Van Berkel, T. J. C., Kruit, T. K., Koster, J. F., and Hulsmann, W. C. (1976). *Biochem. Biophys. Res. Commun.* **72**, 917–925.
Van Berkel, T. J. C., Kruijt, J., and Koster, J. (1977a). *Eur. J. Biochem.* **81**, 423–432.
Van Berkel, T. J. C., Kruijt, J., and Koster, J. (1977b). *Biochim. Biophys. Acta* **500**, 267–276.
Van de Werve, G., Hué, L., and Hers, H. G. (1977). *Biochem. J.* **162**, 135–142.
Varadanis, A. (1977). *J. Biol. Chem.* **252**, 807–813.
Veloso, D., Guynn, R. W., Oskarsson, M., and Veech, R. L. (1973). *J. Biol. Chem.* **248**, 4811–4819.
Von Glutz, G., and Walter, P. (1976). *FEBS Lett.* **72**, 299–303.
Wakat, D., and Haynes, R. C., Jr. (1977). *Arch. Biochem. Biophys.* **184**, 561–571.
Walajtys, E. I., Gottesman, D. P., and Williamson, J. R. (1974). *J. Biol. Chem.* **249**, 1857–1865.
Walsh, D. A., and Chen, L.-J. (1971). *Biochem. Biophys. Res. Commun.* **45**, 669–675.
Walsh, D. A., Ashley, C. D., Gonzalez, C., Calkins, D., Fisher, E. H., and Krebs, E. G. (1971). *J. Biol. Chem.* **246**, 1977–1985.
Weber, G. (1969). *Adv. Enzyme Regul.* **7**, 15–40.
Weber, G., Shinghal, R. L., and Srivastava, S. K. (1965). *Adv. Enzyme Regul.* **3**, 43.
Weinhouse, S. (1976). *Curr. Top. Cell. Regul.* **11**, 1–50.
Whitehouse, S., and Randle, P. J. (1973). *Biochem. J.* **134**, 651–653.
Whitehouse, S., Cooper, R. H., and Randle, P. J. (1974). *Biochem. J.* **141**, 761–774.
Wicks, W. D., Lewis, W., and McKibbin, T. B. (1972). *Biochim. Biophys. Acta* **264**, 177–185.

Wieland, O. H. (1969). *Hoppe-Seyler's Z. Physiol. Chem.* **350**, 329–334.

Wieland, O. H., and Siess, E. A. (1970). *Proc. Natl. Acad. Sci. U.S.A.* **65**, 947–954.

Wieland, O. H., and Van Jagow-Westermann, B. (1969). *FEBS Lett.* **3**, 271–274.

Wieland, O. H., Evertz-Prusse, E., and Stukowski, B. (1968). *FEBS Lett.* **2**, 26–28.

Wieland, O. H., Siess, E., Schulze-Wethmar, F. H., von Funcke, H. G., and Winton, B. (1971). *Arch. Biochem. Biophys.* **143**, 593–601.

Wieland, O. H., Patzelt, C., and Loffler, G. (1972a). *Eur. J. Biochem.* **26**, 426–433.

Wieland, O. H., Siess, E. A., von Funcke, H. J., Patzelt, C., Schirmann, A., Loffler, G., and Weiss, L. (1972b). *In* "Metabolic Interconversion of Enzymes" (A. Wieland, E. Helmreich, and H. Holzer, eds.), pp. 293–309. Springer-Verlag, Berlin and New York.

Wieland, O. H., Siess, E. A., Weiss, L., Loffler, G., Patzelt, C., Portenhauser, R., Hartmann, U., and Schirmann, A. (1973). *Symp. Soc. Exp. Biol.* **27**, 371–400.

Williamson, J. R. (1966). *Biochem. J.* **101**, 11c–14c.

Williamson, J. R., Garcia, A., Renold, A. E., and Cahill, G. F., Jr. (1966a). *Diabetes* **15**, 183–187.

Williamson, J. R., Herczeg, B., Coles, H., and Danish, R. (1966b). *Biochem. Biophys. Res. Commun.* **24**, 437–442.

Williamson, J. R., Kreisberg, R. A., and Felts, P. W. (1966c). *Proc. Natl. Acad. Sci. U.S.A.* **56**, 247.

Williamson, J. R., Browning, E. T., and Scholz, R. (1969a). *J. Biol. Chem.* **244**, 4607–4616.

Williamson, J. R., Scholz, R., and Browning, E. T. (1969b). *J. Biol. Chem.* **244**, 4617–4627.

Williamson, J. R., Browning, E. T., Thurman, R. G., and Scholz, R. (1969c). *J. Biol. Chem.* **244**, 5055–5064.

Williamson, J. R., Anderson, J., and Browning, E. T. (1970). *J. Biol. Chem.* **245**, 1717–1726.

Willms, B., Kleineke, T., and Söling, H. D. (1970). *Biochim. Biophys. Acta* **215**, 438–448.

Wimhurst, J. M., and Manchester, K. L. (1970). *Biochem. J.* **120**, 79–93.

Wojtczak, A. B., Enartowicz, E., Rodionova, M. A., and Duszynski, J. (1972). *FEBS Lett.* **28**, 253–258.

Yamazaki, R. K. (1975). *J. Biol. Chem.* **250**, 7924–7930.

Yamazaki, R. K., and Haynes, R. C., Jr. (1975). *Arch. Biochem. Biophys.* **166**, 575–583.

Yamazaki, R. K., Sax, R. D., and Graetz, G. S. (1977a). *Arch. Biochem. Biophys.* **178**, 19–25.

Yamazaki, R. K., Sax, R. D., and Hauser, M. A. (1977b). *FEBS Lett.* **75**, 295–299.

Zahlten, R. N., Hachberg, A. A., Stratman, F. W., and Lardy, H. A. (1972). *Proc. Natl. Acad. Sci. U.S.A.* **69**, 800–804.

Zahlten, R. N., Stratman, F. W., and Lardy, H. A. (1973). *Proc. Natl. Acad. Sci. U.S.A.* **70**, 3213.

Zalitis, J. (1976). *Biochem. Biophys. Res. Commun.* **70**, 323–330.

Zetterqvist, O., Rognaisson, U., Humble, E., Berglund, L., and Engström, L. (1976). *Biochem. Biophys. Res. Commun.* **70**, 696–703.

Gonadotropin Receptors and Regulation of Steroidogenesis in the Testis and Ovary

MARIA L. DUFAU AND KEVIN J. CATT

Endocrinology and Reproduction Research Branch, National Institute of Child Health and Human Development, National Institutes of Health, Bethesda, Maryland

I. Introduction

The regulation of testicular and ovarian function by gonadotropic hormones is mediated by specific, high-affinity receptors that are located in the plasma membrane of the respective target cells. The receptor sites for luteinizing hormone (LH) and follicle-stimulating hormone (FSH) in testis and ovary have been identified and characterized by *in vivo* and *in vitro* binding studies with various labeled forms of the hormones, most commonly the radioactive derivatives formed by radioiodination or tritiation of highly purified gonadotropin preparations. Similarly, receptors for prolactin have been demonstrated in the mammary gland and the gonads, as well as in a variety of less obvious target tissues including liver, adrenal, and male accessory organs. In each of these target tissues, the binding sites identified with radioactive hormones have been shown to possess the characteristics of receptors for the labeled ligands, i.e., specificity, high affinity, saturability, and temperature-dependent kinetics. In the case of gonadotropins, coupling between hormone binding and an appropriate cellular response, such as cyclic AMP (cAMP, adenosine 3′,5′-monophosphate) formation and testosterone biosynthesis, has also been demonstrated. Thus, there is little reason to doubt that the sites detected by labeled hormones are those responsible for mediating the biological actions of the gonadotropins on their target cells. The situation for prolactin receptors is less completely studied, since the early cellular response to prolactin has yet to be clarified in most target tissues, but the binding sites identified with the labeled hormone almost certainly correspond to the receptors through which prolactin exerts its varied biological actions.

A common feature of receptors for gonadotropins and other protein hormones is their extremely high affinity for the respective ligands, with association constants of about $10^{10} M^{-1}$. Such high binding constants are commensurate with the relatively low concentrations of gonadotropins in plasma, usually only a few nanograms per milliliter. These values are equivalent to molar concentrations of about $10^{-11} M$ and emphasize the extreme specificity of receptor sites that can selectively bind the appropriate hormones in the presence of a millionfold excess of other proteins in the extracellular fluid. For localization and binding studies on the gonadal receptors for LH, labeled human chorionic gonadotropin (hCG) has been more frequently employed than labeled LH. The placental gonadotropin is more readily available in highly purified form and exhibits higher stability and binding activity after labeling with radioactive iodine. The biological properties of hCG appear to be almost identical with those of LH, and the two glycoprotein hormones bind to the same receptor sites in the testis and ovary. Therefore, receptor sites identified by binding studies with labeled hCG will be referred to as LH or LH/hCG receptors.

The initial demonstration of gonadotropin receptors in the rat testis and ovary by isotopic tracer methods was performed by *in vivo* localization of radioiodinated LH or hCG upon the LH receptor sites. In these studies, administration of the labeled hormone was followed by autoradiographic localization of the radioactive tracer at the expected target cells (Lunenfeld and Eshkol, 1967; Espeland *et al.*, 1968; De-Kretser *et al.*, 1969, 1971). These included the Leydig cells of the testis and the corpus luteum of the ovary. Morphological analysis of gonadotropin uptake in the testis was also performed by immunohistochemical and ferritin-labeling approaches, which gave evidence for the *in vivo* uptake of LH and FSH in Leydig and Sertoli cells, respectively (Mancini *et al.*, 1967; Castro *et al.*, 1972). More recent morphological studies employing topical autoradiography have shown that LH receptors of the rat ovary are present in the interstitial tissue and theca cells of the developing follicle, and that LH receptors also begin to appear in granulosa cells at the time of antrum formation (Midgley, 1973). In contrast with the ovary, LH/hCG receptors in the testis are confined to a single cell type, being demonstrable only in the Leydig cells. In the adult rat, no binding of labeled hCG to seminiferous tubules can be detected when the tubule preparation has been adequately freed of interstitial cells. It is of interest to note that the development of LH receptors in the fetal testis occurs at an extremely early stage of embryonic life. Thus, specific gonadotropin binding sites for LH/hCG appear in the fetal rabbit testis on about day 18 of development, concomitant with the morphological and biochemical maturation of the Leydig cell (Catt *et al.*, 1975a).

The morphological evidence for the existence of gonadotropin receptor sites in the gonads has been complemented by a considerable body of *in vitro* data demonstrating that specific hormone binding sites are present in slices, cell suspensions, and homogenates of the testis and ovary. By such methods, LH receptors have been demonstrated in the testes of rat, mouse, rabbit, pig, ram, and bull and in the corpus luteum of the rat, mouse, pig, cow, rhesus, and human ovary. *In vitro* binding studies have commonly been performed upon homogenates of the whole gonad, an approach that appears to be satisfactory for the initial characterization of receptor sites and for the development of radioligand-receptor assays. For preparation of more homogeneous particulate receptors in cell fractions, fragmented interstitial cells and membrane preparations from homogenates of testis and corpus luteum have been employed. The structure of the rat testis permits extensive dissection of the tubule and interstitial elements, and simply teasing apart the seminiferous tubules causes the release of large numbers of intact and fragmented Leydig cells. The interstitial cell particles obtained by this procedure are rich in plasma membrane and provide a convenient source of LH receptors for binding studies and solubilization procedures (Catt *et al.*, 1971, 1972a,b; Dufau and Catt, 1973; Dufau *et al.*, 1973a). The testes of certain other species, notably the pig, contain a much higher proportion of Leydig cells than the rat testis, and are of potential value for large-scale preparation of receptor sites (Catt *et al.*, 1974). However, the ability to obtain a relatively membrane-rich preparation of fragmented Leydig cells from the rat testis has made this tissue particularly useful for studies on the LH receptor. During characterization of ovarian LH receptors, although corpora lutea from livestock such as the cow or pig have the advantages of size and homogeneity (Gospodarowicz, 1973; Rao, 1974), many studies have been carried out on the rat ovary, most frequently utilizing the heavily luteinized gonads of immature female rats which have been pretreated with pregnant mare serum gonadotropins (PMSG) and hCG (Lee and Ryan, 1971, 1972, 1973). Quantitative analysis of LH/hCG binding sites has also been performed in isolated target cells, an approach that permits comparisons of receptor occupancy with the subsequent rate and extent of hormone-dependent cell responses (Catt *et al.*, 1973a,b; Channing and Kammerman, 1974; Mendelson *et al.*, 1975a).

The demonstration of receptor sites for FSH in the testis and ovary has been performed by binding studies with tritiated or, more commonly, radioiodinated human FSH (Means and Vaitukaitis, 1972; Schwartz *et al.*, 1973; Reichert and Bhalla, 1974; Ketelslegers and

Catt, 1974). In the immature rat testis FSH, receptors are confined to the seminiferous tubule and are probably localized exclusively in the Sertoli cells (Means and Huckins, 1974; Desjardins *et al.*, 1974). The ovarian receptors for FSH are situated upon the granulosa cells (Midgley, 1973), an appropriate location to mediate the characteristic actions of FSH on follicular growth and maturation. This location is also analogous to the distribution of FSH receptors in the testis, since the granulosa cells are functionally similar to the Sertoli cells in maintaining the developing germ cells. In the rat, FSH receptors have been demonstrated in the granulosa cells of small follicles, prior to the development of LH receptors, and treatment with FSH has been followed by the induction of LH receptors in the maturing granulosa cells (Zeleznik *et al.*, 1974).

II. Characteristics of Receptors for Gonadotropins and Prolactin

As noted above, the binding sites demonstrated by studies with radioiodinated gonadotropins and prolactin have displayed many of the properties that should be present in the biologically important receptor sites for an active hormonal ligand. These include high affinity and structural specificity for the ligand, saturability and limited binding capacity, and functional coupling of the binding process to a characteristic target-cell response. In addition, the concentration of the respective receptor sites in target tissues has been shown to change in an appropriate fashion with the functional state of the gonad, and with the sex, species, and degree of maturation of the animal host.

A. Gonadal Receptors for Luteinizing Hormone (LH) and Human Chorionic Gonadotropin (hCG)

The location of LH receptors in the plasma membrane of the Leydig cell of the testis and the luteinized cells of the corpus luteum has been shown by density-gradient centrifugation followed by electron microscopy (EM) and marker enzyme studies (Catt *et al.*, 1972a, 1974; Rajaniemi and Vanha-Perttula, 1972, 1973; Gospodarowicz, 1973; Rajaniemi *et al.*, 1974) and also by EM-autoradiography (Han *et al.*, 1974). The distribution of LH receptors on the surface of the Leydig cell has also been demonstrated by an indirect immunofluorescence procedure, after saturation of the sites with hCG and sequential incubation with rabbit antiserum to hCG and fluorescein-conjugated goat antiserum to rabbit γ-globulin (Hsueh et al., 1976a). Other evidence for the surface location of LH receptors has been provided by the biological activity of agarose-bound LH (Dufau et al., 1971a), by the ability to elute bound gonadotropin from the testis at low pH (Dufau et al., 1972c), and by the action of trypsin upon binding of labeled hCG to intact Leydig cells (Catt et al., 1974). The association between LH or hCG and the receptor site shows marked temperature dependence and proceeds more rapidly at 37°C than at lower temperatures. However, many binding studies with labeled LH or hCG have been performed at 20°–24°C, to minimize the effects of degradation of hormone and/or receptors upon the binding reaction. The rate of the interaction between receptor sites and hormone is also concentration dependent, and follows the expected kinetics of a second-order reaction until excess hormone is present, when the reaction becomes pseudo-first-order (Ketelslegers et al., 1975). The binding characteristics of gonadotropin receptors in isolated intact Leydig cells have been found to be identical with those determined in testis homogenates and interstitial cell membranes, and about 15,000 receptors per Leydig cell have been measured by quantitative binding studies with labeled hCG. The equilibrium binding constant of the LH receptor is $4 \times 10^{10} M^{-1}$, and a single class of receptors with no interaction between sites has been indicated by the consistent derivation of linear Scatchard plots, and Hill plots with a slope of 1.0. The rate of dissociation of bound hormone from gonadotropin receptors is quite slow, particularly at lower temperatures. The half-life of the hormone–receptor complex is about 24 hours at 24°C, and the dissociation reaction proceeds even more slowly at 4°C. This property of the gonadotropin-receptor sites has been of considerable value during solubilization and physical characterization of the receptors. The slow dissociation of the LH receptor–hormone complex has made it possible to analyze the soluble complex by relatively lengthy fractionation procedures, including gel filtration and density-gradient centrifugation. The applications of LH/hCG receptors to radioligand-receptor assay and to structural studies on the binding properties of native and modified gonadotropins and subunits are described below (Sections III and IV).

B. GONADAL RECEPTORS FOR FOLLICLE-STIMULATING HORMONE (FSH)

Until recently, relatively few studies have been performed upon the FSH receptors, and these were mainly of the type designed to analyze the changes in FSH receptors that occur in the ovary during functional changes (Midgley, 1973) or hormonal treatment (Goldenberg et al., 1972). An important finding from such studies has been the stimulating effect of estrogen upon FSH receptors in the granulosa cells of the immature rat ovary. In the testis, FSH receptors have been demonstrated in plasma membrane fractions from the seminiferous tubule (Means and Vaitukaitis, 1972) and are predominantly concentrated upon the Sertoli cells (Means and Huckins, 1974). The binding of labeled FSH to homogenates of testes from immature rats with tubules comprised almost entirely of Sertoli cells (produced by irradiation during fetal life) is similar in magnitude to that observed in testes of normal immature rats (Means and Huckins, 1974). The interactions between FSH and testis receptors have been studied in both immature and adult rats (Means and Vaitukaitis, 1972; Reichert and Bhalla, 1974; Schwartz et al., 1973; Ketelslegers and Catt, 1974; Means and Huckins, 1974). The kinetic and equilibrium properties of the FSH receptors are generally similar to those of the LH receptor, with the exception that the association constant (K_a) is almost an order of magnitude lower than that of the LH/hCG receptor. In consequence, the binding of labeled FSH to testicular receptor sites is usually considerably lower than observed for hCG, a feature that is magnified by the greater susceptibility of FSH to loss of biological activity during the iodination procedure. However, in the calf testis, the binding affinity of FSH receptors analyzed in membrane-enriched fractions was found to be higher than in rat testis, with K_a of $10^{10} M^{-1}$ (Cheng, 1975a).

For quantitative studies on FSH binding sites, the preparation of tracer hormone should preferably be performed by the lactoperoxidase method to minimize labeling damage. In our experience, purification of the tracer is most effectively performed by group-specific chromatography on Sepharose–concanavalin A (Dufau et al., 1972a) followed by receptor-affinity purification of the labeled FSH (Ketelslegers and Catt, 1974). The latter can be achieved by adsorption of the active hormone to particulate testis receptors, with elution of the selectively bound active hormone by heat or exposure to low pH. Such tracer displays markedly enhanced binding to FSH receptors in testis homogenates, up to 50% of the total added hormone being bound by an excess of receptor sites. This degree of binding is important for the purification and quantitation of solubilized FSH receptor sites, which cannot be adequately monitored by binding assays performed with tracer FSH that shows only a few percent of specific binding to particulate receptors.

C. Prolactin Receptors

The presence of binding sites with high specificity and affinity for prolactin and other lactogenic hormones has been demonstrated in many tissues—mammary gland, liver, kidney, adrenal, testis, and male accessory organs (Posner *et al.*, 1974a). The distribution of prolactin receptors shows species variations and differs quite markedly between the sexes, as well as with age and hormonal status. Analysis of the binding properties of prolactin receptors has shown considerable overlap with the behavior of growth hormone receptors, in particular with that of human growth hormone (hGH). It now appears clear that specific receptors for lactogenic hormones and growth hormone can be distinguished in liver, and that human growth hormone reacts with each of these sites (Posner, 1976a). In addition, a specific receptor for hGH is present in human cells, at least in liver and cultured lymphocytes, and this site does not interact with other growth hormones or prolactin (Lesniak *et al.*, 1973; Carr and Friesen, 1976). Thus, hGH can bind to three distinct sets of receptors, and this is consistent with its actions on lactation and on growth in animals and man. The selectivity of the hGH receptor is consistent with the weak or absent activities of animal somatotropin and lactogenic hormones in man and with the low growth activity of human placental lactogen. The prolactin receptors have been most thoroughly studied in liver, though their function in this tissue remains unknown. The location of the prolactin receptors is predominantly at the plasma membrane (Shiu and Friesen, 1974), but intracellular sites have also been demonstrated and appear to reside in the Golgi apparatus (Nolin and Witorsch, 1976). Whether this reflects the biosynthesis of receptors, or the turnover and endocytotic processing of membrane receptors, has yet to be established.

Although quite marked differences in the specificity of lactogen and GH receptors have been noted, the affinities of the various tissue receptors are quite similar (about $10^9 M^{-1}$), and each appears to consist of a single order of binding sites. Whereas the GH receptor in human tissues is specific for hGH, the lactogen receptors in rodent or rabbit livers bind prolactins, placental lactogens, and primate growth hormones, but do not react with nonprimate growth hormones. Conversely, the GH receptors in nonprimate liver bind GH from many species, but not prolactins and placental lactogens. Binding studies on prolactin receptors were originally performed with labeled prolactin, usually ovine prolactin labeled with ^{125}I and purified by gel filtration or ion-exchange chromatography. However, the greater stability of [125I]hGH has led to the use of this tracer to identify and analyze "lactogenic" receptors in a wide variety of tissues. However, it should be recognized that labeled hGH will also bind to "growth hormone" receptors in certain tissues, such as liver, and the contributions of the two sites to hGH binding should be recognized and quantitated by appropriate binding-inhibition studies.

III. Techniques for Gonadotropin Receptor Analysis

A. Preparation and Characterization of Labeled Hormones

1. Radioiodination of Gonadotropins

Although the chloramine-T method for radioiodination of proteins has been applied to the preparation of labeled hLH and hCG for receptor-binding studies and radioligand-receptor assays, this procedure is less satisfactory for iodination of FSH and LH preparations. A more generally satisfactory procedure for preparation of labeled gonadotropins for binding studies is based upon the lactoperoxidase method for radioiodination of proteins (Marchalonis, 1969; Thorell and Johansson, 1971). This labeling procedure can be applied with advantage to hFSH and prolactin, as well as to LH and hCG (Catt et al., 1976). It usually results in a higher proportion of biologically active molecules in the tracer preparation, due to less extensive oxidation of the peptide or glycoprotein hormone. However, relatively little difference in the receptor-binding properties of the more stable glycoprotein hormones, such as hCG, can be detected after labeling by either procedure.

2. Purification of Radioiodinated Hormones

After labeling of peptide or glycoprotein hormones by either method of radioiodination, the radioactive hormone can be isolated from the reaction mixture by a number of purification procedures. Gel filtration of the iodination mixture on Sephadex G-50 provides an adequate separation of labeled protein from free iodine, but does not always resolve "damaged" hormone from the intact labeled molecules. If gel filtration is performed, the most effective fractionation of the labeled tracer is achieved by chromatography on a 100-cm column of Sephadex G-100 or BioGel P60. Adsorption and elution performed on cellulose powder has also been applied to purification of tracer hormone, with partial separation of labeled hormone from components damaged during the iodination procedure (Catt et al., 1971). A more selective method for purification of radioiodinated glycoprotein hormones has been based upon the use of concanavalin A coupled to agarose beads, to achieve group-specific affinity chromatography of glycoprotein hormones. During this separation technique, the labeled glycoprotein is bound to a small column of Sepharose–concanavalin A, while free iodide, damaged components, and nonglycoproteins pass freely through the gel bed (Dufau et al., 1972a). After the gel has been washed with carbohydrate-free buffer, the labeled glycoprotein is eluted by a solution of 0.2 M glucopyranoside or mannopyranoside (Fig. 1). This procedure is less rapid than gel filtration or cellulose adsorption-elution, but provides tracer hormone that exhibits high binding activity and low nonspecific binding to gonadal receptor preparations. The combination of lactoperoxidase radioiodination and chromatographic purification on DEAE-cellulose for prolactin (Frantz and Turkington, 1972) or on Sepharose–concanavalin A for LH, hCG, and FSH (Dufau *et al.*, 1972a; Ketelslegers and Catt, 1974; Dufau and Catt, 1976a) provides a highly effective procedure for the preparation of labeled gonadotropic hormones for receptor-binding studies.

The most highly selective procedure for purification of labeled gonadotropic hormones is based upon the finding that tracer hormone bound to gonadal receptor sites displays high biological activity after elution by appropriate techniques (Dufau *et al.*, 1972c; Ketelslegers and Catt, 1974). The dissociation of bound active hormone from receptor sites can be achieved by reduction of pH, or elevation of temperature, both of which elute the receptor-bound molecules with minimal release of nonspecifically bound material. The ability of receptors to combine with the most biologically active labeled molecules can be

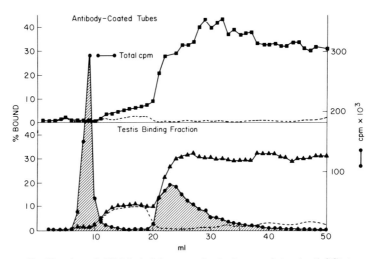

FIG. 1. Purification of ^{125}I-labeled human chorionic gonadotropin (hCG) tracer. The elution profile from an agarose–concanavalin A column is expressed in counts per minute (●——●). Two radioactive peaks are shown: at fractions 6–11 and at fractions 20–30. The binding of tracer from each fraction to plastic tubes coated with antihuman chorionic gonadotropin serum is shown above (■——■), and binding to rat testis receptors is shown below (▲——▲). Displacement of binding to the solid-phase antibody or to the rat testis binding fraction in the presence of excess hCG (100 IU) is shown above and below by the dashed line (----).

utilized to extract the active species from radioiodinated hormone preparations containing a mixture of native and inactivated gonadotropin molecules. This method has been applied to purification of ^{125}I-labeled hCG and hFSH tracers prepared by the lactoperoxidase method, and yields radioactive hormones with considerably enhanced binding activity and biological activity (Catt *et al.*, 1976). It is particularly useful when the tracer preparation shown an unacceptably low level of specific binding, as frequently seen with radioiodinated FSH. For hormones such as human LH and hCG, which usually show maximum binding activities of 40 to 75%, further purification by receptor affinity chromatography is not usually necessary.

3. *Measurement of Specific Activity*

The determination of specific activity for tracer hormones used in receptor analysis should preferably be performed by bioassay or radioligand-receptor assay of the labeled hormone. The relatively imprecise calculations of specific activity which have been applied to tracers for radioimmunoassay are not adequate for the characterization of labeled hormones to be employed for quantitative binding studies. Measurement of tracer specific activity can also be performed by the "self-displacement" method in a specific radioimmunoassay, but the values obtained in this manner may not be valid in terms of the biological activity of the labeled hormone.

The most convenient and valid method to measure specific activity of labeled gonadotropins for receptor-binding studies is by self-displacement assay of increasing concentrations of the tracer in the radioligand-receptor assay. In this way, the single isotopically labeled hormone can be employed both as "tracer" and "sample" during radioreceptor assay against standards of the original unlabeled hormone. Parallel dose-response curves are obtained for binding-inhibition by the labeled and unlabeled hormones, and accurate calculation of specific activity can be performed in terms of the native hormone employed for iodination.

The specific activity of radioactive tracer gonadotropins can also be determined by bioassay, provided that a sufficiently sensitive and specific method is available. The most convenient and precise bioassay procedures are provided by *in vitro* methods that employ the steroidogenic response of testicular or ovarian cells to gonadotropic stimulation. Such methods are comparable to radioimmunoassay in terms of sensitivity and are extremely useful for measurement of the biological activity of gonadotropins that stimulate steroidogenesis in gonadal target cells (Catt *et al.*, 1976).

4. *Determination of Receptor-Binding Activity*

Each labeled hormone preparation should be subjected to binding assay in the presence of excess receptor sites, to determine the proportion of radioactivity that represents "active" hormone with the capacity to interact with specific receptor sites. This value represents the content of biologically active hormone in the labeled preparation and provides an important correction factor for use during calculation of receptor-binding constants. Thus, if 60% of the tracer is bound to excess receptors, the remaining 40% of the total radioactivity will be present as inactive tracer in the "free" fraction. The presence of inactive labeled material in radioactive hormone preparations requires that both bound and free hormone concentrations should be corrected accordingly during analysis of quantitative binding data, as described in the following section.

B. DETERMINATION OF BINDING CONSTANTS AND RECEPTOR CONCENTRATION

For optimal determination of the binding constants of the hormone-receptor interaction, the tracer preparations should be adequately characterized in terms of their specific activity and maximum binding activity. The specific activity of labeled gonadotropin, measured in a bioassay or in a radioligand-receptor assay, is an expression of the radioactivity corresponding to a given amount of biologically active hormone. This value can be used to calculate the total concentration of tracer hormone added to the incubation media during receptor studies. However, if the maximum binding activity of the tracer is less than 100%, only the "bindable" fraction of the total radioactivity will correspond to the bioactive hormone. It has been shown that the radioactive hormone specifically bound to the receptor preparation represents only intact, biologically active gonadotropin. Therefore, the values for specific activity that are used to compute the bound hormone concentrations should be divided by the fraction of the tracer preparation that corresponds to the active labeled molecules. This correction factor is determined by measurement of the proportion of the tracer hormone that is bound by an excess of receptor sites. Failure to apply this correction will lead to underestimation of the bound-hormone concentrations, and overestimation of the free-hormone concentrations if these are calculated by subtracting bound from total hormone.

For example, if 100,000 cpm of labeled hormone corresponds to 1 ng of unlabeled hormone in the radioligand-receptor assay, the uncorrected specific activity is 100,000 cpm/ng. However, if the maximum binding activity of the labeled preparation is 50%, the correct specific activity of the *biologically active* tracer is 50,000 cpm/ng, not 100,000 cpm/ng, since 50% of the radioactivity represents inert material. Then, specific uptake of 20,000 cpm from a total tracer dose of 100,000 cpm corresponds to 0.4 ng of bound (B) hCG, and 0.6 ng of free (F) hCG, with B/F ratio of 0.67. If the maximum binding activity of the labeled hormone preparation is not taken into account, it would be erroneously concluded that only 0.2 ng of hormone was bound, and that 0.8 ng was free, with B/F ratio of 0.25. The use of a correction factor for maximum binding activity provides a more realistic estimate of the true binding constants of peptide hormone receptors. It is important to note that the measurement of maximum binding activity of the tracer hormone should be performed under conditions that minimize or avoid the additional complication of tracer degradation during incubation with the particulate receptor preparation employed for binding studies.

A further correction is necessary when molar concentrations of hormones are computed in binding studies, because the highly purified gonadotropins used for labeling and binding analysis are rarely of maximum attainable bioactivity. When the specific activities of labeled gonadotropins are expressed in terms of such preparations, calculations of the molar hormone concentration should be corrected for their theoretical maximum bioactivity. In practice these are usually not known with great accuracy, since they depend upon the currently best available estimates of the biological potency of the purified hormone. For hCG, we have taken the value of 15,000 IU/mg, as a reasonable approximation to the "true" biological activity of pure hCG, when converting to molar concentrations of the hormone.

Detailed accounts of the mathematical and statistical aspects of the analysis of receptor–hormone interactions, affinity constants, and kinetic parameters have been described elsewhere (Rodbard, 1973; Ketelslegers *et al.*, 1975; Catt *et al.*, 1976). In general, adequate derivations of equilibrium binding constants for gonadotropins and other protein or glycoprotein hormones can be performed by direct analysis of binding curves or by Scatchard analysis. In practice, such analyses are frequently performed on data derived originally from binding-inhibition studies, with subsequent conversion to saturation curves or Scatchard plots. These approaches are based on the assumption that the labeled and unlabeled hormones behave identically, and are present in homogeneous form. Although Scatchard plots provide a convenient graphical picture and simplified calculation of binding constants and receptor concentrations, direct analysis of the saturation curve by curve-fitting has the advantage of avoiding errors introduced by transforming the binding data to forms suitable for linear regression analysis. For this reason we have preferred to employ curve-fitting by the use of computer analysis of binding data according to the appropriate equations for a saturation curve (Ketelslegers *et al.*, 1975). The derivation of rate constants is usually performed by nonlinear curve-fitting of data from kinetic studies with tracer hormone, employing the second-order rate equation for association constants and the first-order rate equation for dissociation constants. There are very few published reports of rigorously validated binding constants for peptide hormone receptors. In most cases the analyses have been performed over a limited range of conditions, and corrections for tracer hormone activity and degradation of hormone and receptors are rarely applied. The difficulty of correcting for the numerous variables involved in peptide hormone-receptor interactions is clearly responsible for the range of binding constants reported in the literature and for the paucity of thermodynamic data in this area. Despite this, there is reasonably close agreement on the apparent binding constants for gonadotropins and prolactin, and experimental variations probably account for the disparities sometimes seen between results obtained in different laboratories. A feature of many gonadotropin–receptor interactions, particularly those of the LH/hCG receptors, is the very slow dissociation rate observed at reduced temperatures. Thus, at 24°C the dissociation of bound hCG occurs over several days, and the reaction is effectively irreversible over shorter time periods. This feature of the LH receptors has been of value in the fractionation and solubilization of receptor sites, since the complex remains intact for long periods at the low temperatures employed for protein fractionation.

IV. RADIOLIGAND-RECEPTOR ASSAYS

The measurement of FSH, LH, hCG and prolactin in plasma by radioimmunoassay has become a routine procedure in the diagnosis and management of endocrine disorders and in physiological investigations. In comparative studies, differences in the immunological and biological potency of gonadotropins have sometimes been noted, and the species specificity of most radioimmunoassays indicates that the antigenic site is not usually identical with the biologically active site. However, the demonstration that occasional gonadotropin antisera show wide species crossreactivity and the development of several heterologous radioimmunoassay systems have indicated that the species specificity of antibodies to gonadotropins is sometimes less absolute than previously believed. Despite the several advantages of radioimmunoassay, there has remained a need for highly sensitive assays that give a measure of the biological activity of peptide hormones. Conventional bioassays provide valuable information about the potency of gonadotropin preparations in the whole animal, but are of relatively low sensitivity and precision in comparison to radioimmunoassay. Recently, the introduction of radioligand-receptor assays for peptide hormones has begun to bridge the gap between radioimmunoassay and the traditional *in vivo* bioassays. In addition, this approach has been extended by the development of highly sensitive *in vitro* bioassays that employ isolated target cells or tissues to quantitate the biological response to nanogram levels of the hormonal ligand.

The specific high-affinity binding sites in homogenates of rat testis and ovary provide an abundant source of material for radioligand-receptor assays of LH, hCG, and FSH. Such receptor assays combine the high precision, reproducibility, and convenience of radioligand assay with the biological specificity of conventional bioassays performed in the intact animal. The sensitivity of radioligand-receptor assays for gonadotropins is somewhat less than that of radioimmunoassays, but is very much higher than that of *in vivo* bioassays. For these reasons, radioreceptor procedures are particularly useful for assay of gonadotropin preparations and of fractions derived during purification and isolation of pituitary and chorionic gonadotropins. Such methods are also of considerable value for structure–function studies on the interactions of chemically modified gonadotropins and derivatives with hormone-receptor sites *in vitro*.

A. RADIOLIGAND-RECEPTOR ASSAYS FOR LH AND hCG

The radioligand-receptor assay for LH and hCG is most simply established by the use of rat testis homogenate and [^{125}I]hCG as the binding system, with standards appropriate for the gonadotropin to be assayed (Catt *et al.*, 1971, 1972a; 1976; Leidenberger and Reichert, 1972). Human LH, both pituitary and urinary preparations, hCG, and primate gonadotropins give parallel binding-inhibition curves in the rat testis [^{125}I]hCG assay. LH from other species, including rat, rabbit, pig, cow, and sheep, and the equine pregnancy gonadotropin PMSG, give less steep assay slopes than those of the human hormones (Fig. 2).

For binding assays, the conditions of incubation can be chosen according to the sensitivity desired in the assay system. In the simplest assay, incubation of the 1500 g sediment of adult rat testis homogenate

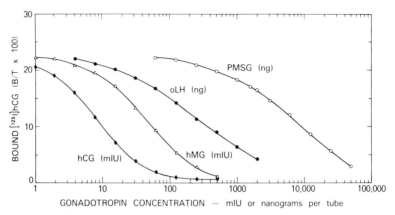

FIG. 2. Radioligand-receptor assay of the Second International Standard human chorionic gonadotropin (hCG), the Second International Reference Preparation for Human Menopausal Gonadotropin (hMG), ovine luteinizing hormone (oLH) (NIH S18), and pregnant mare serum gonadotropin (PMSG).

(equivalent to 1/50 testis) with [^{125}I]hCG (50,000 cpm) is performed in a volume of 1 ml at 24°C for 16 hours, followed by centrifugation and determination of the particle-bound radioactivity by gamma counting. When the incubation is performed in a volume of 1 ml, the effective sensitivity of the assay is 0.5–1 ng of hCG per tube, and the dose for 50% inhibition of binding is about 10 ng of hCG. For higher sensitivity, smaller aliquots of testis homogenate (equivalent to 1/100 testis) are incubated in a total volume of 0.25 ml. For the assay, 100 μl of testis homogenate is incubated with 100 μl of gonadotropin standards (e.g., 0.1–20 ng hCG) or the samples to be assayed, in Dulbecco's phosphate buffer saline–bovine serum albumin (PBS–BSA) (1 mg/ml), and 50 μl of [^{125}I]hCG tracer (50,000 cpm) in PBS–BSA containing 0.05% Neomycin sulfate.

Nonspecific binding is determined in the presence of 100 IU (10 μg) of hCG per assay tube. After mixing and incubation at room temperature for 16 hours, 3 ml of ice-cold PBS are added to each tube and the diluted receptor suspension is either filtered or centrifuged at 1500 g for 20 minutes to isolate the receptor-bound radioactive hormone. If more rapid assays are to be performed, incubation at 37°C for 1–3 hours is sufficient to achieve adequate binding and satisfactory displacement curves. The detection limit of the assay is then about 50 pg of hCG, and the dose level for 50% binding-inhibition is less than 1 ng of hCG. For small numbers of assay tubes, particularly if kinetic studies are to be performed, filtration through albumin-soaked 0.45 μm

Millipore cellulose filters can be employed. Potency estimates can be derived with high precision by computer programs for analysis of parallel-line bioassay data.

It is also possible to perform binding assays with the total particulate fraction sedimented by centrifugation of the testis homogenate at 20,000 g. After overnight incubation, the whole of the 20,000 g aliquot used for binding assay can be recovered by filtration, or more simply by centrifugation at 1500 g. The latter step is effective in sedimenting all the binding particles originally obtained by centrifugation at 20,000 g, since aggregation of the smaller particles occurs during prolonged incubation and the particulate binding sites can then be completely recovered in the 1500-g pellet. When the total testis homogenate is employed for radioligand-receptor binding assays, as little as 1 mg of the homogenate can be used per assay tube, giving initial binding of about 20% of the added tracer hormone. The effective sensitivity of the latter forms of the assay approaches that of radioimmunoassay, but the method cannot be applied to direct assay of low plasma gonadotropin levels, due to nonspecific interference by plasma proteins. However, it is possible to use the radioligand-receptor assay for the measurement of LH peaks and hCG in pregnancy plasma when concentrations of the hormone exceed a few nanograms per milliliter, affording a 1 : 10 dilution of unextracted plasma.

Although radioligand-receptor assay of LH and hCG can also be performed with homogenates of luteinized ovaries from PMS/hCG-treated rats (Lee and Ryan, 1975a) or bovine corpora lutea (Saxena, 1976) the original method based upon rat testis homogenate provides a simple and convenient form of the assay for general use. No pretreatment of the animals is required, and the binding particles obtained from one adult rat are adequate for about 200–500 assay tubes. The specificity and sensitivity of binding assays performed with testicular or ovarian homogenates are similar, and the methods are equally applicable to measurement of a wide variety of LH and chorionic gonadotropin preparations. Satisfactory binding of ^{125}I-labeled LH or hCG can also be obtained with homogenates of testes from other species (pig, mouse, etc.). However, the rat testis provides an abundant source of LH/hCG receptors for radioligand assay, and the isolated testis or prepared testis homogenate can be stored frozen with adequate retention of binding activity. The extent of hormone binding is highest when fresh testis homogenates are employed, but satisfactory assays can be performed with homogenates of rat testes obtained from bulk suppliers and stored frozen at −60°C. Storage of frozen testis at −15°C is accompanied by a more significant loss of binding activity over a period of several months. Once prepared, testis homogenates can be stored on ice for several days with little change in binding activity.

B. RADIOLIGAND-RECEPTOR ASSAY FOR FSH

There is now general agreement that FSH interacts primarily with the Sertoli cells of the seminiferous tubules. Particulate receptor fractions for FSH binding studies and radioassay can be prepared from homogenates of the testes from immature or adult rats (Schwartz et al., 1973; Reichert and Bhalla, 1974; Ketelslegers and Catt, 1974) and calves (Cheng, 1975a,b). In general, FSH binding is higher in testes from immature rats than from adult animals, and on the basis of wet testis weight, the binding of FSH is maximum in gonads from animals between 10 and 15 days of age (Ketelslegers et al., 1977). For optimal assay conditions, and when high binding is required, the use of immature rat testis is sometimes an advantage. However, satisfactory results can also be obtained with homogenates of adult rat testis. This method has the advantage that less time is required to prepare relatively large amounts of homogenate and can be used when routine assays are to be performed for derivation of potency estimates of pituitary, urinary, or plasma extracts. After removal of the capsule, the testes are weighed and homogenized in a ground-glass tissue grinder (15–20 strokes) in ice-cold PBS. The homogenate is filtered through nylon mesh and centrifuged at $20,000\,g$ for 20 minutes. The supernatant is discarded and the pellets are resuspended by gentle homogenization in an appropriate volume of cold PBS. For routine assays, the homogenate is diluted to contain the equivalent of 100–200 mg of wet tissue per milliliter of PBS. For the assay, 100 μl of testis homogenate are incubated with 100 μl of gonadotropin standards (e.g., 0.25–100 ng of FSH) or the samples to be assayed, in PBS–BSA (1 mg/ml), and 50 μl of [^{125}I]hFSH (40,000–50,000 dpm) in PBS–BSA containing 0.05% Neomycin sulfate.

Nonspecific binding is determined in triplicate tubes containing 1–2 IU of Pergonal. After brief application to a vortex mixer, the assay tubes are incubated at 24° or 37°C for 18 hours with continuous shaking. Bound and free hormone are separated by filtration through Millipore filters (0.45 μm), previously soaked in 3% PBS–BSA to reduce nonspecific binding of tracer FSH to the cellulose filter. Filtrations are performed immediately after addition of 3 ml of ice-cold PBS to each incubation tube, and the filters are washed once with the same buffer. Each filter is then transferred to a plastic scintillation counting vial, and its radioactivity is determined in a gamma-spectrometer.

The sensitivity of the assay is 0.5 ng of hFSH per assay tube, and the dose for 50% binding-inhibition is between 5 and 8 ng of hFSH. The specificity of the assay has been demonstrated by the low crossreaction of hLH and hCG in this system, at doses, respectively, 100 and 750 times higher than hFSH. Parallel dose-response curves are obtained with highly purified hFSH and the Second International Reference Preparation for Human Menopausal Gonadotropin (2nd IRP hMG). Purified hFSH, ovine FSH, and PMSG reacted with parallel slopes. When 15-day-old rat testis homogenates are used, the binding of [^{125}I]hFSH is significantly higher at 37°C than at 24°C; the binding-inhibition curve is somewhat more sensitive, and its slope is steeper. In contrast, when adult testis homogenate is used, the binding is lower at 37°C. This could be attributable to higher degradative activity in adult testis homogenates than in those prepared from immature animals. Therefore, if adult testis homogenates are employed for the binding assays, the incubation should be performed at room temperature. Satisfactory assays can be performed with homogenates kept on ice for several days, and the particulate receptors can be stored at −60°C for several weeks without significant loss of binding activity.

C. RADIOLIGAND-RECEPTOR ASSAY FOR PROLACTIN

The development of receptor assays for prolactin and related hormones has been of particular value in the identification and study of lactogenic hormones for which radioimmunoassays were not available. Since radioligand-receptor assays recognize hormonal ligands according to their biological activities, it was not unexpected that prolactin of various species could be detected and measured by this method, and that other lactogenic hormones (placental lactogens and human growth hormone) could also be assayed in prolactin receptor systems. The tissues employed for radioligand-receptor assay have included rabbit mammary gland (Shiu et al., 1973) and rodent liver (Posner, 1975). Application of radioligand-receptor assays to plasma and tissue analysis has permitted the identification and assay of prolactin in 9 species (Kelly et al., 1977) and has been employed in the detection and purification of placental lactogen in sheep, cow, goat, and rat. The behavior of ovine prolactin was of particular interest since it shows both lactogenic and somatotropic activity in receptor assays and in bioassays, and also interacts in the specific hGH assay using human liver particles (Carr and Friesen, 1976). This finding suggests that ovine placental lactogen is more similar to hGH than are nonprimate growth hormones, which are ineffective in man and do not interact with the specific hGH receptors in human tissues. Thus, the use of radioligand-receptor assay has revealed a growth-hormone-like effect of ovine placental lactogen in human tissue, a finding with obvious implications for the potential of this protein in the treatment of clinical disorders of growth in man (Friesen and Shiu, 1977).

D. APPLICATIONS OF RECEPTOR ASSAYS FOR GONADOTROPINS

The use of the radioligand-receptor assay procedure for measurement of LH and chorionic gonadotropin has been described in detail elsewhere (Catt et al., 1971, 1972a, 1973a, 1976; Catt and Dufau, 1973a, Catt and Dufau, 1975). An example of the binding-inhibition curves given by a number of gonadotropin preparations is shown in Fig. 2. The difference in slope between human LH or hCG and the LH of other species (Catt et al., 1972a, 1973a) has been shown to extend over a wide range of animal LH preparations, with least steep binding-inhibition curves in rabbit, chicken, porcine, and canine LH (Leidenberger and Reichert, 1973). In related studies on the formation and properties of native and hybrid molecules of LH and hCG, the slope of the binding inhibition curve was found to be determined by the nature of the β-subunit employed for reassociation studies (Reichert et al., 1973).

The potency estimates for gonadotropins derived by receptor assay are usually commensurate with, or somewhat higher than, those obtained by conventional bioassay. The only notable exception to this general finding has occurred with desialylated gonadotropins prepared by treatment with neuraminidase (Dufau et al., 1971b; Tsuruhara et al., 1972a,b). Such modified gonadotropins are characterized by high binding affinity for gonadotropin receptors in vitro, but display low biological activity during in vivo bioassay due to rapid hepatic clearance and removal from the circulation (Tsuruhara et al., 1972a). This characteristic of desialylated gonadotropins has been demonstrated with enzymically modified hCG and LH, but probably does not occur to a significant degree in pituitary extracts containing LH or in purified urinary hCG preparations. The formation of variably desialylated hCG molecules may occur during urinary excretion of the hormone in pregnancy, though the extent of such a change has not been determined. Owing to the rapid hepatic clearance of asialoglycoproteins in vivo, it is unlikely that significant quantities of desialylated gonadotropin molecules will ever be present in circulating blood and plasma samples. For these reasons, the application of receptor assay to measurement of naturally occurring gonadotropins can be regarded as a valid method for in vitro estimation of the biological activity of gonadotropic hormones. However, gonadotropins that exhibit a short plasma half-life in *vivo* will commonly exhibit higher biological activity by any *in vitro* assay method, including radioligand-receptor assay. This is a notable feature of ovine LH, which contains no sialic acid and is characterized by rapid clearance from plasma during *in vivo* bioassays, with consequent difficulty in comparison with standard hormone preparations of more prolonged half-life, e.g., the 2nd IRP hMG. For such hormones, *in vitro* bioassay or receptor assay methods provide a more accurate measure of the intrinsic biological activity of the molecule at the target cell level.

Although not yet widely applied to measurements of plasma gonadotropin levels, radioligand-receptor procedures have been satisfactory for determination of the relatively high concentrations of pregnancy gonadotropins that occur in human and equine plasma (Catt *et al.*, 1974, 1975b; Rosal *et al.*, 1975; Tomoda *et al.*, 1975; Lee and Ryan, 1975a; Stewart *et al.*, 1976). Measurement of basal gonadotropin levels in plasma of nonpregnant subjects by receptor assay is rendered more difficult by nonspecific interference from plasma proteins, and by the low basal levels of circulating gonadotropins in comparison to the detection limit of the assay system. Such interference prevents the accurate measurement of LH or hCG in plasma below levels of 5–10 ng/ml, and can be minimized if the serum or plasma content of all assay tubes is equalized by addition of hormone-free serum. Alternatively, extraction of gonadotropins from plasma samples by the agarose-concanavalin A method (Dufau *et al.*, 1972a) can be employed to avoid interference and to concentrate the hormone prior to radioligand assay. Fractionation of serum with ethanol or ammonium sulfate has also been employed to avoid nonspecific interference during assay of luteinizing hormone in human serum (Leidenberger *et al.*, 1976). As noted above, direct assay of LH at the midcycle peak and hCG in untreated pregnancy plasma is not a problem, and the latter has been employed as a rapid and sensitive method of early diagnosis of pregnancy (Landesman and Saxena, 1976). Also, the measurement of PMSG in equine serum has been performed by radioreceptor assays for LH and FSH (Stewart *et al.*, 1976). The determination of FSH in serum by receptor assay has been performed in postmenopausal samples measured either directly (Cheng, 1975b) or after dialysis to reduce interference by nonhormonal serum factors (Reichert *et al.*, 1975).

V. Bioassay of Serum LH

The measurement of biologically active gonadotropin levels in serum has been rendered difficult by the extremely low circulating concentrations of such hormones and by the relatively insensitive nature of conventional bioassay techniques. As noted above, the development of radioligand-receptor assays for LH and hCG has improved the sensitivity of methods for determining the biological potency of small quantities of these hormones. However, such radioligand-receptor assays have been mainly of value for studies on the activity of native and modified gonadotropic hormones *in vitro* and for assay of the relatively high levels of gonadotropins in pregnancy plasma. For biological assay of the low levels of LH present in plasma of nonpregnant human subjects, more sensitive methods based on a specific target-cell response have been found to be necessary (Watson, 1972; Dufau *et al.*, 1974a, 1976a,b, 1977f; Quazi *et al.*, 1974; Beitins *et al.*, 1977). Earlier observations on the steroidogenic response of intact rat testes to LH and hCG had demonstrated the high sensitivity and potential value of this approach for bioassay of extremely low concentrations of these gonadotropins (Dufau *et al.*, 1971a, 1972b).

A. THE RAT INTERSTITIAL CELL-TESTOSTERONE (RICT) ASSAY

A highly sensitive bioassay for plasma LH and hCG has been developed by utilizing the testosterone response of collagenase-dispersed rat interstitial cells to gonadotropin stimulation *in vitro*. The *in vitro* bioassay procedure has been abbreviated to the RICT assay (rat interstitial cell-testosterone assay). Testosterone production by dispersed interstitial cells is stimulated by human, ovine, bovine, porcine, rat, rabbit, and monkey LH (Dufau *et al.*, 1974a, 1976a,b, 1977b,f) and hCG, monkey CG, and PMSG (Catt *et al.*, 1975b; Dufau *et al.*, 1976a,b, 1977b,f). The RICT assay gives parallel dose-response curves for all steroidogenic gonadotropins tested, and thus permits cross-species comparison of the intrinsic biological activities of native and modified gonadotropins. This bioassay has been extensively validated and utilized for the measurement of hLH activity in human serum (Dufau *et al.*, 1974a, 1976a,b).

The optimum conditions for bioassay of serum gonadotropins were provided by incubation of collagenase-dispersed interstitial cells in the presence of 0.125 mM 1-methyl-3-isobutylxanthine (MIX), and sodium heparin (100 IU/ml), with addition of gonadotropin-free serum or 5% BSA to ensure a constant proportion of serum protein in all assay samples and standards. Normal female and male serum samples were assayed by the incubation of 25- to 100-μl aliquots with dispersed interstitial cells. When high levels of gonadotropin were expected, the serum samples were diluted with gonadotropin-free serum or 5% BSA.

In the case of postmenopausal females, and luteinizing hormone releasing hormone (LHRH)-stimulated subjects, sample aliquots equivalent to 0.1 to 0.5 μl of serum were used, after dilution of the sample in gonadotropin-free serum or 5% BSA. Serum samples were assayed in duplicate at 3 dose levels in the RICT bioassay. After incubation for 3 hours, testosterone production was determined by radioimmunoassay of appropriate aliquots of the incubation medium (Dufau et al., 1972b, 1974a). The testosterone production in the sample vials was compared with that of standard LH or hCG preparations by a parallel-line bioassay computer program.

The specificity of the RICT assay method was shown by the absence of significant LH activity in purified preparations of FSH, TSH, and GH and by undetectable biological activity in serum from hypopituitary patients and women on oral-contraceptive therapy. The biological activity of hormone standards and plasma samples was neutralized by antisera to LH and hCG, and no LH activity was detectable in serum from hypophysectomized rats. The LH levels in normal subjects were consistent with the physiological condition of the subjects and were always measurable with good precision. The within-assay coefficient of variation (C.V.) for measurement of a normal male plasma pool (30 mIU/ml) was $\pm 10\%$ ($n = 90$), and the between-assay reproducibility of the method was $\pm 15\%$ (C.V.). The precision of the assay (λ) was 0.035 ± 0.015 ($n = 72$), and Finney's g factor was 0.004.

B. HUMAN SERUM LH CONCENTRATIONS MEASURED BY RICT ASSAY

Serum samples from normal cycling females, postmenopausal females, and male subjects gave dose-response curves parallel to the standard curves obtained with standards such as the 2nd IRP hMG and LER 907 (Figs. 3 and 4). The normal circulating LH values determined by the RICT bioassay in terms of milliunits of the 2nd IRP hMG per milliliter of serum (mean $\pm$ SD) were as follows: premenopausal women: 29 ± 16 ($n = 42$); postmenopausal women: 223 ± 92 ($n = 10$); and normal men: 37 ± 19 ($n = 17$). The ranges of serum LH at various stages of the menstrual cycle in normal women were as follows: follicular phase, 10 to 91 mIU/ml; luteal phase, 6 to 79 mIU/ml; and midcycle peak, 98 to 250 mIU/ml. In normal premenopausal women, the mean bio:immuno (B:I) ratio was 1.2 ± 0.32 and did not change significantly throughout the menstrual cycle, though higher values were sometimes observed in the late follicular phase. Higher B:I ratios of 2.6 ± 0.6 and 2.5 ± 0.4 were obtained for basal serum LH values in postmenopausal women and normal men, respectively (Dufau et al.,

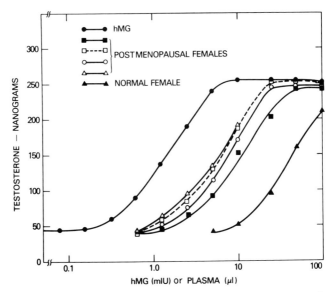

F<small>IG</small>. 3. Testosterone production by dispersed Leydig cells during incubation with human menopausal gonadotropin (hMG) standards and plasma samples from normal female and postmenopausal subjects.

1974a, 1976a). Thus, the serum LH values obtained by RICT assay in human subjects were generally higher than those measured by radioimmunoassay, though the two values were frequently similar in normal premenopausal women. The higher B:I ratio observed in men and postmenopausal women were also apparent during fractionation of serum samples by gel filtration. In such experiments, the peaks of immunoreactive and bioactive hormone were coincident with each other, and with ^{125}I-labeled hLH (Fig. 5).

During the normal menstrual cycle the values of serum LH measured by bioassay were always highly correlated with those measured by radioimmunoassay. The absolute values determined by bioassay were usually equal to or slightly higher than those measured by radioimmunoassay, and the B:I ratio in multiple samples was between 1 and 2 in 3 subjects studied throughout the cycle. Although individual differences in B:I ratio were noted during studies performed throughout the cycle, as exemplified by the ratio above unity in the subject illustrated in Fig. 6, these were usually within the expected range for B:I ratio in normal women based on the 95% confidence limits of 0.5 to 1.8 determined in single samples from a group of 42 premenopausal women.

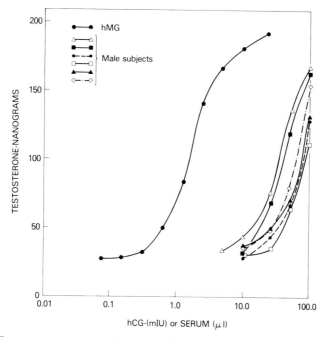

Fig. 4. Testosterone production by dispersed Leydig cells during incubation with hMG standards and plasma samples from normal men.

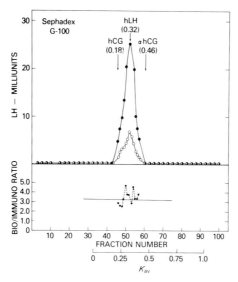

Fig. 5. Elution pattern of a pool sample of human postmenopausal serum subjected to gel filtration on Sephadex G-100. LH measurements were performed on aliquots from samples by RICT assay (●——●) and radioimmunoassay (○——○), upper panel; B:I ratio is indicated in the lower panel.

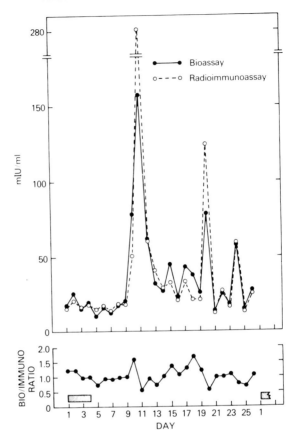

FIG. 6. Serum LH measured by RICT bioassay and radioimmunoassay during the normal menstrual cycle. The B : I ratios are indicated in the lower panel, and menses are shown by the hatched rectangles.

C. Effect of Luteinizing Hormone Releasing Hormone (LHRH) on Bioactive Serum LH Levels

The effects of LHRH stimulation on plasma LH levels measured by bioassay and radioimmunoassay were examined during the normal menstrual cycle, and in normal men and postmenopausal women (Dufau *et al.*, 1976b, 1977f; Beitins *et al.*, 1977). After administration of 100 μg of LHRH by subcutaneous injection during the early follicular phase, a 2.7-fold rise in bioactive serum LH to 58 ± 18 mIU/ml at 30 to 60 minutes was accompanied by an equivalent rise in immunoreactive LH, with unchanged bio : immuno (B : I) ratio of 0.9 ± 0.2 (SD). During the late follicular phase, bioactive serum LH rose 7.6-fold to 306 ± 160 mIU/ml at 30 to 180 minutes, and the B:I ratio was significantly increased from 1.7 to 2.7. During the luteal phase, bioactive LH values rose 8-fold to 223 ± 97 mIU/ml at 30 to 60 minutes, with increase in B:I ratio from 1.1 to 1.8. The LHRH-stimulated serum levels declined more rapidly in the early follicular phase than during the late follicular and luteal phases. Elevations of circulating LH concentrations following LHRH administration during the normal menstrual cycle were usually accompanied by a significant rise in B:I ratio, except during the early follicular phase, when the LH responses were small and the B:I ratio did not change. After LHRH, stimulation of serum LH levels in men (Fig. 7) and postmenopausal women were relatively small, and inconstant elevations of B:I ratio were observed above the basal value of 2.9. Although the B:I ratio was usually close to unity in cycling women, the ratio was from 2 to 3 in men and postmenopausal women and during LHRH stimulation of normal women at the late follicular and luteal phases of the menstrual cycle. Thus, the increased LH secretion rate of postmenopausal women and LHRH-stimulated cycling women was frequently accompanied by a rise in the B:I ratio, suggesting a change in the properties of LH secreted under these conditions.

D. Characteristics of the RICT Assay

The RICT method, based on the highly sensitive and precise response system provided by dispersed rat interstitial cells, has been standardized as a routine method for bioassay of normal LH values in male and female serum. The use of serum samples, and the inclusion of a constant proportion of serum protein, has given the most reproducible conditions for assay of circulating LH concentrations in normal subjects. The assay sensitivity is quite high, permitting the measurement of LH levels in small aliquots of serum from normal male and female subjects. In all studies performed with the RICT assay, the circulating levels of bioactive LH were consistent with the physiological condition of the subjects from whom serum samples were obtained. Thus, LH bioactivity was absent in states of gonadotropin deficiency, and was markedly elevated when gonadotropin secretion was increased, i.e., at the midcycle LH peak, in postmenopausal subjects, after LHRH administration, and during pregnancy (Dufau et al., 1974a; Catt et al., 1975b, 1976). The value of the RICT assay has been clearly demonstrated in two separate areas. First, for the assay of the biological potency of pituitary and urinary LH preparations, and placental gonadotropins from a variety of animal species, the method has unique advantages in

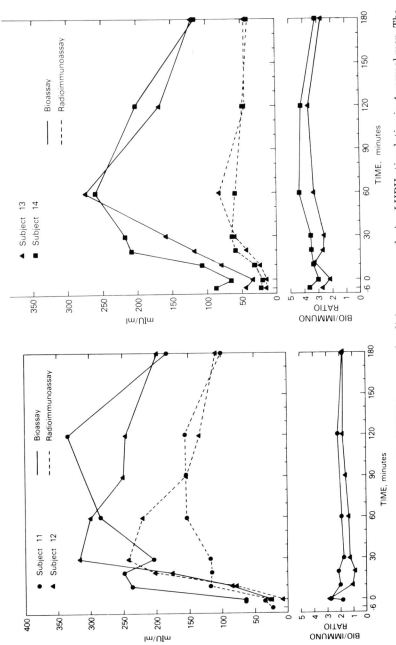

FIG. 7. Serum LH values measured by RICT bioassay and radioimmunoassay during LHRH stimulation in 4 normal men. The B:I ratio for each subject is shown in the lower panels.

terms of both sensitivity and the parallel dose-response curves obtained with all forms of LH and chorionic gonadotropin. The parallel standard curves obtained for human, ovine, porcine, rabbit, and rat LH (Dufau et al., 1974a, 1976a), as well as hCG and PMSG, are illustrative of this feature of the assay. For this reason, the RICT assay permits valid cross-species comparisons to be performed between the intrinsic biological activities of a wide variety of human and animal gonadotropins. Second, the RICT assay permits bioassay of circulating LH and hCG in human serum under all physiological circumstances, and basal levels can be easily measured in normal males and premenopausal females.

The plasma LH values obtained in human subjects have been generally higher than those measured by radioimmunoassay, although the two values are frequently similar in normal premenopausal females. When urinary LH (2nd IRP hMG) was employed as standard, the bio:immuno potency ratio in cycling females was usually close to unity, although occasional subjects gave ratios of 1.5 to 2.0. No consistent change in B:I ratio was observed during the menstrual cycle, and the bioactive serum LH profiles were always identical with those derived by radioimmunoassay. This finding confirmed the validity of immunoreactive LH values as an index of the biologically active LH present in circulation. In male and postmenopausal subjects, the B:I ratio was consistently elevated, with bioassay values 2.5 times higher than those measured in the same samples by radioimmunoassay. Despite this increase in B:I ratio, the profiles of bioactive and immunoactive LH concentrations were always identical, each change of serum LH in the RICT assay being concomitant with the change measured simultaneously by radioimmunoassay. Thus, the two completely different methods of assay, one based on competition with labeled hormone for antibody, and the other on activation of steroidogenesis in isolated target cells, gave identical profiles for serum LH activity, and relatively close absolute values for LH concentration in serum samples.

The presence of a dissociation between bioactive and immunoactive serum LH values in certain groups of human subjects has been clearly indicated above. The possible reasons for the B:I difference between normal cycling women and other human subjects have been recently reviewed (Dufau et al., 1976a,b, 1977g), but the exact mechanism of this dissociation and its distribution have not yet been elucidated. The existence of such a difference in bio- and immunopotency of circulating LH indicates that separate structural properties of the molecule are being recognized by the LH receptor and the antibody employed for radioimmunoassay. The gonadal status of the subject may influence the biological or immunological characteristic of circulating LH, and such an effect could be related to the prevailing levels of estrogen secretion. It is also possible that the rate of gonadotropin secretion could influence the properties of serum LH, accounting for the consistently elevated B : I ratio in serum LH of postmenopausal women. The higher B : I ratio of serum LH in normal men might also be related to gonadotropin secretion rate, since there is evidence to suggest that the production rate of LH is higher in men than in premenopausal women (McArthur et al., 1958; Pepperell et al., 1975).

The use of steroidogenic cells for the bioassay of LH in human serum has also been employed by the incubation of serum samples with luteinized ovarian tissue (Watson, 1972) and interstitial cells from the mouse testis (Van Damme et al., 1973, 1974; Quazi et al., 1974). The ovarian-tissue progesterone assay showed a broad peak of LH activity over 3–5 days at midcycle, and required plasma samples of 2 ml for determination of LH content (Watson, 1972). The mouse-cell testosterone assay is of comparable sensitivity with the RICT assay, but gives a relatively steep dose-response curve and does not appear to be directly applicable to the bioassay of plasma LH in male subjects. However, the values obtained for plasma LH in postmenopausal women (Quazi et al., 1974) were very close to those determined by RICT assay (Dufau et al., 1974a, 1976a,b), indicating that the use of in vitro bioassay could provide more uniform potency estimates that those given by radioimmunoassay. The extent of the bio : immuno discrepancy for plasma LH was much more marked than that observed in our studies, with B : I ratios from 2 to 14. It is likely that the radioimmunoassay methods employed by different laboratories will prove to be the major source of such variations observed in the B : I ratio, since measurements of LH in plasma samples by several radioimmunoassay methods have shown quite marked interlaboratory variations (Albert et al., 1968; Parlow, 1968). Now that in vitro bioassay methods, based upon a defined biological action of the trophic hormone, have achieved adequate sensitivity and precision for the measurement of circulating LH, more satisfactory standardization of the methods and normal values for plasma LH and hCG assays should become possible. Important factors in this improvement are the biological specificity and uniformity of the target cell response to LH, and the parallel dose-response curves for serum samples and various LH standards. The standards employed in the assay can include those prepared from urine extracts (the 2nd IRP), pituitary standards such as LER 907 or 69/104 and the more highly purified 68/40 preparation, and postmenopausal plasma (69/176), all of which are distributed by the Division of Biological Standards, London (Bangham *et al.*, 1973). In contrast, individual antisera can be regarded as unique biological reagents and sometimes show quite marked differences in reactivity with serum LH and the various standards used in radioimmunoassay. The degree of variability between radioimmunoassay methods, and of B : I ratios based upon data from such assays, should be reduced by the use of purified LH standards to avoid the interference in immunoassays of components such as hormone subunits that are not biologically active. The use of such a purified standard (68/40) during biological and immunological characterization of LH in human pituitary extracts has been shown to reduce the B : I ratio to about 1, from the values of 3 and 12 observed when standards of 2nd IRP and 60/104 were employed, respectively (Robertson and Diczfalusy, 1977). These findings are attributable to the presence of immunoreactive material that is biologically inactive (predominantly α-subunit) in the unpurified standards, causing an artificially low estimate for the hormone present in samples assayed against these standards. The recognition that impurities in standards composed of crude extracts can seriously interfere in immunoassay estimations may initiate a return to the more logical viewpoint that standards for gonadotropins (and other substances) should be as pure as possible.

The *in vitro* bioassay method has not only confirmed the biological relevance of immunoassay measurements in human plasma, but provides the additional advantages of a more absolute and well-standardized measure of biologically active LH in serum. This method can be also applied for the bioassay of serum LH in species for which satisfactory radioimmunoassays are either not developed or of limited availability. An example of the value of the procedure for bioassay of plasma LH in a nonhuman primate species is described in the following section.

E. BIOACTIVE SERUM LH IN THE RHESUS MONKEY

The application of RICT bioassay for measurement of LH concentration in rhesus monkey serum has been recently demonstrated under a variety of physiological conditions (Dufau *et al.*, 1977b,g; Neill *et al.*, 1977). Human menopausal gonadotropin was used as a standard for routine bioassay of monkey serum LH, and gave dose-response curves that provided a working range in serum of 1–25 mIU/ml. A laboratory standard of crude monkey pituitary gonadotropin (LER 909-2) gave a dose-response curve parallel to the hMG standard, with relative potency of 15.7 $\pm$ 0.42 IU/mg. Serum samples from normal cycling females, postmenopausal or castrated females, and adult male monkeys (Fig. 8) gave dose-response curves that were parallel to those obtained with the human and rhesus gonadotropin standards. Conversely, serum samples from hypophysectomized female monkeys contained no detectable LH activity (Dufau *et al.*, 1977b). However, immunoreactive serum "LH" values in these animals were 0.8, 2.0, and 2.7 μg of LER-1909-2 per milliliter, equivalent to 12, 32, and 43 mIU/ml based on the bioassay potency of the standard. Low or undetectable bioactive serum LH levels were also observed in immature male and female monkeys. In addition, immunoreactive "LH" was detected in serum of all immature animals examined, at concentrations of 0.6–2.2 μg/ml. The absence of nonspecific interference by plasma factors during assay of serum samples by the RICT method was indicated by the virtual absence of LH activity in plasma or serum samples from hypophysectomized and immature monkeys, as indicated above. The suppression of markedly elevated serum LH levels in castrated females to undetectable levels by estrogen/progesterone treatment provided further evidence that the assay is not subject to nonspecific interference. The LH-like immunoreactive material observed in sera of hypophysectomized, immature, and steroid-suppressed animals (Niswender *et al.*, 1971) was not detected during bioassay of serum by the RICT method.

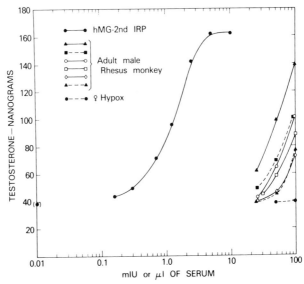

FIG. 8. Dose-response curves from serum samples of adult male rhesus monkeys. Curves for human gonadotropin standard and for hypophysectomized female monkey are included for comparison.

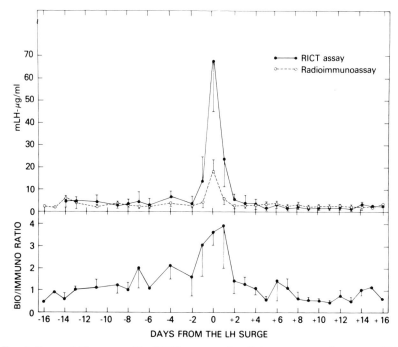

F<small>IG</small>. 9. Serum LH measured by RICT assay and radioimmunoassay (in terms of LER 1909-2; μg/ml) in 4 ovulatory menstrual cycles. The individual values were combined by defining the day of the LH surge as day zero. Vertical bars indicate the standard deviation of the mean; when fewer than 4 values were combined, no deviation is indicated. The mean ± SD of the B : I ratio is shown in the lower panel.

This finding indicates that such material does not represent biologically active LH and is probably an artifact of the heterologous radioimmunoassay of rhesus LH. Measurement of serum LH by the RICT assay throughout the rhesus menstrual cycle revealed follicular phase levels of 76 ± 52 mIU/ml (mean ± SD, $n = 7$) and luteal phase levels of 35 ± 5 mIU/ml ($n = 5$), with usually symmetrical midcycle peaks and maximum LH values ranging from 500 to 2100 mIU/ml (Fig. 9). When bioassay values were compared with results obtained by radioimmunoassay in 4 complete cycles (Fig. 9, lower panel) and from 3 other monkeys, the LH levels observed during follicular and luteal phases were similar, and the corresponding B : I ratios in a large number of individual samples were close to unity. The midcycle LH peaks measured by each assay were coincident, but the bioactive LH surges were broader and 3 to 4 times higher than those detected by radioimmunoassay, with B : I ratios across the midcycle peak ranging from 1.4 to 6.3 (3.1 ± 1.5, $n = 18$). At the maximum of the bioactive LH peak, which was coincident with the maximum of the immunoactive LH peak in each cycle, the B : I ratio ranged from 3.6 to 6.3.

By comparison with LH concentrations measured by bioassay in human serum (Dufau *et al.*, 1974a, 1976a,b) the values for LH in rhesus monkey serum were similar during the follicular and luteal phases of the menstrual cycle, but were markedly higher than the human levels at midcycle and in postmenopausal and oophorectomized animals. The rhesus LH values were 5- to 10-fold higher than the bioactive LH concentrations observed in the human under similar conditions, and 2 to 3 times higher than the maximum LH levels observed in the human during LHRH stimulation (Dufau *et al.*, 1976b). There was an accompanying rise of 3- to 6-fold in the B : I ratio of circulating rhesus monkey LH during the midcycle peak, perhaps reflecting the release of LH from a pituitary pool other than that responsible for tonic secretion of LH during the follicular and luteal phases of the cycle (Dufau *et al.*, 1977b). Such a change is analogous to the responses of the human female to LHRH stimulation near midcycle, when the B : I ratio was elevated by about 2-fold above the basal value (Dufau *et al.*, 1976b). The marked increase in B : I ratio of rhesus monkey serum LH at midcycle, and in the perimenopausal monkeys, could be related to a change in the carbohydrate composition of the LH molecules synthesized at these times. Desialylation of hLH and hCG has been shown to reduce the actions of these hormones upon stimulation of steroidogenesis *in vitro* (Dufau *et al.*, 1971b), and it is possible that *increases* in sialylation could have the opposite effect upon bioactivity *in vivo* and *in vitro*. The metabolic clearance rates of glycoprotein molecules are inversely related to their contents of sialic acid (Morell *et al.*, 1971), and it is of interest that the plasma LH of ovariectomized rhesus monkeys exhibits larger apparent molecular size and lower metabolic clearance rate than LH from intact female monkeys (Peckham and Knobil, 1976). Whichever of these mechanisms is responsible for the higher bioactive LH values observed in the rhesus monkey at midcycle, and in postmenopausal women, will need to be resolved by more detailed analysis.

VI. RECEPTOR STRUCTURE AND HORMONE BINDING

A. CHEMICAL AND PROTEOLYTIC MODIFICATIONS

The structural features of gonadotropin receptors that are essential for hormone binding have been examined by chemical and enzymic modification of particulate and soluble receptor preparations from the testis and ovary. Like all hormone receptors, those for gonadotropins are proteins and lose their specific binding properties after treatment with trypsin and other proteolytic enzymes (Dufau et al., 1973a). This property of the receptors is consistent with their nature as predominantly protein components of the cell membrane. It should be noted that brief exposure to proteolytic enzymes does not necessarily destroy gonadotropin receptors and that preparation of dispersed cells from testis (Mendelson et al., 1975a) and ovary (Papaionnou and Gospodarowicz, 1975) by collagenase digestion did not alter the binding properties of LH receptors in these tissues. Also, treatment of particulate receptors for insulin (Kono and Barham, 1971) and LH (Catt et al., 1974) with low concentrations of trypsin caused an initial increase in receptor-binding activity, followed by a progressive decrease during more extensive destruction of the receptor sites.

A further indication of the importance of peptide conformation in receptor binding is provided by the effects of disulfide bond cleavage upon the gonadotropin receptor. Specific binding of [^{125}I]hCG by testicular LH receptors was abolished by reduction and alkylation of particulate and soluble receptors with dithiothreitol and N-ethylmaleimide. This indicates that intrachain disulfide bonds are essential for maintenance of receptor conformation and determine the ability to exhibit specific binding of gonadotropins. By contrast, the retention of bound gonadotropin by the preformed hormone–receptor complex was not influenced by reducing agents, suggesting that the conformational stability of the complex is maintained by hormone binding despite the reduction of disulfide bonds which are necessary for hormone binding by the unoccupied form of the receptor (Dufau et al., 1974c, 1977e).

Nitration of the exposed tyrosines of the α-subunit in native LH decreased both biological potency and receptor binding of the hormone (Liu et al., 1974; Catt et al., 1974). Depending on the conditions employed for nitration, derivatives containing from 1 to 5 nitro groups may be obtained. When a single tyrosine group was nitrated, the biological activity of LH was decreased by approximately 50%; if more than one tyrosine group was nitrated, biological activity dropped by more than 90%. All the exposed tyrosines were located on the α-subunit and were required for recombination with the β-subunit, but nitration of both β-subunit tyrosines did not destroy recombining activity (Liu et al., 1974). Acylation studies indicated that the NH$_2$-terminal and 10 of the 12 lysine-ζ-amino groups were readily reactive and peripherally located in the LH molecule, while only 2 were buried and did not react during acylation. One of the 10 lysine residues of the α subunit was unavailable for acylation, and the 2 lysine residues of the β-subunit could be readily acylated. The charge of the β-subunit did not seem to be important for recombination, but a neutral or positive charge was necessary for biological activity in the recombined LH molecule. Acylation of the β-subunit showed that all or part of the amino groups on this subunit with positive charge were essential for biological activity (Liu *et al.*, 1974).

B. EFFECTS OF PHOSPHOLIPASE TREATMENT

In addition to the obvious importance of protein structure and conformation in binding activity, there is considerable evidence that phospholipids have a significant influence on gonadotropin receptor function. Thus, treatment of particulate and soluble receptors from the rat testis with phospholipase A markedly reduced the binding activity of the free receptors. These and other studies on the effects of phospholipases on hormone binding have indicated an important function of phospholipids in the biological activity of the gonadotropin receptor (Dufau *et al.*, 1973a). Also, the interaction of phospholipids with ovine LH or its β-subunit has been shown to cause conformational changes that are detectable during circular dichroism studies. Since the phospholipid effect was confined to the tertiary structure of the β-subunit, a specific amino acid sequence may be involved in this interaction (Ward *et al.*, 1974).

The lipid content of the testis gonadotropin receptor is probably quite small, in view of the high density of the solubilized binding sites, but appears to play a significant role in hormone binding (Dufau *et al.*, 1973a). The effects of phospholipase treatment upon receptor function appear to depend upon the physical state and occupancy of the sites during exposure to the enzyme. Thus, phospholipases A and C had no effect upon the hormone–receptor complex formed *in vitro* between [125I]hCG and soluble receptors extracted with Triton X-100 from testis particles. However, treatment of prelabeled testis particles with these enzymes before extraction with Triton X-100 caused considerable aggregation of the solubilized hormone–receptor complexes. The soluble hormone–receptor complex extracted with nonionic detergents from prelabeled particulate fractions was also aggregated by exposure to phospholipase C, while phospholipase A had no effect (Charreau *et al.*, 1974). These various studies indicated that phospholipase A has a more pronounced effect upon the free or unoccupied LH/hCG binding sites, whether soluble or particulate, than on the corresponding receptors during occupancy by gonadotropin. The effects of phospholipase C on receptor aggregation are apparent whether receptors are in the soluble or particulate form during exposure to the enzyme.

In the ovary, treatment of plasma membranes from bovine corpus luteum with phospholipases A and C caused a reduction in the binding of [^{125}I]hCG to its receptors, whereas phospholipase D had no effect on hormone binding (Gospodarowicz, 1973; Azhar and Menon, 1976). Analysis of the hydrolysis products released by phospholipase C into the incubation medium showed that phosphatidylcholine and phosphatidylethanolamine were hydrolyzed more rapidly than phosphatidylserine. These reaction products were found to have no effect on receptor-binding activity. However, changes in the membrane phospholipid environment could be responsible for the decreased binding activity, which was partially restored by detergent solubilization of phospholipase-C-treated membranes (Azhar et al., 1976a). In contrast, the end products of phospholipase A action, such as lysophosphatides and fatty acids, remained associated with the plasma membrane. Such reaction products were found to inhibit both membrane-associated and solubilized receptor activities (lysophosphatidylcholine < lysophosphatidylethanolamine < lysophosphatidylserine). The inhibitory effect of phospholipase A on gonadotropin binding was reversed upon removal of membrane-bound hydrolysis products by washing the membranes with defatted BSA.

The specific binding of [^{125}I]FSH to testicular receptors was abolished by pretreatment with phospholipases A and C, but not by phospholipase D. In this case, addition of phosphatidylserine or a phospholipid fraction obtained from the whole testis partly restored the receptor-binding capacity of the enzyme-treated membranes (Abou-Issa and Reichert, 1976). Treatment of particulate and soluble receptors with neuraminidase, RNase, and DNase did not alter the binding of labeled hCG to gonadotropin binding sites in the testis (Charreau et al., 1974).

C. STRUCTURE–FUNCTION RELATIONSHIPS OF GONADOTROPINS

The analysis of gonadotropin binding to particulate receptor preparations has proved to be a useful technique for the study of structure–function relations in modified and derivatized forms of the gonadotropic hormones. For example, removal of sialic acid from hCG is known to cause almost complete loss of biological activity when the desialylated hormone is evaluated by in vivo bioassay (Van Hall et al., 1971a). However, desialylated hCG has been shown to be rapidly cleared from the circulation, with a half-life of minutes (Van Hall *et al.*, 1971b; Tsuruhara *et al.*, 1972a,b), and such rapid metabolism is the main reason for the low biological activity of the asialo-hCG derivative *in vivo*. Thus, asialo-hCG is only about 3% as effective as intact hCG in competing with [125I]hCG for binding to the ovary *in vivo*, whereas the receptor-binding activity of the modified hormone *in vitro* is usually significantly higher than that of the native hormone (Dufau *et al.*, 1971b; Tsuruhara *et al.*, 1972b). Removal of the adjacent galactose residues from the hCG molecule is also accompanied by retention of binding activity, indicating that neither of the major terminal carbohydrate residues is essential for interaction of the hormone with the receptor sites in testis and ovary (Tsuruhara *et al.*, 1972a,b). However, the *in vitro* activities of the modified glycoprotein upon stimulation of cAMP and testosterone production are significantly less than those of the intact hormone. Although the asialo- and asialo-agalacto derivatives of hCG can elicit a full steroidogenic response in testis and Leydig cells *in vitro*, the relative potencies of asialo-hCG and asialo-agalacto-hCG are about 50% and 15%, respectively, of that of the native hormone (Catt and Dufau, 1973a). Furthermore, the ability of the modified hormones to elicit cAMP production in the Leydig cell is even more markedly impaired, such that neither preparation can elicit a full cAMP response *in vitro* (Catt *et al.*, 1974). Thus, the asialo- and asialo-agalacto derivatives act as weak agonists in terms of steroid production, and as partial agonists for cAMP production. Such hCG derivatives which retain binding activity and show reduced agonistic activity are potential competitive antagonists, and may prove to be of value as inhibitors of gonadotropin activity *in vitro*. The ability of such derivatives to act as *in vitro* antagonists of hCG under suitable conditions has been demonstrated in dispersed interstitial cells (Moyle *et al.*, 1975), confirming the partially agonistic properties of hCG lacking the terminal carbohydrate residues.

In addition to studies on the role of carbohydrate residues in receptor binding and activation, radioligand-receptor systems have been used to evaluate the biological activity of isolated gonadotropin subunits (Catt *et al.*, 1973a). The existence of a common α-subunit and specific β-subunits in the glycoprotein hormones had suggested that the α-subunit could be responsible for a common action of the various hormones, such as activation of adenylate cyclase, while the β-subunit is responsible for the specific recognition of the hormone by the receptor site. Initial reports on the biological properties of glycoprotein hormone subunits indicated that the isolated LH subunits may exhibit specific biological activities, most clearly those of lipolysis in isolated fat cells (Gospodarowicz, 1971) and ovulation in the hamster (Yang *et al.*, 1972). However, evidence for specific actions on steroidogenesis in the mammalian testis or ovary was less convincing during a number of studies performed to determine the true biological activity of the isolated subunits upon mammalian gonadotropin receptors. Application of the rat testis radioligand-receptor assay to a variety of α- and β-subunits showed that the biological activities of such preparations were very low, and equivalent only to that given by conventional bioassays. Identical values were obtained by *in vitro* bioassay of subunits with isolated rat testes, indicating that the apparent activity of certain subunit preparations was attributable to contamination with intact hormone (Catt *et al.*, 1973a). No enhancement of specific functions, either receptor binding or target cell activation, was detectable with either α- or β-subunits. The absence of biological activity in hCG subunits was also demonstrated by the results of bioassay combined with neutralization studies with specific antisera (Rayford *et al.*, 1972). Subunits of FSH have also been shown to exhibit binding activity commensurate only with the degree of contamination with undissociated hormone (Reichert and Bhalla, 1974).

The recombination of homologous and heterologous pairs of gonadotropin subunits has also been evaluated by the radioligand-receptor assay, which provides a rapid and convenient system for kinetic studies of subunit combination and dissociation. The characteristic binding-inhibition slopes of human and nonhuman LH preparations in the rat testis/hCG radioligand assay were found to be determined by the respective β-subunits of these hormones (Reichert *et al.*, 1973). Also, the β-subunit of hCG conferred higher binding affinity upon the hormone formed by recombination with α-subunits of LH (Leidenberger and Reichert, 1973), reflecting the generally higher binding potency of hCG in comparison to LH in receptor assay systems (Catt *et al.*, 1972a,b). In most reports, recombination of the α- and β-subunits of LH or hCG has not completely restored receptor-binding and biological activity. This suggests that subunit dissociation and preparation irreversibly disrupts a unique conformation of the native hormone required for high receptor affinity (Liu *et al.*, 1977) and that the subunits derived by current procedures may undergo partial denaturation during isolation. The radio-ligand-receptor assay has also been useful in the analysis of effects of chemical modification of functional groups upon receptor-binding activity of gonadotropin derivatives (Catt *et al.*, 1974; Liu *et al.*, 1974, 1977; Cheng, 1976).

VII. CHARACTERIZATION OF SOLUBLE GONADOTROPIN AND PROLACTIN RECEPTORS

A. SOLUBILIZATION OF LH/hCG RECEPTORS OF TESTIS AND OVARY

Solubilization of the particulate high-affinity gonadotropin receptors for LH and hCG in testis and ovary has been performed by extraction of homogenates and membranes with nonionic detergents such as Triton X-100, Lubrol PX, and Lubrol WX (Dufau and Catt, 1973; Dufau *et al.* 1973a, 1974b, 1975a,b; Charreau *et al.*, 1974), Brij-35, Ipegal-630 (Saxena, 1976), and Eumolophogene (Bellisario and Bahl, 1975). Extraction of gonadal particles with Triton X-100 was found to provide soluble LH/hCG receptors with uniform and reproducible binding properties, and these have been utilized for determination of the physical characteristics of the soluble receptor site. To this end, the gonadotropin receptors of the rat testis and ovary were solubilized by detergent extraction of the 120–27,000 g binding fraction of fragmented interstitial cells, or ovarian homogenates from the gonads of PMS/hCG-treated immature female rats, by dispersion of the 27,000 g pellets in 1% Triton X-100 for 30 minutes at 4°C. The binding activity of the soluble receptor preparation was assayed by equilibration with [^{125}I]hCG tracer for 16 hours at 4°C, followed by separation of bound and free tracer by precipitation of the bound complex with polyethylene glycol (PEG, Carbowax 6000). A study on the effect of increasing polyethylene glycol concentration upon precipitation of the soluble receptor–hormone complex showed that optimal separation was obtained at 12% polyethylene glycol, whereas higher concentrations caused increasing precipitation of the free gonadotropin (hCG, LH, or FSH) (Fig. 10). The most satisfactory separation of receptor-bound and free tracer hormone was obtained by redissolving the precipitate in 0.1% Triton X-100 and performing a second precipitation at 12% PEG. By this method, specific binding of up to 40% of the added [^{125}I]hCG tracer was demonstrable, and nonspecifically bound radioactivity was reduced to less than 1% of the added tracer hormone.

The tracer hormone employed for binding studies with soluble receptors required careful preparation to minimize nonspecific binding in the soluble fraction. The most consistently satisfactory method for tracer preparation was by radioiodination of the glycoprotein hormones with ^{125}I by the lactoperoxidase technique, to a specific activity of about 40 μC/μg (approximately 1 atom per molecule). For purification of ^{125}I-labeled hCG, LH, or FSH, the iodination mixture was fractionated by elution from cellulose powder, or by gel filtration, followed by group-

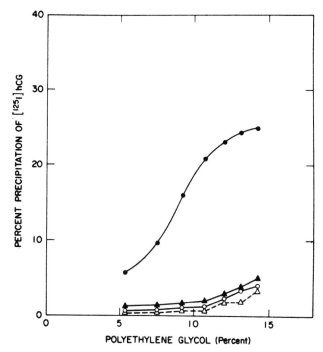

FIG. 10. Separation of receptor-bound and free [^{125}I]hCG by precipitation of bound complex with increasing concentrations of polyethylene glycol. In the presence of excess unlabeled hCG, binding of ^{125}I-labeled hormone is reduced to the level of the blank value observed in the absence of soluble receptor. ●——●, Soluble receptor; ▲——▲, soluble receptor + 10^{-7} M hCG; ○——○, reagent blank, △——△, reagent blank + 10^{-7} M hCG.

specific affinity chromatography on Sepharose–concanavalin A. Alternatively, the radioactive hormone could be purified directly by Sepharose–concanavalin A chromatography (Dufau *et al.*, 1972a, 1973a; Dufau and Catt, 1976a). The tracer hormone isolated by the combination of the two procedures gave the highest specific uptake by testicular and ovarian soluble receptors, and the lowest blank or "nonspecific" value (Table I). However, for the majority of binding studies, tracer hormone purified by chromatography on concanavalin A has been found to be satisfactory.

B. Properties of Soluble LH/hCG Receptors from Rat Testis

Specific binding of ^{125}I-labeled hCG by soluble gonadotropin receptors increased serially with rising concentrations of the solubilized re-

TABLE I

BINDING OF TRACER PREPARATIONS, [125I]hCG, BY SOLUBLE GONADOTROPIN RECEPTORS

Method of preparation	Cellulose purification				Sepharose–concanavalin A purification		Cellulose followed by Sepharose–concanavalin A	
					Fraction A	Fraction B	A	B
Column fraction no.	5	6	7	8	(18–24)	(25–33)	A	B
Content of labeled tracer (%)[a]	12	49	29	14	81	19	80	20
(a) Bound to soluble receptor	22	18	20	21	17	24	19	27
(b) Bound to soluble receptor + 10 μg hCG	10	3	3	3	1	1	1	1
Specific binding[a]	12	15	17	18	16	23	18	26

[a] Bound [125I]hCG as percent of total contents per minute.

ceptor preparation. At high protein concentrations, a decrease in binding was sometimes observed owing to increased tracer degradation. Saturation of soluble LH receptor sites by increasing quantities of labeled and/or unlabeled hCG was readily demonstrable, with approximate binding capacity of 1.5×10^{-12} mol mg^{-1} of soluble protein. The effect of pH on equilibrium binding of hCG by the soluble gonadotropin receptors was investigated over a wide pH range, and showed that maximum binding was attained at pH 7.4 upon incubation with [^{125}I]hCG for 16 hours at 4°C. The rate and extent of hormone binding were markedly influenced by temperature, but not by moderate variations in ionic strength of the assay medium (Dufau et al., 1973a).

1. Binding Constants of Soluble Testicular Receptors

The initial rate of hormone association with soluble receptors was more rapid at 24°C and 34°C than at 4°C, whereas maximum binding was much higher at 24°C and 4°C. This difference was shown by preincubation studies to result from increased receptor degradation at the higher temperature. Such binding studies indicated that the interaction between testis receptors and [^{125}I]hCG followed second-order kinetics at the concentrations used for binding assay, with association rate constant (K_a) of 6.1×10^5 M^{-1} min^{-1} at 4°C. Dissociation of the receptor–hormone complex was extremely slow, with first-order dissociation rate constant of 1.2×10^{-4} min^{-1} at 4°C. The slow dissociation of the complex facilitated fractionation and physicochemical studies of the soluble hormone–receptor complex (Dufau et al., 1973a, 1974b, 1975b; Charreau et al., 1974). The equilibrium binding constant of the Triton-solubilized receptors, determined from the association and dissociation rate constants at 4°C, was 0.5×10^{10} M^{-1}.

Equilibrium binding of [^{125}I]hCG by soluble testis receptors after incubation for 16 hours at 4°C, 24°C, and 34°C showed progressive binding inhibition in the presence of increasing concentrations of the unlabeled gonadotropin. The binding capacity of the soluble receptor preparation was significantly reduced when incubations were performed at 34°C, presumably as a result of the receptor degradation that occurred at the higher temperature. Analysis of the binding-inhibition curves, by conversion to Scatchard plots or saturation curves, showed the soluble testis receptors to behave as a single order of binding sites with association constant (K_a) of $0.6–1 \times 10^{10}$ M^{-1} at 4°C and 24°C, and 0.2 to 0.4×10^{10} M^{-1} at 34°C (Dufau et al., 1973a). Binding-inhibition curves obtained with the soluble receptor were similar to those observed during incubation of [^{125}I]hCG with rat testicular homogenate, and with the interstitial cell fraction from which the soluble receptor was extracted by treatment with Triton X-100. However, the association constant of the soluble receptor was reduced to about 50% of that of the original particulate preparation, and the binding capacity was also significantly reduced.

When the soluble free receptor preparation was stored for several hours, either by standing at 4°C for 16 hours or by dialysis against buffer containing 0.1% Triton, subsequent binding studies gave Scatchard plots consistent with two sets of binding sites. The major site was of similar affinity to that observed in the freshly prepared soluble receptors, with K_a of $0.6 \times 10^{10} M^{-1}$. However, a marked reduction of total binding sites occurred during storage, revealing the presence of a small number of high-affinity receptor sites with association constant of 3 to $4 \times 10^{10} M^{-1}$, similar to that of the original particulate receptor preparation. If aging of the preparation was extended for a further period of time, the lower-affinity site completely disappeared, leaving only a small quantity of high-affinity sites. This was demonstrated by binding studies on a preparation aged for 48 hours at 4°C which contained only receptors with (K_a $3 \times 10^{10} M^{-1}$) (Dufau and Catt, 1975). The lability of the solubilized receptor preparations during storage was much more marked for the free receptors than for the hormone–receptor complex. However, with further purification the free receptors were found to be relatively stable when kept at 0–4°C.

2. Physical Characteristics of Soluble Testicular Receptors

Extraction of particulate binding fractions of the rat testis was performed with various detergents, both before and after labeling the particulate receptor sites with [^{125}I]hCG *in vitro*. The soluble receptors and receptor–hormone complexes remaining in solution after centrifugation at $360,000 \times g$ for 1 hour were analyzed by gel filtration and sucrose density gradient centrifugation. The results of these studies and the physical properties of the solubilized testis receptors are summarized in Table II.

Fractionation of free receptors, and equilibrium mixtures of the hormone-receptor complex and free [^{125}I]hCG, was performed on columns of Sephadex G-200 and Sepharose 6B, equilibrated with Tris · HCl buffer containing 0.1% Triton X-100. The soluble receptor and receptor–hormone complex showed adsorption to Sepharose 6B during gel filtration, and were quantitatively bound by blue Dextran, presumably due to ionic interaction with the chromophore. For these reasons, blue Dextran could not be used as a front marker during gel filtration studies, and 0.01% bovine serum albumin was included in buffers employed for chromatography on Sepharose 6B. The distribu-

TABLE II

PHYSICAL CHARACTERISTICS OF DETERGENT-SOLUBILIZED GONADOTROPIN RECEPTORS[a]

Extraction procedure	Preparation	Sedimentation constant (S)	K_{av} Sepharose 6B	Stokes radius (Å)	Frictional ratio	Apparent MW
Triton X-100	Free receptor	6.5 ± 0.12 (3)	0.32 (3)	64	1.65	194,300
	Equilibrated receptor–hCG complex	7.5 ± 0.35 (5)	0.32 (5)	64	1.56	224,000
	Dialyzed 7.5 S receptor–hCG complex	8.8 (3)	0.27 (3)	74	—	—
	Preformed particulate hCG–receptor complex	8.8 ± 0.09 (10)	0.31 (3)	64	1.47	270,000
Lubrol WX	Preformed complex	7.0 (4)	0.26 (3)	77	1.87	236,200
Lubrol PX	Preformed complex	7.0 (3)	0.32 (3)	64	1.64	196,000
Triton X-100	hCG	2.9	0.56 (10)	34	1.4	38,000

[a] Values are the mean (±SD) of the number of observations in parentheses.

tion coefficient (K_{av}) of the receptor–hormone complex on Sephadex G-200 was 0.09, and that of free hCG was 0.33. On columns of Sepharose 6B, the K_{av} of the free receptors and the receptor–hormone complex was 0.32, and that of free hCG was 0.56 (Fig. 11). By reference to the behavior of standard proteins during gel filtration on Sepharose

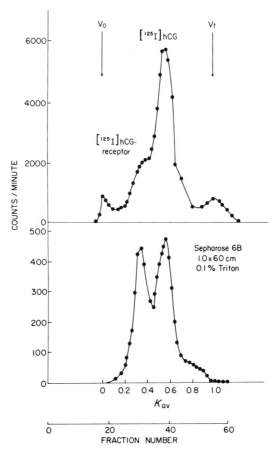

FIG. 11. Elution profile of hCG-receptor complex and free ^{125}I-labeled hCG during gel filtration on Sepharose 6B of the equilibrium mixture of soluble receptors and labeled hormone. A small peak of radioactivity was present at the void volume, coincident with a minor and constant peak of aggregated protein. The hCG receptor protein was eluted as a shoulder preceding the major peak of free hCG (below). Fractions corresponding to the hCG-receptor peak were pooled and concentrated 5-fold with Sephadex G-25. An aliquot was then subjected to gel filtration on Sepharose 6B. The elution profile shows two clearly separated radioactive peaks corresponding to free hCG and the hormone–receptor complex.

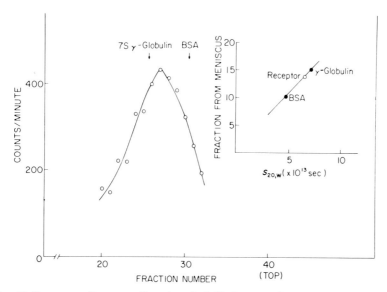

FIG. 12. Sucrose gradient centrifugation of soluble free gonadotropin receptor [^{125}I]hCG binding by gonadotropin receptor after sucrose gradient centrifugation (5–20% in 0.1% Triton). Bound radioactivity was determined by precipitation with polyethylene glycol. BSA, bovine serum albumin.

6B, the hydrodynamic radius of the receptor was calculated to be 64 Å. Sucrose density-gradient centrifugation showed that the sedimentation constant of the free receptor was 6.5 S (Fig. 12), and that of the hormone–receptor complex was 7.5 S (Fig. 13). Dialysis of the complex to reduce the concentration of Triton X-100 caused conversion to an 8.8 S form, but no aggregation of the complex was observed. The apparent molecular weights of the 6.5 S (free) and 7.5 S (combined) forms of the receptor, calculated by the method of Siegel and Monty (1966) were 194,000 and 224,000, respectively. The difference between the free and combined forms was consistent with binding of one molecule of gonadotropin by each molecule of the receptor. The frictional ratios of the receptor and the receptor–hormone complex were calculated to be 1.65 and 1.56, corresponding to prolate axial ratios of 12.0 and 10.2. These values suggest that the solubilized forms of the gonadotropin receptor exist in solution as highly asymmetric molecules (Dufau *et al.*, 1973a).

In addition to analysis of the unoccupied or free receptors described above, the properties of the receptor–hormone complex formed by incubation of testis particles with [^{125}I]hCG *in vitro* were also determined

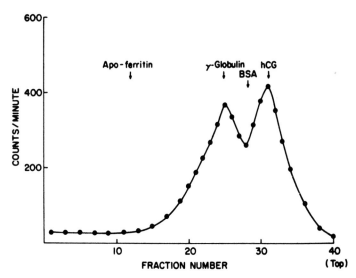

F‍IG. 13. Sucrose gradient centrifugation of the hormone–receptor complex previously fractionated on Sepharose 6B (see Fig. 11). Two discrete peaks of radioactivity were resolved, corresponding to free hCG (2.9 S) and the hormone–receptor complex (7.5 S), which was 98% precipitable with polyethylene glycol. Conditions: 3–20% gradient; 50 mM Tris-HCl buffer, 0.1% Triton; 16 hours at 170,000 g.

following extraction with Triton X-100, Lubrol PX, and Lubrol WX. Extraction of prelabeled testis particles with Triton X-100 gave only the 8.8 S form observed after dialysis of the 7.5 S complex formed in 0.1% Triton. However, the 8.8 S complex extracted from prelabeled particles aggregated during dialysis, and was converted to the 8.8 S form when reequilibrated with 0.1% Triton X-100. The increased sedimentation velocity of the 8.8 S form solubilized from prelabeled testis particles was indicative of a larger or less asymmetric species than that extracted from unlabeled particulate receptors (Charreau et al., 1974).

When the 8.8 S hormone–receptor complex was subjected to electrophoresis in 5% polyacrylamide gels containing 0.1% Triton X-100, a major symmetrical peak of radioactivity was observed with R_f of 0.30 (Fig. 14, left). The small peak of radioactivity at R_f 0.60 corresponded to [^{125}I]hCG dissociated from soluble receptor during the extraction and fractionation procedures. By this method, resolution of the receptor–hormone complex and free hormone could be obtained during electrophoresis of equilibrium mixtures, as shown in the right panel of Fig. 14. Such separations are of potential value to complement the results of

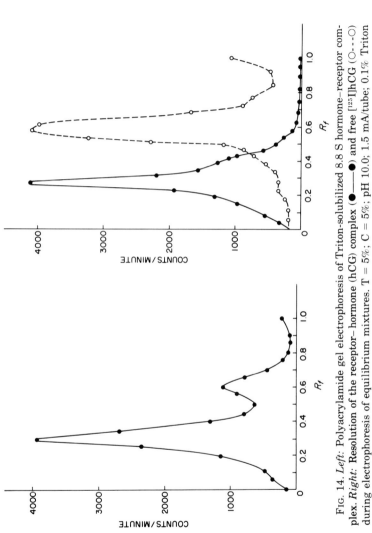

Fig. 14. *Left*: Polyacrylamide gel electrophoresis of Triton-solubilized 8.8 S hormone–receptor complex. *Right*: Resolution of the receptor–hormone (hCG) complex (●——●) and free [^{125}I]hCG (○--○) during electrophoresis of equilibrium mixtures. T = 5%; C = 5%; pH 10.0; 1.5 mA/tube; 0.1% Triton X-100.

sucrose density-gradient centrifugation and gel filtration, to provide a further estimate of the molecular radius and valence of the receptor, and to monitor the homogeneity of isolated receptor preparations. Staining procedures for proteins and glycoproteins in Triton-containing gels were complicated by the excessive background staining caused by dye binding to the detergent. The most satisfactory protein staining was achieved with Amido Schwarz followed by electrolytic destaining to remove the background dye-detergent complex.

Treatment of the 8.8 S form of the hormone–receptor complex with 0.5 M KCl did not dissociate the hormone from the soluble receptor, and did not cause the receptors to dissociate into smaller forms or subunits. However, exposure of the hormone–receptor complex to pH 3.5 or below for 1–5 minutes, by addition of acetic acid, immediately dissociated the hormone from the receptor sites. After exposure to pH 3.5 for 1 minute to dissociate the hormone–receptor complex, substantial reassociation occurred after neutralization to pH 7.4 and reincubation for 16 hours. The resulting hormone–receptor complex clearly differed from the original 8.8 S preparation, having acquired the sedimentation characteristics of the 7.5 S hormone–receptor complex. These results were of value in experiments on the purification of receptors, by providing a rapid and effective step for the dissociation of the free receptor from affinity columns with retention of hormone-binding activity. Exposure of the complexes to 2 M urea or guanidine HCl also caused complete dissociation of the hormone from receptor sites as determined by sucrose density-gradient centrifugation.

Extraction of prelabeled testis particles with Lubrol PX or WX yielded a 7 S complex which also aggregated reversibly upon dialysis. If extraction with detergents of the Lubrol series was performed as with Triton X-100, i.e., by incubation for 30 minutes with 1% solution of detergent, followed by dilution to 0.1%, the receptor–hormone complex underwent aggregation. The minimal detergent concentration required to prevent aggregation of the Lubrol-extracted receptor–hormone complex was 0.3%; at this concentration, the extracted complex showed sedimentation behavior identical with that of the preparation obtained using 1% Lubrol. Since the density of the 7 S Lubrol-extracted form of receptor complex was greater than that of the Triton-solubilized form, and the apparent fractional ratio was higher (1.6 versus 1.4 for the 8.8 S form), the lower sedimentation velocity of the Lubrol form in sucrose gradients probably reflected the extraction of a more highly asymmetric or lower molecular weight form of the receptor.

Extraction of the prelabeled testis particles with an ionic detergent, such as sodium deoxycholate, gave a hormone-receptor complex with sedimentation coefficient of 8.8–9 S, similar to that obtained by Triton X-100 extraction of prelabeled particles. When sodium dodecyl sulfate (SDS) (0.1–1%) was used for extraction, the sedimentation behavior of the soluble "hormone–receptor complex" in sucrose gradients could not be differentiated from that of the free hormone. Similar results were obtained using gel chromatography at several concentrations of SDS, suggesting that much or all of the SDS-extracted radioactivity represented free hCG, rather than a true hormone–receptor complex (Dufau *et al.*, 1974d).

The presence of a carbohydrate component in the solubilized receptors was suggested by the ability of concanavalin A to combine with the Triton-solubilized binding sites. When the soluble testicular preparation was applied to a column of Sepharose–concanavalin A (0.4 × 14 cm), binding activity was completely adsorbed by the gel. Initial washing of the column with PBS eluted most of the contaminating protein with only a minor fraction (5%) of the binding activity. The remainder of the free receptor could be eluted subsequently with 0.2 *M* methyl mannopyranoside as a broad peak of binding activity. This result indicated that the soluble receptors possess carbohydrate residues, such as mannose or other sugars with binding affinity for concanavalin A (see also Section VIII, D).

C. Solubilized Ovarian Gonadotropin Receptors

1. *Detergent-Solubilized Ovarian Receptors*

The properties of ovarian receptors solubilized with Triton X-100 and Lubrol PX have also been determined by gel filtration and sucrose density-gradient centrifugation (Dufau *et al.*, 1974b). The physical characteristics of the soluble ovarian receptors were almost identical with those of the testis receptors (Table III). In each case, the receptor behaved as an asymmetric molecule of about MW 200,000 and appeared to contain phospholipid and carbohydrate moieties in addition to the major binding protein. The ovarian receptors have been employed for comparative studies on the properties of the receptor–hormone complex labeled *in vivo* and *in vitro* with [^{125}I]hCG (Dufau *et al.*, 1975b). For these studies, PMSG/hCG-treated female rats with heavily luteinized ovaries were given 10 μCi of [^{125}I]hCG by intravenous injection. After 2 hours, when ovarian uptake of the tracer was 30–50%, the ovaries were removed and homogenized, and the 200–20,000 *g* fraction was extracted with 1% Triton X-100 or Lubrol PX.

TABLE III

COMPARISON OF PHYSICOCHEMICAL CHARACTERISTICS OF SOLUBILIZED
TESTICULAR AND OVARIAN RECEPTORS

Parameter	Ovarian receptors	Testicular receptors
Association constant (K_a)	$0.66 \times 10^{10}\,M^{-1}$	$0.60 \times 10^{10}\,M^{-1}$
Binding capacity	0.15×10^{-12} mol/mg protein	0.12×10^{-12} mol/mg protein
Stokes radius		
Free receptor	60 Å	64 Å
hCG-receptor complex formed after extraction	60 Å	64 Å
hCG-receptor complex extracted from prelabeled particles	71 Å	64 Å
Sedimentation constant		
Free receptor	6.0–6.8 S	6.5 S
hCG-receptor complex formed after extraction	7.5 S	7.5 S
hCG-receptor complex extracted from prelabeled particles	8.8 S	8.8 S
Density		
7.5 S hCG-receptor complex	1.283	1.289
8.8 S hCG-receptor complex	1.273	1.278
Binding to concanavalin A–Sepharose		
Free receptor	60% adsorbed	100% adsorbed

After centrifugation at 360,000 g for 1 hour, the clear supernatant solution was subjected to gel filtration on Sepharose 6B and to density-gradient centrifugation in 5–20% sucrose.

The elution pattern on Sepharose 6B of soluble *in vivo*-labeled receptors extracted by Lubrol PX was similar to that of the complex formed *in vitro*. No significant difference was observed between the K_{av} values of the two complexes, which corresponded to Stokes radii of 64 and 60 Å, respectively. Furthermore, the sucrose gradient centrifugation pattern of the *in vivo*-labeled Lubrol-extracted complex was identical with that of the complex formed *in vitro,* with sedimentation constant of 7 S (Fig. 15). The Triton-extracted form of the *in vivo*-labeled receptors also showed identical sedimentation behavior to that of the complex formed *in vitro,* with a sedimentation constant of 8.8 S (Fig. 16). The elution pattern on Sepharose 6B of the soluble *in vivo*-labeled receptor extracted with Triton X-100 gave a K_{av} of 0.32, similar to the *in vitro* form obtained with Triton X-100, and corresponding to a radius of 64 Å. These studies demonstrated that the physical forms of the gonadotropin receptor–hormone complex derived by solubilization of homoge-

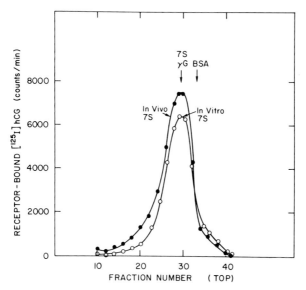

Fig. 15. Sucrose density-gradient (5–20%) centrifugation of the *in vivo* prelabeled ovarian receptors extracted with 0.5% Lubrol PX. The soluble complex migrated with a sedimentation constant of 7.0 S and was precipitable with 12% polyethylene glycol.

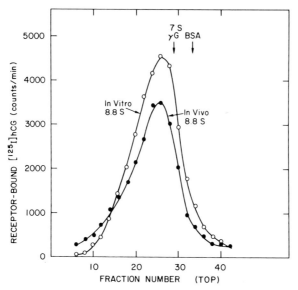

Fig. 16. Sucrose density-gradient (5–20%) centrifugation of the "*in vivo*" prelabeled ovarian receptors extracted with 0.1% Triton X-100. The soluble complex migrated with a sedimentation constant of 8.8 S and was precipitable with 12% polyethylene glycol.

nates labeled *in vivo* showed close identity with those formed by labeling the receptor sites with radioiodinated hCG *in vitro*.

The properties of Triton X-100 or Lubrol PX-solubilized ovarian receptors were also examined during fractionation on agarose-concanavalin A. In contrast with the behavior of the testis receptors, two species of the ovarian receptor were observed during the lectin-affinity chromatography step. About 50% of the binding activity was not adsorbed to the gel and was eluted by the washing buffer with most of the protein; the remainder of the receptors were adsorbed to the column and could be eluted with the competing sugar. Upon re-chromatography of the two fractions, the first peak again passed unadsorbed through the column, while the second peak that was initially adsorbed to the column had lost affinity for the lectin and was eluted by the washing buffer. The binding affinity of the two receptor species for hCG was almost identical, but the carbohydrate composition of these two species of receptors appeared to be different.

A notable feature of the detergent solubilization studies was the reproducibility with which the several forms of the receptor complex labeled *in vitro* or *in vivo* could be extracted under defined conditions by various detergents. Interpretation of the various forms of the gonadotropin receptors extracted from testis or ovarian particles was complicated by the differential effects of detergent binding and molecular conformation upon sedimentation velocity during density-gradient centrifugation in sucrose solutions. It is likely that changes in the symmetry or degree of association of the complexes are responsible for the multiplicity of forms detected under different conditions of detergent extraction. The glycoprotein nature of the ligand and a degree of asymmetry in the receptor molecule also contribute to the observed disparity between Stokes radius and sedimentation velocity, and combine to exaggerate the apparent asymmetry of the receptor–hormone complex as calculated from the hydrodynamic properties of the molecule.

2. *Lipid-Associated Ovarian Receptors*

In addition to the receptors solubilized from luteinized ovaries by detergents, ovarian homogenates prepared in the absence of detergents have also been found to contain a small proportion (<10%) of spontaneously soluble receptor sites (Conti *et al.*, 1976a, 1978). Such soluble receptors were present in the floating lipid fraction of the 360,000 *g* supernatant of homogenates prepared from luteinized ovaries, and could not be detected in similar fractions prepared from interstitial cells or homogenates of the rat testis. The physicochemical properties were, in general, similar to those of the detergent-solubilized receptors extracted with Triton X-100. The affinity constant of the spontaneously soluble ovarian receptor sites for [^{125}I]hCG was $0.70 \times 10^{10} M^{-1}$, and that of the receptors solubilized by Triton X-100 was $0.72 \times 10^{10} M^{-1}$. When the equilibrium mixture of soluble receptors and [^{125}I]hCG was subjected to Millipore filtration, no significant binding activity was retained on the filter, in contrast to the significant activity obtained by polyethylene glycol precipitation. The maximum binding capacity varied, as for the particulate and detergent-soluble gonadotropin receptor, with the time after treatment with gonadotropin to induce ovarian luteinization. The maximum binding capacity of 59 fmol/mg protein was reached 8–10 days after injection of PSMG. The sedimentation pattern of the soluble receptors during sucrose gradient centrifugation showed extensive aggregation into rapidly sedimenting forms. However, centrifugation of the spontaneously soluble receptor in the presence of Triton X-100 gave a single 6.5 S component, similar to the solubilized receptors previously characterized in detergent extracts of rat ovary and testis.

The lipid-associated soluble receptors appeared to be distinct from the predominant population of membrane-bound ovarian receptors. No increase in the ratio of soluble to particulate receptors was observed with progressively increasing degrees of homogenization, suggesting that the soluble receptors do not represent binding sites released from the membrane by homogenization. In fact, a slight decrease in ratio was observed, indicating that while the recovery of accessible particulate receptors was raised by increasingly vigorous homogenization, the number of soluble receptors remained fairly constant. This finding also indicated that the conditions of cell disruption did not significantly affect the release of the receptor molecules from the plasma membrane. When the presence of membrane contamination was evaluated by measuring the activity of membrane associated enzymes, it was not possible to demonstrate adenylate cyclase activity in the lipid-associated receptor fraction. The lipid-associated receptors could be derived from newly synthesized receptors in the process of incorporation into the plasma membrane. This explanation would be consistent with the increase in relative concentration of the soluble receptors soon after hormone treatment, and with the finding that they are not labeled *in vivo* by administered [^{125}I]hCG. Alternatively, the lipid-soluble receptors could represent binding sites that have been internalized from the plasma membrane and are undergoing metabolism or being otherwise processed within the cytoplasm. Perhaps the most likely origin is from the solubilizing effects of ovarian lipids upon the plasma membranes of the luteal cells during homogenization, leading to the formation of liposome-like particles that contain receptor-bearing regions of the cell membrane.

The presence of soluble receptor activity in the ovarian cytosol fraction could be relevant to the observation that gonadotropin binding-inhibition activity is present in the soluble fraction of the luteinized rat ovary (Yang et al., 1976). Since the soluble receptors remained in the free fraction during the procedure for the separation of the hormone bound to the particulate receptors, they can compete for gonadotropin during the binding reaction and thus behave as apparent inhibitors of gonadotropin binding activity. However, the quantitative contribution of the soluble receptors to the binding-inhibition activity of the cytosol must be quite small, and it is probable that hormone degradation and other factors are more significant in this regard.

D. PURIFICATION OF SOLUBILIZED LH/hCG RECEPTORS

Soluble gonadotropin receptors for purification studies were prepared from interstitial cell particles by extraction with 1% Triton X-100 for 30 minutes at 4°C. The suspension was then diluted to 0.1% Triton with phosphate-buffered saline pH 7.4 (PBS), and centrifuged at 360,000 g for 1 hour at 4°C. The clear supernatant solution contained the majority (about 90%) of the gonadotropin binding sites solubilized from particulate fractions previously equilibrated with I-hCG. However, when particulate receptor sites in the free or unoccupied form were solubilized with detergents, only 10–20% of the original activity was detectable in the supernatant solution. Thus, the yields of soluble receptors from the original content of about 1 pmol per testis were usually about 150 fmol per testis (Dufau et al., 1975a).

Affinity chromatography media for isolation of the LH/hCG receptors were prepared by coupling partially purified hCG to agarose beads by a number of conjugation procedures. In experiments performed with hCG coupled directly to cyanogen bromide-activated Sepharose or to Sepharose–concanavalin A, the uptake of gonadotropin receptors from solution by hCG substitute gel was almost complete. However, relatively poor recovery of receptor-binding activity was obtained during subsequent elution of agarose-hCG under a variety of dissociating conditions. In the case of receptors adsorbed by Sepharose–concanavalin A, elution of receptor sites from the gel was readily performed with mannopyranoside, but a considerable quantity of contaminating protein was eluted together with the peak of binding activity. In addition, a significant proportion of the binding activity was lost during this procedure, and only a modest degree of purification was achieved (Dufau and Catt, 1976b). The most satisfactory medium for affinity chromatography was the gel–gonadotropin complex prepared by conjugation of hCG to agarose beads bearing a 10 Å aliphatic chain terminating in N-hydroxysuccinimide ester (Affigel 10, Bio-Rad). Of the elution procedures tested, dissociation of the hormone–receptor complex at low pH, previously observed to release gonadotropin bound to particulate and soluble testis receptors (Dufau et al., 1972c; Charreau et al., 1974), was found to give the highest and most consistent yield of soluble gonadotropin receptor sites. An example of the elution of receptor sites from the gel–gonadotropin conjugate is shown in Fig. 17.

By contrast with the original crude receptor solution, the purified LH receptors were quite stable and showed no loss of binding activity during storage in solution for 3 days at 4°C (Fig. 18). In addition, the purified receptors retained full binding activity after lyophilization and storage at −60°C for up to 8 weeks. Binding studies performed upon the lyophilized receptors showed retention of specificity for LH and hCG, and no significant crossreaction with other peptide and

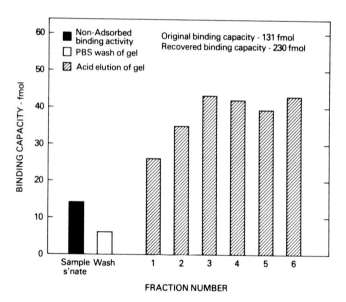

FIG. 17. Adsorption and elution of gonadotropin receptors on agarose–hCG. The first two columns show the binding capacities of the unadsorbed applied fraction and the buffer eluate, respectively. The hatched bars represent the binding activity of receptors eluted with 0.025 M acetic acid.

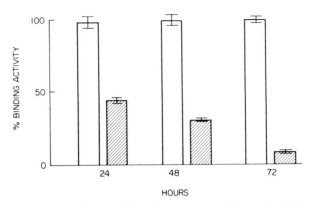

F<small>IG</small>. 18. Stability of binding activity of affinity-purified receptor (open bars) and solubilized particulate receptor (hatched bars).

glycoprotein hormones. Analysis of equilibrium binding data by direct fitting of the saturation curve, or by Scatchard plots, confirmed the presence of a single order of binding sites with high affinity ($10^{10}\,M^{-1}$) for hCG. The sedimentation constant of the complex formed after binding of ^{125}I-labeled hCG by the purified receptor was determined to be 7.5 S, by sucrose density-gradient centrifugation performed in the presence or the absence of 0.1% Triton. The receptor purified by affinity chromatography showed no aggregation during density-gradient centrifugation in the absence of Triton X-100, by contrast with the crude receptor, which consistently aggregated into more rapidly sedimenting forms after reduction of detergent concentration by extensive dialysis (Charreau *et al.*, 1974).

The hCG binding capacity of the receptors recovered by acid elution from the hCG-agarose medium was about 220 pmol/per milligram of protein. However, the anticipated binding capacity of the purified receptors, based on a molecular weight of 200,000, would be close to 5000 pmol/mg. Thus a further purification of 20- to 25-fold would be necessary to approach homogeneity. Analytical gel electrophoresis of the first two acid-eluted fractions revealed the presence of contaminating proteins that were not present in the subsequent receptor-containing eluates. When the initial fractions were discarded to remove these nonreceptor proteins, the specific activity of the pooled subsequent fractions rose to 2500 pmol/mg, corresponding to a purification factor of about 15,000 from the original material (Table IV). This degree of purification is equivalent to 50% homogeneity of the receptor isolated by affinity chromatography and illustrates the value of this procedure for isolation of hormone receptor sites (Dufau *et al.*, 1975a). The most highly purified receptor preparation was demonstrated by SDS–polyacrylamide gel electrophoresis to migrate as a single component, with appropriate MW of 90,000 by comparison with standard proteins and correction for the possible effects of hydrophobicity. This finding suggests that the detergent-extracted free receptor, of MW 194,200, could consist of a dimer composed of two 90,000 MW subunits. Further analysis of the properties of the receptor sites purified by affinity chromatography should provide insight into the mechanisms of receptor activation during hormone occupancy and the functional relationship between binding sites and membrane-associated enzyme systems.

An identical procedure was amenable for purification of ovarian LH receptors. However, with this tissue only a final 3000-fold purification was achieved after a single passage through the affinity chromatographic column. The K_a of the purified ovarian receptor for hCG was $0.29 \times 10\ M^{-1}$ (Fig. 19, right) comparable to the affinity observed for the original particulate receptors, of $0.75 \times 10^{10}\ M^{-1}$ (Fig. 19, left). The abundance of LH receptors in the luteal tissue (1 luteinized ovary being equivalent to 5 testes) suggests that this tissue may be preferable for large-scale purification. In contrast, the spontaneously lipid-soluble receptor was poorly adsorbed to the affinity column, probably owing to interference by lipid in the interaction between receptors and matrix-bound hormone (Conti *et al.*, 1975, 1978). In any case, the spontaneously soluble sites constituted only a small proportion of the total receptor population and cannot be regarded as a potential source of receptor for purification.

E. Properties of Soluble FSH Receptors

Extraction and fractionation of FSH receptors has been rendered difficult by the relatively low binding observed in particulate and solu-

TABLE IV
LH/hCG Receptor Purification

Receptor preparation	Specific activity (cpm/mg)	Binding capacity (pmol/ml)
Triton-solubilized particles	2.07×10^3	0.15
From affinity column	3.13×10^7	2546[a]
Pure receptor		5000[b]

[a] Purification factor: 15,000.
[b] For complete purity: 30,000.

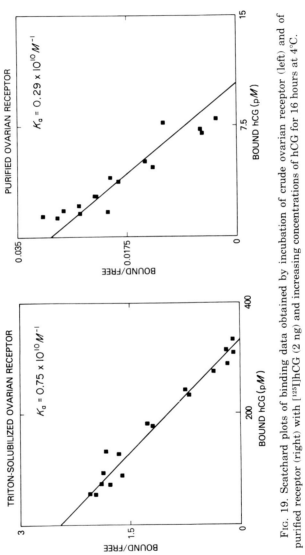

FIG. 19. Scatchard plots of binding data obtained by incubation of crude ovarian receptor (left) and of purified receptor (right) with [^{125}I]hCG (2 ng) and increasing concentrations of hCG for 16 hours at 4°C.

ble FSH preparations. Solubilization of rat testis FSH receptors has been most efficiently performed by extraction of the 27,000 g homogenate from 21-day-old rats with 1% Triton X-100 (Catt et al., 1976; Dufau et al., 1977d). This detergent extracted 20–40% of the prelabeled FSH receptor sites, whereas other nonionic detergents, such as Lubrol PX or WX, and ionic detergents, such as sodium deoxycholate, were less effective. For binding studies, the soluble receptor preparation was incubated for 16 hours at 22°C, and separation of hormone–receptor complex and free hormone was performed by polyethylene glycol precipitation as described for soluble LH/hCG receptor-binding studies. The detergent-solubilized receptors exhibited a 5-fold increase in binding affinity for [^{125}I]hFSH, to a mean K_a of 8.5×10^9 M^{-1}, and the concentration of sites was 8.2×10^{-15} mol mg^{-1} protein. In addition to the receptors solubilized by detergent treatment, water-soluble high-affinity receptors for [^{125}I]FSH were demonstrated in the testis homogenates. The K_a of the water-soluble receptor was $1.17 \times 10^9 M^{-1}$, similar to that of the particulate receptor (1.55 ± 0.6 [SD] $\times 10^9 M^{-1}$) and their concentration was 4.6×10^{-15} mol mg^{-1} protein. Such receptors represented about 20% of the total receptor population and were not retained during filtration through 0.45 μm Millipore membranes.

The detergent-extracted FSH receptors from rat testis could not be analyzed by gel filtration in the free form, but were readily observed as the hormone–receptor complex when extracted from particles previously labeled with [^{125}I]hFSH. The partition coefficient of the Triton-soluble hormone–receptor complex on 6% agarose was 0.30 with Stokes radius of about 65 Å, similar to that of detergent-solubilized receptors for luteinizing hormone (Fig. 20). The dissociation of free ^{125}I-labeled hFSH from the hormone–receptor complex during gel filtration was in contrast with the tight binding observed during analytical studies of the testicular and ovarian LH receptors (Dufau et al., 1973a; 1975b; Charreau et al., 1974). Since the equilibrium binding constants of the two solubilized receptors were quite similar, the more rapid dissociation of the FSH-receptor complex implied a significantly higher dissociation rate constant for the FSH receptor site.

Recent studies have indicated that immature calf testes are a rich source of FSH receptors (Cheng, 1975a; Abou-Issa and Reichert, 1977). The particulate receptors had a binding capacity of 5.2×10^{-13} mol mg^{-1} protein. These values were considerably higher than those of the developing calf, 1.6×10^{-13} mol mg^{-1} protein; mature beef 1.2×10^{14} mol mg^{-1} protein and immature 1.7×10^{-14} mol mg^{-1} protein. Solubilization of this receptor was achieved as in the rat by extraction with Triton X-100. The detergent-solubilized receptors had a high affinity

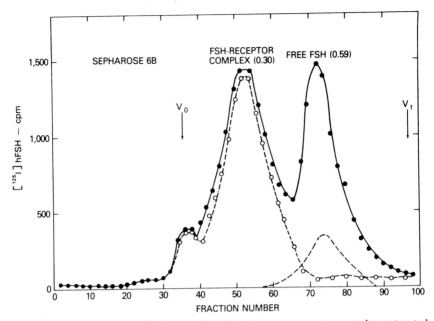

Fig. 20. Gel filtration on Sepharose 6B of the hormone–receptor complex extracted with Triton X-100 from testis receptors labeled with [^{125}I]hFSH. Two discrete peaks of radioactivity were resolved: (●) corresponding to free [^{125}I]FSH (K_{av} 0.59) and the hormone–receptor complex (K_{av} 0.30), which was 98% precipitable by polyethylene glycol (○). The hormone–receptor complex was not present when the preceding incubation with ^{125}I-labeled FSH was performed in the presence of excess FSH (–).

for hFSH ($K_a = 2.1 \times 10^9\ M^{-1}$), about 2-fold greater than the association constant for the particulate receptor in this species. A marked reduction of binding capacity, to 35% of the capacity of the starting particulate fraction, was observed upon detergent solubilization. The Stokes radius of the solubilized receptor was estimated to be 47 Å and that of the hormone–receptor complex was 50 Å, with sedimentation coefficients of 6.3 S and 7.4 S, respectively. The sedimentation behavior of the calf FSH receptor was quite similar to that observed for the LH/hCG receptors of the Leydig cells, but the Stokes radius was somewhat different from that of the rat FSH and LH hormone–receptor complexes. The calculated molecular weight was 146,000 for the free receptor and 183,000 for the hormone–receptor complex. Addition of millimolar concentrations of nucleotides was found to reduce the binding of ^{125}I-labeled hFSH and to enhance the dissociation of bound hormone form from its receptor in both particulate and soluble calf testis preparations (Abou-Issa and Reichert, 1977).

The detection and analysis of soluble FSH receptors depends upon the use of optimal tracer preparations for binding studies. These can be obtained by lactoperoxidase radioiodination and concanavalin A fractionation, followed by receptor-affinity chromatography, i.e., binding of [^{125}I]hFSH to particulate FSH receptor sites followed by elution of the active tracer at low pH (Ketelslegers and Catt, 1974). The use of less purified tracer preparations is attended by considerable difficulty in the demonstration of soluble FSH receptors (Dufau et al., 1977d). A common feature of soluble FSH receptors from rat or calf testis is their increase in affinity by 5- and 2-fold upon solubilization in the presence of detergent. Such increases have been described also for the prolactin receptors solubilized with Triton X-100 from rabbit mammary glands and liver (Shiu and Friesen, 1974). In contrast, the LH/hCG receptors solubilized from rat testis (Dufau et al., 1973a) and ovary (Dufau et al., 1974b) exhibited lower affinity for hCG than the original particulate receptors. Another common feature of the rat and calf FSH receptors is their binding characteristics, with maximal binding at 24°C and attainment of equilibrium at 4–6 hours. Also, binding remained maximum for up to 20 hours without indication of tracer or receptor degradation. In contrast, binding at 4°C was quite low and did not reach equilibrium when incubation was continued for up to 48 hours. In all cases, low binding was observed during incubations at 37°C owing to receptor and tracer degradation.

The water-soluble FSH receptor described above has only been described in the rat testis, and the nature of the water-soluble sites has yet to be determined. This minor fraction of the receptor population could represent newly synthesized molecules in the process of being incorporated in the cell membrane, or membrane receptors that have undergone internalization as a consequence of membrane turnover. It is also possible that these receptors are loosely attached to the membrane and are rendered soluble during the initial homogenization procedure. Further analysis of these receptors could be complicated by their relatively low association constant and low concentration in the testis. However, the detergent-solubilized FSH receptors are more amenable to further characterization, and should be of value for more detailed studies on the molecular interaction between FSH and specific receptor sites. The calf testis is the most abundant source of FSH receptors yet described and should be particularly suitable for purification of the FSH receptor sites.

F. PROPERTIES AND PURIFICATION OF PROLACTIN RECEPTORS

Prolactin and lactogenic hormone receptors have been solubilized by Triton X-100 from crude membrane fractions isolated from pregnant rabbit mammary glands (Shiu and Friesen, 1974). During studies on receptor solubilization, the ^{125}I-ovine prolactin tracer used in particulate receptor binding studies was found to be altered by Triton X-100. This change was attributed to binding of detergent and micelle formation, and gave an apparent molecular weight of 80,000 instead of the 23,000 exhibited by prolactin in aqueous solution. Also, the iodinated ovine prolactin was found to be precipitated by polyethylene glycol. For these reasons, ^{125}I]hGH was employed as tracer during equilibrium binding studies of soluble prolactin receptors and during characterization of the receptor–hormone complex. The sedimentation and gel filtration properties of hGH were not affected by detergent, and the double polyethylene glycol precipitation initially described for LH/hCG receptors (Dufau and Catt, 1973) could be employed for separation of bound and free tracer.

The soluble receptor was found to retain the specificity of the particulate receptor, and Scatchard analysis demonstrated that the affinity of the soluble receptors (K_a $16 \times 10^9 M^{-1}$) was 5-fold increased above that of the particulate receptor. Binding studies were performed at 23°C, since at this temperature the specific binding reached equilibrium at 6 hours and no degradation of receptors or tracer was observed. In contrast, binding studies performed at 4°C did not reach equilibrium until almost 60 hours had elapsed. Most of the characterization studies were performed on partially purified receptors prepared by affinity chromatography on hGH–Affigel 10, in parallel to the crude soluble receptor preparation. During fractionation of partially purified receptors on Sepharose 6B, the hormone–receptor complex and free receptors were eluted with K_{av}'s of 0.38 and 0.40, and similar elution patterns were observed with the crude soluble material. Molecular weights were calculated on the basis of gel filtration properties to be 220,000 and 240,000 for the free and hormone-bound receptors, respectively. The mammary glands of pseudopregnant rabbits were quite abundant in prolactin receptors, with binding capacity of 2.5×10^{-14} mol mg^{-1} protein. The availability of large quantities of tissue, with receptors distributed in most of the mammary gland, facilitated the purification of this receptor.

For isolation of soluble prolactin receptors, Triton X-100 extracts of membranes prepared from 100 gm of fresh mammary tissue were passed through a 5-ml column bed of the adsorbent, hGH–Affigel 10. The column was initially washed with 20 bed volumes of buffer containing detergent (0.1% Triton), which eluted most of the protein and none of the adsorbed receptor activity. The receptors attached to the affinity gel were eluted by 5 M MgCl$_2$ in buffer-detergent, followed by extensive dialysis and concentration of the pooled receptor preparation. Purification of 140- to 200-fold was achieved in a single column purification and a final purification of 1100- to 1600-fold was obtained with a yield of approximately 8%. Analysis of the purified receptor by gel electrophoresis revealed several bands of stained protein, one of which was coincident with the peak of receptor activity at R_f 0.12. The presence of several protein bands on gel electrophoresis, and the final binding capacity, revealed that the purified receptor was less than 10% pure. However, such preparations were employed successfully to raise antibodies to the receptor sites by immunization of guinea pigs (Shiu and Friesen, 1976).

Such guinea pig antiserum to prolactin receptors, purified from rat mammary glands of pregnant rabbit by affinity chromatography, inhibited binding of ^{125}I-labeled prolactin to its membrane receptor and of ^{125}I-labeled growth hormone to soluble prolactin receptor preparations. The antireceptor sera also blocked the effect of prolactin on incorporation of [3H]leucine into casein of mammary tissue in organ culture. The same antibodies had no effect on insulin-stimulated amino acid transport and glucose oxidation in mammary tissue and did not appear to bind prolactin. Also, the prolactin-dependent transport of [14C]aminoisobutyric acid was completely abolished by the receptor antiserum, as shown by blockade of the additive effect of prolactin on stimulation of amino acid uptake induced by insulin. The ability of the antiserum to inhibit these actions of prolactin indicated that the specific antibody was directed only to the prolactin receptor and did not have a general effect on membrane-mediated functions.

VIII. Detergent-Solubilized Adenylate Cyclase and Receptors

A. Properties of Gonadal Adenylate Cyclase

In testis homogenates or Leydig-cell particles, adenylate cyclase activity was readily demonstrable by fluoride stimulation, yet the responses to LH and hCG were relatively small and inconstant. That testicular adenylate cyclase is highly responsive to gonadotropin in the intact Leydig cell is shown by the marked cAMP responses of testis tissue and dispersed interstitial cells to picogram and nanogram concentrations of gonadotropin in vitro (Catt and Dufau, 1973a; Dufau et al., 1973b, 1977c; Catt et al., 1974; Mendelson et al., 1975a). The response of ovarian homogenates to gonadotropin stimulation is more readily demonstrable than that of testis particles and is consistently evoked under assay conditions in which testicular preparations show a small or negligible response to LH and hCG. However, the ovarian cyclase is also quite sensitive to physical treatment, and enzyme activity is reduced unless homogenization is kept to a minimum during tissue disruption.

Studies on the activation of adenylate cyclase in particulate testis preparations showed increases of 8- to 10-fold over basal levels in the presence of 10 mM fluoride. The stimulation of adenylate cyclase produced by hCG or ovine LH was usually quite small in comparison to the fluoride response, but was statistically significant and demonstrable by both conversion from [α-^{32}P]ATP and by radioimmunoassay of cAMP produced from unlabeled ATP (Dufau *et al.*, 1977a). The possibility that vesicle formation during preparation of the particulate fraction could limit the availability of substrate during the enzyme assay was examined. For this purpose, Leydig-cell particles were prepared in the presence and absence of 5 mM MgATP. When assayed in the presence of ATP in the standard incubation system, each preparation showed a small but significant stimulation of adenylate cyclase in the presence of ovine LH (1 μg/ml) while a 50-fold stimulation was observed in the presence of fluoride. That the preparation of testis particles in the presence of ATP did not improve the subsequent response to gonadotropin indicated that the small response to LH was not attributable to inaccessibility of substrate during the enzyme assay.

B. SOLUBILIZATION OF GONADAL· ADENYLATE CYCLASE

Exposure of particulate gonadal fractions to nonionic detergents, including Triton X-100, Lubrol PX, and Lubrol WX, caused significant enhancement of the adenylate cyclase activity of the testicular preparations, both basal and fluoride-stimulated. This enhancement was clearly more marked with Lubrol WX and Lubrol PX than with Triton X-100. The soluble fraction obtained by centrifugation of the detergent-treated particles at 360,000 g for 3 hours contained a major proportion (about 60%) of the enzyme activity originally demonstrable in the particles assayed in the presence of detergent. However, the solubilized testicular adenylate cyclase was no longer stimulated by trophic hormone. When the effect of various Lubrol PX concentrations upon the basal and fluoride-stimulated activities of the soluble enzyme was examined, the optimal detergent level was found to be 0.5%, and this concentration was used for most of the subsequent studies. An increase in basal enzyme activity and a marked elevation of fluoride-stimulated activity was also observed in soluble preparations in the presence of 0.25–1% Lubrol PX (Fig. 21). The recovery of fluoride-stimulated adenylate cyclase activity in soluble gonadal extracts prepared with 0.5% Lubrol PX ranged from 50 to 70% of the enzyme activity of particles assayed in the presence of the detergents.

In experiments carried out with ovarian particles prepared from the luteinized gonads of PMSG/hCG-treated immature female rats, detergent treatment and solubilization did not consistently increase adenylate cyclase activity over the values obtained with the original particulate fraction, in contrast to the marked detergent effect upon testis preparations. A small but significant degree of stimulation of enzyme activity by LH was demonstrable in the 360,000 g supernate after solubilization of ovarian particles with Lubrol PX. The retention of hormone-responsiveness in the detergent-solubilized ovarian preparation was not constant, being demonstrable in 5 of 10 experiments performed with solubilized ovarian particles (Dufau *et al.*, 1976b, 1977a). Since retention of hormone responsiveness by detergent-solubilized adenylate cyclase is relatively uncommon, the soluble ovarian preparation may be useful for studies of the ovarian receptor complex, particularly suitable for analysis of the physical and functional relationships between peptide hormone binding sites and adenylate cyclase in solution.

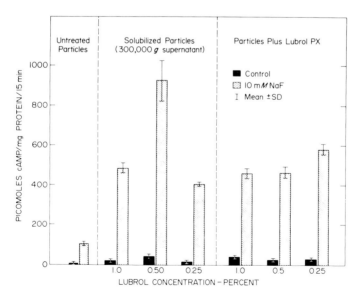

FIG. 21. Extraction of adenylate cyclase from testis by various concentrations of Lubrol PX.

The ability of nonionic detergents to extract soluble adenylate cyclase has been previously noted in several tissues (Sutherland *et al.*, 1962; Levey, 1970; Stansfield and Franks, 1971; Johnson and Sutherland, 1971). Such detergents have been found to enhance the activity of the particulate enzyme from cerebellum and cerebral cortex (Johnson and Sutherland, 1971; Perkins and Moore, 1971). However, in contrast to the interstitial cell enzyme, the activity of detergent-treated enzyme of the rat cerebral cortex was not stimulated by sodium fluoride (Perkins and Moore, 1971).

The mechanism by which adenylate cyclase activity is increased in certain tissues by detergent treatment or extraction is not known, but at least part of the effect could be due to an inhibitory action upon substrate degradation by ATPase during enzyme assay. Testicular particles possess high ATPase activity, which is inhibited or destroyed by detergents and by storage at 2–4°C, and can cause rapid loss of the ATP substrate during adenylate cyclase assay. For this reason, it is possible that the enzyme reaction could become substrate-dependent if ATP levels decreased during the reaction, even though such a reduction was not severe enough to cause nonlinearity of the initial velocity curve. Therefore, the possibility that a proportion of the detergent effect upon adenylate cyclase activity in testis particles resulted from inhibition of ATPase activity cannot be excluded. Likewise, the stimulation of detergent-treated particles and solubilized enzyme by sodium fluoride could also contain a component attributable to further inhibition of ATPase activity by fluoride. However, the effect of 10 mM sodium fluoride in this regard is probably very small, since the ATPase activity of testicular particles is only partially inhibited by sodium fluoride concentrations as high as 100 mM.

Other reports on the hormonal responsiveness of solubilized adenylate cyclase preparations have indicated that retention of hormone sensitivity is a variable and unpredictable phenomenon. Studies upon soluble adenylate cyclase derived from cat myocardium have shown that responsiveness to hormonal stimulation by glucagon or epinephrine was lost after solubilization, but could be regained after removal of detergent and addition of specific phospholipids (Levey, 1972; Levey *et al.*, 1974). In addition, observations on solubilized adenylate cyclase from the renal medulla (Neer, 1973) have shown that the enzyme in detergent did not respond to stimulation with vasopressin. However, removal of Lubrol PX with DEAE-cellulose partially restored the hormone responsiveness, and addition of purified phospholipids was not required for the response of the soluble enzyme to vasopressin. Reports on the properties of solubilized liver membranes (Ryan and Storm,

1974) and renal cortex membranes (Queener *et al.*, 1975) have described stimulation of soluble adenylate cyclase in the presence of detergents by glucagon and calcitonin, respectively.

C. EFFECTS OF MAGNESIUM AND MANGANESE ON GONADAL ADENYLATE CYCLASE

The effects of increasing concentrations of Mg^{2+} and Mn^{2+} on basal and fluoride-stimulated adenylate cyclase were evaluated in particulate and soluble gonadal preparations (Dufau *et al.*, 1976b, 1977a). In testis particles, addition of Mn^{2+} produced a marked increase in both basal and fluoride-stimulated adenylate cyclase activities, by comparison with incubations performed in the presence of Mg^{2+}. Also, when detergent-solubilized testis particles were incubated with Mn^{2+}, both basal and fluoride-stimulated cyclase activities were again much higher than those observed with Mg^{2+}. The adenylate cyclase response to fluoride activation was maximum over the range 1–2 mM Mn^{2+} and showed a significant decrease at higher concentrations (Fig. 22). By contrast, fluoride-stimulated enzyme activity increased progressively in the presence of increasing concentrations of Mg^{2+}, but did not reach the levels measured in the presence of Mn^{2+}. No response of testicular adenylate cyclase to LH was demonstrable in the presence of detergent.

The rate of cAMP formation in testis preparations exposed to detergent (both detergent-treated particulate and soluble preparations), studied over a period of 30 minutes in the presence or absence of fluoride or trophic hormone in the presence of 2 mM Mn^{2+}, showed a marked increase of enzyme activity after 2 minutes of incubation, and the reaction remained linear for at least 30 minutes. The K_m of the basal and fluoride-stimulated enzyme for ATP in the Lubrol-treated particulate preparations was 0.40 and 0.43 mM, respectively, and was 0.20 and 0.23 mM for the completely soluble preparations.

In contrast with the testis preparation, ovarian adenylate cyclase activity in particulate and solubilized fractions did not show a marked enhancement of basal activity when Mn^{2+} was added to the incubation mixture. Increasing Mn^{2+} concentrations produced a progressive increase in fluoride-stimulated enzyme activity, which was optimal from 4 to 8 mM Mn^{2+} (Table V). Although low concentrations of Mn^{2+} (0.5–1 mM) were as effective as higher concentrations of Mg^{2+} (2–4 mM), the effects of both cations were similar at concentrations of 4–8 mM. Hormonal activation of particulate adenylate cyclase was again consistently observed in the presence of ovine LH (1 μg/ml, about 10^{-7} M), and was of similar extent in the presence of either Mn^{2+} or Mg^{2+}. The

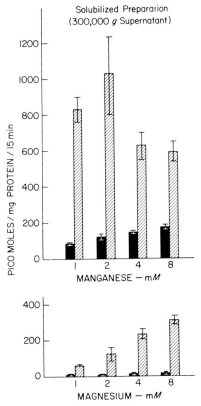

FIG. 22. Effects of Mn^{2+} and Mg^{2+} upon adenylate cyclase activity in particulate and solubilized testicular preparation.

TABLE V

ADENYLATE CYCLASE ACTIVITY IN OVARIAN PARTICULATE HOMOGENATES[a]

Cation concentration (mM)	Control		10 mM NaF		oLH (1 μg/ml)	
	Mg^{2+}	Mn^{2+}	Mg^{2+}	Mn^{2+}	Mg^{2+}	Mn^{2+}
0.5	—	36 ± 5	—	132 ± 6	—	93 ± 4
1	17 ± 4	61 ± 8	63 ± 9	247 ± 27	39 ± 4	127 ± 8
2	41 ± 3	58 ± 10	269 ± 26	262 ± 11	76 ± 8	93 ± 10
4	52 ± 5	72 ± 11	395 ± 30	344 ± 10	116 ± 10	127 ± 2
8	73 ± 10	78 ± 2	398 ± 19	454 ± 20	81 ± 8	95 ± 8
No cation	25 ± 8		71 ± 6		84 ± 7	

[a] Picomoles of cAMP per milligram of protein in 15 minutes (mean $\pm$ SD, $n = 4$).

soluble ovarian enzyme was also equally responsive to Mn^{2+} and Mg^{2+}, and showed an inconsistent response to ovine LH as noted above (Dufau et al., 1977a).

It is of interest that, in all experiments with the testis enzyme, addition of Mn^{2+} produced a marked increase in the basal and fluoride-stimulated activities when compared with incubations performed in the presence of Mg^{2+}. The replacement of Mg^{2+} by Mn^{2+} as a divalent cation requirement of adenylate cyclase is well recognized, and in certain tissues the enzyme activity at low Mn^{2+} concentrations is higher than that obtained with comparable Mg^{2+} concentrations. However, Mn^{2+} does not enhance hormone-stimulated enzyme activity, and in some cases inhibits activation of adenylate cyclase by peptide hormones (Perkins, 1973).

D. FRACTIONATION OF RECEPTORS AND ADENYLATE CYCLASE

To examine the physical relationship between solubilized adenylate cyclase and gonadotropin receptors, Lubrol-solubilized extracts from rat testis and ovary were analyzed by gel filtration on Sepharose 6B, and by other fractionation techniques. After gel filtration in the presence of the detergent, the fractions eluted from the column were assayed for receptor-binding activity with ^{125}I-labeled hCG, and for adenylate cyclase activity in the presence of 2 mM Mn^{2+} or 8 mM Mg^{2+} for testicular and ovarian soluble preparation, respectively. In this way, the elution profile of "free" or unoccupied receptor sites could be compared with that of the soluble enzyme activity. In all cases, recovery of adenylate cyclase activity after gel filtration was relatively small, unless fractionation was performed in the presence of 10 mM NaF. However, in several experiments with solubilized testis or ovarian particles, a peak of binding activity with K_{av} of 0.32–0.33 was consistently accompanied by a small peak of adenylate cyclase activity. Also, a minor peak of enzyme and binding activity was eluted at the void volume. The enzyme activity in column eluates was not further stimulated by fluoride (Fig. 23). An additional peak of gonadotropin binding activity was eluted with K_{av} of 0.51. This binding peak of lower molecular weight was not accompanied by adenylate cyclase activity. The presence of such smaller molecular species of the binding site was not observed during earlier studies on solubilization of testis and ovary receptors by Triton X-100 which demonstrated only a single peak with K_{av} 0.36 on Sepharose 6B and sedimentation constant of 6.5 S on sucrose density-gradient centrifugation. The second peak of binding activity could result from a dissociating effect of Lubrol during extraction of

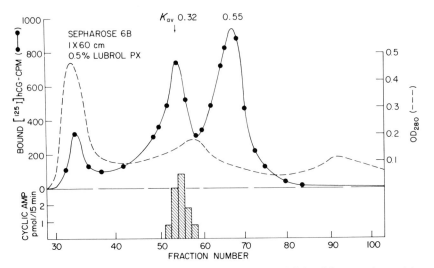

F_IG. 23. Gel filtration on Sepharose 6B of free receptor solubilized from testis particles in the absence of NaF with 0.5% Lubrol PX. Binding activity of the column profile (●), and adenylate cyclase activity in the presence of 8 mM Mg (crosshatched bars) were simultaneously determined in aliquots of eluent fraction.

the unoccupied gonadotropin receptors, and possibly represents a receptor subunit bearing the hormone binding site that became separated from the receptor dimer during detergent extraction and gel filtration of the soluble preparation. During Sepharose 6B fractionation of Lubrol-solubilized preparations, prepared in the presence of fluoride to preserve adenylate cyclase activity, the lower molecular weight peak of receptor-binding activity was not observed (Fig. 24). Instead, most of the binding activity was eluted as a broad peak of K_{av} 0.31 that embraced the narrow and symmetrical peak of enzyme activity with K_{av} 0.29. As in the column fractionations performed in the absence of fluoride, a smaller peak of binding and enzyme activity was eluted at the void volume. However, the more retarded peak of binding activity was not observed in fluoride-pretreated soluble receptors.

   The coincident elution of gonadotropin receptors and adenylate cyclase activity during gel filtration suggested that the soluble receptor molecule may exist as a loose complex containing both the hormone binding site and the cyclase enzyme. Alternatively, the receptor-binding site and adenylate cyclase activity could be physically separate but coincident during gel filtration on Sepharose 6B. To examine these possibilities, further resolution of soluble testicular and ovarian preparations was pursued by additional fractionation techniques (Dufau *et al.*, 1978b). During group-specific affinity chromatography on concanavalin A, testicular receptor sites were eluted separately from the corresponding adenylate cyclase activity. The enzyme was not adsorbed by the affinity column, and it eluted with most of the protein in the soluble preparation, while all of the receptor binding activity was adsorbed to the column and could be subsequently eluted by the competing sugar (Fig. 25). Both adenylate cyclase and gonadotropin receptor activities were recovered with high yield, because column fractionation was performed rapidly and the gonadal particles were treated with 10 mM sodium fluoride prior to solubilization. In previous experiments, the enzyme was found to be extremely labile, and recovery of cyclase activity was small after fractionation on Sepharose 6B; also, the soluble adenylate cyclase lost its responsiveness to sodium fluoride during such fractionation.

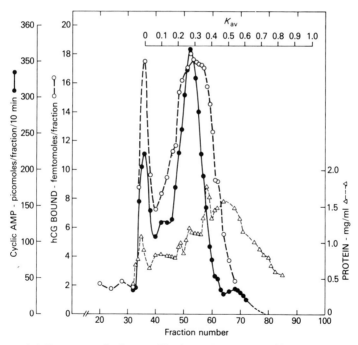

FIG. 24. Gel filtration on Sepharose 6B column (1 × 60 cm) of free receptor solubilized from ovarian particles in the presence of 10 mM NaF with 0.5% Lubrol PX. Binding activity of the column profile (O- - -O), adenylate cyclase activity in the presence of 8 mMMg^{2+} (●——●), and protein elution pattern, OD$_{280}$ (△---△) were simultaneously determined in aliquots of the eluent fractions.

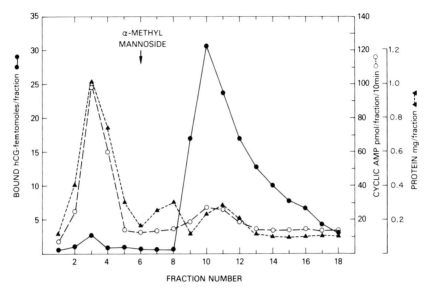

FIG. 25. Chromatography of Lubrol-solubilized LH/hCG receptor and adenylate cyclase from testis interstitial cell fraction on Sepharose–concanavalin A. After elution, each fraction was incubated with [^{125}I]hCG in the presence or the absence of 10^{-7} M hCG for 16 hours at 4°C to determine binding activity (●——●); other aliquots were assayed for adenylate cyclase activity (○——○) and protein (▲---▲).

During chromatography of soluble ovarian preparations on agarose–concanavalin A, two peaks of receptor binding activity were observed (Fig. 26A). The unadsorbed receptor peak that eluted with most of the protein contained all of the adenylate cyclase activity in the preparation. A second receptor fraction was adsorbed to the affinity column and could be subsequently eluted with 0.2 M α-methyl mannoside as a broad peak of binding activity. This finding was consistently observed in soluble ovarian preparations and indicated the presence of two species of the ovarian receptor sites, one containing mannose residues, and the other presumably devoid of sugars responsible for interaction with the lectin. Equilibrium binding analysis of the two forms of the ovarian receptor revealed that both species had similar binding affinities for chorionic gonadotropin.

When the first receptor peak was rerun on the affinity column, it exhibited an almost identical elution profile, but had lost more than 50% of its binding activity (Fig. 26B). The adenylate cyclase activity that coeluted with the first receptor peak, as previously shown, had also lost about 50% of its activity during the second fractionation step.

Rechromatography of the second receptor peak from agarose-concanavalin A showed this species to be much more labile. Thus, little or no activity was found to adsorb to the column on subsequent affinity chromatography, when the small amount of residual activity was eluted with the sugar-free buffer, similar to the first peak seen on initial chromatography (Fig. 26C). These findings indicated that the major receptor species was labile, and probably became converted to a mannose-free form that was not adsorbed by the affinity column. The appearance of two species of the ovarian receptors was also noted during fractionation of solubilized ovarian preparations on DEAE-cellulose, when the individual receptor peaks were eluted by 175 and 255 mM sodium chloride, respectively, while the adenylate

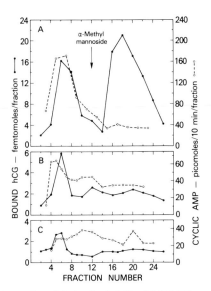

FIG. 26. (A) Chromatography of Lubrol-solubilized LH/hCG receptors and adenylate cyclase from homogenates of pseudopregnant ovaries on Sepharose–concanavalin A. After elution each fraction was incubated with [^{125}I]hCG in the presence or the absence of 10^{-7} M hCG for 16 hours at 4°C to determine receptor-binding activity (●——●); other aliquots were assayed for adenylate cyclase activity (○---○). (B) Fractions corresponding to the first peak of receptor binding and enzyme activity eluted by buffer (see A) were pooled and concentrated 5-fold and subjected to further chromatography on Sepharose–concanavalin A. The elution profile showed identical distribution of the receptor binding and enzyme activity as in (A). A marked decrease on binding and enzyme activity was observed after rechromatography. (C) Fractions corresponding to the second peak of receptor-binding activity were pooled and concentrated. Upon rechromatography it was observed that receptor-binding activity was not adsorbed to the concanavalin A column and was eluted by the phosphate buffer.

cyclase activity was eluted as a sharp peak at 220 mM sodium chloride. The origin, function, and coupling properties of these two forms of the soluble ovarian receptor are yet to be determined.

E. TRANSFER OF GONADOTROPIN RECEPTORS TO ADRENAL CELLS

The preceding studies have indicated that the gonadotropin receptor and adenylate cyclase activity are physically separate entities and can be readily resolved during appropriate fractionation procedures. The finding that detergent-solubilized receptor and enzyme activities can be resolved by chromatographic procedures does not exclude the possibility that the two species are associated in some manner in the lipid bilayer of the plasma membrane. However, there is other evidence to show that hormone receptors and adenylate cyclase exist as separate entities within the cell membrane. In recent studies, Schramm *et al.* (1977) have employed cell fusion to examine the relationship between β-adrenergic receptors and adenylate cyclase. In this approach, cells bearing β-adrenergic receptors but devoid of adenylate cyclase activity were fused by treatment with Sendai virus to cells containing only adenylate cyclase activity. Subsequently, activation of adenylate cyclase in such cell hybrids upon exposure to the adrenergic ligand could be demonstrated. Such experiments strongly support the view that receptor and adenylate cyclase molecules exist independently as mobile species within the cell membrane and can readily achieve functional contact that mediates receptor-cyclase coupling upon occupancy of receptor sites by the appropriate ligand.

Another procedure for the transfer of receptor sites to heterologous cells involves the use of lipid particles or liposomes in which the appropriate receptors have been incorporated. For this purpose, we have recently employed a lipid-rich fraction of ovarian luteal cells to transfer the LH-hCG receptors to isolated adrenal cells (Dufau *et al.*, 1978b). Homogenization of luteinized rat ovaries has been previously shown to provide a lipid-rich fraction that contains about 5% of the total ovarian gonadotropin receptor content (Conti *et al.*, 1978). This fraction can be recovered after centrifugation of ovarian homogenates at 360,000 *g*, as a floating layer containing lipid globules that are associated with the receptors. Such "spontaneously soluble" receptors are in fact associated with lipid and are analogous to liposomes formed by more conventional procedures. It has been possible to incorporate the receptors present in such lipid preparations into isolated adrenal cells prepared from the fasciculata zone of the rat adrenal cortex. The number of receptor sites that could be incorporated into each adrenal cell by this procedure was relatively small, ranging from 12 to 200 sites per cell as determined by binding studies with [^{125}I]hCG. During subsequent incubation of such treated cells with hCG *in vitro*, significant increases in cAMP production were observed, indicating that the transferred receptors were able to establish functional coupling with the adenylate cyclase in the plasma membrane of the recipient cell. That the cAMP produced during stimulation of such adrenal cells by hCG was available for stimulation of intracellular processes characteristic of the adrenal cell was shown by the stimulation of corticosterone production in adrenal fasciculata cells incubated with human chorionic gonadotropin (Dufau *et al.*, 1978b). The amounts of cAMP and steroid produced in response to hCG were much less than those evoked by supramaximal concentrations of ACTH, but the degree of corticosterone elevation was proportional to the small increases in cAMP produced, and was commensurate with the steroid production observed during equivalent degrees of cAMP stimulation by low concentrations of ACTH (Sala *et al.*, 1978a). The results of these studies on gonadotropin receptor transfer by liposome-like particles derived from the ovary demonstrate the potential application of this approach to analysis of the relationships between receptors and adenylate cyclase in the plasma membrane of a wide variety of hormone target cells.

IX. Gonadotropin Binding and Regulation of Gonadal Cell Responses

A. Receptor Occupancy, Cyclic AMP, and Steroidogenesis

In addition to analysis of the binding properties and physical characteristics of LH/hCG receptors, it has been of interest to evaluate the functional relationships between gonadotropin binding and the subsequent events that express the biological actions of the trophic hormones upon the target cell. Measurement of gonadotropin binding in relation to cAMP production by isolated rat testis and collagenase-dispersed interstitial cells, and more recently by Leydig cells purified on Metrizamide gradients to about 90% homogeneity (Conn *et al.*, 1977), showed that the mature rat testis contains a large excess of specific gonadotropin receptors that bind much higher quantities of hCG than required for maximum stimulation of steroidogenesis. It has been estimated that occupancy of about 1% of the receptors should be adequate to stimulate a full steroidogenic response (Catt and Dufau, 1973b). Since each Leydig cell possesses 15,000 to 20,000 receptors (assuming equal cell distribution of receptors) only about 200 receptors need be occupied to evoke a maximal testosterone response.

In earlier studies on isolated testes and dispersed interstitial cells, cAMP formation was not detectably increased by low concentrations of LH or hCG which stimulated steroidogenesis, but rose *pari passu* with increasing gonadotropin binding to a level in considerable excess of that required for a full steroid response (Dufau *et al.*, 1973b; Mendelson *et al.*, 1975a). There is no doubt that most of the excess or spare binding sites of the testis are receptors with the potential to be activated, since their occupancy by increasing gonadotropin concentrations leads to increasing cAMP production up to extremely high levels. The presence of excess gonadotropin receptors in the testis probably represents a general phenomenon in endocrine tissues, and is comparable to the "spare" receptors described in drug-responsive tissues by Stephenson (1956), and in the adrenal by Beall and Sayers (1972). Such spare receptors may increase the sensitivity of the target cell to circulating trophic hormones by enhancing the probability that a given gonadotropin level will result in an adequate degree of receptor occupancy to initiate steroidogenesis. As discussed in more detail below, such receptors also serve as a reservoir of sites to replace those lost by processing or internalization after hormone–receptor interaction at the cell surface.

An association between hormone binding and cAMP responses has also been demonstrated for FSH in the tubules of the testis (Means and Huckins, 1974) and for hCG in slices and cell suspensions from the luteinized and immature rat ovary (Koch *et al.*, 1974; Clark and Menon, 1975). In the porcine ovary, the number of LH receptors per granulosa cell increases about 35-fold during follicle maturation (Kammerman and Ross, 1975) and a corresponding increase takes place in the gonadotropin-sensitive adenylate cyclase activity of the same cells (Lee, 1976). LH and hCG scarcely stimulate adenylate cyclase in testis particles (Dufau *et al.*, 1977a), despite the marked effect of these hormones on cAMP formation in the intact cell (Dufau *et al.*, 1973b; Catt and Dufau, 1973a,b; Catt *et al.*, 1973b; Moyle and Ramachandran, 1973; Mendelson *et al.*, 1975a). Although such rises in cAMP could also be due to changes in the rate of nucleotide degradation, gonadotropins do not appear to have a significant effect upon phosphodiesterase activity in the Leydig cell. Thus, gonadotropin-induced rises in cAMP production in the Leydig cells are attributable to activation of adenylate cyclase, despite the small hormonal effects upon enzyme activity in broken-cell preparations.

In the testis, discrepancies between cAMP formation and steroidogenesis has been observed in intact testis or isolated Leydig cells during stimulation of low concentrations of trophic hormone. In such experiments, gonadotropin levels capable of eliciting steroidogenesis *in vitro* (0.1 to 2 pM) caused no detectable change in cAMP production. Also, the formation of cAMP by decapsulated testes and isolated interstitial cells did not begin to rise until maximum testosterone production had been achieved. Similar discrepancies have been observed in several hormonal target cells (Beall and Sayers, 1972; Moyle and Ramachandran, 1973; Cooke *et al.*, 1976; Ling and Marsh, 1977), but the dissociation between cAMP and cell responses was particularly marked in the Leydig cell.

B. ROLE OF CYCLIC AMP AND PROTEIN KINASE IN GONADOTROPIN ACTION

The absence of a rise in cAMP during the steroidogenic response of interstitial cells had queried the intermediate role of cAMP in the acute steroidogenic response to physiological concentrations of gonadotropin. Such discrepancies were less marked or not apparent when the target tissues studied (isolated cells, tissue slices, or intact organs) were less sensitive to trophic hormone, with dose responses at hormone concentrations above the physiological range (Marsh *et al.*, 1966; Grahame-Smith *et al.*, 1967). However, there is much indirect evidence to suggest that cAMP acts as an intermediate in the acute steroidogenic response to peptide hormones. Thus, testosterone production by interstitial cells or intact testes was stimulated by cAMP or dibutyryl cAMP (Catt and Dufau, 1973b). In addition, an increase in the sensitivity of the steroid response-curve to gonadotropin was observed when incubations were performed in the presence of phosphodiesterase inhibitors such as theophylline or MIX (Dufau *et al.*, 1974a; Mendelson *et al.*, 1975a). In the absence of a detectable rise in cAMP, these indirect observations raised the possibility that steroidogenesis is activated by extremely low concentrations of cAMP. Such activation could also occur by translocation of cAMP within a small intracellular pool, or by a mechanism involving increased turnover of the nucleotide. It might be expected that stimulation of protein kinase activity by minute amounts of cAMP formed in target cells during hormone action should provide an additional, and perhaps more sensitive, index of the intermediate role of cyclic AMP.

However, only minor changes in enzyme activity have been observed during gonadotropic stimulation of interstitial cells (Cooke *et al.*, 1976; Dufau *et al.*, 1977c) (Table VI) and ovarian tissue slices (Ling and

TABLE VI

ACTIVATION OF LEYDIG-CELL PROTEIN KINASE BY GONADOTROPIN
STIMULATION DURING INCUBATION FOR 60 MINUTES[a]

Concentration of hCG (pM)	Protein kinase activity ratio (−cAMP/+cAMP)
0	0.14 ± 0.01
0.2	0.20 ± 0.03
0.5	0.22 ± 0.01
1	0.37 ± 0.01
2	0.31 ± 0.01
5	0.38 ± 0.03
10	0.58 ± 0.02
100	0.51 ± 0.02
1000	0.58 ± 0.02

[a] Results are expressed as mean ± SD of quadruplicate determinations.

Marsh, 1977), sometimes in the absence of a detectable rise in cAMP. More recent studies have clearly demonstrated that hormonal stimulation of purified Leydig cells, by gonadotropin concentrations in the range that produces a graded testosterone response, is accompanied by a simultaneous increase in endogenous cAMP bound to its major intracellular receptor protein, the regulatory subunit of protein kinase (Fig. 27). In addition, a concomitant decrease of free cAMP receptors was demonstrable during occupancy by endogenous cAMP (Fig. 28). All the cAMP receptors related to the steroidogenic response appear to be confined to the cytoplasm, implying that activation of protein kinase during hormone action on steroidogenesis is mainly a cytoplasmatic event (Table VII) (Dufau et al., 1977c).

In addition, only a small fraction (15–25%) of the cAMP receptors need be occupied by endogenous cAMP to produce a full steroidogenic response, and occupancy of more cAMP receptors did not produce further increases in steroidogenesis (Fig. 29). The level of receptor occupancy was 20–40% in control incubations performed in the presence of a phosphodiesterase inhibitor (MIX), and increased by 16–25% over the gonadotropin concentration range that evoked a graded steroid response. The number of cAMP receptors in the purified cell preparations ranged from 3×10^5 to 6×10^5 sites per cell, and less than 10% of these receptors were located in the particulate cell fraction.

The finding of moderate levels of receptor-bound cAMP in control incubations is consistent with previous observations that partial dissociation (i.e., activation) of protein kinase in unstimulated Leydig

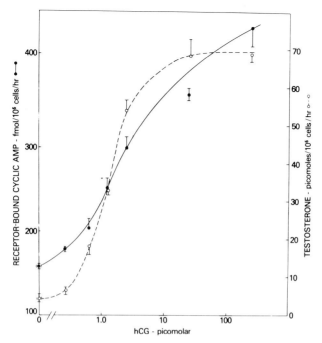

Fig. 27. Comparison of receptor occupancy by endogenous cAMP (●) with testosterone production (○) in Leydig cells incubated with low concentrations of hCG.

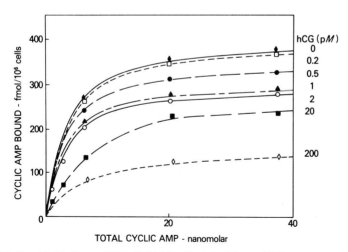

Fig. 28. Specific binding of [³H]cAMP (10 pM–0.1 μM) to cAMP receptors of Leydig cells stimulated with hCG concentrations that elicited a dose-dependent increase of testosterone production (0–2 pM), and with supramaximal hCG concentrations (20 and 200 pM).

TABLE VII

BINDING AFFINITY AND CONCENTRATION OF cAMP RECEPTORS
IN LEYDIG CELL FRACTIONS WITHOUT AND WITH hCG[a]

Preparation	Treatment	Affinity constant, K_a $(10^9 M^{-1})$	Receptor concentration (fmol/10⁶ cells)
Cytosol	Control	1.8 ± 0.3	520 ± 49
	+ hCG	1.6 ± 0.7	222 ± 28[b]
Particulate fraction	Control	2.1 ± 0.4	25 ± 1.3
	+ hCG	1.8 ± 0.6	28 ± 1.8

[a] Samples were incubated for 60 minutes without and with 200 pM hCG as indicated.
[b] $P < 0.001$.

cells is detectable during fractionation by ion-exchange chromatography, gel filtration, and sucrose gradient centrifugation. Thus, during
ion-exchange chromatography on DEAE-cellulose, a small peak of
cAMP-independent protein kinase activity was consistently eluted at

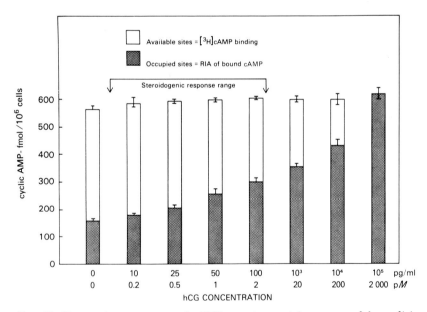

FIG. 29. Progressive occupancy of cAMP receptor protein, measured by radioimmunoassay of bound cAMP after Leydig-cell stimulation with increasing concentrations
hCG (0–200 pM). The dose-dependent decrease of available cAMP receptors during hCG
stimulation was measured with saturating concentrations of [³H]cAMP and expressed as
the binding capacity of cAMP receptors per 10⁶ cells.

low salt concentration (Dufau *et al.*, 1977e). Gel filtration and sucrose gradient centrifugation studies (Podesta *et al.*, 1976a) have also demonstrated that free regulatory and catalytic subunits are present in Leydig cell extracts. These indices of partial activation of protein kinase in unstimulated cells were not attributable to the use of a phosphodiesterase inhibitor during cell incubations. Thus, experiments performed in the absence of MIX showed that intracellular cAMP and cAMP bound to receptors in control cells were identical with the levels observed in the presence of the phosphodiesterase inhibitor. Also, no significant changes were observed in receptor-bound and intracellular cAMP in the presence or absence of MIX; stimulation was confined to the extracellular compartment and increases on the ED_{50} for hCG of 5- to 10-fold in the stimulation of testosterone responses (Dufau *et al.*, 1977c). These findings could indicate that the changes in cAMP are extremely small or undetectable with the present method or, alternatively, that MIX has an extra-cAMP effect that increases the sensitivity of the steroid response to hormone stimulation. Similar findings have also been observed in the adrenal and ovary, though in these tissues MIX produces only small changes in ED_{50}, of about 2-fold as compared to the 5- to 10-fold increase observed in the Leydig cell (Sala *et al.*, 1978a,b).

The estimation of free receptors by [³H]cAMP binding assay was made possible by the relatively high binding affinity of the testicular cAMP receptor ($K_a\ 10^9\ M^{-1}$). The slow dissociation rate constant of the receptor-cAMP complex at low temperature permitted assay of free sites with [³H]cAMP during increasing degrees of receptor occupancy by endogenous cAMP, in the absence of significant effects due to exchange of the labeled and unlabeled nucleotide. The degree of endogenous occupancy could be measured with good precision, when performed by radioimmunoassay following rapid cellulose filtration and quantitative recovery of endogenous cAMP from the filters (Dufau *et al.*, 1977c,e).

These observations have provided an explanation for the apparent dissociation between cAMP and testosterone production during stimulation of Leydig cells by gonadotropic hormones *in vitro*. The presence of a small but significant increase in cAMP formation and binding to specific receptors, in parallel with the steroid response to hormone stimulation, is important evidence for the role of cAMP as a mediator of gonadotropin-induced steroidogenesis. The much greater production of cAMP at higher hormone concentrations reflects the considerable quantity of excess LH/hCG receptors, and accompanying adenylate cyclase, that characterize the rat Leydig cells (Catt and Dufau, 1973a,b; Catt *et al.*, 1973b, 1974; Mendelson *et al.*, 1975a). Although the presence of coincident changes in cAMP and steroid production does not prove that cAMP is the sole mediator of the steroidogenic responses, there remains little doubt that cAMP plays a major role in this process. It is likely that apparent dissociations between cAMP and hormone-induced responses in other target tissues are also due to the extremely small changes in cAMP production that serve to transmit signals arising from hormonal activation of the receptor–cyclase complex in the target cell membranes.

Almost identical results have been recently observed in adrenal and ovarian cells stimulated with ACTH and hCG, respectively (Sala *et al.* 1978a,b). Studies performed in luteal cells from pseudopregnant rat ovaries have shown increased occupancy of cAMP receptor sites by endogenous cAMP during dose-related stimulation of progesterone responses by hCG (Fig. 30). In the ovary, unlike the testis and adrenal gland, most of the cAMP receptor sites (75%) are occupied during dose-related stimulation of progesterone by the trophic hormone. In keeping with this finding, it was also evident that the dose-response curve of steroid production occurred over a wider concentration range

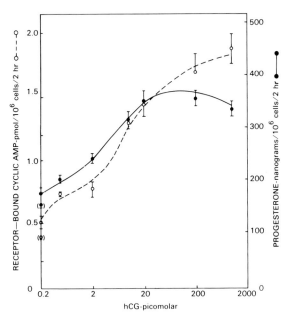

FIG. 30. Comparison of receptor occupancy by endogenous cAMP (○) with progesterone production (●) in ovarian luteal cells incubated with hCG. The increasing occupancy of cAMP receptor protein by cAMP was parallel with the increased progesterone production evoked by low hCG concentrations.

of gonadotropin than that characteristic of the testis response to hCG.

The effects of changes in ionic environment on the steroidogenic effects of LH in the testis have also been investigated in dispersed Leydig cells. Binding of hCG to the gonadotropin receptors of Leydig cells was not altered in the absence of Ca^{2+} or K^+, and the production of testosterone was relatively unaffected by changes in Ca^{2+} concentration (Mendelson *et al.*, 1975a). In the absence of K^+, testosterone responses to trophic hormone were abolished, and cAMP production was reduced by 50% (Fig. 31). Ouabain concentrations as low as $10^{-7} M$ significantly reduced the cAMP and testosterone responses to hCG, with a major fall in extracellular nucleotide levels and maintenance of the intracellular cAMP response (Figs. 32 and 33). Thus, the effects of ouabain on membrane function result in decreased activity of adenylate cyclase and/or

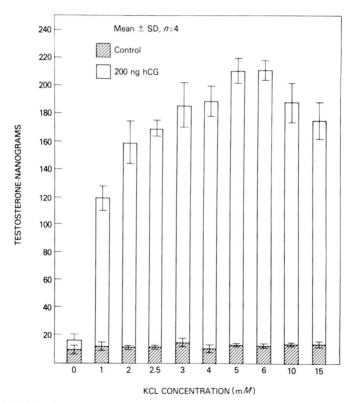

FIG. 31. Effect of potassium concentration on the stimulation of testosterone production by hCG (100 ng/ml) in collagenase-dispersed interstitial cells.

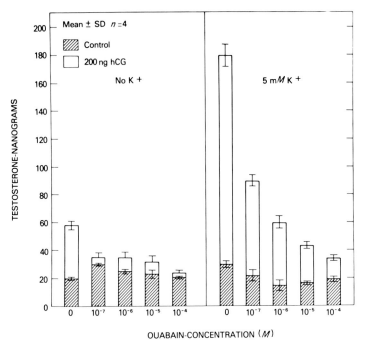

FIG. 32. Effect of ouabain (10^{-7} to $10^{-4} M$) on hCG-stimulated testosterone production by interstitial cells incubated in the absence of potassium (left) and in the presence of 5 mM potassium (right).

impaired extrusion of cAMP from the cells, with associated reduction in steroidogenesis (Dufau *et al.*, 1977e).

C. FUNCTIONAL COMPARTMENTALIZATION OF HORMONE-ACTIVATED CYCLIC AMP RESPONSES

The role of cAMP in the steroidogenic response to physiological concentrations of gonadotropin has been further analyzed by comparative studies on the actions of hCG and choleragen upon the acute metabolic responses of purified Leydig cells. This comparison was performed to gain insight into the selective ability of low concentrations of gonadotropin to produce maximum steroidogenic responses while activating only a minute change in cAMP production. These effects of gonadotropin suggested the occurrence of functional compartmentalization of the cAMP response during hormone action.

In isolated Leydig cells, the dose-response curve for stimulation of intracellular and extracellular cAMP by choleragen was biphasic, with

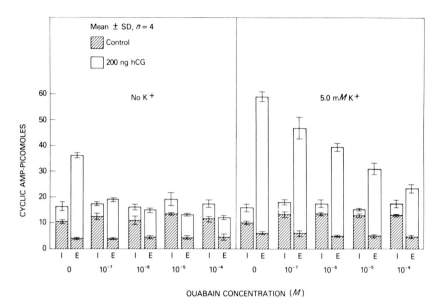

FIG. 33. Effect of ouabain (10^{-7} to 10^{-4} M) on hCG-stimulated cAMP production by interstitial cells incubated in the absence of potassium (left) and in the presence of 5 mM potassium (right) The intracellular (I) and extracellular (E) concentrations of cAMP are shown at each ouabain concentration.

an initial response over the concentration range from 10^{-12} to 10^{-9} M and a second response up to 10^{-7} M choleragen (Fig. 34). Equilibrium binding studies showed 2 sets of choleragen receptor sites with affinity constants of 10^{10} M^{-1} and 10^8 M^{-1} (Fig. 35), corresponding to the first and second components of the dose-dependent choleragen activation curve for cAMP production. During stimulation by choleragen, occupancy of protein kinase receptor sites by cAMP paralleled the initial rise of intracellular cAMP and showed saturation at 10^{-10} M choleragen (Fig. 36). The subsequent secondary rise in cAMP production at higher choleragen concentrations caused no further increase in binding of cAMP to intracellular receptor sites. The higher-affinity choleragen site was responsible for the stimulation of cAMP-dependent metabolic responses in the Leydig cells and for mediating the gonadotropin-like effects of choleragen. Low concentrations of choleragen were found to increase the production and receptor binding of cAMP without a corresponding effect upon testosterone production. This discrepancy, and the higher sensitivity of steroidogenesis to hCG ($ED_{50} = 10^{-12}$ M) than to choleragen ($ED_{50} = 10^{-10}$ M) in the presence of equivalent changes in cAMP production, are consistent with intracellular compartmentaliza-

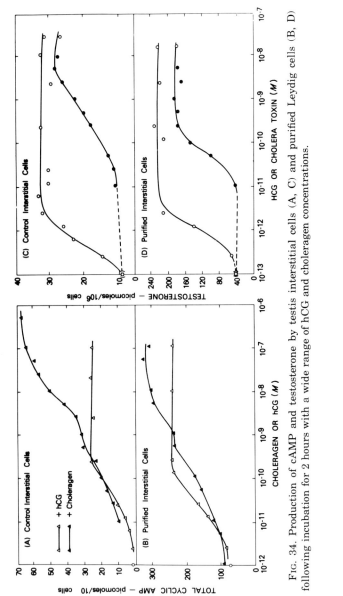

Fig. 34. Production of cAMP and testosterone by testis interstitial cells (A, C) and purified Leydig cells (B, D) following incubation for 2 hours with a wide range of hCG and choleragen concentrations.

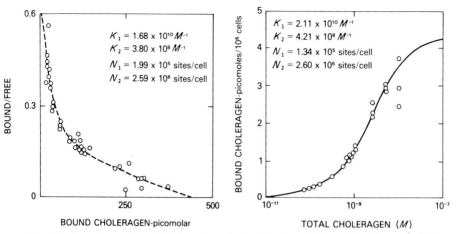

FIG. 35. Scatchard plot of binding data obtained by incubation of Leydig cells with
^{125}I-labeled choleragen and increasing concentrations of choleragen for 1 hour at 24°C
(left). Semilogarithmic plot of specific binding of choleragen to Leydig cells obtained by
computer analysis employing a two-site weighted-fit analysis of "total" and specifically
bound toxin (right).

tion of the hormonal pathway for activation of steroidogenesis (Dufau
et al., 1978a).

The presence of a biphasic activation pattern for cAMP during incubation of collagenase-dispersed interstitial cells with choleragen suggested that two sets of toxin binding sites are present in the Leydig
cell. Direct evidence for heterogeneity of the choleragen binding sites
was provided by binding studies with labeled toxin. In addition, there
was a close correlation between the dose-response curves for choleragen activation of intracellular and receptor-bound cAMP, and the
dose-related choleragen inhibition of ^{125}I-labeled choleragen binding to
isolated Leydig cells. During toxin stimulation, testosterone dose-
response curves occurred when 75–100% of cAMP receptors were filled,
in contrast to the 25% occupancy needed during hormonal stimulation
to evoke maximum steroidogenic levels (Dufau *et al.*, 1977c, 1978a).

These observations suggest that cAMP produced during hormonal
stimulation has more ready access to cAMP receptors in the vicinity of
key steroidogenic enzymes which depend upon activation of protein
kinase to effect increased testosterone production. After binding of
choleragen, and nonspecific stimulation of adenylate cyclase at multiple sites in the cell membrane, the cAMP produced could also occupy
cAMP receptors not directly related to the protein kinase involved in
the activation of steroidogenesis. This would explain the finding that a
major proportion of the available cAMP receptors needs to be occupied

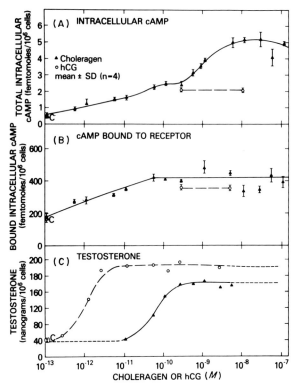

FIG. 36. Correlation between intracellular cAMP (A), receptor-bound cAMP (B), and testosterone production (C) during stimulation of Leydig cells with a wide range of choleragen concentrations, from 10^{-13} to $10^{-7}\,M$. Incubation time for (A) and (B) was 60 minutes and for (C) was 180 minutes. Stimulation of cAMP by a maximally effective hCG dose ($10^{-10}\,M$) and a supramaximal dose ($10^{-8}\,M$) are also shown (○). Study of testosterone production during incubation of Leydig cell with choleragen (▲) or hCG (10^{-13} to $10^{-8}\,M$) (○). Each point represents the mean of quadruplicate incubation.

to mediate the maximal steroidogenic response to choleragen, whereas a much smaller degree of cAMP receptor occupancy is adequate for maximum responses to hormonal stimulation. In the testis, only 25% or less of receptor sites need to be occupied by endogenous cAMP to obtain a full testosterone response, while with choleragen most of cAMP receptors needed to be filled to attain equal stimulation of testosterone production despite cAMP responses markedly elevated upon initial occupancy of receptors as the result of choleragen stimulation. It is therefore possible that there is compartmentalization of a specific group of cAMP receptors within the protein kinase of the Leydig cell, with a small proportion of the holoenzyme adjacent to regulated steroidogenic enzymes and the rest at locations that do not affect the immediate steroidogenic response.

D. PROPERTIES OF LEYDIG-CELL PROTEIN KINASE

The presence of cAMP-dependent protein phosphokinase in the testis was first demonstrated in homogenates of testes from trout (Jergil and Dixon, 1969) and rat (Reddi *et al.*, 1971; Means *et al.*, 1974; Bernard and Wasserman, 1974). In the rat testis, AMP-dependent protein kinase was demonstrated in the cytosol fraction of adult testis homogenates and shown to enhance phosphorylation of certain histones (Reddi *et al.*, 1971). The testicular protein kinase activity of prepuberal and adult rats also demonstrated preferential phosphorylation of histones, and enzyme activity increased during development at 35 to 45 days of age (Bernard and Wasserman, 1974). In this report, protein kinase activity was detected in the interstitial tissue as well as in the seminiferous tubules, and the rise in enzyme activity during maturation was more marked in the tubules. However, no increase in protein kinase activity of testicular homogenates from immature rats was demonstrable after *in vivo* treatment with LH or FSH. In contrast, Means *et al.* (1974) found that exposure to FSH *in vitro* increased the cAMP-dependent protein kinase of seminiferous tubules and that enzyme activity was correlated with the intracellular accumulation of cAMP. This study also demonstrated that incubation of intact testes with LH or hCG caused activation of protein kinase *in vitro*, whereas no effect of these hormones was observed in isolated seminiferous tubules.

A detailed characterization of the protein kinase of the interstitial cells has been performed by Podesta *et al.* (1976a,b) and Cooke *et al.* (1976) during analysis of the role of the adenylate cyclase–protein kinase pathway in the activation of target-cell responses by LH and hCG in gonadal tissues. These studies, and those of Dufau *et al.* (1977c) demonstrated the presence of two forms of cAMP-dependent protein kinase in unstimulated Leydig cells. In addition, a small amount of cAMP-dependent protein kinase was detected in the Leydig cells, corresponding to the catalytic subunit common to the two holoenzymes. Complete activation of both holoenzymes by low concentration of hCG (1 to 2×10^{-10} M) led to formation of a common catalytic subunit, which eluted as a peak of cAMP-independent activity at 0.05 M NaCl during ion-exchange chromatography on DEAE-cellulose at pH 7.4 (Fig. 37) (Dufau *et al.*, 1977e). The two holoenzymes were also resolved by density-gradient centrifugation, as 6.2 S and 4 S species (Podesta *et*

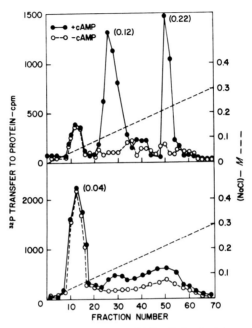

FIG. 37. Ion-exchange chromatography (DEAE-cellulose) of interstitial cell protein kinase activity from unstimulated control cells (above) and cells exposed to 10 ng of hCG *in vitro* (below).

al., 1976a) (Figs. 38 and 39), and could be eluted from DEAE-cellulose as individual peaks of cAMP-dependent activity at 0.125 and 0.220 M NaCl (see Fig. 37). The two enzymes could also be separated by stepwise gradient elution on DEAE-Sephadex A-50. From these values, and the Stokes radii of 47.7 and 37.9 Å derived from gel filtration on Sephadex G-200, the molecular weights of the holoenzymes were estimated to be 116,400 and 59,600, respectively (Podesta *et al.*, 1978a). The regulatory subunits of the protein kinase holoenzymes were identified by cAMP binding analysis, after gel filtration and sucrose density centrifugation, as 4.2 S and 3 S components with estimated molecular weights of 66,300 and 35,000. The molecular weight of the catalytic subunit was calculated from its sedimentation constant (2.9 S) and Stokes radius (29 Å) to be 33,000 (Podesta *et al.*, 1976a, 1978a).

Incubation of purified Leydig cells with low concentrations of hCG (from 10^{-13} to 10^{-10} M) caused progressive activation of protein kinase *in vitro* (Table VI), with conversion to the 2.9 S catalytic subunit (Fig. 40). The testicular enzymes exhibited relatively high binding affinity for cAMP (1×10^{9} M^{-1}) by comparison with values observed in other

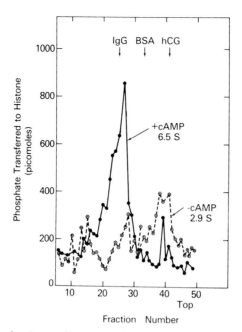

FIG. 38. Sucrose density-gradient centrifugation of interstitial cell protein kinase eluted with >200 mM NaCl from DEAE-Sephadex A-50. Sedimentation analysis was performed in 5–20% sucrose by centrifugation at 105,000 g_{av} (45,000 rpm in an SW 40 rotor) for 19 hours at 4°C. After fractionation of the gradient, aliquots were assayed for protein kinase activity in the presence and in the absence of cAMP.

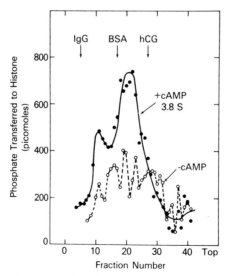

FIG. 39. Sucrose gradient centrifugation of interstitial cell protein kinase eluted by 0.2–0.4 M NaCl fractions from DEAE-Sephadex.

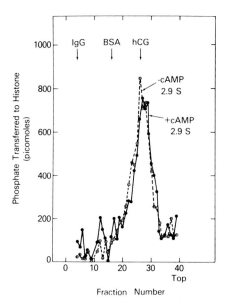

FIG. 40. Sucrose density-gradient centrifugation of protein kinase from hCG-stimulated interstitial cells after elution from Sephadex A-50 with >150 mM NaCl.

tissues. The major 6.2 S holoenzyme accounted for about 70% of the total cAMP-dependent protein kinase activity of the Leydig cell, and exhibited properties comparable with those of the type I protein kinase described in other tissues. However, the 4 S holoenzyme eluted by 200 mM NaCl did not correspond to the type II holoenzyme of other tissues and appeared to arise from the 6.2 holoenzyme during storage *in vitro* (Podesta *et al.*, 1978a). Thus, a portion of the smaller enzyme may be derived by breakdown or dissociation of the 6.2 enzyme during *in vitro* analysis of the Leydig cell extracts. However, it is also present in cells, presumably as an endogenous product of the larger holoenzyme, since the 4 S holoenzyme was consistently demonstrable in Leydig cell extracts, even when protease inhibitors were present during cell disruption and/or Sephadex G-200 fractionation (Podesta *et al.*, 1978a). The finding that partially purified preparations of the larger holoenzyme could yield the three forms of protein kinase (i.e., the 6.2 and 4 S holoenzyme and the free catalytic subunit) suggests that the larger form (6.2 S) exists as an R_2C_2 complex and the smaller (4 S) as an RC form of protein kinase (Table VIII). In addition, the 6.2 S holoenzyme has been detected only in the cytosol, while the 4 S species was present in a particulate membrane-rich fraction as well as in the cytosol. The presence of a smaller form of protein kinase that is presumably derived

TABLE VIII

PHYSICAL PROPERTIES OF LEYDIG-CELL PROTEIN KINASE
HOLOENZYMES AND REGULATORY SUBUNITS[a]

	Sedimentation coefficient ($\times 10^{-13}$ sec)	Stokes radius ($\times 10^{-8}$ cm)	Molecular weight ($\times 10^{-3}$) mean (99% C.L.[b])
Holoenzyme I	6.2 ± 0.1 (3)	47.7 ± 1.6 (9)	116 (112– 120)
Holoenzyme II	4.0 ± 0.1 (4)	37.9 ± 1.0 (5)	59 (57– 61)
Regulatory subunit I	4.2 ± 0.2 (4)	42.1 ± 1.5 (5)	66 (63– 69)
Regulatory subunit II	3.0 ± 0.1 (4)	30.1 ± 1.9 (5)	35 (32– 38)
Catalytic subunit	2.9 ± 0.1 (3)	29.0 ± 1.5 (4)	33 (30– 35)

[a] Values were derived from gel filtration on Sephadex G-200, G-100, and density-gradient centrifugation. Values are mean ± SD; (n) Number of determinations.
[b] Confidence limits.

from the larger holoenzyme has also been described in the calf ovary, where a proteolytic conversion of the larger to the smaller enzyme has been proposed (Talmadge et al., 1977).

If the 4.0 S and 6.2 S protein kinase holoenzymes in the Leydig cell were equally and readily accessible to receptor-generated cAMP, then both enzymes would be activated simultaneously during gonadotropin action. Alternatively, one of the enzymes could be located at a site that favors selective activation by minute changes or translocation of cAMP. Preferential activation of cytosolic protein kinase has been suggested by the recent demonstration that occupancy of cAMP binding sites in the cytosol follows minute increases in cAMP production evoked by physiological concentrations of hCG (10^{-13} to 10^{-12} M) (Dufau et al., 1977c). This finding, with the location of the 6.2 S holoenzyme exclusively in the cytosol of the Leydig cells, indicates that the larger holoenzyme participates in the biochemical events that mediate hormonal activation of steroidogenesis. Dose-dependent occupancy of the 6.2 S holoenzyme by endogenous cAMP in Leydig cells stimulated by low concentrations of hCG (10^{-13} to 10^{-11} M) has been recently demonstrated (Podesta et al., 1978b) during polyacrylamide gel electrophoresis studies by resolution of the regulatory subunits. Such experiments have specifically localized the increase of occupied sites and the decrease of free cAMP sites to the regulatory subunit of the larger holoenzyme. Furthermore, supramaximal hCG concentrations also affected the smaller holoenzyme, manifested as a marked decrease of free sites on the 3 S regulatory subunit, with a simultaneous increase in bound endogenous cAMP. This was demonstrated by polyacrylamide electrophoresis of extracts from hCG-stimulated Leydig cells after

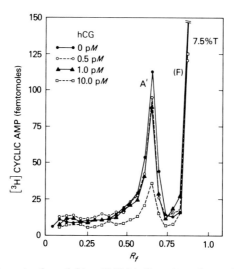

Fig. 41. Electrophoresis of available cAMP binding sites of protein kinase (after dissociation to the regulatory subunits by [³H]cAMP) from rat Leydig cells stimulated *in vitro* with increasing concentrations of hCG for 1 hour at 34°. After incubation, cell sonicates were equilibrated with 10^{-7} M [³H]cAMP for 1 hour at 4°. On subsequent polyacrylamide gel electrophoresis, the radioactivity bound to the regulatory subunits indicated the amount of dissociable holoenzyme remaining after trophic hormone stimulation.

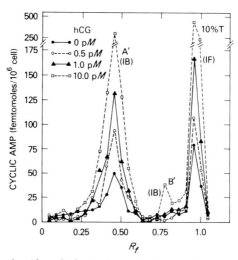

Fig. 42. Polyacrylamide gel electrophoresis and radioimmunoassay of endogenous cAMP bound to the regulatory subunits of protein kinase after activation of rat Leydig cells by hCG *in vitro* (0–10 pM). Extracts of control and hormone-stimulated cells were subjected to electrophoresis in 10% gels, then cAMP was eluted from the gel slices and measured by radioimmunoassay. The results are expressed as femtomoles per 10^6 cells of intracellular cAMP bound to regulatory subunits (IB) and free (IF) after stimulation in increasing concentrations of hCG.

equilibration with [³H]cAMP under nonexchange conditions and by radioimmunoassay of endogenous cAMP bound to the regulatory subunit isolated by gel electrophoresis (Figs. 41 and 42). These observations have confirmed that the cAMP binding proteins of the Leydig cell correspond to the regulatory subunits of protein kinase and have indicated that preferential activation of the larger, cytosolic holoenzyme occurs during stimulation of Leydig cells by low concentrations of gonadotropin (Podesta *et al.*, 1978a).

E. Actions of LH on Early Steps in Steroid Biosynthesis

Since the major locus of action of both ACTH and LH upon steroidogenesis is at the conversion of cholesterol to pregnenolone (Karaboyas and Koritz, 1965; Behrman and Armstrong, 1969), the proteins phosphorylated by protein kinase are probably concerned with this step in steroid biosynthesis. Also, the labile proteins synthesized in Leydig cells and necessary to sustain the actions of gonadotropin upon steroidogenesis (Mendelson *et al.*, 1975a; Cooke *et al.*, 1975a) are likely to function at this level of the steroid biosynthetic pathway. Such proteins could be necessary for cholesterol transport into mitochondria and for the activation of the side-chain cleavage system. The precise step that is stimulated by LH in the biosynthetic sequence between cholesterol and pregnenolone probably involves increased conversion of cholesterol to 20- and 22α-hydroxycholesterol (Burstein *et al.*, 1975). In the testis and ovary, both LH and prolactin have been reported to influence cholesterol ester synthesis and metabolism. The activities of cholesterol ester synthetase and cholesterol esterase are, respectively, decreased and increased in the gonads by LH treatment (Behrman and Amstrong, 1969; Flint *et al.*, 1973; Moyle *et al.*, 1973). In the mouse testis, prolactin treatment promotes the accumulation of cholesterol esters and leads to increased production of testicular androgens in the presence of LH (Hafiez *et al.*, 1972).

Once formed in the cytoplasm, free cholesterol moves to the outer mitochondrial membrane, probably by combination with a carrier protein (Kan and Ungar, 1973). Since the side-chain cleavage complex is situated on the inner mitochondrial membrane, cholesterol must move into the mitochondria for conversion to pregnenolone. In the adrenal, ACTH has been shown to promote binding of cholesterol to the cytochrome P-450 enzyme system, which mediates the side-chain cleavage reaction. There are probably two steroid binding sites on the cytochrome P-450 that participates in the cholesterol side-chain cleavage reaction (Jefcoate, 1975). This enzyme reaction is a rate-limiting step in steroid biosynthesis and depends upon a complex series of mixed-function oxidases, which insert C-20 and C-22 hydroxyl groups into the cholesterol molecule prior to cleavage of the side chain to yield pregnenolone. Hypophysectomy of male rats causes a marked decrease of testicular cytochrome P-450, and long-term administration of LH prevents this decline (Purvis and Menard, 1975). Phosphorylation of the reconstituted enzyme system by ovarian cAMP-dependent protein kinase has been reported to increase side-chain cleavage enzyme activity *in vitro* (Caron *et al.*, 1975). The cholesterol esterase in crude extracts of adrenal cortex is activated in a reaction that is dependent on MgATP and is stimulated by cAMP or its derivatives (Trzeciak and Boyd, 1973, 1974; Naghshineh, 1974; Beckett and Boyd, 1975). The reaction is stimulated by addition of exogenous cAMP-dependent protein kinase and can be blocked by the protein inhibitor and seems likely to involve phosphorylation. Recently it has been reported that highly purified cholesterol esterase can be phosphorylated and activated by cAMP. The degree of activation, however, was quite small when compared to stimulation of hormone production evoked by ACTH (Beckett and Boyd, 1975). Also, cAMP-dependent protein kinase has been reported to increase side-chain cleavage activity *in vitro* (Caron *et al.*, 1975). Such effects could obviously be important control points for the regulation of steroid synthesis by LH.

The subsequent conversion of pregnenolone to testosterone in the smooth endoplasmic reticulum (Tamaoki *et al.*, 1975) requires at least 5 enzymic reactions: 17α-hydroxylase, 17-20 lyase (desmolase), 17β-hydroxysteroid dehydrogenase, and 3β-hydroxysteroid dehydrogenase, Δ^5-3-ketoisomerase. The enzyme sequence and relative contributions of Δ^4 and Δ^5 pathways differ according to species, but all steps of androgen biosynthesis can be stimulated by prolonged treatment with LH and hCG. However, such long-term effects of gonadotropins are manifestations of the trophic action of LH in the testis, and probably operate through mechanisms other than those involved in the acute regulation of steroid secretion by the interstitial cell.

In the Leydig cell, gonadotropin action upon testosterone production is dependent upon continuous synthesis of RNA and protein (Mendelson *et al.*, 1975b). However, gonadotropins do not appear to exert direct effects upon RNA and protein synthesis during acute stimulation of steroidogenesis *in vitro* (Rebar *et al.*, 1977). The rapid and marked blockade of gonadotropin-induced steroidogenesis in the testis by inhibitors of protein synthesis has indicated that a labile protein is essential for hormonal activation of testosterone production (Shin and Sato, 1971; Mendelson *et al.*, 1975b; Cooke *et al.*, 1975a,b), and that its effect is located at a step before pregnenolone formation (Cigorraga *et al.*, 1978a). Recent work has shown that two proteins appear to be synthesized in rat testis Leydig cells during LH action, and at least one of these could be important in the regulation of testosterone production by LH (Janszen *et al.*, 1976). However, since the LH-induced protein was detected only 2 hours after the addition of LH or dibutyryl cAMP to Leydig cells and had a half-life longer than 30 minutes, it seems unlikely to be the labile protein involved in the acute stimulation of steroidogenic responses by gonadotropin.

X. Hormonal Regulation of Gonadotropin Receptors

The concentration of gonadotropin receptor sites in testis and ovary show quite marked changes during development and during cyclical or seasonal variations in gonadal function. Although LH is the major trophic hormone of the interstitial cells of the testis and ovary, and acts on the maturing granulosa cells of the ovary, there is little evidence for positive effects of LH upon receptor content except during the process of luteinization that follows spontaneous or induced ovulation. Hypophysectomy is followed by a decrease in testicular LH receptors (Frowein and Engle, 1975), but postoperative treatment with LH, while maintaining Leydig-cell function, has not yet been shown to restore the receptor population of the testis. Rather, administration of exogenous LH or hCG has been commonly followed by occupancy and/or loss of gonadal LH receptors, as described below (see also Section IX, B). However, heterologous regulation of LH receptors during maturation or differentiation of target cells under the influence of FSH and prolactin has been clearly demonstrated in both testis and ovary.

A. Regulation of Gonadotropin Receptors by Heterologous Hormones

1. *Follicle-Stimulating Hormone*

The endocrine function of the testis is well recognized to be influenced by FSH, as well as by LH and to some extent by prolactin and growth hormone. The LH receptors of the rat testis show a marked rise before and during the pubertal rise in testosterone secretion, and increase coincidently with rising FSH levels from 15 to 35 days of age. Also, FSH treatment of immature hypophysectomized rats causes an increase in the LH receptors per testis, as well as in the sensitivity and magnitude of the steroidogenic response to LH (Ketelslegers *et al.*,

1977). These changes are consistent with a role of FSH in regulating the formation of LH receptors during development in the rat, an action that may be the major mechanism of sexual maturation in the male in certain species (Odell and Swerdloff, 1976).

In the ovary, the induction of LH receptors in preantral follicles by exogenous FSH has been demonstrated by Zeleznik et al., (1974). This study showed that treatment of estrogen-primed immature hypophysectomized rats with FSH for 2 days caused a marked increase in binding of radioiodinated hCG by granulosa cells. This in vivo effect of FSH upon LH receptors has also been demonstrated in vitro with cultured porcine granulosa cells (Channing, 1975) and with cultured ovarian fragments from estrogen-treated hypophysectomized rats (Nimrod et al., 1977).

2. Prolactin

Synergistic effects of prolactin and growth hormone upon the actions of FSH on testicular responsiveness to LH have been observed in the hypophysectomized male rat (Odell and Swerdloff, 1976). Also, prolactin is known to enhance the effects of LH upon spermatogenesis, and testosterone synthesis and secretion (Bartke, 1977). Recently, specific receptors for prolactin have been demonstrated in the interstitial cells of the rat testis (Aragona and Friesen, 1975; Charreau et al., 1977). Also, prolactin has been shown to increase LH receptors in the mouse testis (Bohnet and Friesen, 1976) and in the regressed testes of light-deprived hamsters (Bex and Bartke, 1977). These several reports have clearly indicated that prolactin has important effects on testis function via interaction with specific receptors in the interstitial cells, and that induction of LH receptors is one of these effects.

The actions of prolactin in the ovary are more clearly apparent than in the testis, but are also more complex. The luteotrophic action of prolactin is exerted in conjunction with LH, and the relative contributions of each hormone varies between species, and also within a species during the course of pregnancy and lactation (Cowie and Forsyth, 1975). In rodents, prolactin has a major luteotrophic action, but requires LH and FSH for its full effect. As in the testis, prolactin acts on steroidogenesis in the rat ovary by increasing cholesterol ester turnover and providing cholesterol for the early steps of steroid hormone biosynthesis that are regulated by the actions of LH.

Specific binding sites for prolactin have been demonstrated in large antral follicles and corpora lutea of the rat ovary (Midgley, 1973). The process of luteinization is accompanied by a decrease in LH and FSH receptors and a marked increase in prolactin receptors. Also, treatment with prolactin causes an increase in the LH receptor content of luteal cells (Richards and Williams, 1976), and the presence of endogenous prolactin during luteinization appears to be necessary for full expression of LH receptors in the corpus luteum (Holt et al., 1976). In rats with established corpora lutea, inhibition of prolactin secretion with ergocryptine is followed by decreased LH receptor content, and this effect is blocked by treatment with prolactin (Grinwich et al., 1976). In the same study, the loss of LH receptors and luteal function caused by prostaglandin $F_{2\alpha}$ ($PGF_{2\alpha}$) was prevented by prolactin administration. Also, the maintenance of LH receptors in luteinized ovaries by estrogen-induced prolongation of pseudopregnancy (Lee and Ryan, 1975b) is probably related to the concomitant increase in prolactin secretion. These observations demonstrate that prolactin increases the number of LH receptors in the rat corpus luteum, and suggest that the recognized synergism between LH and prolactin upon progesterone formation in the ovary could operate through this mechanism. However, there is evidence that LH receptor induction by prolactin is not a requirement for the stimulating effect of prolactin on progesterone production, and that altered intracellular mechanisms are more important in determining the luteal cell response to prolactin (Richards and Williams, 1976). The extent to which prolactin regulates the development of LH receptors in the ovary during the normal estrous cycle and pregnancy has yet to be established.

The tissue distribution of prolactin receptors shows quite marked variations between species, and major sex variations have been observed within species. The prolactin content of different tissues also varies with age with physiological changes and is influenced by several modulators of prolactin receptors (Posner et al., 1974a; Kelly et al., 1974). Lactogen binding sites in liver closely resemble those in mammary tissue (Shiu and Friesen, 1974). Studies on the hepatic lactogenic receptors have shown that the binding activity is high in adult female rats, considerably augmented by pregnancy, and low or absent in adult male rats (Posner et al., 1974a; Kelly et al., 1974). Marked increases in hepatic prolactin receptors could be induced in male rats by estrogen treatment (Posner et al., 1974b) while hypophysectomy in the male abolished the response to estrogen (Posner et al., 1974b). Hypophysectomy of the female resulted in a rapid and marked decrease of hepatic sites, and implantation of the pituitary under the renal capsule prevented loss of prolactin binding sites in the liver and restored the sensitivity to estrogen administration (Posner et al., 1975a,b; Posner, 1977).

With this background, and the knowledge that the marked increase of lactogenic sites consequent to pituitary transplantation was preceded by sustained elevation of serum prolactin, it was suggested that prolactin regulated the increases of its own receptor (Posner, 1976b). Subsequently, several attempts to induce lactogen binding sites with ovine prolactin injections in combination with other hormones in estrogen-treated hypophysectomized rats were unsuccessful. The failure of such replacement therapy to induce prolactin receptors has been attributed to the inability of prolactin injections to produce chronic and sustained levels of circulating prolactin (Posner, 1976a,b). However, in one report the administration of large single doses of prolactin was found to increase prolactin receptors in the liver of hypophysectomiced female rats (Costlow et al., 1975). The autoregulatory effects of prolactin upon receptors in the liver have been also observed in those of the rat mammary gland during pregnancy and in the early postpartum period and lactation (Holcomb et al., 1976).

It is apparent that many factors influence prolactin binding sites. Estrogens have been found to be a major modulator of prolactin receptors, producing a marked increase of prolactin receptors in the rat liver while decreasing receptors in the kidney and prostate, and showing no effect in other tissue. The former effects are now ascribed to the ability of estrogens to stimulate prolactin secretion from the pituitary, but may also reflect a direct action of estrogen upon the liver in the presence of an intact hypophysis. Androgens have been found to produce the opposite effects to estrogens upon prolactin receptors. Following castration of male rats, there is a major increase in specific binding of prolactin to liver membrane preparations. The magnitude of receptor increase varied with the age of the animals and the time after castration and was most marked in 80-day-old rats. Treatment with testosterone propionate at the time of castration prevented the subsequent increase in prolactin receptors, and administration of estradiol enhanced the rise in prolactin receptors (Aragona et al., 1976a,b). The increase in prolactin binding sites in the male rat liver following castration does not seem to be mediated by an increase in serum prolactin levels (Shin et al., 1974; Friesen and Shiu, 1977) and cannot be reproduced by the administration of prolactin (Posner, 1976b). The enhancement of prolactin binding activity in the liver of male rats after castration appears to require not only the presence of adequate concentrations of prolactin, but also a functioning pituitary gland (Aragona et al., 1976b).

B. REGULATION OF GONADOTROPIN RECEPTORS BY HOMOLOGOUS HORMONES

Several hormonal and other ligands have been shown to regulate the concentration of their specific receptor sites on the surface of target cells (Gavin et al., 1974; Kebabian et al., 1975; Mukherjee et al., 1975, 1976; Hinkle and Tashjian, 1975; Lesniak and Roth, 1976; Raff, 1976). This phenomenon was initially recognized as antigenic modulation of surface immunoglobulins, and later as homologous regulation of peptide hormone receptors (Kahn et al., 1973; Kahn and Roth, 1976). This regulation most commonly leads to loss of receptor sites with little or no change in the binding properties of the residual receptors. Recently, gonadotropins such as LH and hCG have been shown to cause marked loss of specific receptor sites in their target cells in the testis and ovary (Hsueh et al., 1976b, 1977; Sharpe, 1976, 1977a,b; Conti et al., 1976b, 1977a,b; Tsuruhara et al., 1977; Haour and Saez, 1977; Auclair et al., 1977; Cheng and Payne, 1977). The consequence of hormone-induced receptor loss upon target cell function have not been examined in detail, though several reports have established that "desensitization" of adenylate cyclase to hormonal stimulation is correlated with reduction of specific receptors (Kebabian et al., 1975; Mukherjee et al., 1975). The desensitizing effects of gonadotropin upon ovarian adenylate cyclase (Hunzicker-Dunn and Birnbaumer, 1976a,b,c; Bockaert et al., 1976; Conti et al., 1976b, 1977a) have been shown to possess two components: an early loss of enzyme activity and a later loss of LH receptors. Also, the negative regulation of testicular and ovarian LH receptors by gonadotropin is accompanied by reduced responses of cAMP and testosterone production in excised tissues during hormone stimulation in vitro (Conti et al., 1976b; Hsueh et al., 1977; Sharpe, 1977a,b; Haour and Saez, 1977; Tsuruhara et al., 1977).

Studies performed on testis tissue, and more recently in purified Leydig cells of animals treated with gonadotropins, have demonstrated that important functional consequences occur as a result of the receptor regulation induced by LH and hCG (Hsueh et al., 1977; Tsuruhara et al., 1977; Cigorraga et al., 1978a). Administration of a single dose of hCG or ovine LH, as analogs of the endogenous luteinizing hormone, caused marked loss of LH receptors and responsiveness of the testis in vitro. Loss of LH receptors was not observed when the dose of hCG was as low as 100 ng, but became detectable at 200 ng of hCG and increased in a serial manner after 1 μg and 10 μg of hCG (Fig. 43). The fall in LH receptors was dose-dependent and was evident a few hours after injection of a low dose (0.2 μg) of hCG. Loss of LH receptor binding capacity was also observed after treatment with the more rapidly metabolized gonadotropin, ovine LH. Prior to the above-cited initial decreases of receptors, there was a noticeable increase in LH receptors from 2 to 18 hours after hCG injection, occurring between 2 and 6 hours with the higher doses of the hormone and somewhat later with the lower doses (Fig. 44). Occupancy of a small number of binding sites several hours

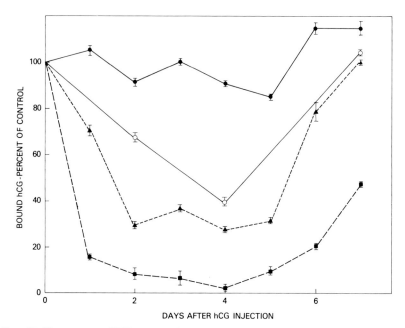

FIG. 43. Time course of LH receptor loss in Leydig cells of hCG-treated animals. The dose-dependent decrease and return of LH receptors during 6 days after single injections of hCG (●——●, 0.1 μg; ○——○, 0.2 μg; ▲---▲, 1.0 μg; and ■——■, 10 μg) was measured by equilibration with saturating concentrations of ^{125}I-labeled hCG, and expressed as a percentage of the binding capacity of control cells. Each point represents the mean ± SD of 6 determinations for the 0.1 ,1, and 10 μg groups, and of 4 determinations for the 0.2 μg group.

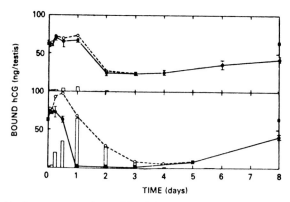

FIG. 44. Testicular concentrations of LH/hCG receptors and tissue-bound hCG after injection of 10 IU (upper panel) or 200 IU (lower panel) of hCG. The total testicular content of LH/hCG receptors (---) was determined by summation of the number of available receptors (—) and the occupied sites represented by tissue-bound hCG (open bars). Each point represents the mean ± SE of 3 or more testes per determination.

after administration of 1 or 10–20 μg of hCG was consistently accompanied by an initial increase in total receptor sites. This finding suggests that initial binding of hCG may induce early changes in membrane conformation that lead to the unmasking of surface receptors with an early increase in total receptor content (Hsueh *et al.*, 1977; Sharpe, 1977a).

The level of receptor occupancy caused by the lowest effective hCG dose (200 ng) was not detectable at 48 hours by elution and assay of the bound hormone, yet led to 60% loss of receptors on day 4 after injection. The intermediate dose (1 μg) caused about 8% occupancy after 24 hours, and produced more extensive receptor loss (see Fig. 44). After the highest dose (10 μg), which caused near-maximum receptor occupancy at 24 hours, the degree of occupancy was still significant at 48 hours, and declined over the next few days (Fig. 45). The consequent loss of receptors from isolated Leydig cells was maximum at day 4, and returned almost to the normal level by day 8. The loss of receptors in each of the lower-dose groups (0.2 and 1 μg hCG) was clearly in considerable excess of the level of occupancy caused by the administered hormone, and the major fall in receptors occurred when occupancy was undetectable or minimal (Tsuruhara *et al.*, 1977). This indicates that an active process of receptor regulation was initiated at the cell mem-

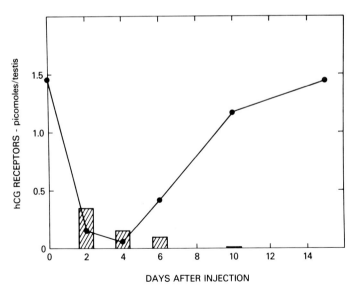

FIG. 45. Changes in the testicular concentration of free LH receptors (●——●) and tissue-bound hCG (hatched bars) after treatment with 10 μg of hCG. Data are expressed as picomoles per testis, and each point is the mean of 3 determinations.

brane level when a small proportion of the receptor population had been occupied by the homologous hormone or its active analog. In the animals treated with the highest dose of hCG, the initial loss of available receptors was largely due to occupancy by the administered hormone (Hsueh *et al.*, 1977), and by the second day a major loss of total receptor sites was evident, as shown in Figs. 44 and 45.

The loss of LH receptors after hCG treatment was less marked in detergent-extracted preparations than in the corresponding membrane-rich particulate fraction (Table IX) (Tsuruhara *et al.*, 1977). This difference in available sites suggests that a proportion of the declining receptor population is masked or occluded with the membrane, and rendered free for interaction with hormone when solubilized with nonionic detergent. It is likely that the initial occlusion of receptor sites at the membrane level is followed by internalization of the complexes by endocytosis and subsequent degradation after association with lysosomes, similar in sequence and also probably in mechanism to the process of adsorptive pinocytosis by which solutes bound to specific recognition sites are interiorized while bound to the pinocytic vesicle membrane (Steinman and Cohn, 1976). Thus, recent studies have suggested that some of the LH bound to Leydig cells was internalized and eventually degraded by lysosomes (Ascoli and Puet, 1977), and similar changes were observed in ovarian tissue where the trophic hormone has been identified with luteal cells (Petrusz, 1973) and localized by autoradiography to the plasma membrane and cytoplasmic dense bodies regarded as lysosomes (Chen *et al.*, 1977).

Further observations in lutejnized ovarian cells have revealed that the hormone–receptor complexes initially formed at the cell membrane are later internalized and become associated with a particulate fraction of the cytoplasm (Conn *et al.*, 1977). Evidence has also been pre-

TABLE IX
RECEPTOR CONCENTRATION

Preparation	Leydig cell (no. of binding sites per cell)	Soluble receptor (fmol/mg protein)
Control	13,000 (100)[a]	98 (100)
hCG		
0.2 μG	6,562 (48)	83 (85)
1 μG	4,242 (31)	51 (52)
10 μG	934 (6.8)	24 (24)

[a] Percentage of control.

sented for the internalization of cell-bound epidermal growth factor, and loss of the specific receptors after endocytosis of the growth factor–receptor complex (Carpenter and Cohen, 1976). These various examples of endocytosis of hormone–receptor complexes are part of the more general activity of the vacuolar system responsible for pinocytosis followed by processing, digestion, and recycling of the ingested components (Steinman and Cohn, 1976). The extent to which this process is specifically activated by hormonal ligands, and whether it represents more than the expression of a general cell response to membrane-binding of extracellular ligands, has yet to be established. However, the function of such a process to effect feedback regulation of the receptor population has been clearly demonstrated in studies on the low-density lipoprotein receptor of cultured fibroblasts (Brown and Goldstein, 1976), and could account for the chronic lowering of receptor concentration in cells exposed to high hormone levels from prolonged periods.

C. Hormone Responses of Desensitized Target Cells

The changes in hCG-induced cell responses following receptor loss were generally in keeping with the expected effects of impairment of the hormone activation sequence. Thus, cAMP production was proportional to receptor content, and closely followed the loss of receptors at days 2 and 4 (Hsueh et al., 1977; Tsuruhara et al., 1977). The acute desensitization of the cAMP response occurred a few hours after hCG treatment, and corresponded to the initial phase of receptor occupancy, prior to the actual loss of receptors and responses which occurred from 2–6 days after the administration of hCG. The recovery phase of the cAMP response was relatively slow, and lagged behind the return of the LH receptors. Thus, after 6 days the maximum cAMP responses of cells from the groups given 0.2 and 1 μg hCG had not returned to normal, despite complete recovery of the LH receptor population (Fig. 46). Since stimulation of cAMP responses by cholera toxin was normal or increased throughout the period of receptor loss and recovery, it is possible that a coupling defect exists between newly formed receptors and adenylate cyclase during the initial phase of the recovery process.

The corresponding changes in testosterone responses of cells after hCG-induced receptor loss were more complex, and also bore a more interesting relationship to the known physiological action of the trophic hormone in maintaining Leydig-cell function and androgen secretion. An important finding in this regard was the increased testosterone responses seen at 2 and 4 days in cells of rats treated with the

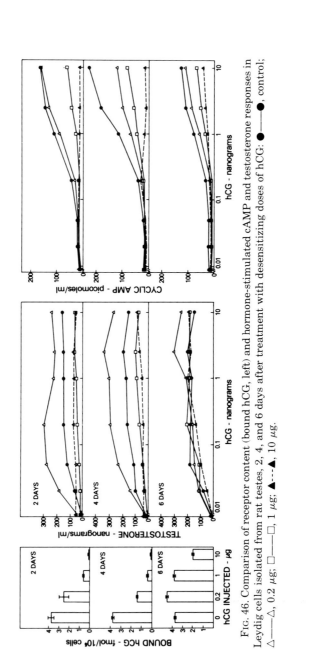

FIG. 46. Comparison of receptor content (bound hCG, left) and hormone-stimulated cAMP and testosterone responses in Leydig cells isolated from rat testes, 2, 4, and 6 days after treatment with desensitizing doses of hCG: ●——●, control; △——△, 0.2 μg; □——□, 1 μg; ▲---▲, 10 μg.

lowest dose of hCG (200 ng) despite the significant fall of hCG receptors and cAMP responses of these cells (Fig. 46). This effect reveals that the process of receptor regulation that occurs at all levels of occupancy is followed by enhancement of the steroidogenic pathway when small doses of hormones are given to simulate physiological gonadotropin levels *in vivo*. By contrast, Leydig cells from animals treated with higher doses of hCG showed marked reduction of maximum steroid responses at 2 and 4 days. At 6 days the steroid dose-response curves had returned to normal in animals treated with 1 μg hCG, and showed a 2-fold higher ED_{50} in cells from rats treated with 10 μg of hCG.

Since the Leydig cell has an abundance of spare receptors (Catt and Dufau, 1973a,b) such marked reductions in receptors would be expected to cause a shift to the right in the dose-response curve, with increased ED_{50} for hCG reflecting a decrease in sensitivity to gonadotropin hormone. However, maximum testosterone levels were not attained at higher stimulatory doses of trophic hormone, and this obscured the anticipated change in sensitivity, such that a shift in ED_{50} was evident only during the recovery phase of cells from rats treated by the higher doses of hCG. The failure to achieve the maximum steroid responses to gonadotropin in hCG-desensitized cells could arise from a defect at one of several levels in the biochemical sequence leading to testosterone production. These include the possibility that the cAMP produced was not available for stimulation of subsequent responses, that a marked reduction of the relevant protein phosphokinase had taken place, or that a more distal lesion had occurred in one or more of the enzymes regulating the steroidogenic pathway.

Stimulation of the Leydig cells with choleragen elicited cAMP responses that were comparable with that of control groups, but despite such cAMP increases the production of testosterone remained markedly reduced (Fig. 47). Also, the steroidogenic lesion was not overcome by stimulation with dibutyryl cAMP in concentrations that evoked steroidogenesis in normal Leydig cells (Tsuruhara *et al.*, 1977). Since cAMP binding studies showed no loss of cAMP-dependent phosphokinase in the desensitized cells (Fig. 48), it appears unlikely that cAMP and protein kinase are limiting factors in impaired steroid response. Further, the finding that hormone stimulation *in vitro* in the presence of spironolactone and cyanoketone produced a significant increase in pregnenolone synthesis in the group given 1 μg of hCG, leading to loss of 70% of the LH receptors, indicates the adequate availability of cholesterol side-chain cleavage enzyme activity (Fig. 49). Therefore, the gonadotropin-induced second lesion in the steroidogenic pathway lies beyond the side-chain cleavage enzyme in cells with moderate degrees of receptor depletion (Tsuruhara *et al.*,

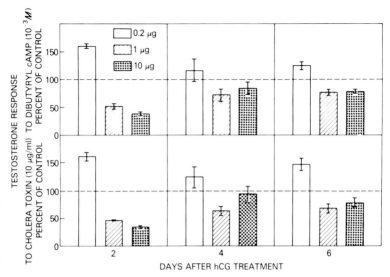

FIG. 47. Testosterone response of Leydig cells to 1 mM dibutyryl cAMP (above) and 10 μg of choleragen (below) at 2, 4, and 6 days after hCG treatment (0.2, 1, 10 μg). Values are expressed as a percentage of the control value (mean ± SD, n = 6).

1977; Cigorraga *et al.*, 1978a). However, more extensive receptor loss (~99%) produced by higher hCG doses was accompanied by abolition of both testosterone and pregnenolone responses to hCG (Fig. 49). This indicates that the most extensive loss of receptors, and presumably of coupled responses, is accompanied by loss of the processes necessary to maintain steroidogenic enzymes including the cholesterol side-chain cleavage enzyme. More recent studies have localized the steroidogenic lesion that follows trophic hormone stimulation (by 2–4 days after the intravenous desensitizing injection of hCG) to a partial block of the 1̇7–20 lyase and 17-hydroxylase steps in androgen biosynthesis. These biosynthetic defects led to accumulation of progesterone, 17α-hydroxyprogesterone, pregnenolone and 17α-hydroxypregnenolone, whereas accumulation and/or formation of dehydroepiandrosterone, Δ⁵-androstenediol, androstenedione, and testosterone was not apparent. In control cells incubated with hCG, dibutyryl cAMP, or choleragen in the absence of inhibitors (Fig. 50), the major androgen accumulated was testosterone, with minor quantities (1 : 4) of androstenedione (Cigorraga *et al.*, 1978a).

    In contrast to the effect of intravenous hCG on subsequent steroid responses, no loss of the maximum response was observed after subcutaneous administration of a dose of hCG (10 μg) that caused loss of

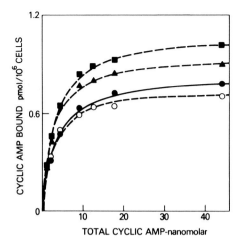

FIG. 48. Specific binding of [³H]cAMP ($10^{-11}\,M$ to $10^{-7}\,M$) to cAMP receptors of Leydig cells during incubation with cell extracts for 16 hours at 6°C. hCG: ■---■, 0.2 μg; ▲---▲, 1 μg; ●——●, none; ○---○, 10 μg.

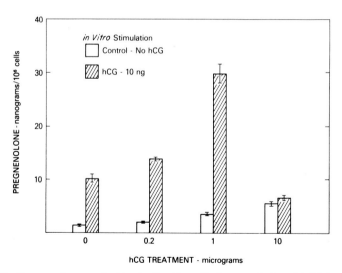

FIG. 49. Pregnenolone production by Leydig cells from control and hCG-treated animals, determined 2 days after treatment with 0.2, 1, and 10 μg of hCG. Synthesis of pregnenolone from endogenous precursors was measured during stimulation with hCG in the presence of caynoketone. Results are the mean ± SD of quadruplicate determinations.

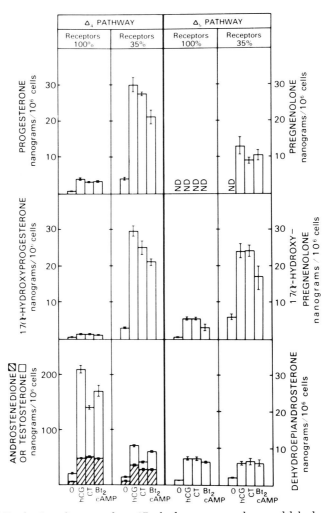

Fig. 50. Production of pregnenolone, 17 α-hydroxypregnenolone, and dehydroepiandrosterone (Δ^5 pathway, right) and progesterone, 17α-hydroxyprogesterone, androstenedione, and testosterone (Δ^4 pathway, left) by Leydig cells with 100% and 35% receptors during stimulation in the absence of inhibitors with hCG (100 ng, 2 nM) choleragen
(CT, 50 μg), and dibutyryl cAMP (Bt$_2$ cAMP, 1 mM).

85% of the LH receptor population at 3 days. However, a marked decrease in the *sensitivity* of the testosterone response to hCG was evident
in such experiments, with ED_{50} about 20- and 40-fold lower than that of
control Leydig cells during incubation in the presence or in the absence
of 1-methyl-3-isobutylxanthine (MIX), respectively (Fig. 51, Left: A
and B). Incubation with the phosphodiesterase inhibitor caused a 4.5-

and 2.1-fold reductions in the ED_{50} for hCG in the controls and desensitized groups, respectively. This small difference could indicate that the desensitized cells have somewhat lower phosphodiesterase activity than the controls. However, the differences observed during the experiment with MIX are more related to the high basal levels of the desensitized group, and less to the stimulated values (i.e., basal values were increased 2-fold). The reduction of receptors was accompanied by a marked reduction in cAMP (basal and hCG-stimulated) with only minor changes in the ED_{50} in the presence or the absence of the phosphodiesterase inhibitor (Fig. 51, right). The basal cAMP values in the desensitized cells in the presence of MIX were significantly higher than in control cells, indicating that the increased basal testosterone levels observed in the desensitized group could be caused by the changes observed in cAMP formation. Thus, the receptor loss induced by subcutaneous injections of hCG was not accompanied by the prominent steroidogenic block seen in cells from rats with a comparable degree of receptor loss induced by intravenous doses of gonadotropin. Instead, such cells clearly showed the decrease in sensitivity that would be expected of target tissues after receptor depletion without major impairment of the enzymic steps that mediate the specific response to hormonal stimulation.

However, the finding of a concomitant small accumulation of progesterone and 17α-hydroxyprogesterone indicated the presence of minor defects in 17α-hydroxylase and 17–20 lyase activities, analogous to the more severe defects seen in Leydig cells after intravenous desensitizing doses of hCG, that probably contribute to the decrease in sensitivity to gonadotropin after subcutaneous hCG treatment.

The cause of the marked decline in 17–20 lyase activity in gonadotropin-desensitized Leydig cells following intravenous injection of hCG has yet to be elucidated, but there are at least two major mechanisms that could be responsible for the enzymic lesion. First, previous studies have indicated that estrogen administration produces a rapid decrease in testicular and plasma testosterone levels, apparently with no effect on plasma LH (Tcholakian et al., 1974). Also, addition of estradiol or diethylstilbestrol (50 μg/ml) was found to reduce the accumulation of testosterone in the medium by 50–80% during incubation of decapsulated mouse and rat testes in vitro, though lower doses of estrogens were ineffective (Bartke et al., 1975). These results obtained with decapsulated mouse testes were in agreement with earlier findings of Samuels et al. (1964), which demonstrated a direct effect of estrogen implants upon androgen synthesis, with suppression of 17α-hydroxylase and 17–20 lyase activities in the testes of BALB/c mice. Similar results were reported in the same studies for

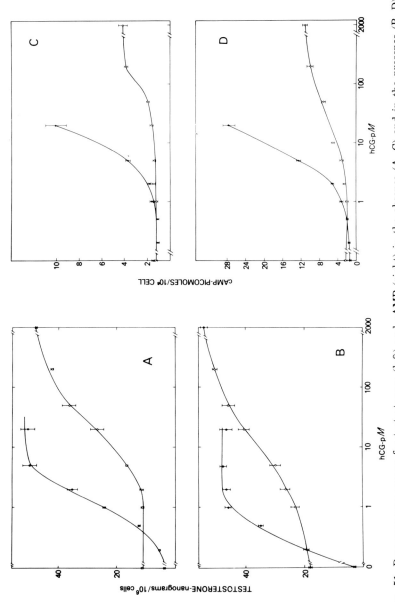

FIG. 51. Dose-response curves for testosterone (left) and cAMP (right) in the absence (A, C) and in the presence (B, D) of 1-methyl-3-isobutylxanthine (MIX). Data were derived by *in vitro* stimulation (0–2000 pM hCG) of control Leydig cells and cells from rats given a single subcutaneous injection of 10 μg of hCG. Data points are the mean ± SE of 3 determinations. The LH receptor content of the cells prepared 3 days after the hCG treatment was reduced to 15% of the control value in cells from untreated rats. ●——●, Control; ○——○, 10 μg of hCG.

intact mice, and in hypophysectomized mice replaced with gonadotropin to exclude the effects of gonadotropin suppression by estrogen. In addition, recent studies performed by measurement of plasma testosterone (Kalla *et al.*, 1977) and androgen production in testes of hypophysectomized gonadotropin-treated rats (Hsueh *et al.*, 1978) have confirmed the direct suppression of androgen biosynthesis described by Samuels *et al.* (1964).

A direct effect of estrogens on the endocrine function of the testis is not unexpected, since Leydig cells isolated from rat testes contain estradiol receptors (Mulder *et al.*, 1976). Also, production of estradiol by the testis has been demonstrated in testicular venous plasma after acute treatment with hCG and in testicular tissue after more prolonged subcutaneous administration of hCG (de Jong *et al.*, 1973, 1974). Thus, it is likely that stimulation of local estrogen production in the testis by the intravenous desensitizing dose of hCG could have caused the block in steroidogenesis, as a parallel phenomenon to the loss of LH receptors induced by gonadotropin. A related defect in steroidogenesis may arise from the increased formation of progesterone, 17α-hydroxyprogesterone and/or 20α-dihydroprogesterone in the testes of estrogen-treated male rats (Dorner *et al.*, 1975), since this steroid has been previously proposed to inhibit the activity of 17–20 lyase, and thus to exert an inhibitory effect on androgen biosynthesis (Inano *et al.*, 1967). However, the latter effects were observed at extremely high concentrations of the progestins (Samuels *et al.*, 1964) and do not operate at the levels normally present in the testis. In addition to the well-defined effects of estrogen on testicular steroidogenesis, it is possible that androgens and other steroid intermediates could directly influence steroid biosynthesis during the acute testosterone response induced by the desensitizing dose of gonadotropin.

Second, the general effects of withdrawal or sudden reduction of trophic hormone support for differentiated Leydig cell functions could be an additional factor in the appearance of biosynthetic defects in desensitized cells. The extent to which estrogen-induced defects in steroidogenesis contribute to the biosynthetic lesion observed in the studies in gonadotropin-desensitized Leydig cells will need to be resolved in further studies on the magnitude and effects of estrogen formation in gonadotropin-stimulated Leydig cells. Preliminary studies have demonstrated that administration of an estrogen antagonist, tamoxifen, at the same time as the intravenous desensitizing dose of hCG, prevented the development of the steroidogenic lesion while the loss of LH receptors was similar to that observed in the absence of the antagonist (Cigorraga *et al.*, 1978b).

Such studies have shown that the responses of target cells after hormone-induced receptor loss undergo a series of changes that result in the overall process referred to as desensitization. The earliest change is the rapid loss of adenylate cyclase responsiveness to hormone, which has been best demonstrated in the ovary (Conti *et al.*, 1976b), with consequent loss of cAMP production in the intact cell (Conti *et al.*, 1977b; Tsuruhara *et al.*, 1977). After the low dose of hCG (1 μg), which caused no change in basal cAMP production, the cAMP response during incubation with hCG fell markedly and reached a minimum at 24 hours, then recovered over the next few days (Hsueh *et al.*, 1977; Tsuruhara *et al.*, 1977). Thus, the initial rate of fall of the cAMP response to gonadotropin was much more rapid than the initial fall in receptors (Conti *et al.*, 1976b).

The initial desensitization of adenylate cyclase is an immediate consequence of receptor occupancy, and occurs much earlier than the true loss of receptors, i.e., within the first hours of hCG injection (Conti *et al.*, 1977a,b; Hsueh *et al.*, 1977). This process of enzyme desensitization has been described in the luteal cells of the ovary (Marsh *et al.*, 1973; Hunzicker-Dunn and Birnbaumer, 1976a,b; Bockaert *et al.*, 1976; Conti *et al.*, 1976b) and in several other tissues (Kebabian *et al.*, 1975; Mukherjee *et al.*, 1975, 1976) as well as the Leydig cells of the testis (Hsueh *et al.*, 1977). The later consequences of receptor occupancy include the loss of receptors noted in many reports, and the related impairment of cAMP and more distal responses in the target cell. Two components of this delayed effect can be distinguished and probably operate to different extents in specific target cells. The first and most obvious of these is the loss of ability to activate adenylate cyclase and cAMP production, in proportion to the loss of receptor sites which mediate the hormonal signal. This change probably occurs in all receptor-depleted target cells, and in the absence of other changes in cell function would result mainly in a relative loss of sensitivity of responses to the homologous hormone. However, a second effect of receptor depletion occurs in certain target cells, such as those of the testis and ovary (Tsuruhara *et al.*, 1977; Conti *et al.*, 1977a,b; Cigorraga *et al.*, 1978a, Dufau *et al.*, 1978c). In these tissues, additional changes occur at more distal points in the cellular metabolic pathways and modify the capacity of the cells to respond to hormonal stimuli. Such a change is the defect in steroidogenesis that resulted in loss or reduction of the maximum steroid response to saturating hormone concentrations. This defect will possibly prove to be characteristic of target cells for trophic peptide and protein hormones that regulate the state of differentiation as well as the acute responses of the target cell. By this reasoning, the loss of steroidogenesis in receptor-depleted Leydig cells would represent the result of impaired trophic action by LH *in vivo* during the initial phases of desensitization and receptor loss. Alternatively, the hormone-induced block in steroidogenesis could be the result of increased production of steroids such as estradiol, which is known to exert direct inhibitory effects upon androgen synthesis in the testis (Samuels *et al.*, 1964; Tcholakian *et al.*, 1974; Dorner *et al.*, 1975).

Hormone-induced loss of specific receptors in target cells is now a well-recognized property of several peptide hormones. As noted above, insulin and growth hormone regulate their own receptors *in vivo* and *in vitro;* also, thyrotropin-releasing hormone and catecholamines induce receptor loss after ligand–hormone interaction. Since tissue-bound hormone was not measured in earlier reports, estimates of receptor loss were based upon the assumption of negligible occupancy during subsequent assay of binding sites. In at least one of these systems, the interaction between catecholamines and β-adrenergic receptors, dissociation of the agonist from receptors has since been recognized to occur slowly, and it probably contributes to the observed loss of available sites (Lefkowitz and Williams, 1977). In the rat testis and ovary measurement of tissue-bound hormone by radioimmunoassay provided direct evidence of the decrease in both total and available LH receptors after hCG treatment *in vivo* (Conti *et al.*, 1976b, 1977a,b; Hsueh *et al.*, 1976b, 1977; Tsuruhara *et al.*, 1977).

Desensitization of cAMP production and steroidogenesis in target cells after hormonal treatment *in vivo* offers a unique opportunity to study the relationships between hormone receptors and hormone-induced responses. Comparison of the time courses of receptor loss and desensitization of the cAMP response revealed that 2 separate processes were involved. The occupancy of a small fraction of receptor sites by hCG *in vivo* rapidly caused inhibition of the cAMP response, probably via desensitization at the level of adenylate cyclase. Receptor loss took place at a later time, after initial occupancy and presumably through processes involving receptor degradation and/or inhibition of synthesis of new receptors. Desensitization of adenylate cyclase activity has also been demonstrated in adrenergic systems and could be correlated with loss of ligand binding capacity (Mukherjee *et al.*, 1975; Kebabian *et al.*, 1975). In addition, hCG-induced receptor loss and desensitization of adenylate cyclase activity has been observed in the luteinized rat ovary, as described below.

Relatively low levels of circulating LH are present in male rats, and interstitial cells are probably rarely exposed to the high concentrations of hormone used to induce receptor loss in the studies described above.

However, it is likely that desensitization by circulating gonadotropin is important in certain pathological and physiological states. For example, men with choriocarcinoma sometimes exhibit extremely high levels of plasma hCG without a corresponding increase in testosterone secretion (Kirschner et al., 1970). Our findings support the view that this lack of testicular response to high gonadotropin levels could be due to negative regulation of the interstitial cell receptors for LH and hCG (Gavin et al., 1974), though the decreased secretion of FSH in such patients probably plays an important part in their impaired testosterone responses (Reiter and Kulin, 1971). In the ovary, desensitization of adenylate cyclase has been observed in Graafian follicles and corpus luteum after endogenous elevations of gonadotropin secretion during the estrous cycle and pregnancy in rats and rabbits, as well as after injection of hCG (Marsh et al., 1973; Hunzicker-Dunn and Birnbaumer, 1976a,b,c). Also, inhibition of ovarian function (Johnson et al., 1976a), ovulation (Bowers and Folkers, 1976), and endocrine-dependent mammary tumors (Johnson et al., 1976b) in rats treated with agonist analogs of LHRH has been proposed to result from desensitization of ovarian H receptors and gonadal responses by sustained high concentrations of endogenous LH (Hsueh et al., 1977). A similar effect has been recently demonstrated in the testes of male rats treated with a potent LHRH agonist for several days (Auclair et al., 1977), which caused a marked reduction in testis weight and testicular LH receptors.

The effects of treatment of male rats with single doses of the native LHRH molecule has also been shown to cause loss of testicular LH receptors, a process that reaches its maximum about 2 days after the surge of endogenous LH evoked by administration of LHRH (Catt et al., 1978). The effect of increasing doses of LHRH on plasma LH, plasma testosterone, and testicular LH receptors are shown in Fig. 52. The magnitude of the LHRH-induced peak in plasma LH is dose-dependent, and reaches a substantial value within 15 minutes. The maximum level of plasma LH occurs from 15 to 60 minutes after LHRH injection, and the return to baseline values is complete within 1 to 4 hours. The corresponding testosterone responses are slightly delayed and in general similar to the plasma LH profiles. After each dose of LHRH, from 100 ng to 10 μg, there was a dose-related fall in testicular LH receptors that was evident within 24 hours, became maximum at 48 hours, and returned to the normal value in 5–6 days. The delayed loss of LH receptors in the testis was most evident 2 days after LHRH treatment and the ensuing transient LH peak, and was not attributable simply to occupancy of the lost sites by endogenous hormone. Also, direct measurement of receptor occupancy, by elution and assay of the

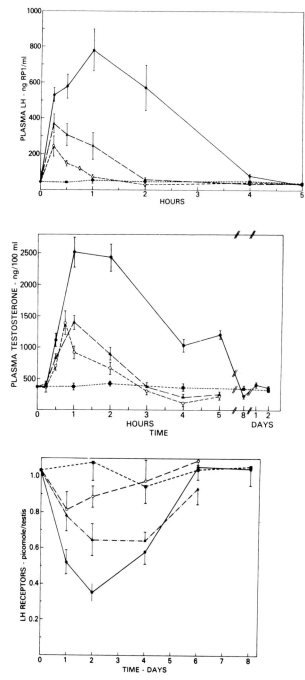

FIG. 52. Effects of increasing subcutaneous doses of LHRH (○, 0.1 μg; ▲, 1.0 μg; ●, 10 μg; ■, control) upon plasma LH (above) plasma testosterone (middle) and testicular LH receptors (below) in adult male rats.

bound endogenous LH, revealed that the total extent of receptor occupancy was low or undetectable with the smaller doses of LHRH, though more apparent after the highest dose. Therefore, the process of LH receptor regulation by the homologous hormone is initiated by relatively minor degrees of receptor occupancy during the phase of Leydig-cell stimulation, then proceeds over the subsequent 24–48 hours to cause a much more extensive loss of receptors, presumably a majority of free sites as well as the small number involved in the original hormone–receptor interaction. The sequence of receptor loss and recovery is similar to that observed after treatment with exogenous gonadotropins, either hCG or ovine LH, and illustrates that elevations of endogenous LH initiate the same process of receptor regulation.

The loss of LH receptors induced by LHRH-evoked rises in plasma LH was accompanied by changes in the *in vitro* responses of Leydig cells to hormone stimulation, analogous to those seen after densensitization by hCG treatment (Fig. 53). Thus, cAMP production was proportional to receptor content, and followed the decline in LH receptors observed at 2 and 4 days. As in the hCG-desensitized cells, testosterone reponses to gonadotropin *in vitro* also varied with the degree of receptor depletion. At low levels of receptor loss, steroid responses were sometimes increased above control values, while moderate to severe receptor loss was consistently accompanied by a fall in testosterone production in response to saturating concentrations of hCG, as well as to choleragen and dibutyryl cAMP. The latter finding indicated the presence of a post-cAMP block, as in cells from hCG-desensitized animals. Once again, there was no change in the availability of cAMP receptors, and incubation in the presence of cyanoketone showed no loss of the pregnenolone response to gonadotropin. However, elevations of progesterone and 17α-hydroxyprogesterone revealed the presence of enzymatic defects beyond pregnenolone formation, at the same loci (17α-hydroxylase and 17,20 desmolase) at which steroidogenesis is impaired after treatment with desensitizing doses of exogenous gonadotropin. In addition, accumulation of steroid intermediates was observed in the blood of LHRH-treated animals, consistent with the partial steroidogenic block detected *in vitro*.

It is important to note that more prolonged treatment with LHRH analogs probably accentuates the testicular lesion by an additional desensitizing action at the pituitary level, causing the functional regression of the receptor-depleted gonad to be succeeded by regression due to impaired gonadotropin release. These findings have obvious implications during the therapeutic use of LHRH to stimulate gonadal function, as well as in the analysis of physiological mechanisms re-

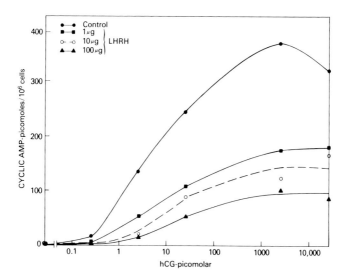

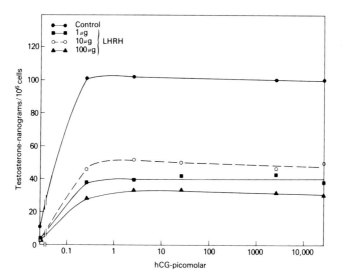

FIG. 53. Effects of LHRH on Leydig cell responses to gonadotropin (hCG) *in vitro*. The cAMP responses (top) were reduced to 37, 32, and 25% of the control value, while LH receptors were 33, 26, and 11%, respectively. The testosterone responses (bottom) were decreased at each LHRH dose, with a loss in maximum production due to enzymatic defects in the steroidogenic pathway (see text).

sponsible for the regulation and integration of pituitary–gonadal function.

The relatively constant nature and function of testicular interstitial tissue, with well-defined hormonal responses in the absence of changing cell differentiation, offers a useful model for analysis of the mechanisms by which peptide hormones regulate receptor concentration and specific responses in their target cells.

A similar relationship between gonadotropin-induced loss of LH receptors and desensitization of hormonal responses is seen in the ovary. Treatment with LH or hCG *in vivo* or *in vitro* has been shown to abolish subsequent adenylate cyclase responses of ovarian homogenates to hormonal stimulation *in vitro* (Marsh *et al.*, 1973; Bockaert *et al.*, 1976; Zor *et al.*, 1976; Hunzicker-Dunn and Birnbaumer, 1976c). The desensitization of adenylate cyclase in the luteinized rat ovary induced by treatment with hCG was recently shown to be accompanied by a reversible loss of LH receptors during the hormone-refractory state (Conti *et al.*, 1976b, 1977a). After administration of hCG, gonadotropin binding capacity and hormonal stimulation of adenylate cyclase declined rapidly to reach a minimum at 6–12 hours, remained depressed for 4 days, then returned to the control level at 5–7 days. Total adenylate cyclase activity measured in the presence of fluoride fell by 50% within a few hours but returned to normal by 24 hours (Fig. 54). As in the testis, assay of receptor-bound hormone showed that the initial loss of binding capacity and hormone sensitivity was associated with occupancy of the LH receptor sites, whereas the more prolonged changes were attributable to a decrease in hormone receptor sites in the luteal cell (Conti *et al.*, 1976b, 1977a). The presence of a hormone-specific desensitization of ovarian adenylate cyclase, in the absence of a change in LH receptors, has also been demonstrated in the preovulatory follicles of the rat ovary (Lamprecht *et al.*, 1977). Thus, the initial phase of the desensitization phenomenon appears to be a result of receptor occupancy and target-cell activation by the agonist, whereas the more prolonged loss of responsiveness is caused by a subsequent loss of specific receptor sites. The loss of LH receptor sites that follows gonadotropin-induced desensitization in male and female rats effectively extends the period of hormone refractoriness by imposing a secondary barrier on the ability of hormone to activate the receptor–adenylate cyclase complex.

The marked reduction of receptor and corresponding cAMP responses to trophic hormone in luteal cells from desensitized ovaries was accompanied by a corresponding reduction of progesterone formation upon incubation with hCG (Conti *et al.*, 1977b). The decrease in progesterone production was not simply a consequence of the reduced

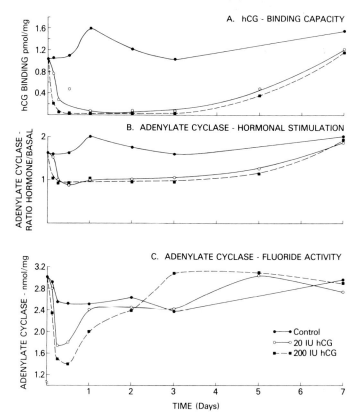

Fɪɢ. 54. The time course of changes in gonadotropin binding capacity and adenylate cyclase in luteinized rat ovaries following injection of hCG. Luteinized rats were injected with 20 or 200 IU of hCG (2 or 20 μg of hCG) and killed at intervals up to 7 days. The 20,000 g fraction was assayed for binding capacity and adenylate cyclase activity. (A) Receptor capacity as measured by [¹²⁵I]hCG binding per milligram of protein. (B) Hormonal responsiveness of adenylate cyclase, expressed as a ratio of hormone to basal activity. (C) Total adenylate cyclase activity measured in the presence of sodium fluoride. The basal activity of adenylate cyclase in all experimental groups did not vary over the 7-day period of the experiment.

cAMP formation in desensitized luteal cells. As in the testis, steroid production in response to dibutyryl cAMP or cholera toxin was also diminished, whereas both agents stimulated progesterone production as effectively as hCG in control cells. The impairment of the steroidogenic responses to endogenous and exogenous cAMP in the ovary was analogous to the situation previously described in the testis and indicated the existence of an additional lesion in the progesterone biosynthetic pathway beyond the level of cAMP production (Conti *et al.*, 1977b). The desensitized state could also be accompanied by increased metabolism of progesterone by enzymes such as 20α-hydroxysteroid dehydrogenase or 5α-reductase, with accumulation of 20α-dihydroprogesterone and/or 5α-pregnane-3,20-dione (allopregnandione). Alternatively, the enzymic lesion could be located at steps prior to progesterone formation (i.e., at the level of cholesterol esterase, side-chain cleavage enzyme, or 3β-hydroxysteroid dehydrogenase).

The steroidogenic lesion was transitory, and recovered more rapidly than the loss of hormone receptors. Production of cAMP and nucleotide-stimulated progesterone responses returned to normal levels over 7 days; by day 5 the progesterone response was fully recov-

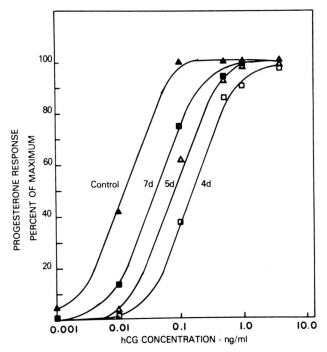

Fig. 55. The changing dose-response curve for hCG-stimulated progesterone production in isolated luteal cells during recovery from desensitization. Primed immature rats were desensitized with 2.0 μg of hCG and sacrified 2, 4, 5, and 7 days later. Progesterone production by isolated luteal cells was assayed after incubation with increasing doses of hCG, and the control curve represents the response at day 2. Points are the mean of duplicate incubations. The data have been expressed as percentage of the maximum response obtained on each day after treatment, to illustrate the shift in sensitivity during reappearance of LH receptors.

ered, before the complement of receptors had returned to control levels. The recovery phase was characterized by a shift in the steroidogenic dose-response curve, with reduced sensitivity to stimulation by hCG during cell incubation (Fig. 55). At this time, in the presence of fewer LH receptors, maximum progesterone production could still be evoked when the hormone concentration was sufficiently increased.

These findings illustrate the ability of gonadotropins to impair target cell responses at several sites in the steroid activation pathway, in both luteal and Leydig cells. In addition to causing decreased sensitivity to hormone stimulation, as would be expected from partial receptor lost in cells with abundant "spare" receptors, hormone-induced loss of LH receptors is accompanied by additional lesions at the cell membrane and beyond. These include desensitization of adenylate cyclase and independent defects in the steroidogenic pathway. It is the summation of these changing effects that determines the cellular capacity for steroid secretory responses during the period in which the hormone-induced refractory state is the dominate influence on target cell function.

REFERENCES

Abou-Issa, H., and Reichert, L. E. (1976). *J. Biol. Chem.* **251,** 3326.

Abou-Issa, H., and Reichert, L. E. (1977). *J. Biol. Chem.* **252,** 4166.

Albert, A., Rosemberg, E., Ross, G. T., Paulsen, C. A., and Ryan, R. J. (1968). *J. Clin. Endocrinol. Metab.* **28,** 1214.

Aragona, C., and Friesen, H. G. (1975). *Endocrinology* **97,** 677.

Aragona, C., Bohnet, H. G., Fang, F. S., and Friesen, H. G. (1976a). *Endocr. Res. Commun.* **3,** 199.

Aragona, C., Bohnet, H. G., and Friesen, H. G. (1976b). *Endocrinology* **99,** 1017.

Ascoli, M., and Puett, D. (1977). *FEBS Lett.* **75,** 77.

Auclair, C., Kelly, P. A., Labrie, F., Coy, D. H., and Schally, A. V. (1977). *Biochem. Biophys. Res. Commun.* **76,** 855.

Azhar, S., and Menon, K. M. J. (1976). *J. Biol. Chem.* **251,** 7398.

Azhar, S., Hajra, A. K., and Menon, K. M. J. (1976a). *J. Biol. Chem.* **251,** 7405.

Bangham, D. R., Berryman, J., Burger, H., Cotes, P. M., Furnival, B. E., Hunter, W. M., Midgley, A. R., Musset, M. V., Reichert, L. E., Rosemberg, E., Ryan, R. J., and Wide, L. (1973). *J. Clin. Endocrinol. Metab.* **36,** 647.

Bartke, A. (1977). *In* "The Testis in Normal and Infertile Men" (P. Troen and H. R. Nankin, eds.), p. 367. Raven, New York.

Bartke, A., Williams, K. I. H., and Dalterio, S. (1975). *Biol. Reprod.* **17,** 645.

Beall, R., and Sayers, G. (1972). *Arch. Biochem. Biophys.* **148,** 70.

Beckett, G. J., and Boyd, G. S. (1975). *Biochem. Soc. Trans.* **3,** 892.

Behrman, H. R., and Armstrong, D. T. (1969). *Endocrinology* **85,** 474.

Beitins, I. Z., Dufau, M. L., O'Loughlin, M., Catt, K. J., and McArthur, J. (1977). *J. Clin. Endocrinol. Metab.* **45,** 605.

Bell, J. J., and Harding, B. W. (1974). *Biochim. Biophys. Acta* **348**, 285.

Bellisario, R., and Bahl, O. P. (1975). *J. Biol. Chem.* **250**, 3837.

Bernard, E. A., and Wasserman, G. F. (1974). *Can. J. Biochem.* **52**, 563.

Bex, F. J., and Bartke, A. (1977). *Endocrinology* **100**, 1223.

Bockaert, J., Dunn, M. H., and Birnbaumer, L. (1976). *J. Biol. Chem.* **251**, 2653.

Bohnet, H. G., and Friesen, H. G. (1976). *J. Reprod. Fertil.* **48**, 307.

Bowers, C. Y., and Folkers, K. (1976). *Biochem. Biophys. Res. Commun.* **72**, 1003.

Brown, M. S., and Goldstein, J. L. (1976). *Science* **191**, 150.

Burstein, S., Middleditch, B. S., and Gut, M. (1975). *J. Biol. Chem.* **250**, 9028.

Caron, M. G., Goldstein, S., Savard, K., and Marsh, J. M. (1975). *J. Biol. Chem.* **250**, 5137.

Carpenter, G., and Cohen, S. (1976). *J. Clin. Endocrinol. Metab.* **71**, 159.

Carr, D., and Friesen, H. G. (1976). *J. Clin. Endocrinol. Metab.* **42**, 482.

Castro, A. E., Alonso, A., and Mancini, R. E. (1972). *J. Endocrinol.* **52**, 129.

Catt, K. J., and Dufau, M. L. (1975). *In* "Methods in Enzymology" (B. W. O'Malley and J. G. Hardman, eds.), Vol. 37, Part B, p. 167. Academic Press, New York.

Catt, K. J., and Dufau, M. L. (1973b). *Nature (London)*, *New Biol.* **244**, 219.

Catt, K. J., and Dufau, M. L. (1975). *In* "Methods in Enzymology" (B. W. O'Malley and J. G. Hardman, eds.), Vol. 37, Part B, p. 167. Academic Press, New York.

Catt, K. J., Dufau, M. L., and Tsuruhara, T. (1971). *J. Clin. Endocrinol. Metab.* **32**, 860.

Catt, K. J., Dufau, M. L., and Tsuruhara, T. (1972a). *J. Clin. Endocrinol. Metab.* **34**, 123.

Catt, K. J., Tsuruhara, T., and Dufau, M. L. (1972b). *Biochim. Biophys. Acta* **279**, 194.

Catt, K. J., Dufau, M. L., and Tsuruhara, T. (1973a). *J. Clin. Endocrinol. Metab.* **36**, 73.

Catt, K. J., Watanabe, K., and Dufau, M. L. (1973b). *Nature (London)* **239**, 280.

Catt, K. J., Tsuruhara, T., Mendelson, C., Ketelslegers, J.-M., and Dufau, M. L. (1974). *In* "Hormone Binding and Target Cell Activation in the Testis" (M. L. Dufau and A. R. Means, eds.), p. 1. Plenum, New York.

Catt, K. J., Dufau, M. L., Neaves, W. B., Walsh, P. C., and Wilson, J. D. (1975a). *Endocrinology* **97**, 1157.

Catt, K. J., Dufau, M. L., and Vaitukaitis, J. (1975b). *J. Clin. Endocrinol. Metab.* **40**, 537.

Catt, K. J., Ketelslegers, J.-M. and Dufau, M. L. (1976). *In* "Methods in Receptor Research" (M. Blecher, ed.), Part I, p. 175. Dekker, New York.

Catt, K. J., Baukal, A., Davies, T. F., and Dufau, M. L. (1978). *Endocrinology* (in press).

Channing, C. P. (1975). *Proc. Soc. Exp. Biol. Med.* **149**, 238.

Channing, C. P., and Kammerman, S. (1974). *Biol. Reprod.* **10**, 179.

Charreau, E. H., Dufau, M. L., and Catt, K. J. (1974). *J. Biol. Chem.* **294**, 4189.

Charreau, E. H., Attramadal, A., Torjesen, P. A., Purvis, K., Calandra, R., and Hansson, V. (1977). *Mol. Cell. Endocrinol.* **6**, 303.

Chen, T. T., Abel, J. H., McClellan, M. C., Sawyer, H. R., Dickman, M. A., and Niswender, G. D. (1977). *Cytobiologie* **14**, 412.

Cheng, K. W. (1975a). *Biochem. J.* **149**, 123.

Cheng, K. W. (1975b). *J. Clin. Endocrinol. Metab.* **41**, 581.

Cheng, K. W. (1976). *Biochem. J.* **159**, 71.

Cheng, Y. D. I., and Payne, A. H. (1977). *Biochem. Biophys. Res. Commun.* **74**, 1589.

Cigorraga, S., Dufau, M. L., and Catt, K. J. (1978a). *J. Biol. Chem.* **253**, 4297.

Cigorraga, S., Dufau, M. L., and Catt, K. J. (1978b). Submitted for publication.

Clark, M., and Menon, K. M. J. (1975). *Fed. Proc., Fed. Am. Soc. Exp. Biol.* **34**, Abstr. 2067, 534.

Conn, P. M., Tsuruhara, T., Dufau, M. L., and Catt, K. J. (1977). *Endocrinology* **101**, 639.

Conti, M., Dufau, M. L., and Catt, K. J. (1976a). *Clin. Res.* **24**, 426A.

Conti, M., Harwood, J. P., Hsueh, A. J. W., Dufau, M. L., and Catt, K. J. (1976b). *J. Biol. Chem.* **251**, 7729.

Conti, M., Harwood, J. P., Dufau, M. L., and Catt, K. J. (1977a). *Mol. Pharmacol.* **13**, 1024.

Conti, M., Harwood, J. P. Dufau, M. L., and Catt, K. J. (1977b). *J. Biol. Chem.* **252**, 8869.

Conti, M., Dufau, M. L., and Catt, K. J. (1978). *Biochim. Biophys. Acta* **541**, 35.

Cooke, B. A., Janszen, F. H. A., Clotscher, W. F., and van der Molen, H. J. (1975a). *Biochem. J.* **150**, 413.

Cooke, B. A., Janszen, F. H. A., and van der Molen, H. (1975b). *Acta Endocrinol. Suppl. (Copenhagen)* **199**, 104.

Cooke, B. A., Lindh, M. L., and Janszen, F. H. A. (1976). *Biochem. J.* **160**, 446.

Costlow, M. E., Buschow, R. A., and McGuire, W. L. (1975). *Life Sci.* **17**, 1457.

Cowie, A. T., and Forsyth, I. A. (1975). *Pharmacol. Ther.* **1**, 437.

de Jong, F. H., Hey, A. H., and van der Molen, H. J. (1973). *J. Endocrinol.* **57**, 277.

de Jong, F. H., Hey, A. H., and van der Molen, H. J. (1974). *J. Endocrinol.* **60**, 409.

DeKretser, D. M., Catt, K. J., Burger, H. G., and Smith, G. C. (1969). *J. Endocrinol.* **43**, 105.

DeKretser, D. M., Catt, K. J., and Paulsen, C. A. (1971). *Endocrinology* **88**, 332.

Desjardins, C., Zeleznik, A. J., Midgley, A. R., and Reichert, L. E. (1974). *In* "Hormone Binding and Target Cell Activation in the Testis" (M. L. Dufau and A. R. Means, eds.), p. 221. Plenum, New York.

Dorner, G., Stahl, F., Rohde, W., and Schnorr, L. (1975). *Endokrinologie* **66**, 221.

Dufau, M. L., and Catt, K. J. (1973). *Nature (London), New Biol.* **242**, 246.

Dufau, M. L., and Catt, K. J. (1975). *FEBS Lett.* **52**, 273.

Dufau, M. L., and Catt, K. J. (1976a). *In* "Concanavalin A as a Tool" (H. Bittiger and H. P. Schnebli, eds.), p. 339. Wiley New York.

Dufau, M. L., and Catt, K. J. (1976b). *In* "Cell Membrane Receptors for Viruses, Antigens and Antibodies, Polypeptide Hormones, and Small Molecules (R. F. Beers and E. G. Bassett, eds.), pp. 135–163.

Dufau, M. L., Catt, K. J., and Tsuruhara, T. (1971a). *Biochim. Biophys. Acta* **252**, 574.

Dufau, M. L., Catt, K. J., and Tsuruhara, T. (1971b). *Biochem. Biophys. Res. Commun.* **44**, 1022.

Dufau, M. L., Tsuruhara, T., and Catt, K. J. (1972a). *Biochim. Biophys. Acta* **278**, 281.

Dufau, M. L., Catt, K. J., and Tsuruhara, T. (1972b). *Endocrinology* **90**, 1032.

Dufau, M. L., Catt, K. J., and Tsuruhara, T. (1972c). *Proc. Natl. Acad. Sci. U.S.A.* **69**, 2414.

Dufau, M. L., Charreau, E. H., and Catt, K. J. (1973a). *J. Biol. Chem.* **248**, 6973.

Dufau, M. L., Watanabe, K., and Catt, K. J. (1973b). *Endocrinology* **92**, 6.

Dufau, M. L., Mendelson, C., and Catt, K. J. (1974a). *J. Clin. Endocrinol. Metab.* **39**, 610.

Dufau, M. L., Charreau, E. H., Ryan, D., and Catt, K. J. (1974b). *FEBS Lett.* **39**, 149.

Dufau, M. L., Ryan, D. W., and Catt, K. J. (1974c). *Biochim. Biophys. Acta* **343**, 417.

Dufau, M. L., Charreau, E. H., Ryan, D. W., and Catt, K. J. (1974d). *In* "Hormone Binding and Target Cell Activation in the Testis" (M. L. Dufau and A. R. Means, eds.), p. 47. Plenum, New York.

Dufau, M. L., Ryan, D., Baukal, A., and Catt, K. J. (1975a). *J. Biol. Chem.* **250**, 4822.

Dufau, M. L., Podesta, E., and Catt, K. J. (1975b). *Proc. Natl. Acad. Sci. U.S.A.* **72**, 1272.

Dufau, M. L., Pock, R., Neubauer, A., and Catt, K. J. (1976a). *J. Clin. Endocrinol. Metab.* **42**, 958.

Dufau, M. L., Beitins, I. Z., McArthur, J. W., and Catt, K. J. (1976b). *J. Clin. Endocrinol. Metab.* **43**, 658.

Dufau, M. L., Baukal, A., Ryan, D., and Catt, K. J. (1977a). *Mol. Cell. Endocrinol.* **6**, 253.

Dufau, M. L., Hodgen, G. D., Goodman, A. L., and Catt, K. J. (1977b). *Endocrinology* **100**, 1557.

Dufau, M. L., Tsuruhara, T., Horner, K. A., Podesta, E. J., and Catt, K. J. (1977c). *Proc. Natl. Acad. Sci. U.S.A.* **74**, 3419.

Dufau, M. L., Ryan, D. W., and Catt, K. J. (1977d). *FEBS Lett.* **81**, 359.

Dufau, M., Podesta, E., Tsuruhara, T., Hsueh, A., Harwood, J., and Catt, K. (1977e). *Endocrinol., Proc. Int. Congr. Endocrinol., 5th, 1976* Excerpta Med. Found. Int. Congr. Ser. No. 402, Vol. I, pp. 441–445.

Dufau, M. L., Beitins, I. Z., McArthur, J., and Catt, K. J. (1977f). *In* "Proceedings of the Third Testis Conference" (P. Troen and H. Nankin, eds.), pp. 309–325. Raven, New York.

Dufau, M. L., Hodgen, G. D., and Catt, K. J. (1977g). *Endocrinol., Proc. Endocrinol., 5th, 1976* Abstract No. 158.

Dufau, M. L., Horner, A. E., Hayashi, K., Tsuruhara, T., Conn, P. M., and Catt, K. J. (1978a). *J. Biol. Chem.* **253**, 3721.

Dufau, M. L., Hayashi, I., Sala, G., Baukal, A., and Catt, K. J. (1978b). *Proc. Natl. Acad. Sci. U.S.A.* **75**, 4769.

Dufau, M. L., Hsueh, A. J. W., Cigorraga, S. B., and Catt, K. J. (1978c). *Int. J. Andrology, Suppl.* **2**, 193.

Espeland, D. H., Naftolin, F., and Paulsen, C. A. (1968). *In* "Gonadotropins 1968" (E. Rosemberg, ed.), pp. 177–184. Geron-X Inc., Los Altos, California.

Flint, A. P. F., Grinwich, D. L., and Armstrong, D. T. (1973). *Biochem. J.* **132**, 313.

Frantz, W. L., and Turkington, R. W. (1972). *Endocrinology* **91**, 1545.

Friesen, H. G., and Shiu, R. P. C. (1977). *Endocrinol., Proc. Int. Congr. Endocrinol., 5th, 1976* Excerpta Med. Found. Int. Congr. Ser. No. 403, Vol. II, pp. 1–6.

Frowein, J., and Engel, W. J. (1975). *J. Endocrinol.* **64**, 59.

Gavin, J. R., Roth, J., Neville, D. M., De Meyts, P., and Buell, D. N. (1974). *Proc. Natl. Acad. Sci. U.S.A.* **71**, 84.

Goldenberg, R. L., Vaitukaitis, J. L., and Ross, G. T. (1972). *Endocrinology* **90**, 1492.

Gospodarowicz, D. (1971). *Endocrinology* **89**, 669.

Gospodarowicz, D. (1973). *J. Biol. Chem.* **248**, 5042.

Grahame-Smith, G. B., Butcher, R. W., Ney, R. L., and Sutherland, E. W. (1967). *J. Biol. Chem.* **242**, 5535.

Grinwich, D. L., Hichens, M., and Behrman, H. R. (1976). *Biol. Reprod.* **14**, 212.

Hafiez, A. A., Bartke, A., and Lloyd, C. W. (1972). *J. Endocrinol.* **53**, 223.

Han, S. S., Rajaniemi, H. J., Cho, M. I., Hirshfield, A. N., and Midgley, A. R. (1974). *Endocrinology* **95**, 589.

Haour, F., and Saez, J. M. (1977). *Mol. Cell. Endocrinol.* **7**, 17.

Hinkle, P. M., and Tashjian, A. H., Jr. (1975). *Biochemistry* **14**, 3845.

Holcomb, H. H., Costlow, M. E., Buschow, R. A., and McGuire, N. L. (1976). *Biochim. Biophys. Acta* **428**, 104.

Holt, J. A., Richards, J. S., Midgley, A. R., and Reichert, L. E. (1976). *Endocrinology* **98**, 1005.

Hsueh, A. J. W., Dufau, M. L., Katz, S. I., and Catt, K. J. (1976a). *Nature (London)* **261**, 710.

Hsueh, A. J. W., Dufau, M. L., and Catt, K. J. (1976b). *Biochem. Biophys. Res. Commun.* **72**, 1145.

Hsueh, A. J. W., Dufau, M. L., and Catt, K. J. (1977). *Proc. Natl. Acad. Sci. U.S.A.* **74**, 592.

Hsueh, A. J. W., Dufau, M. L., and Catt, K. J. (1978). *Endocrinology* **103**, 1096.

Hunzicker-Dunn, M., and Birnbaumer, L. (1976a). *Endocrinology* **99**, 185.

Hunzicker-Dunn, M., and Birnbaumer, L. (1976b). *Endocrinology* **99**, 198.

Hunzicker-Dunn, M., and Birnbaumer, L. (1976c). *Endocrinology* **99**, 211.

Inano, H., Nakano, H., Shikita, M., and Tamaoki, B. (1967). *Biochim. Biophys. Acta* **137**, 540.

Janszen, F. H. A., Cooke, B. A., Van Driel, M. J. A., and van der Molen, H. J. (1976). *FEBS Lett.* **71**, 269.

Jefcoate, C. R. (1975). *J. Biol. Chem.* **250**, 4663.

Jergil, B., and Dixon, G. H. (1969). *J. Biol. Chem.* **245**, 425.

Johnson, E. S. Gendrich, R. L., and White, W. F. (1976a). *Fertil. Steril.* **27**, 853.

Johnson, E. S., Seeley, J. H., White, W. F., and DeSombre, E. R. (1976b). *Science* **194**, 329.

Johnson, R. A., and Sutherland, E. W. (1971). *J. Biol. Chem.* **248**, 5114.

Kahn, C. R., and Roth, J. (1976). *In* "Isolation of Hormone Receptors" (G. S. Levey, ed.), pp. 1–29. Dekker, New York.

Kahn, C. R., Neville, D. M., Jr., and Roth, J. (1973). *J. Biol. Chem.* **248**, 244.

Kalla, N. R., Nisula, B. C., Menard, R. H., and Loriaux, D. L. (1977). *Endocrinology* **100**, Suppl., 82 (abstr.).

Kammerman, S., and Ross, J. (1975). *J. Clin. Endocrinol. Metab.* **41**, 546.

Kan, K. W., and Ungar, F. (1973). *J. Biol. Chem.* **248**, 2868.

Karaboyas, G. C., and Koritz S. B. (1965). *Biochemistry* **43**, 462.

Kebabian, J. W., Zatz, M., Romero, J. A., and Axelrod, J. (1975). *Proc. Natl. Acad. Sci. U.S.A.* **72**, 3735.

Kelly, P. A., Rosner, B. I., Tsushima, T., and Friesen, H. G. (1974). *Endocrinology* **95**, 532.

Ketelslegers, J.-M., and Catt, K. J. (1974). *J. Clin. Endocrinol. Metab.* **39**, 1159.

Ketelslegers, J.-M., Knott, G. D., and Catt, K. J. (1975). *Biochemistry* **14**, 3075.

Ketelslegers, J.-M., Hsueh, A. J. W., Hetzel, W. D., and Catt, K. J. (1977). *Endocrinol., Proc. Int. Congr. Endocrinol., 5th, 1976* Abstract 519.

Kirschner, M. A., Wider, J. A., and Ross, G. T. (1970). *J. Clin. Endocrinol. Metab.* **30**, 504.

Koch, Y., Zor, U., Chobsieng, P., Lamprecht, S. A., Pomerantz, S., and Lindner, H. R. (1974). *J. Endocrinol.* **61**, 179.

Kono, T., and Barham, T. W. (1971). *J. Biol. Chem.* **246**, 6210.

Lamprecht, S. A., Zor, U., Salomon, Y., Koch, Y., Ahren, K., and Lindner, H. (1977). *J. Cyclic Nucleotide Res.* **3**, 69.

Landesman, R., and Saxena, B. B. (1976). *Fertil. Steril.* **27**, 357.

Lee, C. Y. (1976). *Endocrinology* **99**, 42.

Lee, C. Y., and Ryan, R. J. (1971). *Endocrinology* **89**, 1515.

Lee, C. Y., and Ryan, R. J. (1972). *Proc. Natl. Acad. Sci. U.S.A.* **69**, 3520.

Lee, C. Y., and Ryan, R. J. (1973). *Biochemistry* **12**, 4609.

Lee, C. Y., and Ryan, R. (1975a). *J. Clin. Endocrinol. Metab.* **40**, 228.

Lee, C. Y., and Ryan, R. J. (1975b). *Endocrinology* **95**, 1691.

Lefkowitz, R. J., and Williams, L. T. (1977). *Proc. Natl. Acad. Sci. U.S.A.* **74**, 515.

Leidenberger, F. A., and Reichert, L. E. (1972). *Endocrinology* **91**, 901.

Leidenberger, F. A., and Reichert, L. E. (1973). *Endocrinology* **92**, 646.

Leidenberger, F. A., Willaschek, R., Pahnke, V. G., and Reichert, L. E. (1976). *Acta Endocrinol. (Copenhagen)* **81**, 54.

Lesniak, M. A., and Roth, J. (1976). *J. Biol. Chem.* **251**, 3720.

Lesniak, M. A., Roth, J., and Gordon, P. (1973). *Nature (London), New Biol.* **241**, 22.

Levey, G. S. (1970). *Biochem. Biophys. Res. Commun.* **38**, 86.

Levey, G. S. (1972). *Ann. N.Y. Acad. Sci.* **185**, 449.

Levey, G. S., Fletcher, M. A., Klein, I., Ruiz, E., and Schenk, A. (1974). *J. Biol. Chem.* **249**, 2665.

Ling, W. Y., and Marsh, J. M. (1977). *Endocrinology* **100**, 1571.

Liu, W.-K., Yang, K.-P., Burleigh, B. D., and Ward, D. N. (1974). In "Gonadotropin Binding and Target Cell Activation in the Testis" (M. L. Dufau and A. R. Means, eds.), p. 89. Plenum, New York.

Liu, W.-K., Furlong, N. B., and Ward, D. N. (1977). *J. Biol. Chem.* **252**, 522.

Lunenfeld, B., and Eshkol, A. (1967). *Vitam. Horm.* (*N.Y.*) **25**, 137–190.

McArthur, J. W., Ingersoll, F. M., and Worcester, J. (1958). *J. Clin. Endocrinol. Metab.* **18**, 460.

Mancini, R. E., Castro, A., and Seigeur, A. C. (1967). *J. Histochem. Cytochem.* **15**, 516.

Marchelonis, J. J. (1969). *Biochem. J.* **113**, 299.

Marsh, J. M., Butcher, R. W., Savard, K., and Sutherland, E. W. (1966). *J. Biol. Chem.* **241**, 5436.

Marsh, J. M., Mills, T. M., and Lemaire, W. J. (1973). *Biochim. Biophys. Acta* **304**, 197.

Means, A. R., and Huckins, C. (1974). In "Hormone Binding and Target Cell Activation in the Testis" (M. L. Dufau and A. R. Means, eds.), p. 145. Plenum, New York.

Means, A. R., and Vaitukaitis, J. L. (1972). *Endocrinology* **90**, 39.

Means, A. R., MacDougall, Soderling, T. R., and Corbin, J. D. (1974). *J. Biol. Chem.* **249**, 1231.

Mendelson, C., Dufau, M. L., and Catt, K. J. (1975a). *J. Biol. Chem.* **250**, 8818.

Mendelson, C., Dufau, M., and Catt, K. J. (1975b). *Biochim. Biophys. Acta* **411**, 222.

Midgley, A. R. (1973). In "Receptors for Reproductive Hormones" (B. W. O'Malley and A. R. Means, eds.), p. 365. Plenum, New York.

Morell, A. G., Gregoriadis, G., Scheinberg, I. H., Hickman, J., and Ashwell, G. (1971). *J. Biol. Chem.* **246**, 1461.

Moyle, W. R., and Ramachandran, J. (1973). *Endocrinology* **93**, 127.

Moyle, W. R., Jungas, R. L., and Greep, R. O. (1973). *Biochem. J.* **134**, 407.

Moyle, W. R., Bahl, O. P., and Marz, L. (1975). *J. Biol. Chem.* **25**, 9163.

Mukherjee, C., Caron, M. G., and Lefkowitz, R. J. (1975). *Proc. Natl. Acad. Sci. U.S.A.* **72**, 1945.

Mukherjee, C., Caron, M. G., and Lefkowitz, R. J. (1976). *Endocrinology* **99**, 347.

Mulder, E., Peters, M. J., van Beurden, W. M. O., Galdier, M., Rommerts, F. F. G., Janszen, F. H. A., and van der Molen, H. J. (1976). *Biochem. J.* **70**, 331.

Naghshineh, S. (1974). *Biochem. Biophys. Res. Commun.* **61**, 1076.

Neer, E. J. (1973). *J. Biol. Chem.* **218**, 3742.

Neill, J. D., Dailey, R. A., Tsou, R. C., and Reichert, L. E. (1977). *Endocrinology* **100**, 856.

Nimrod, A., Tsafriri, A., and Lindner, H. R. (1977). *Nature* (*London*) **267**, 632.

Niswender, G. D., Monroe, S. E., Peckham, W. D., Midgley, A. R., Knobil, E., and Reichert, L. E. (1971). *Endocrinology* **88**, 1327.

Nolin, J. M., and Witorsch, R. J. (1976). *Endocrinology* **99**, 949.

Odell, W. D., and Swerdloff, R. S. (1976). *Recent Prog. Horm. Res.* **32**, 245.

Papaionnou, S., and Gospodarowicz, D. (1975). *Endocrinology* **97**, 114.

Parlow, A. F. (1968). In "Gonadotropins 1968" (E. Rosemberg, ed.), pp. 57–79. Geron-X Inc., Los Altos, California

Peckham, W. D., and Knobil, E. (1976). *Endocrinology* **98**, 1054.

Pepperell, R. I., DeKretser, D. M., and Burger, H. G. (1975). *J. Clin. Invest.* **56**, 118.

Perkins, J. P. (1973). *Adv. Cyclic Nucleotide Res.* **3**, 1.

Perkins, J. P., and Moore, M. M. (1971). *J. Biol. Chem.* **246**, 62.

Petrusz, P. (1973). *J. Histochem. Cytochem.* **21**, 279.

Podesta, E. J., Dufau, M. L., and Catt, K. J. (1976a). *Mol. Cell. Endocrinol.* **5**, 109.

Podesta, E. J., Dufau, M. L., and Catt, K. J. (1976b). *FEBS Lett.* **70**, 212.

Podesta, E. J., Dufau, M. L., and Catt, K. J. (1978a). *Biochemistry* (in press).

Podesta, E. J., Solano, A., and Dufau, M. L. (1978b). *J. Biol. Chem.* **253** (in press).

Posner, B. I. (1975a). *Can. J. Physiol. Pharmacol.* **53**, 689.

Posner, B. I. (1976a). *Endocrinology* **98**, 645.

Posner, B. I. (1976b). *Endocrinology* **99**, 1168.

Posner, B. I. (1977). *Endocrinol., Proc. Int. Congr. Endocrinol., 5th, 1976* Excerpta Med. Found. Int. Congr. Ser. No. 403, Vol. II, p. 178.

Posner, B. I., Kelly, P. A., Shiu, R. P. C., and Friesen, H. G. (1974a). *Endocrinology* **95**, 521.

Posner, B. I., Kelly, P. A., and Friesen, H. G. (1974b). *Endocrinology* **97**, 1408.

Posner, B. I., Kelly, P. A., and Friesen, H. G. (1975b). *Science* **187**, 57.

Purvis, J. L., and Menard, R. (1975). *In* "Hormonal Regulation of Spermatogenesis" (F. S. French *et al.*, eds.), p. 65. Plenum, New York.

Quazi, M. H., Romani, P., and Diczfaluzy, E. (1974). *Acta Endocrinol. (Copenhagen)* **77**, 655.

Queener, S. F., Fleming, J. W., and Bell, N. H. (1975). *J. Biol. Chem.* **250**, 7586.

Raff, M. (1976). *Nature (London)* **259**, 265.

Rajaniemi, H., and Vanha-Perttula, T. (1972). *Endocrinology* **90**, 1.

Rajaniemi, H., and Vanha-Perttula, T. (1973). *J. Endocrinol.* **57**, 199.

Rajaniemi, H. J., Hirschfield, A. N., and Midgley, A. R. (1974). *Endocrinology* **95**, 579.

Rao, C. V. (1974). *J. Biol. Chem.* **249**, 2864.

Rapaport, B., and Adams, R. J. (1976). *Proc. Natl. Acad. Sci. U.S.A.* **251**, 6653.

Rayford, P. L., Vaitukitis, J. L., Ross, G. T., Morgan, F. J., and Canfield, R. E. (1972). *Endocrinology* **91**, 144.

Rebar, R., Williams, C., and Catt, K. J. (1977). *Horm. Res.* (in press).

Reddi, A. H., Ewing, L. L., and Williams-Ashman, H. G. (1971). *Biochem. J.* **122**, 333.

Reichert, L. E., and Bhalla, V. K. (1974). *Endocrinology* **94**, 483.

Reichert, L. E., Lawson, G. F., Leidenberger, F. L., and Trowbridge, C. G. (1973). *Endocrinology* **93**, 938.

Reichert, L. E., Ramsey, R. B., and Carter, E. B. (1975). *J. Clin. Endocrinol. Metab.* **41**, 643.

Reiter, E. O., and Kulin, H. E. (1971). *J. Clin. Endocrinol. Metab.* **33**, 957.

Richards, J. S., and Williams, J. J. (1976). *Endocrinology* **99**, 1571.

Robertson, D. M., and Diczfalusy, E. (1977). *Mol. Cell. Endocrinol.* **9**, 57.

Rodbard, D. (1973). *In* "Receptors for Reproductive Hormones" (B. W. O'Malley, and A. R. Means, eds.), p. 289. Plenum, New York.

Rodriguez-Rigan, L. J., Tcholakian, R. K., Smith, K. D., and Steinberger, E. (1977). *In* "The Testis in Normal and Infertile Men" (P. Troen and H. Nankin, eds.), p. 457. Raven, New York.

Rosal, T. P., Saxena, B. B., and Sanderman, R. (1975). *Fertil. Steril.* **26**, 1105.

Ryan, J., and Storm, D. R. (1974). *Biochem. Biophys. Res. Commun.* **60**, 304.

Sala, G., Dufau, M. L., and Catt, K. J. (1978a). *Clin. Res.* **26**, 312A.

Sala, G., Dufau, M. L., and Catt, K. J. (1978b). *J. Biol. Chem.* (in press).

Samuels, L. T., Short, G. J., and Huseby, R. A. (1964). *Acta Endocrinol. (Copenhagen)* **45**, 487.

Saxena, B. B. (1976). *In* "Methods in Receptor Research" (M. Blecher, ed.), Part I, p. 251. Dekker, New York.

Schramm, M., Orly, J., Eimerl, S., and Korner, M. (1977). *Nature (London)* **268**, 310.

Schwartz, S., Bell, J., Rechnitz, S., and Rabinowitz, D. (1973). *Eur. J. Clin. Invest.* **3**, 475.
Sharpe, M. (1976). *Nature (London)* **264**, 644.
Sharpe, M. (1977a). *Biochem. Biophys. Res. Commun.* **75**, 711.
Sharpe, M. (1977b). *Biochem. Biophys. Res. Commun.* **76**, 957.
Shin, S., and Sato, G. H. (1971). *Biochem. Biophys. Res. Commun.* **45**, 501.
Shin, S. H., Aiken, R. B., Roberts, R., and Howitz, C. (1974). *J. Endocrinol.* **63**, 257.
Shiu, R. P. C., and Friesen, H. G. (1974). *J. Biol. Chem.* **249**, 7902.
Shiu, R. P. C., and Friesen, H. G. (1976). *Science* **192**, 259.
Shiu, R. P. C., Kelly, P. A., and Friesen, H. G. (1973). *Science* **180**, 968.
Siegel, L. M., and Monty, K. J. (1966). *Biochim. Biophys. Acta* **112**, 346.
Stansfield, D. A., and Franks, D. (1971). *Biochim. Biophys. Acta* **242**, 606.
Steinman, R. M., and Cohn, Z. A. (1976). *In* "Biogenesis and Turnover of Membrane Macromolecules" (J. S. Cook, ed.), p. 1. Raven, New York.
Stephenson, R. P. (1956). *Br. J. Pharmacol.* **11**, 379.
Stewart, F., Allen, W. R., and Moor, R. M. (1976). *J. Endocrinol.* **71**, 371.
Sutherland, E. W., Rall, T. W., and Menon, T. (1962). *J. Biol. Chem.* **237**, 1220.
Talmadge, K. W., Bechtel, E., and Eppenberger, V. (1977). *Eur. J. Biochem.* **78**, 419.
Tamaoki, B., Iano, H., and Suzuki, K. (1975). *In* "Hormonal Regulation of Spermatogenesis" (F. S. French *et al.*, eds.), p. 123. Plenum, New York.
Tcholakian, R. K., Chowdury, M., and Steinberger, E. (1974). *J. Endocrinol.* **63**, 441.
Thorell, J. I., and Johansson, B. G. (1971). *Biochim. Biophys. Acta* **251**, 363.
Tomoda, Y., Miwa, T., and Ishizuka, N. (1975). *J. Clin. Endocrinol. Metab.* **40**, 644.
Trzeciak, W. H., and Boyd, G. S. (1973). *Eur. J. Biochem.* **37**, 327.
Trzeciak, W. H., and Boyd, G. S. (1974). *Eur. J. Biochem.* **46**, 201.
Tsuruhara, T., Dufau, M. L., Hickman, J., and Catt, K. J. (1972a). *Endocrinology* **91**, 296.
Tsuruhara, T., Van Hall, E. V., Dufau, M. L., and Catt, K. J. (1972b). *Endocrinology* **91**, 463.
Tsuruhara, T., Dufau, M. L., Cigorraga, S., and Catt, K. J. (1977). *J. Biol. Chem.* **252**, 9002.
Van Damme, M.-P., Robertson, D. M., Romani, P., and Diczfalusy, E. (1973). *Acta Endocrinol. (Copenhagen)* **74**, 642.
Van Damme, M.-P., Robertson, D. M., and Diczfalusy, E. (1974). *Acta Endocrinol. (Copenhagen)* **77**, 655.
Van Hall, E. V., Vaitukaitis, J. S., Ross, G. T., Hickman, J. W., and Ashwell, G. (1971a). *Endocrinology* **88**, 456.
Van Hall, E. V., Vaitukaitis, J. L., Ross, G. T., Hickman, J. W., and Ashwell, G. (1971b). *Endocrinology* **89**, 11.
Ward, D. N. Jirgensons, B., and Jackson, R. L. (1974). *FEBS Lett.* **45**, 175.
Watson, J. (1972). *J. Endocrinol.* **54**, 19.
Yang, K. P., Samaan, N. A., and Ward, D. N. (1976). *Endocrinology* **98**, 233.
Yang, W. H., Sairam, M. R., Papkoff, H., and Li, C. H. (1972). *Science* **175**, 637.
Zeleznik, A. J., Midgley, A. R., and Reichert, L. E. (1974). *Endocrinology* **95**, 818.
Zor, U., Lamprecht, S. A., Misulovin, Z., Koch, Y., and Lindner, H. R. (1976). *Biochim. Biophys. Acta* **428**, 761.

Subject Index

A

A
B
C
D
E
F
G
H
I
J